SIMULATION AND IMAGING OF THE CARDIAC SYSTEM

DEVELOPMENTS IN CARDIOVASCULAR MEDICINE

Lancée CT, ed: Echocardiology, 1979. ISBN 90-247-2209-8.

Baan J, Arntzenius AC, Yellin EL, eds: Cardiac dynamics. 1980. ISBN 90-247-2212-8.

Thalen HJT, Meere CC, eds: Fundamentals of cardiac pacing. 1970. ISBN 90-247-2245-4.

Kulbertus HE, Wellens HJJ, eds: Sudden death. 1980. ISBN 90-247-2290-X.

Dreifus LS, Brest AN, eds: Clinical applications of cardiovascular drugs. 1980. ISBN 90-247-2295-0.

Spencer MP, Reid JM, eds: Cerebrovascular evaluation with Doppler ultrasound. 1981. ISBN 90-247-2348-1.

Zipes DP, Bailey JC, Elharrar V, eds: The slow inward current and cardiac arrhythmias. 1980. ISBN 90-247-2380-9.

Kesteloot H, Joossens JV, eds: Epidemiology of arterial blood pressure. 1980. ISBN 90-247-2386-8.

Wackers FJT, ed: Thallium-201 and technetium-99m-pyrophosphate myocardial imaging in the coronary care unit. 1980. ISBN 90-247-2396-5.

Maseri A, Marchesi C, Chierchia S, Trivella MG, eds: Coronary care units. 1981. ISBN 90-247-2456-2.

Morganroth J, Moore EN, Dreifus LS, Michelson EL, eds: The evaluation of new antiarrhythmic drugs. 1981. ISBN 90-247-2474-0.

Alboni P: Intraventricular conduction disturbances. 1981. ISBN 90-247-2484-X.

Rijsterborgh H, ed: Echocardiology. 1981. ISBN 90-247-2491-0.

Wagner GS, ed: Myocardial infarction: Measurement and intervention. 1982. ISBN 90-247-2513-5.

Meltzer RS, Roelandt J, eds: Contrast echocardiography. 1982. ISBN 90-247-2531-3.

Amery A, Fagard R, Lijnen R, Staessen J, eds: Hypertensive cardiovascular disease; pathophysiology and treatment. 1982. ISBN 90-247-2534-8.

Bouman LN, Jongsma HJ, eds: Cardiac rate and rhythm. 1982. ISBN 90-247-2626-3.

Morganroth J, Moore EN, eds: The evaluation of beta blocker and calcium antagonist drugs. 1982. ISBN 90-247-2642-5.

Rosenbaum MB, ed: Frontiers of cardiac electrophysiology. 1982. ISBN 90-247-2663-8.

Roelandt J, Hugenholtz PG, eds: Long-term ambulatory electrocardiography. 1982. ISBN 90-247-2664-8.

Adgey AAJ, ed: Acute phase of ischemic heart disease and myocardial infarction. 1982. ISBN 90-247-2675-1.

Hanrath P, Bleifeld W, Souquet, J. eds: Cardiovascular diagnosis by ultrasound. Transesophageal, computerized, contrast, Doppler echocardiography. 1982. ISBN 90-247-2692-1.

Roelandt J, ed: The practice of M-mode and two-dimensional echocardiography. 1983. ISBN 90-247-2745-6.

Meyer J, Schweizer P, Erbel R, eds: Advances in noninvasive cardiology. 1983. ISBN 0-89838-576-8.

Morganroth J, Moore EN, eds: Sudden cardiac death and congestive heart failure: Diagnosis and treatment. 1983. ISBN 0-89838-580-6.

Perry HM, ed: Lifelong management of hypertension. 1983. ISBN 0-89838-582-2.

Jaffe EA, ed: Biology of endothelial cells. 1984. ISBN 0-89838-587-3.

Surawicz B, Reddy CP, Prystowsky EN, eds: Tachycardias. ISBN 0-89838-588-1.

Spencer MP, ed: Cardiac Doppler diagnosis. 1983. ISBN 0-89838-591-1.

Villarreal H, Sambhi MP, eds: Topics in pathophysiology of hypertension. 1984. ISBN 0-89838-595-4.

Messerli FH, ed: Cardiovascular disease in the elderly. 1984. ISBN 0-89838-596-2.

Simoons ML, Reiber JHC, eds: Nuclear imaging in clinical cardiology. 1984. ISBN 0-89838-599-7.

Ter Keurs HEDJ, Schipperheyn JJ, eds: Cardiac left ventricular hypertrophy. 1983. ISBN 0-89838-612-8.

Sperelakis N, ed: Physiology and pathophysiology of the heart. ISBN 0-89838-615-2.

Messerli FH, ed: Kidney in essential hypertension. ISBN 0-89838-616-0.

Sambhi MP, ed: Fundamental fault in hypertension. ISBN 0-89838-638-1.

Marchesi C, ed: Ambulatory monitoring: Cardiovascular system and allied applications. ISBN 0-89838-642-X.

Kupper W, MacAlpin RN, Bleifeld W, eds: Coronary tone in ischemic heart disease. ISBN 0-89838-646-2.

Sperelakis N, Caulfield JB, eds: Calcium antagonists: Mechanisms of action on cardiac muscle and vascular smooth muscle. ISBN 0-89838-655-1.

Godfraind T, Herman AS, Wellens D, eds: Calcium entry blockers in cardiovascular and cerebral dysfunctions. ISBN 0-89838-658-6.

Morganroth J, Moore EN, eds: Interventions in the acute phase of myocardial infarction. ISBN 0-89838-659-4.

Abel FL, Newman WH, eds: Functional aspects of the normal, hypertrophied, and failing heart. ISBN 0-89838-665-9.

Sideman S, Beyar R, eds: Simulation and imaging of the cardiac system. ISBN 0-89838-687-X.

SIMULATION AND IMAGING OF THE CARDIAC SYSTEM

State of the heart

edited by

SAMUEL SIDEMAN D.Sc., Chem.Eng.

R.J. Matas/Winnipeg Professor of Biomedical Engineering
Director, The Julius Silver Institute of Biomedical Engineering
Head, Department of Biomedical Engineering, Technion
Israel Institute of Technology
Haifa 32000, Israel

RAFAEL BEYAR, MD, D.Sc.

The Julius Silver Institute of Biomedical Engineering
Department of Biomedical Engineering, Technion
Israel Institute of Technology
Haifa, 32000, Israel

1985 **MARTINUS NIJHOFF PUBLISHERS**
a member of the KLUWER ACADEMIC PUBLISHERS GROUP
BOSTON / DORDRECHT / LANCASTER

Distributors

for the United States and Canada: Kluwer Academic Publishers, 190 Old Derby
Street, Hingham, MA 02043, USA
for the UK and Ireland: Kluwer Academic Publishers, MTP Press Limited, Falcon
House, Queen Square, Lancaster LA1 1RN, UK
for all other countries: Kluwer Academic Publishers Group, Distribution Center,
P.O. Box 322, 3300 AH Dordrecht, The Netherlands

Library of Congress Cataloging in Publication Data

Main entry under title:

Simulation and imaging of the cardiac system.

   (Developments in cardiovascular medicine)
   Proceedings of the International Henry Goldberg
Workshop, held in Haifa, Israel, March 4-7, 1984,
sponsored by the Technion, Israel Institute of
Technology, Haifa, and others.
   Includes index.
   1. Heart--Models--Congresses. 2. Electrocardio-
graphy--Congresses. 3. Ultrasonic cardiography--
Congresses. I. Sideman, S.   II. Beyar, Rafael.
III. International Henry Goldberg Workshop (1984 :
Haifa, Israel) IV. Tekhniyon, Makhon Tekhnologi
le-Yiśrael. V. Series.
QP111.4.S56 1985   612'.17'0724   84-22824

ISBN-13: 978-94-010-8710-0   e-ISBN-13: 978-94-009-4992-8
DOI: 10.1007/978-94-009-4992-8

Copyright

Dedicated to three wise persons:

JULIUS SILVER

MICHAEL KENNEDY LEIGH

PEARL MILCH

who made the stars shine brighter
over Mt. Carmel ...

Proceedings of the International Henry Goldberg Workshop on 3-D simulation and imaging of the cardiac system, held in Haifa, Israel, March 4–7, 1984.

WORKSHOP OFFICIALS AND SPONSORS

ORGANIZING COMMITTEE	*R. Beyar,* Technion, I.I.T. Haifa (Secretary).
	M.S. Gotsman, Haddassah Heart Center, Jerusalem.
	N. Neufeld, Sheba Heart Center, Tel-Hashomer.
	Y. Palti, Faculty of Medicine, Rappaport Institute, Technion, I.I.T.
	E.L. Ritman, Mayo Clinic, Rochester, MN.
	S. Sideman, Technion, I.I.T. Haifa (Chairman).
SCIENTIFIC ADVISORY COMMITTEE	*R. Plonsey,* Duke University, Durham, NC.
	W. Welkowitz, Rutgers University, Piscataway, NJ.
SPONSORS	Technion, Israel Institute of Technology, Haifa, Israel.
	National Council for Research and Development, Israel.
	Mr. Henry Goldberg, NY.
	Sirkin Visiting Fund, Technion.
	Mr. Elmer Bloch, NY.

Table of contents

X

Welcome address

Professor JOSEPH SINGER, President,
Israel Institute of Technology, Haifa, Israel

The Henry Goldberg Workshop on 3-D Simulation and Imaging of the Cardiac System is an example of co-operation between medicine and engineering that is one of the main developments in recent decades.

The Technion has for many years realized the importance of this co-operation. We were fortunate to have the partnership of a man of foresight like Julius Silver, who made this Institute possible. Since 1976, when the Technion's Biomedical Research was concentrated here, multidisciplinary collaboration and co-operation have increased, not only in form, but in depth as well, under the very active leadership of Professor Sideman.

The rare combination of a Faculty of Medicine and an Institute of Technology at the Technion has played an important role in this advance.

This distinguished gathering marks an important milestone in the development of Biomedical Engineering at Technion – and I am hopeful that it will be followed by more such meetings in the future.

It is a great pleasure to me to welcome you on behalf of the Technion. I hope you will have a chance to get to know us a little better while you are here, and to see something of our compus. I hope it will be a beginning, especially for those of you here for the first time, of a close relationship with our Institution.

I wish you fruitful deliberations.

J.S.

Greetings

DR. GERSHON METZGER, Deputy Director
National Council for Research & Development
Ministry of Science & Development

I am truly pleased to extend to you all the most cordial felicitations of the Ministry of Science & Development and the National Council for Research & Development.

At least three specific reasons can be cited, from the point of view of the National Council for Research & Development (NCRD) for regarding this workshop as a particularly relevant event.

The first and foremost reason is its purpose, to bring substantial benefit to human beings, individually and collectively, by alleviating pain and improving the effectiveness of diagnosis and therapy related to cardiac conditions.

Secondly, the interdisciplinary nature of the subject of the workshop and of its participants, provide a singularly suitable forum to bring together a truly impressive representation of the pertinent scientific, technological and practitioning skills and expertise in a concerted-coordinated effort to assess what has been achieved to date, and what should be done to advance the state of the art even further in the immediate future.

Last, but far from least, the NCRD has a special interest in promoting internation scientific cooperation. From this point of view I am certain that this workshop, in bringing together expert from different countries, will not only make a general contribution to improved international relations per se, but will also make a very significant and specific contribution to the quality of medical practice in the countries represented here.

I wish you all stimulating and productive deliberations and discussions, and to our guests from abroad, a most pleasant stay in Israel.

Introductory remarks

Professor S. SIDEMAN
Head, Biomedical Engineering Department
Technion – Israel Institute of Technology, Haifa, Israel

Two years ago a gathering of the Biomedical Engineering Group here at the Silver Institute of the Technion have birth to a dream: let us combine our diversified expertise in our respective fields of science, engineering and medicine, so as to serve humanity best through a meaningful contribution to the science to the cardiac system; let us join forces and integrate the multidisciplined aspects of the cardiac system into a coherent, quantitative framework so as to better understand the interactions and complicated interrelationships between the numerous parameters affecting the cardiac system. It was a dream based on a strong belief that hard work, some talent, and a huge amount of cooperation and good will, both locally and internationally, can indeed bear fruits so that the sum of the whole will be larger than that of the individual efforts. It was a dream based on the naive belief that in a world besieged with cynicism and evil, there is still a large group of scientists who believe in the importance of sharing their talents in order to improve the world for one and all; that in a world full of selfishness, there are still people who are willing to give of themselves so as to make this dream possible.

Today, we celebrate not only the second birthday of this dream, but also the marvel of scientific cooperation. This distinguished gathering of the most outstanding scientists from all over the world, who excel in their respective fields of learning of the cardiac system, is indeed a living testimonial to the fact that the spirit of pioneering and caring, cooperation and progress still prevails. Let us all remember that once together, the extent of our imagination is the only limit to our potential achievements.

It is with great pleasure that I acknowledge here those who have made this project possible. First and foremost, our dear friends who are not here: Mrs. Pearl Milch, Chairman of the Board of the ATS Women's Division, New York, and the Women's Division Presidium, Miriam Leighton, Ramie Silbert, Rita Wallach, and their Executive Director Mrs. Flo Cohen, who encouraged us with their unshakable trust and provided the means to start the Women's Division Heart System Research Center; Mr. Michael Kennedy-Leigh of London, who trusted us with the support for our initial research program; Professor J. Singer, President of the Technion, who actually believed us that we can indeed make some dreams come true; Professors Walter Welkowitz and Erik Ritman of the United States, who gave us, young toddlers, their trust, council and encouragement in our first steps in this wavy terrain; Professor Y. Palti and Professor D. Front of our Faculty of Medicine who weaved with us the first rough outline of this project; Professor H. Neufeld and Professor M. Gotsman, outstanding cardiologists, who as members of the organizing committee guided us on our way; our colleagues, in the Julius Silver Institute, whose combined medical and engineering education and good common sense kept us on an even keel; Mr. Jacob Sapir, Head, Israel National Council Research and Development, who sponsored the workshop; and finally, last but by no means least, our deep hearted thanks to Mr. Henry Goldberg, a wise young man of 84, and his partner, Elmer Bloch, whose generosity and kindness made this meeting an enjoyable milestone in cardiac research.

Interaction of modern technology and clinical practice

HENRY N. NEUFELD
The Heart Center and The Division of Cardiology The Sheba Medical Center, Tel Hashomer, Israel

The science of medicine and engineering has undergone major progress in recent years. The development of medical science is directed towards better understanding of the physiological processes, deeper understanding of the pathophysiology of diseases, better diagnostic techniques and better solutions for prevention and treatment of diseases. Analytical approaches, new designs and techniques for quantitative measurements of physiological phenomena as well as therapeutic tools are examples of the wide interaction between clinical practice and modern technology.

The dependence of the medical sciences on the engineering sciences is obvious. The field of cardiology and cardiovascular dynamics is a specially challenging area for the interdisciplinary cross fertilization between the medical practice, medical sciences and engineering sciences. As cardiologists we have a large patient base and a broad clinical responsibility and we can offer our patients complete and valued services. Our abilities to arrive at precise anatomic diagnoses, physiological assessment and establish an accurate prognosis, often noninvasively, have grown rapidly thanks to technological advances. Indeed we have seen an impressive decline in cardiovascular mortality in the past one and a half decades. Cardiologists are resourceful and our research programs are vigorous as reflected in the increasing number of our journals. Out of the genius of Einthoven, Roentgen and many others, cardiovascular diagnosis has been brought to the high state of technical perfection for which it has been so admired and of which we may be so proud. The future still holds a promise for the perfection and the exploitation of diagnostic techniques such as ultrasound real-time scanners, nuclear angiography, digital angiography, the computerised CT scan and the NMR. These are recent developments which change the view of cardiovascular diagnosis.

3-Dimensional imaging by various techniques, currently under intense research, will hopefully provide the physician with a more comprehensive picture of the patient pathology. The electrical phenomena of the heart are used as a powerful source of information to the cardiologist. The routine electrocardiogram is being complemented by more sophisticated electro-physiological studies. A new dimension to electrocardiography, body surface potential mapping, may improve the interpretation of the electrical cardiac phenomenon and provide the physician with a more comprehensive picture of bioelectric phenomena.

The deep interrelationship between the basic medical sciences, the mathematical theories and the engineering techniques are of the utmost importance. The development of fast computers in the past years has enabled the application of complicated models of the cardiovascular system to clinical, theoretical and physiological problems. As I have already implied, the vast development of imaging techniques has almost completely changed the cardiovascular diagnosis in the last few years. In medical therapeutics, bioengineering has developed various cardiac assisting devices – cardiac pulmonary bypass machine and other tools to aid cardiologists. These include the PTCA (Percutaneous Transluminal Coronary Angioplasty) a new technique to open stenosis in coronary arteries. Yet another new technique, Laser angioplasty, currently under intensive research will hopefully enable us to open stenosed coronary arteries.

The large numbers of diagnostic techniques used in clinical practice to assess cardiac disease are integrated in each patient by the physician based on his own clinical experience and logical interpretation of the data. Though some of the techniques provide us with firm, accurate data about physiological processes, the integration of various aspects in cardiac physiology is still missing. Although cardiac mechanics is directly related to electrical activation patterns, very little has been done to quantatively relate these intra-cardiac phenomena. The same is true for the interrelationships between the cardiac mechanical processes and the exact pattern of the blood perfusion and energy consuming processes within the heart.

The recent advances in computer and engineering techniques open the way for the idea of the global computerised heart. Such a feasible engineering medical model of the heart will help towards a better understanding of the phenomena which are directly related to the interrelationship between the complex processes within the heart. The bedside physician will never be replaced by such sophisticated tools which will enable him to interrelate different clinical measurements. But, of course, in the right hands and given the right interpretation, these will introduce a quantitative aspect to the qualitative impression of the physician.

I believe that the clinical practice of medicine and cardiology of the future will be influenced more, much more, profoundly by studies of human genetics, molecular biology, cellular physiology and experimental pathology, by studies of problems such as the mechanisms of endocytosis as the mechanisms of ondocystosis, the control of calcium fluxes across the sarcolemma of the colemma of the myocardium and specialised cardiac tissue, the fundamental mechanisms by which platelets adhere to the arterial endothelium or by which adrenalin acts on its receptors and vascular smooth muscle; the renal cortex and other tissues; by all these, and other fundamental studies. It is becoming even clearer that in most forms of heart disease, the heart is an innocent bystander which has been injured by a process that primarily affects the cardiac cells. The most fruitful future research in cardiovascular disease may well not even be focused on the heart.

Be it as it may, the success of medicine in general, in cardiology in particular, greatly depends on the close interaction between clinical practice and modern technology. I can forsee important accomplishments in cardiovascular diagnosis such as noninvasive measurements of intra-cardiac pressures and flows, the elucidation of coronary arterial anatomy, to give only a few examples. The number of successful intervention procedures will also grow steadily thanks to modern technology. The time has come, I believe, to acknowledge that while we may have reached the happy state that allows us to establish an accurate anatomic and physiological diagnosis with reasonable safety in almost all patients with heart disease, we still do not understand the cause of most forms of congenital heart disease, of hypertension, arteriosclerosis, cardiomyopathy, many forms of valvular diseases and most forms of congestive heart failure.

Despite the continuous reduction of cardiovascular mortality in the western world, sudden Cardiac Death remains, unfortunately, a greatly unsolved problem. In October 1966 I had the great pleasure of opening the first Cardiological International Workshop in Israel. The topic was Electrical Regulation of the Heart. (The symposium was published in the Israel Journal of Medical Sciences). Among other things there I said, and I quote, 'one can assume that in the not too distant future, while men walk down the street, that teleelectrocardiogram might be recorded and analysed by central computing stations. Abnormalities will then be detected and prior to the development of an acute catastrophic clinical picture, it will be possible to institute prophylactic treatment. Technological development may lead to ultra-sophistication of electronic devices on the one hand, and new potent anti-arrhythmic drugs on the other hand, in order to prevent Enemy Number One – Sudden Death.' Successful interaction of modern technology in clinical medicine and clinical practice will hopefully realise this dream in the not too distant future. We all hope so.

We must do our best with the means at our disposal. As those are, unfortunately, very limited in many countries, we must develop optimal cooperation which will lead to better understanding of the development of disease processes, for better diagnosis, more effective treatment and finally, successful prevention. Effective control of the major forms of heart diseases will require understanding of their fundamental causes and mechanisms rather than association of the natural history. Stronger links between cardiovascular research and the other biomedical sciences will, I hope, gradually, shift the track of the cardiology of today from the exploitation of technology designed to provide more accurate diagnosis and treatment of existing disease to the cardiology of tomorrow, which I believe, will use the techniques of modern biology and technology to elucidate the fundamental causes of heart disease and then eliminate them. This shift will lead, with the help of modern technology, to new and even more exciting cardiology and I would like to think that this symposium which is very well planned and very well organized will contribute in this direction. Today's clinical practice is the diagnosis and treatment of different cardiovascular conditions. Tomorrow's cardiologists will be, I hope, prevention. We are a very fortunate and a very frustrated medical generation. We are fortunate because the field of cardiology is changing so rapidly, literally in front of our eyes, and we have the privilege to participate and even sometimes to influence these changes. But we are also a sorely frustrated medical generation because the scope and rate of change exceed our adaptation capabilities. To keep abreast with current literature becomes mission impossible; to absorb, classify and store the most important data has become an intellectual nightmare. Hence the great importance of scientific meetings such as this one. There is no better, quicker and more efficient way of transmitting scientific information than direct personal contacts.

Before I finish, I would like to remind all of us that after all the progress and achievements, despite the successful interaction of medicine and technology, our sacred goal is the benefit of our patients. We in our profession have to remember that the cardiologist is a member of a group which deals with technical procedures which are already too complex for one individual to master. But whether the cardiologist is a member of a team having expert knowledge of the different aspect of his role or whether he still works as an individual, he is a professional member of a community for whose welfare and progress he shoulders considerable responsibility. Today, more than ever before, the moral obligation and responsibility of physicians is to extend their influence beyond the catheterization and ECG laboratories towards a real universal acceptance and the understanding of the human values which they represent. Let us not forget, therefore, about these human qualities. Let us all also remember that behind each new machine or gadget there is a suffering human being, a patient who needs badly our help.

Finally, in the name of the Israeli cardiologists, we would like to welcome our very distinguished guests from abroad and to wish you a very pleasant stay in Israel and a very successful meeting. Thank you very much.

Major interacting parameters in a 3–D model of the cardiac system

SAMUEL SIDEMAN*
The Julius Silver Institute and Department of Chemical and Biomedical Engineering, Technion-Israel Institute of Technology, Haifa 32000, Israel

Abstract

An overview of the major parameters which hopefully describe the cardiac system is presented and some of the basic reconstruction elements required to develop a 3–D computer simulation model are discussed. The interactions between cardiac mechanics, hemodynamics and transport phenomena are shown to yield the pressure gradients within the 3–D left ventricle (LV) cavity and the temporal temperature distribution within the myocardium, thus demonstrating the potential power of the envisioned 3–D simulation model.

Introduction

The intense, but highly dispersed, efforts of cardiac researchers during the last decades provide a good understanding and a deep insight into many of the numerous aspects which make up the cardiovascular field. Various variables in the fields of cardiac mechanics, hemodynamics and coronary circulation, myocardial metabolism, geometrial imaging techniques and related topics were extensively studied, However, attempts at interrelating and/or integrating multidisciplined parameters into 'all inclusive', or even a 'partially inclusive', models are rather scarce. Moreover, the attempts at interrelating these different areas have usually been carried out in a qualitative rather than a quantitative way. Figure 1 represents a schematic overview of the interrelated parameters arranged in concentric primary and secondary circles. Obviously, a multi-disciplinary research program, aimed at developing a quantitative simulation model which relates the various cardiac parameters by translating the physiological phenomena of the cardiac system to quantitative engineering relationships, is highly desired. By relating, either directly or indirectly, to clinical problems, the model

* Roy J. Matas/Winnipeg Professor of Biomedical Engineering

will greatly contribute to the knowledge of the heart's function and the understanding of dysfunctions due to various insults to the system. Clearly, before the major areas of interest can be qualitatively interrelated to one another, it is essential to know the 'internal' physiological-engineering laws within each of these areas. Once the quantitative laws in each area are known, the interrelations between the various areas can be developed, and continuously validated, by physiological-clinical measurements.

It is the purpose of this presentation to introduce this highly complex multidisciplinary system; to highlight the major interrelated areas and to discuss some of the important steps in the development of an all inclusive simulation model of

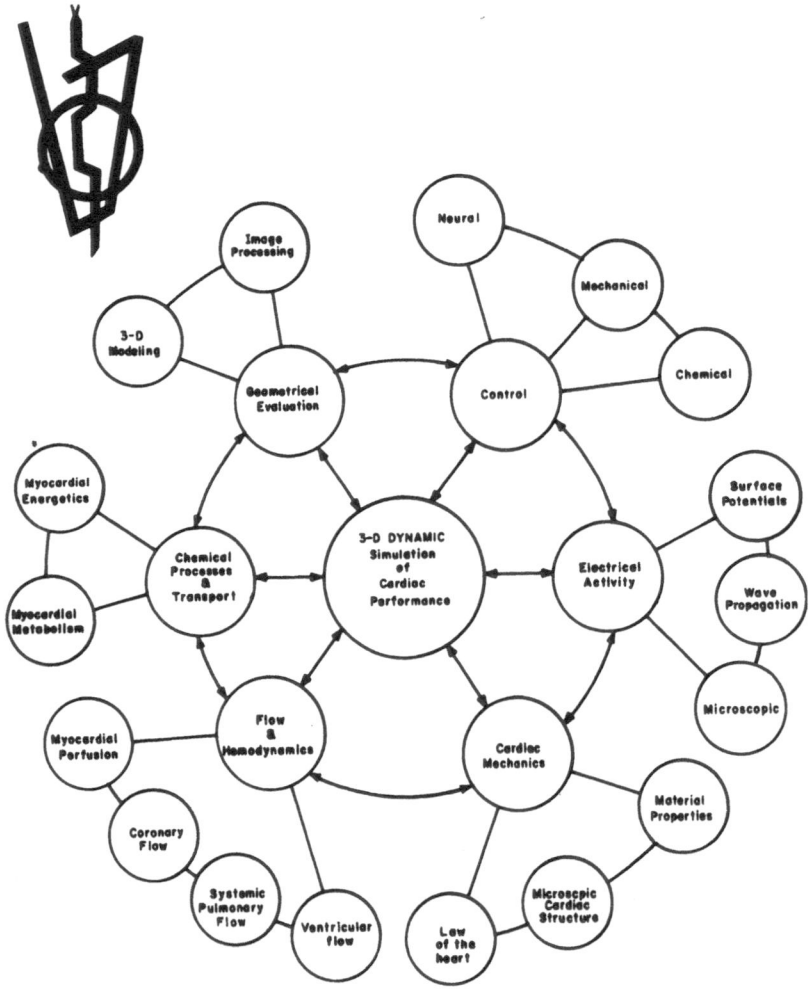

HEART SYSTEM RESEARCH CENTER

Figure 1. An overview of the interrelating parameters constructing the dynamic simulation model.

this system. The major interacting areas of the cardiac system, and some of the potential benefits which may come out once these areas are indeed brought together, are schematically presented in Figure 2. The 'heart of the model' is the dynamic simulation of the interacting cardiac functions. Obviously, representing the correct mechanical aspects entails a correct combination of the microscale muscle structure and the macroscale geometry of the heart (aspects studied by geometrical reconstruction technique); the flow and hemodynamics (which determine the preload and afterload); the electrical activation sequence (which dictates the mechanical activation sequence), as well as the basic heart rate. Not the least important, the simulation must include the coronary perfusion which is instrumental in translating chemical to mechanical energy needed for the cardiac activity. Finally, the model should include the control of the cardiac system, which is governed by a complex dynamic mechanism which adjusts the function of the heart to the body's needs. Needless to say, a model of such a magnitude requires the close cooperation of the outstanding specialists in the various fields.

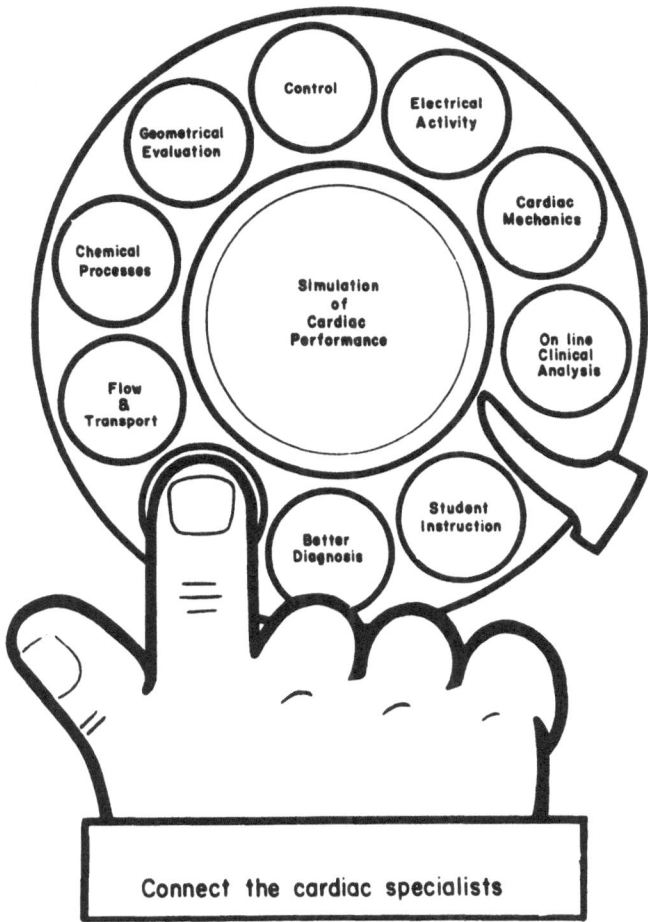

Figure 2. Major interacting parameters in a 3-D model.

The simulation model perceived here represents the so-called 'forward problem' of the heart. Perturbations of different interactions and parameters will help to study the evolution of various diseases and to evaluate different physiological effects on cardiac dysfunction. Also, on-line evaluation of short-term therapeutic, mainly pharmaceutical, procedures can be envisioned. Eventually, the model may help with the most challenging solution of the 'inverse problem', i.e., to help identify the pathology in a specific patient.

Some cardiac mechanics aspects

The major function of the heart muscle is to pump blood from the low pressure venous system to the high pressure arterial pathways. All the systems of the heart serve this special purpose. Therefore, the formulation and solution of the mechanical problem is a basic element in any general model of the cardiac system.

In general, a model can include structural and physiological assumptions, depending on the phenomena to be described. Models describing the cardiac function, and mainly the LV function, have been suggested with various degrees of complexity. Scalaric models describe the interrelationship $f(t)$ between scalaric paremeters, like pressure and volume as a function of time, during the LV contraction (Beyar and Sideman, 1984a). It is noted that valuable physiological diagnostic information can be derived from such simple global models which play a major role in the estimation of cardiac function.

Knowledge of the instantaneous and local functional distribution $f(y,t)$ throughout the LV wall is required for the calculation of various cardiac phenomena (Beyar and Sideman, 1984b). This entails accounting for the anatomic microscopic orientation of the muscles' fibers which hold a direct relation to the distribution of the mechanical properties. A 3-D dynamic model $f(r,\theta,\varphi)$ is needed for a detailed description of the geometry of the cardiac chambers, and to account for the distributed parameters within the myocardium in the spatial inhomogeneities associated with certain diseases, like myocardial infarction.

One obvious application of this multi-variable approach is the calculation of the 3-D flow and pressure field within the LV cavity. Figure 3 represents a first (Horowitz et al., 1984) attempt to evaluate the pressure distribution within the LV. The isobars indicate the corresponding normalized pressures at a systolic phase of 0.3 s at maximum wall displacement, assuming a constant aortic pressure. This 3-D flow analysis was made possible by the courtesy and cooperation of Spalding (1984) utilizing the Phoenics 3-D computer program for heat, mass and momentum transfer (CHAM Corp. London).

The combination of the sarcomere and fiber mechanics with the fine anatomical details of the fiber pathways yields the 'law of the heart'. The material properties of the cardiac muscle, both in the passive and active states, still need to

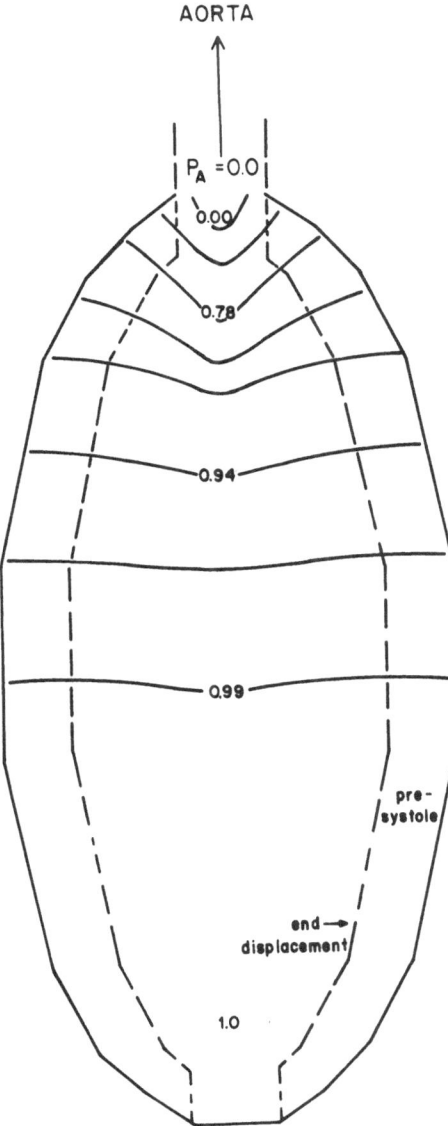

Figure 3. Pressure gradients within the cavity of the contracting LV at a systolic phase of 0.3 s.

the intensely studied. The physiologic parameters can then be translated to stress, strain and strain rate which can be solved by utilizing the theory of elásticity.

The solution of the 3-D elastic problem of a nonlinear nonhomogeneous anisotropic material presents a major engineering challenge. The interaction between the geometry of the moving dynamic muscle and muscle mechanics can be evaluated by different approaches. The obvious difficulty lies in the uncertainty of the spatial values of the material properties in a nonhomogeneous body.

One approach is to start with a given initial state (like, for example, the reference unstressed LV configuration) which is then perturbed by a given interference, say a pressure increment in the cavity, to yield a calculated new shape. The new shape may now be compared to the corresponding measured, real, shape and the 'error' in the prediction of the new shape is used to modify the local characteristics and material properties. In a second approach, one starts with a given measured geometry (before and after the interference) and solves for the stress and pressure distribution by adjusting for the appropriate values of the local material properties. Obviously, the first approach is suitable for the study of given local perturbations whereas the second one is more suitable to identify local anomalities.

The use of finite elements is currently the best method to deal with such a multidimensional problem, although the method is quite cumbersome and requires relatively long computer time. However, future generation computers as well as new techniques utilizing array processors and parallel computers will eventually enable faster handling of this 3-D dynamic problem.

Some geometrical aspects

A clear and well outlined geometry of the LV gives the physician an important tool by providing him with information regarding the location and extension of pathological states. The advantages increase with the increase in the number of the dimensions that can be viewed. Thus, the change from 1-D to 2-D echocardiology supplied the physician with a more powerful tool for the evaluation of diseases. The transformation of local, static 2-D pictures to 3-D reconstructed images is considered as one of the most important recent developments in medical science. The reconstruction of 3-D dynamic geometries fascinates the imagination and is intensively pursued by a number of groups of engineers and physicians. In general, the 3-D images of the cardiac system can be reconstructed from section images (Ultrasound sector scan, DSR) or from projection images (angiography, nuclear radiography). Other imaging techniques, which are currently rather slow for dynamic pictures (CT scan, NMR scan), may play a larger role in the future.

The major steps in the imaging and 3-D reconstruction of the heart from series 2-D section images, of say, ultrasound, are limited by some inherent difficulties. These include:

(a) Exact definition of the location, in space, of the section points taken;
(b) Accurate edge detection of the LV wall borders (by manual, semiautomatic or automatic techniques);
(c) Accurate construction (by interpolation) of an assumed geometry, based on the given set of spatial points defining the endocardial and epicardial surfaces;

(d) Clear graphic presentation (shadowing) and efficient computer manipulation of the reconstructed 3-D image, for better perception in space and clearer identification of deviations from the expected normal pattern.

An example of a 3-D image reconstruction (Brevdo *et al.*, 1984) from a set of 2-D epicardial cross sections is shown in Figure 4. The data, cordially provided by Ritman (1984), was obtained by the DSR technique. The reconstruction procedure involves transformation from cartesian to spherical coordinates and calculation of an interpolation function in order to find coordinates of the grid points on the boundary of a closed body. The basic assumption is that every ray which emanates from the origin (the midpoint of the longest axis) meets the boundary of the body in just one point. The boundary of the body in any spherical coordinate system, coinciding in its origin with the cartesian coordinate system, is given by a single valued function: $r = (\varrho,\theta)$ defined in the rectangle $0<\varrho< \pi$; $0<\theta<\pi$. The measured coordinates $(x_i y_i z_i)$ of the i-th grid point are translated into (r_i,ϱ_i,θ_i). The problem of calculating r_0 for a given (ϱ_0,θ_0) is treated as an interpolation problem for the function $r = r(\varrho,\theta)$. The interpolating value of r was calculated by using IQHSCV subroutine from MSL (IBM library) which utilizes a method for bivariate interpolation and smooth surface fitting for irregularly distributed data points (Akima, 1978).

Some electrophysiological aspects

The electrical activity of the heart is a complex process which includes cellular

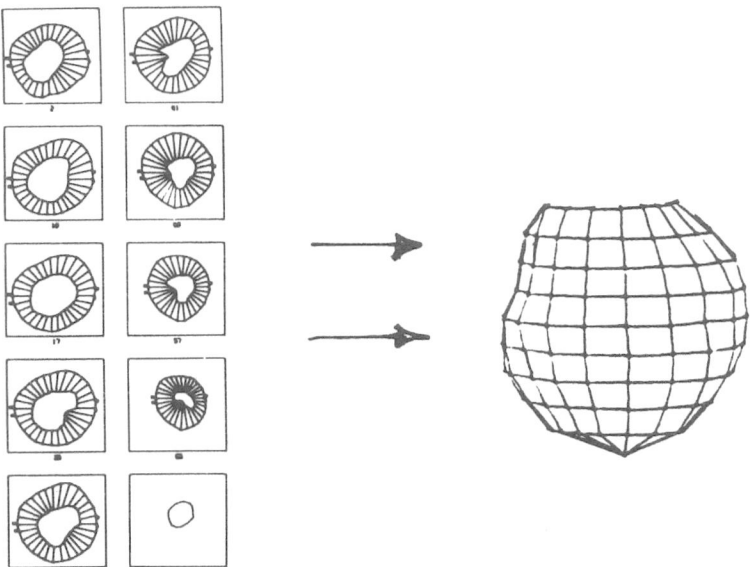

Figure 4. Reconstructed 3-D image based on 2-D epicardial DSR cross sections.

membrane excitation, propagation of the activation wave and transformation of the internal potential sources to epicardial and body surface potentials. The electrical activity of the heart actually dictates its mechanical function and, to some extent, the reverse is true too.

In order to define the interaction between the electrical and mechanical processes, one must relate to the microscopic level. The electromechanical linkage is a complex function of ionic processes within the cardiac fibers. The microscopic electromechanical interaction is embedded within the sequence of activation of the myocardium. Under normal conditions, the endocardium is activated almost uniformly and instantaneously (less than 80 msec) through a conducting network system, followed by a radial propagation wave of the activation signal from the endocardium to the epicardium. This assures an even contraction of the LV and an optimal mechanical function. A small apicobasal component of the activation sequence creates a 'peristaltic' movement of the heart which helps to achieve a minimum energy waste during the contraction processes.

The solution of the pattern of the electrical activation propagation has to bring into account the microscopic electrical properties of the fibers, the anisotropysm in the electrical properties of the fibers, the geometry and structure of the electrical conduction system and the fiber architecture within the heart.

As demonstrated in Table 1, based on a simple model which utilizes a sinusoidal activation wave (Beyar and Sideman, 1984b), the effect of the propagation velocity of the electrical signal on the LV mechanics of a 'normal' homogeneous heart is rather minor. However, the myocardial excitation in hearts with abnormal electrical activation (a block in the conduction system or an ectopic activation occurring out of the conduction system) is non-uniform. The solution of the mechanical problem may thus have to account for regional delayed activation extending beyond 200 ms. It is expected that perturbations of the electrical propagation in a model, which is strongly related to a mechanical model of the heart, will help to understand the causes and effects of various electrical pathologies and cardiac dysfunction.

Another problem which has to be solved in order to achieve the desired integrated view of the global heart is the transfer function from the source potentials of the heart to the body surface potentials which are measured either by routine ECG, vector cardiography, or the new techniques of surface potential mapping (Liebman et al., 1981; Hinsen et al., 1981). The forward problem of transforming known source potentials to surface potential maps, based on electri-

Table 1. Effect of radial propagation velocity on LV mechanics

Velocity of radial spread	dp/dt (mmHg/s)	Ejection fraction [%]	E_{max} (mmHg/ml)
30 cm/s	1959	69	4.1
15 cm/s	1900	67	3.8

cal properties of the volume conductor, i.e. the chest, has been solved in various degrees of success. The inverse problem of solving for the epicardial potentials from the body surface potentials is of great clinical interest, and presents a major theoretical and clinical problem. Some of the intensive work in this field is further discussed in this meeting.

Myocardial energy balance, perfusion and temperature distribution

One of the important parameters in the function of the heart is the energy demand and supply interrelation within the myocardium. The energy needed for the contraction process is dictated by metabolic and mechanical parameters (Beyar and Sideman, 1984c). As most of the cardiac metabolism is aerobic, energy demand can be expressed in terms of oxygen demand without introducing a major error. The coronary perfusion distribution shown in Figure 5 is based on the mechanical data obtained (Effert *et al.*, 1984) from a patient with coronary stenosis. A detailed comparison with a normal heart is presented later in this meeting. It suffices to note that Figure 5 demonstrates the mechanical effects of compression on the blood perfusion during systole and diastole and is an excellent example of the power of a quantitative interaction between LV mechanics and hemodynamics.

The combination of the time dependent wall dimensions, the distributed energy demand parameters (which is associated with oxygen consumption) and the time dependent blood flow distribution provide the basic data needed to

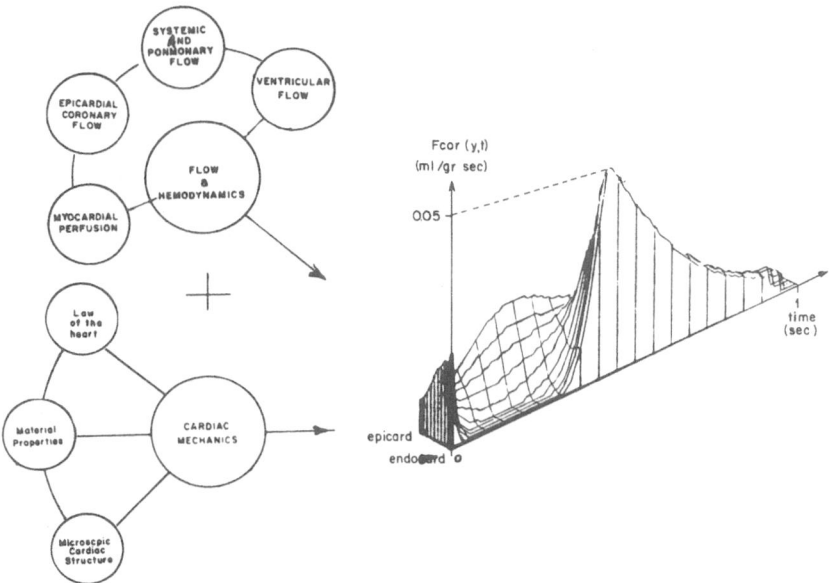

Figure 5. Instantaneous blood flow distribution in the myocardium.

14

calculate the myocardial temperature distribution under various aerobic conditions in man. The instantaneous local temperature T in the myocard is obtained (Barta *et al.*, 1984) by solving the heat balance equation

$$\alpha \frac{\partial T}{\partial T} = \frac{\partial^2 T}{\partial r^2} + \frac{1}{r} \frac{\partial T}{\partial r} + \frac{1}{k} [\dot{q}_m + \dot{m}_b \, \rho_b \, c_b \, (T_b - T)] \tag{1}$$

where $\alpha = \varrho C/k$ is the thermal diffusivity of the muscle, k denotes the thermal conductivity of the muscle, ϱ is the density, C is the scecific heat, $\dot{q}_m$ is the metabolic heat production rate, $\dot{m}$ is mass flow rate per unit muscle weight, and the subscript b denotes the blood.

The solution of Eq. (1) for three different heart rates is presented in Figure 6. Note that the calculations show that the temperature at any given point does *not* change, in any significant sense, during the contraction and relaxation phases.

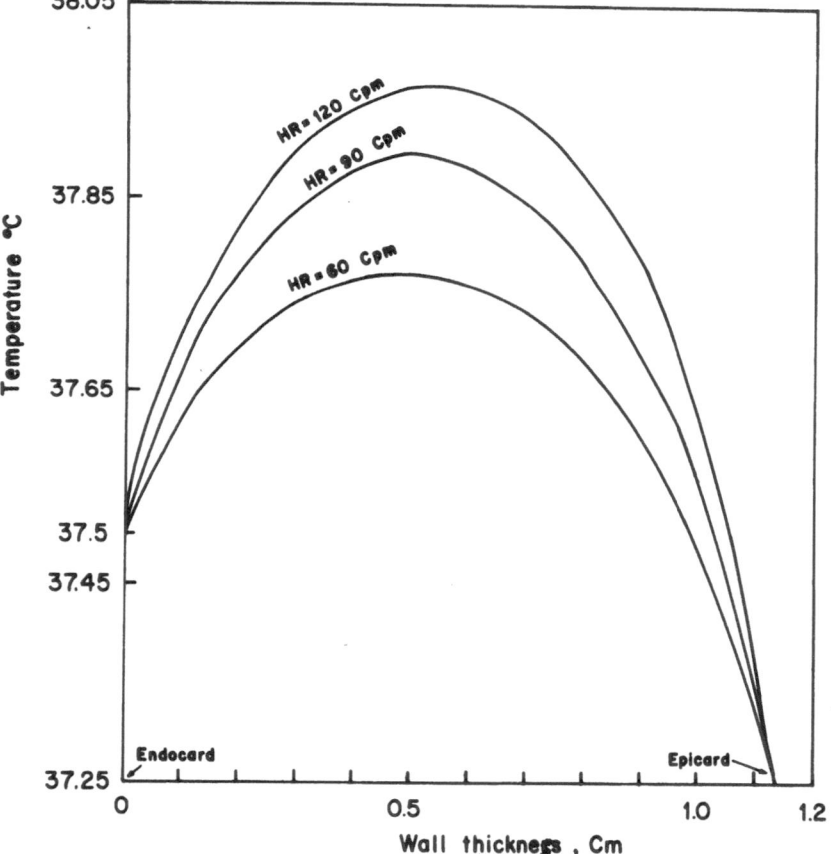

Figure 6. Temperature distribution across the LV wall, at different heart rates. Note that the local temperatures do not change significantly during the cycle.

The results are consistent with experimental data (animals) and represent an excellent example of the complex interaction between cardiac mechanics, energy metabolism, coronary flow and local control loops affecting the coronary perfusion.

Some control aspects

Obviously, the control of the cardiac function is a most important and difficult area encompassing a number of interacting parameters. Figure 7 is a simple representation of some of the major control aspects involved in this highly complicated phenomena which greatly challenge the imagination when attempting to quantify them. Work along these lines is certainly required if a meaningful simulation model is to be developed.

Conclusion

An overview of various major parameters and their interactions in the cardiac system is presented and attempts to relate the geometry to the physiological characteristics are discussed. Particular emphasis is given to the geometrical evaluation of the real heart and the reconstruction of the 3-Dimensional simulated heart. Attempts to evaluate the 3-D pressure distribution within the LV are reported. The application of the spatial and temporal mechanics, coronary perfusion flow and energetics inside the myocardium to the solution of the temperature field inside the wall under various aerobic operating conditions is demonstrated as an example of a step in the quantitative evaluation of the interacting phenomena. The need for a quantitative 3-D model describing the dynamic heart, either as a responding study tool or as an aid to interpret various cardiac dysfunctions is emphasized.

Acknowledgement

This presentation is a part of the intensive research effort currently being carried out in the J. Silver Institute Heart System Research Center. We are greatly indebted to the courageous foresight and support of Mrs. Pearl Milch and the MEP group of the Women's Division, American Technion Society, N.Y. The personal interest and financial support of Mr. and Mrs. Michael Kennedy-Leigh is also warmly acknowledged. Finally, the trust and cooperation of students and colleagues, both in Israel and abroad, is gratefully and gleefully acknowledged.

16

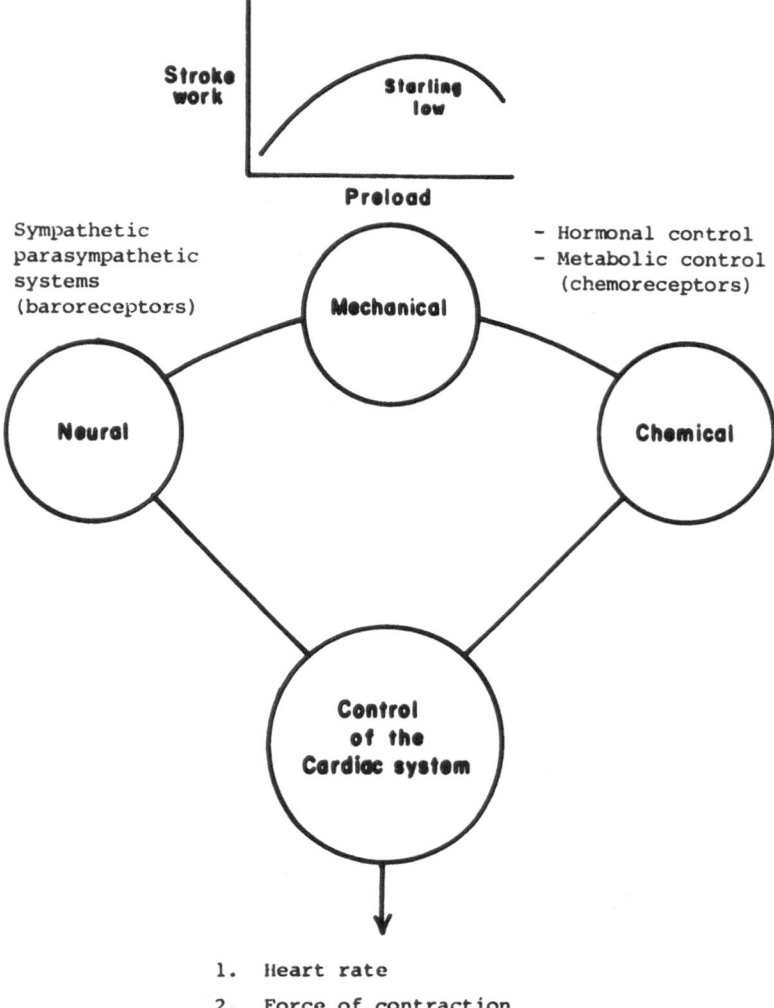

Figure 7. Some control aspects.

References

Akima H (1978) A method of bivariate interpolation and smooth surface fitting for irregularly distributed data points. ACM Trans Math Software 4:148–159

Barta E, Beyar R, Sideman S (1984) A mathematical model for the temperature distribution within the canine and human hearts. Int J Heat and Mass Transfer, in press

Beyar R, Sideman S (1984a) A model for left ventricular contraction combining the force-length-velocity relationship with the time varying elastance theory. Biophys J 45:1167–1177

Beyar R, Sideman S (1984b) A computer study of the left ventricular performance based on the fiber structure, sarcomere dynamics and transmural electrical propagation velocity. Circ Res 55:358–375

Beyar R, Sideman S (1984d) Time dependent coronary blood flow distribution in the left ventricular wall. Submitted for publication

Beyar R, Sideman S (1984c) Spatial energy balance within a structural model of the left ventricle. Submitted to Am J Physiology

Brevdo L, Sideman S, Adam D, Beyar R (1984) Interpolation technique for 3-D reconstruction from a finite number of surface points. In preparation

Effert S, Von Essen R (1984) Pressure-volume data obtained by catherization of a patient with aortic stenosis. Personal Communication

Hinsen R, Von Essen R, Silny J, Merx W, Rau G, Effert S (1981) Computer analysis of multiple lead stress tests for predicting coronary artery disease. In: Budapest Z Antaloczy, I Preda (eds) Electrocardiology

Horowitz A, Perl M, Sideman S, Spalding BD (1984) 3-D cavity flow and pressure distribution, Internal report No. 121. Technion R&D Foundation Project: 130–118

Liebman E, Thomas W, Rudy Y, Plonsey R (1981) Electrocardiographic body surface potential maps of the QRS of normal children. J Electrocardiology 14:249–260

Ritman E (1984) 2-D sections of a canine heart and a corresponding 3-D grid based on DSR. Personal Communication

Spalding BD (1984) Application of the Phoenix 3-D CHAM computer program. Imperial College London. Personal Communication

Some physiological aspects in the development of cardiac models

RAFAEL BEYAR
Julius Silver Institute and Department of Biomedical Engineering Technion – Israel Institute of Technology, Haifa, Israel

Abstract

Appropriate physiological assumptions are the first step in the development of any model of the cardiac system. The use of the physiological laws should be guided by the desired complexity of the model and the phenomena to be described. The physiological laws which are required for a complete description of the mechanical, energetic and perfusion aspects of the cardiac cycle are presented and discussed. The complexities involved in going from global models to multidimensional ones are shown. The development of a 3–D model should be guided by physiological laws which are studied and quantified by lower dimensional models of axial symmetry.

Introduction

The function of the heart is the outcome of a complex combination of the different processes which relate to cardiac mechanics. The basic laws which determine the function of the heart are influenced by the cardiac electrical activity, the coronary perfusion supplying the energy demands of the system, the pathways of metabolism involved in the energetic processes and the general control mechanisms which are aimed to adjust cardiac function to the body needs. Each of the above-mentioned fields has been a subject for intensive investigation for many years. In spite of that, the rules which determine the function of the system are not always clear, and are actually sometimes ambiguous. Furthermore, the interrelationship between different processes have been studied, and quantified, only to a limited extent.

An engineering approach to the cardiovascular system necessitates clearly defined rules as well-as quantification of physiological parameters. A quantitative description of a dynamic three dimensional model of the heart presents a major mathematical problem. It requires a good definition of the various 'laws of the heart' and the identification of the important parameters which should be used in the 3-D model.

It is the purpose of this presentation to consider a quantitative approach to some of the physiological aspects required for the solution of the major cardiac functions and to highlight the missing links and controversial areas which have to be studied in the future for better understanding of the global cardiac performance.

The mechanical problem

The common approaches to the quantitative description of cardiac function ignore the spatial distribution of various parameters and interrelate the global parameters like pressure, volume, flow, average stress, etc. The cardiac mechanics laws which lead to the global characteristics of the LV, are (Figure 1):

(a) The passive exponential (inactive state) pressure-volume (P-V) relationship (Diamond et al., 1971).

(b) The active P-V relationship known as the time varying elastance (Suga et al., 1973).

(c) The relationship between the maximum elastance and the LV volume (Suga et al., 1976).

(d) The force-velocity relationship relating the velocity of contraction to the opposing forces (classical measurements provide us with an hyperbolic force velocity relationship (Hill's 1978) for the fully active state. However the exact relationship for the partially activated state is still a subject for further research).

(e) The mathematical relationship between the LV pressure, geometry and average wall stress (Mirsky, 1974).

A simulation of LV performance based on the above assumption, with linkage to a simple arterial model (Windkessel), is shown in Figure 2. The simulated pressure volume, pressure-time, flow-time, volume-time and stress-time, for different values of the preload are consistent with physiological measurements and show that the global LV function can be adequately described by an average 'zero-dimensional' model.

It is well known that the intramyocardial stress and pressure (Streeter et al., 1970; Mirsky, 1974), the coronary flow pattern, and the energy demand (Gibbs, 1978), are not evenly distributed in the LV wall. Furthermore, the spatial orientation of the muscle fibers is a function of the distance from the endocard (Streeter et al., 1979). Thus, a spatial model which will describe distributed properties is highly desired. A good design of a distributed-parameter model depends on the following data and assumptions:

(a) The selection of a well approximated geometry to describe the LV, Figure 3a.

20

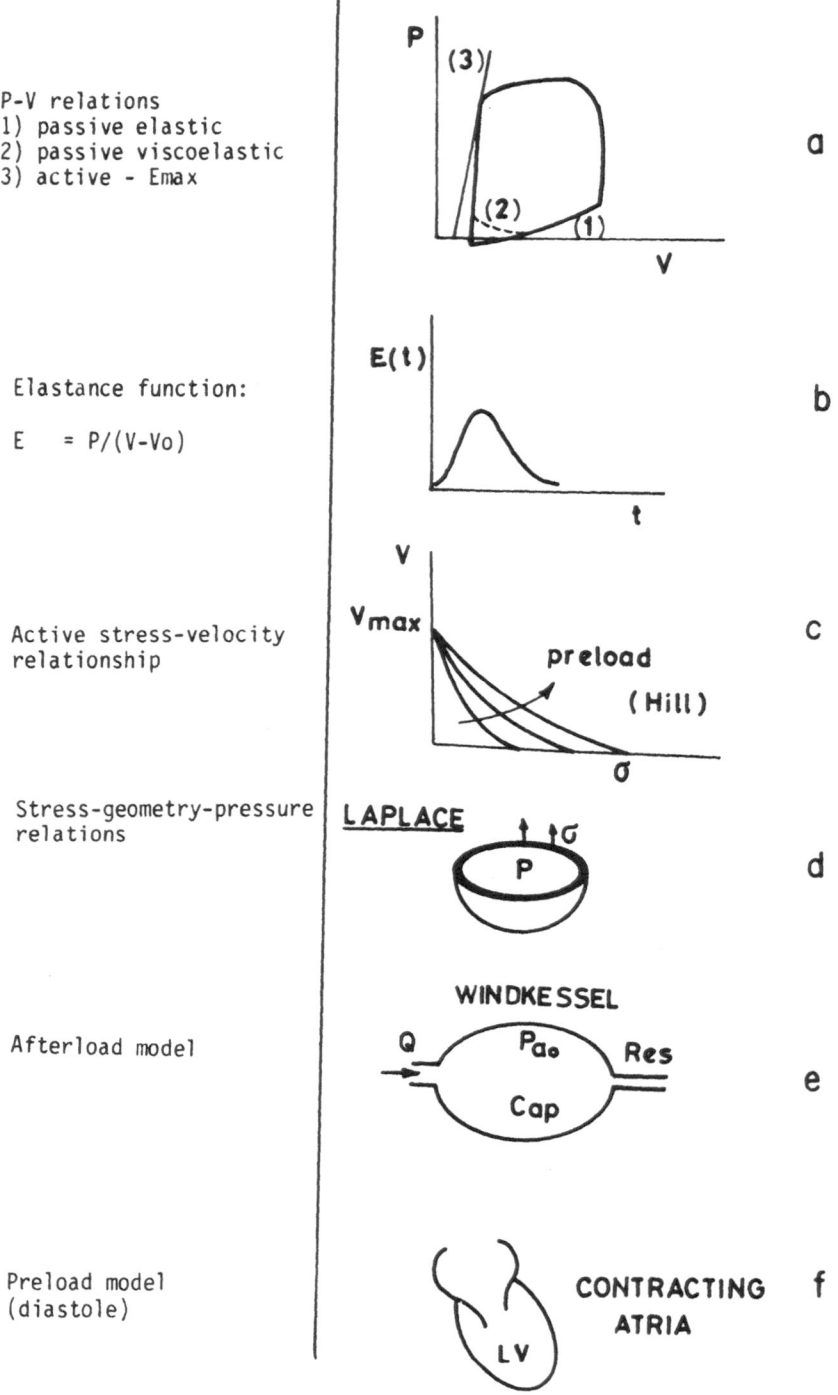

P-V relations
1) passive elastic
2) passive viscoelastic
3) active - Emax

Elastance function:

$E = P/(V-Vo)$

Active stress-velocity
relationship

Stress-geometry-pressure
relations

Afterload model

Preload model
(diastole)

Figure 1. The macroscale interacting parameters and relations for the description of global LV mechanics.

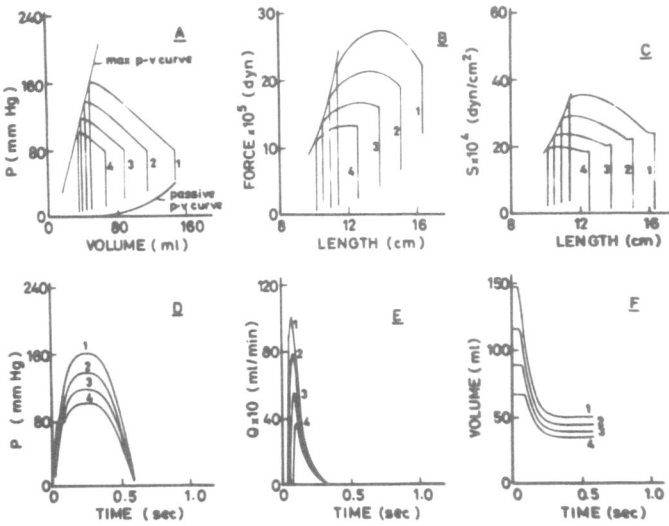

Figure 2. Simulation of LV performance based on the macroscale parameter (Beyar and Sideman, 1984a). A – pressure volume; B – force length; C – stress length; D – pressure time; E – flow time; F – volume time.

(b) A realistic description of the fiber angle distribution throughout the wall, Figure 3b, (Streeter, *et al.*, 1969).

(c) Geometrical considerations which need to be defined. It can be shown mathematically that during LV contraction the strains and strain rates are maximal in the endocardial layers, Figure 3c. Using solely the geometrical assumptions, it can be shown that twisting of the LV along its longitudinal axis, Figure 3d, tends to attenuate the differences between the stresses developed in the endocardial and epicardial sarcomeres. (Beyar and Sideman, 1984b).

(d) A description of the electrical activation propagation pattern. A centripetal electrical activation spread can be assumed in a simple symmetrical model of the LV with sufficient accuracy, Figure 3e. A more precise description of the electrical activation should include a apicobasal component of the activation vector. This pattern of electrical spread is important for the optimization of the flow pattern within the LV cavity.

(e) Estimation of the passive fiber properties, parallel (and later perpendicular) to the fibers direction. The exponential stress-strain law along the fibers is well established, Figure 4a. Some data exist regarding the stiffness perpendicular to the fiber direction. However, the latter is less established due to the difficulties in the measurements of the transfiber properties of the muscle. The viscoelastic properties of the fibers are well recognized and

22

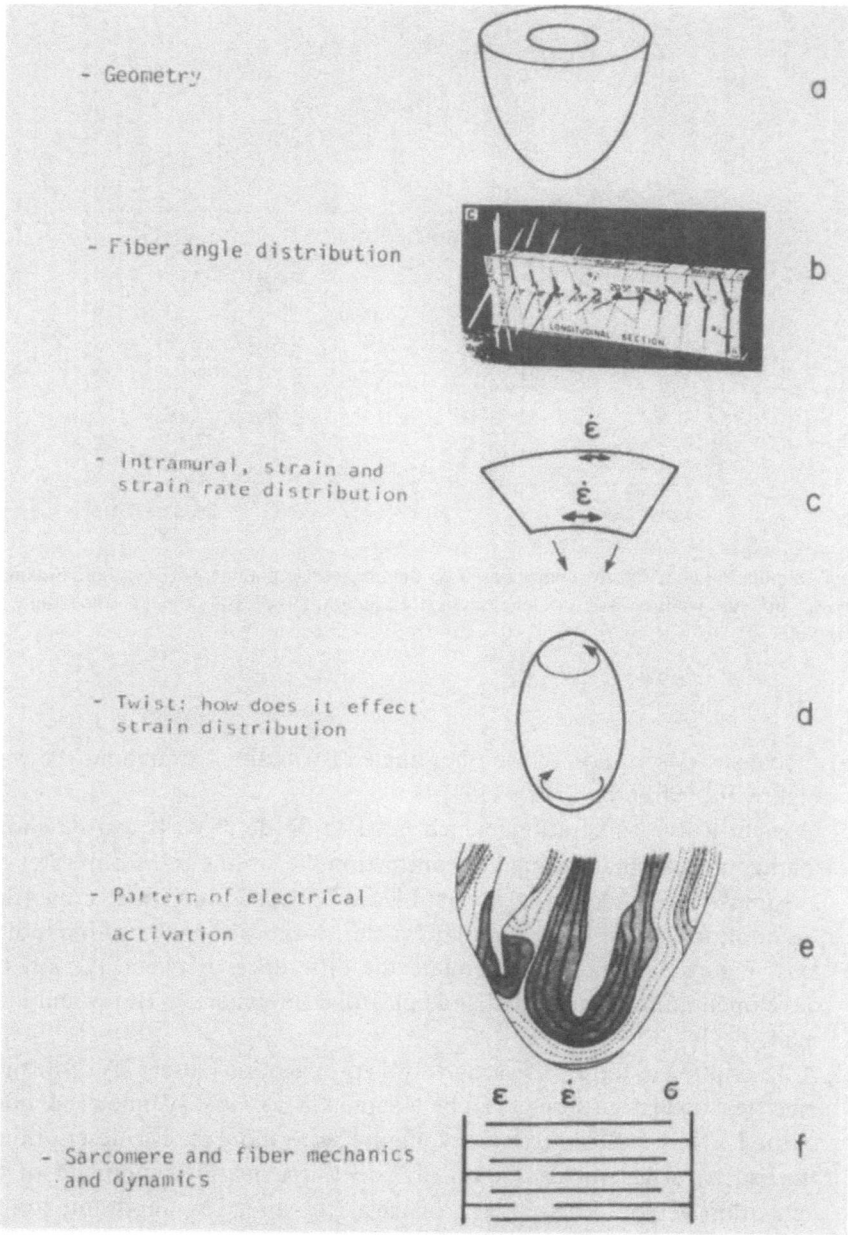

Figure 3. The structural parameters needed for the description of distributed properties within the LV wall.

should be accounted for in the model, especially for the rapid filling period of the ventricles where the highest values of the strain rate are obtained.

(d) A relation between the fiber active force development and the sarcomere length. A linear relation between the length of the sarcomere and the developed stress is well known, Figure 4a, line 2.

(g) A description of the activation function, Fac, which is needed to describe the LV mechanics during systole, Figure 4b. The degree of activation of the fibers is not easily measurable. Based on the classical three-element model of the cardiac muscle (composed of contractile, series and parallel elastic elements) with (a calculated) v_{max} as a parameter for the degree of activity, an activation function of the contractile proteins was suggested. This activation function is characterized by a rapid increase, and a slow decrease, of the degree of activity. These three-element models of the muscle are open to criticism (Pollack and Krueger, 1978) and an approach that the stress-length relationship is applied to the muscle fiber as a whole, and combined with a mechanical activation function is suggested here. In this way the activation function is closer to a sine wave. The long relaxation tail which is frequently observed must eventually account for the rate of the pressure relaxation in the LV.

(h) A description of the electromechanical interactions. This is an important aspect which is still not exactly defined, including the relation between the duration of the electrical systole to the duration of the activation function and to the peak developed stress. Since the maximum elastance is usually

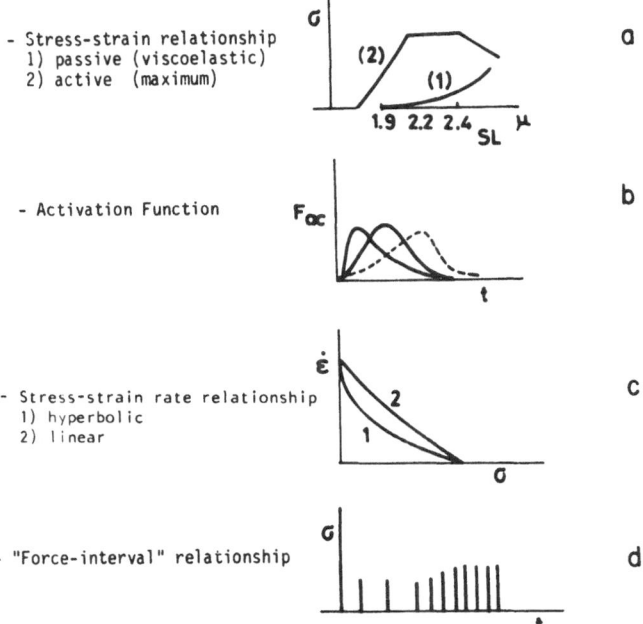

Figure 4. The physiological lays of fiber mechanics.

encountered during end systole, it is suggested that the activation function achieves its maximum value simultaneous with the T wave of the ECG.

(i) Selection of the appropriate stress strain rate relation of the fiber, since the choice between a linear and hyperbolic function is still inconclusive, Figure 4c, (Pollack and Krueger, 1978).

(j) Relating the heart rate and cardiac mechanics. A precise description of the duration of systole for different heart rates. This will be provided by the duration of the activation function which changes with the heart rate.

(h) Relating the force of contraction, i.e. the contractility, to the heart rate, Figure 4d. This is known as the force interval relationship. In a very rude approximation, the contractility increases with the heart rate in an almost linear fashion. However, a more precise approach should include the complex interrelationship which are known for the rapid and slow changes in the force interval relationship.

The application of a model incorporating the above relationships, including only longitudinal fiber stresses, (Beyar and Sideman, 1984b) shows that the global LV performance is adequately described by incorporating all the above assumptions. As shown in Figure 5, the results from the structural approach are similar to the earlier results from the global model. However, a detailed analysis shows that

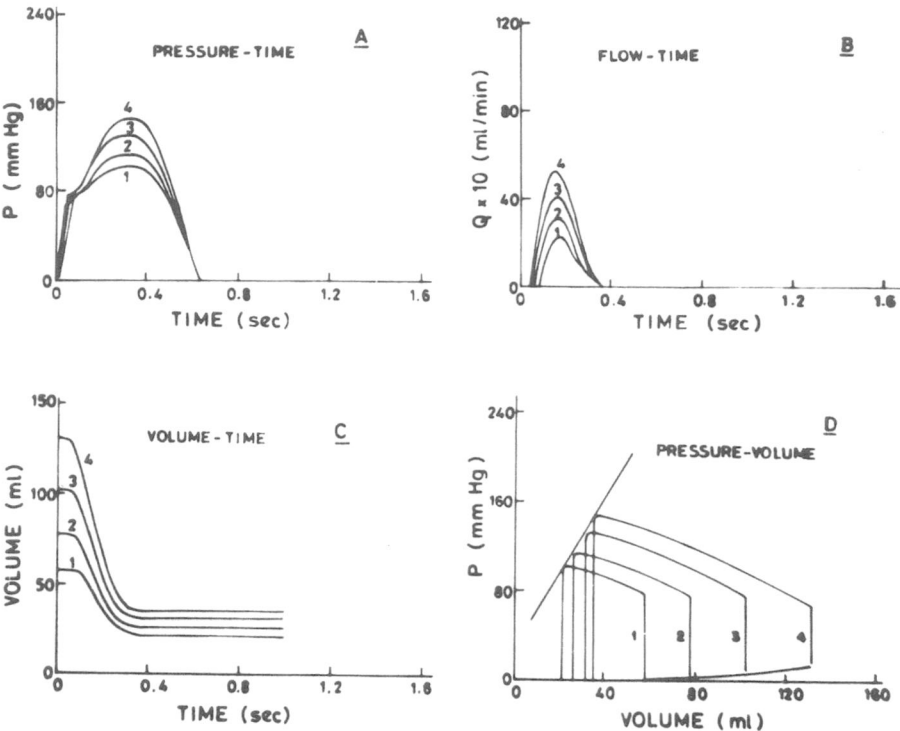

Figure 5. An example of the global pressure-volume-time relationship calculated based on a structural model of the LV (Beyar and Sideman, 1984b).

the slope of the maximum pressure volume relation (maximum elastance), Figure 5d, corresponds to the slope of the stress length relationship of the sarcomere Figure 4a.

An important feature of the 'distributed' model is the stress and pressure distribution within the LV wall, Figure 6, which is an important factor in the determination of the local myocardial perfusion. Note that the strain rate affects the stress distribution when the flow is high, Figure 6b. Note also the change in the sarcomere length distribution from the beginning to the end of systole, Figure 6d.

A detailed sensitivity analysis of the performance of such a model (Beyar and Sideman, 1984b) highlights the following points:

(a) The transfiber stresses play but a minor role in affecting the global LV performance. However, they may modify the stress and pressure distribution within the LV wall, and should be accounted for in future analysis.

(b) The ejection fraction is sensitive to the sarcomere length distribution at the reference configuration. This point should be carefully considered in the adjustment of the model results to experimental or clinical data.

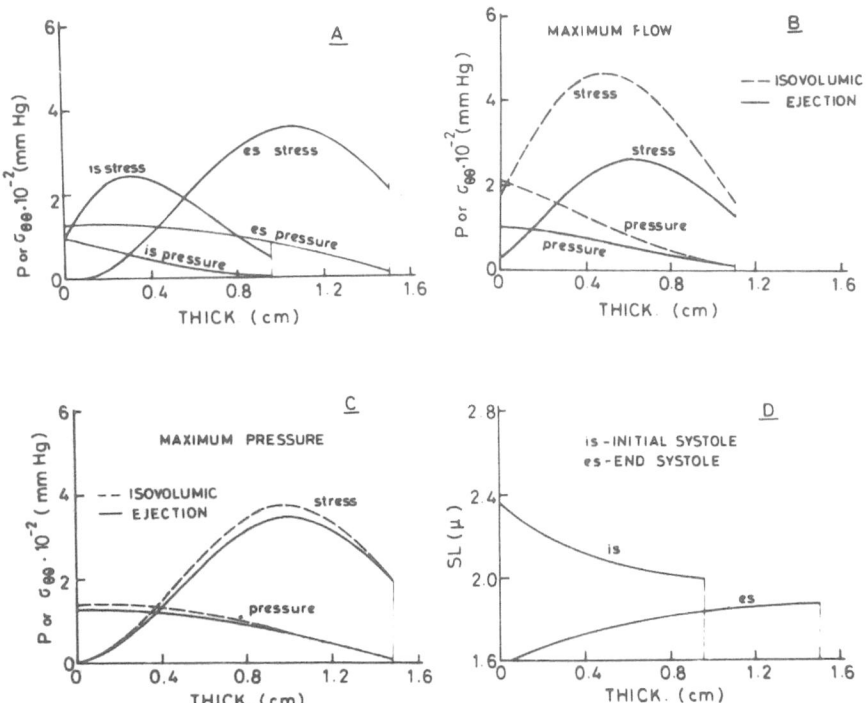

Figure 6. Circumferential stress, pressure distribution and sarcomere length (SL) throughout the myocardium. is – initial systole; es – end systole; thick – distance from the endocard (y). A theoretical isovolumic result (assuming no strain rate effect on the stress), is compared with the 'ejection' result at the same time and volume in two instances corresponding to maximum flow and maximum pressure.

26

(c) The correct mathematical form of the stress-strain rate relationship (hyperbolic vs. linear) cannot be determined based on global LV parameters like the ejection fraction. Direct comparision of the model results with carefully controlled experimental results may help a better definition of this subject *in vivo*.

The coronary perfusion

The coronary perfusion supplied the muscle with the metabolic demand (which is in itself a complex function of mechanical and metabolic parameters which has been lately reviewed by Gibbs, 1978).The coronary circulation is quite unique, being the 'energy supplier' of the tissue which generates the coronary driving pressure. Therefore, the LV is subjected to a strong positive feedback, which reduces the stability of the cardiac system. Thus, a strong negative feedback mechanism is essential for the control of the coronary circulation. This is accomplished by the local autoregulatory mechanism of the coronary bed, which adjusts the coronary flow to the basal metabolic demand. Based on large numbers of experimental data (reviewed by Feigl, 1983 and Berne, 1979), coronary flow can

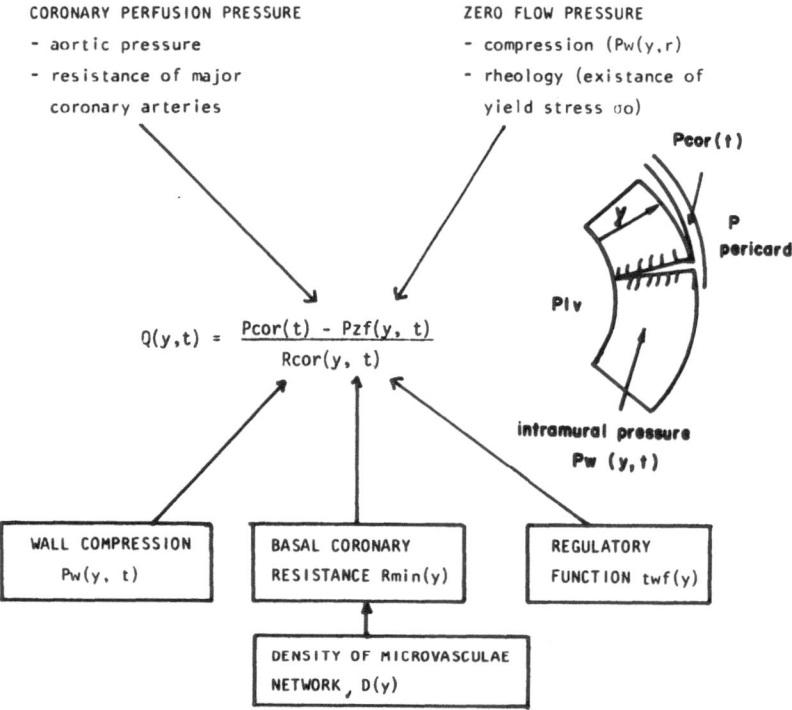

Figure 7. The different parameters effecting the spatial time dependent coronary flow $Q(y, t)$.

be described by the formula shown in Figure 7. The instantaneous local coronary perfusion $F_{cor}(y, t)$, is determined by the coronary perfusion pressure $P_{cor}(t)$, the zero flow pressure $P_{zf}(y, t)$, and the coronary resistance $R_{cor}(y, t)$.

The coronary perfusion pressure, $P_{cor}(t)$, is actually determined by the aortic pressure and the impedance of the coronary conductance vessels. It is well known that, for normal coronary arteries, the pressure drop over the major vessels is minimal and can in fact be neglected. In this case, the coronary perfusion pressure is close to the aortic pressure. Stenosis, resulting from atheroma, spasm or other causes, affects the coronary perfusion when significant pressure gradients are developed over the stenosis, thus reducing the perfusion pressures. It is assumed here that the perfusion pressure $P_{cor}(t)$ is not a function of y, i.e. no pressure drop exists along the penetrating coronary arteries. However, this assumption should be reconsidered in view of the possible compression of the penetrating coronary arteries during systole.

The zero flow pressure, a well known phenomenon in the coronary bed, is commonly known in other vascular beds as the 'critical closing pressure'. Many theories attempt to explain the reason for the existance of the critical closing pressure (Hoffman, 1978; Archie, 1978; Bellamy, 1978). Is this a real physical closure of the micro vessel lumen, or is it a function of the 'yield stress' of the blood attributed to its 'cassonian' rheological properties? The zero flow pressure, P_{zf}, is in fact a combination of the critical closing pressure, the compressive effects and the autoregulating effects.

The compressive effect is due to the transmural pressure drop $P_{cor}(y)-P_w(y, t)$ across the microvessels. A negative transmural pressure drop will generate collapse of the vessel and halt the flow in the vessel. The rigidity of the vessel's wall determines its resistance to collapse and determines the transmural pressure which is associated with the collapse phenomena. The combination of all these parameters determines the well known spatial dependence of P_{zf} on the LV pressure and the coronary tonus (Bellamy, 1978; 1980; Sherman, 1980).

The resistance of the coronary bed $R_{cor}(y)$ is defined by three parameters:

(a) the basal coronary resistance, which is a function of the geometry of the vascular bed, the density of the vessels and the viscosity of blood. This resistance is actually determined *in vivo* by perfusing a non-contracting heart, with maximum vasodilatation accomplished by adenosine infusion.

(b) the autoregulatory function, which changes between zero and unity, corresponding to minimum and maximum vasoconstriction. This function, which defines the coronary resistance, is modulated by changes in the tonus which effects the geometry of the small coronary vessels.

(c) the compressive forces which affect both the coronary resistance and P_{zf}. Assuming that the coronary microvessels are elastic, a higher transmural pressure will enlarge the cross-sectional area of the vessels. The cross-sectional area has an inverse cubic relationship to the flow resistance of the vessel (according to Poiseuille equation). Thus, the coronary resistance decreases as the transmural pressure, $P_{cor}(t)-P_w(y, t)$, increases.

An example of the calculated coronary perfusion flow based on the above relations, is shown in Figure 8. The coronary flow to the endocardial layers is seen to stop during systole (compression) while the flow in the epicardial layers, which are subjected to much lower compression values of $P_w(y, t)$, is seen to reduce only slightly. The autoregulatory effect which adjusts the blood flow to the metabolic demand, is demonstrated by comparing curves *A* and *B* in Figure 8. Lower blood

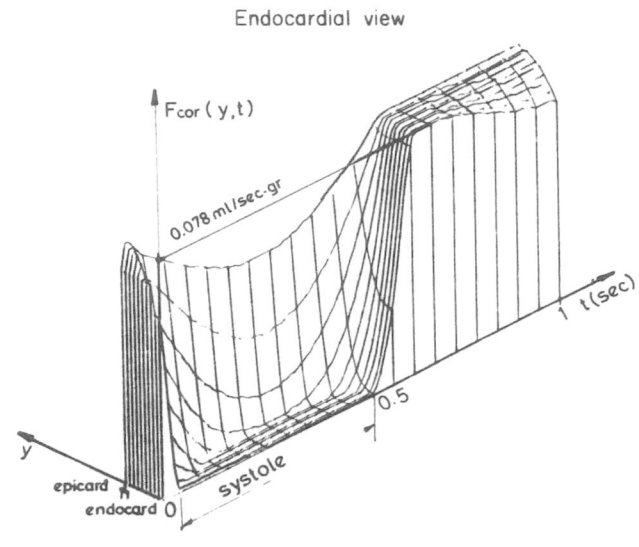

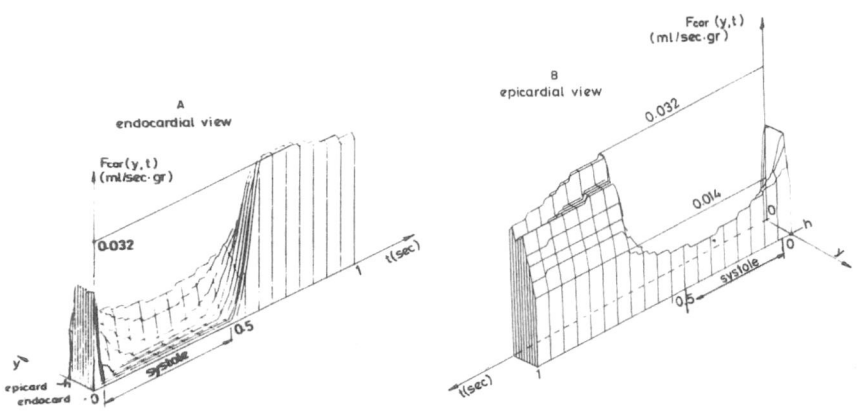

Figure 8. Time dependent coronary blood flow distribution with (lower) and without (upper) introduction of an algorithm for autoregulation. These calculated results are based on integrated model combing mechanical with coronary perfusionarameters (Beyar and Sideman, 1984c)

flow values to the epicardial layers than to the endocardial layers characterises diastolic autoregulated perfusion.

Space and time integration of the coronary perfusion flow yields the total blood flow to the LV. A classical experiment relating the total blood flow to the coronary pressure is simulated in Figure 9. The calculated classical autoregulating range are shown for two metabolic demands. The curvilinearity of the coronary flow pressure relationship, above and below this range, is due to the modification of the resistance by the increase of the coronary transmural pressures.

Energy metabolism

The energy utilization by the cardiac muscle is a complex process which is strongly affected by metabolic and mechanical parameters. The cardiac muscle derives almost all of its energy supply by aerobic metabolism and is thus highly dependent on the oxygen supply. Short cessations of the oxygen supply to the contracting tissues will affect the contraction mechanics within a few seconds.

Intensive work has been done in the past 50 years to find a reliable index of oxygen demand (Gibbs, 1979). The various indexes which were tested include various combinations of pressure, time, stress, external work, and others. However, in view of the large number of proposed indexes, it is obvious that none has been proven to be sufficiently accurate to become universal.

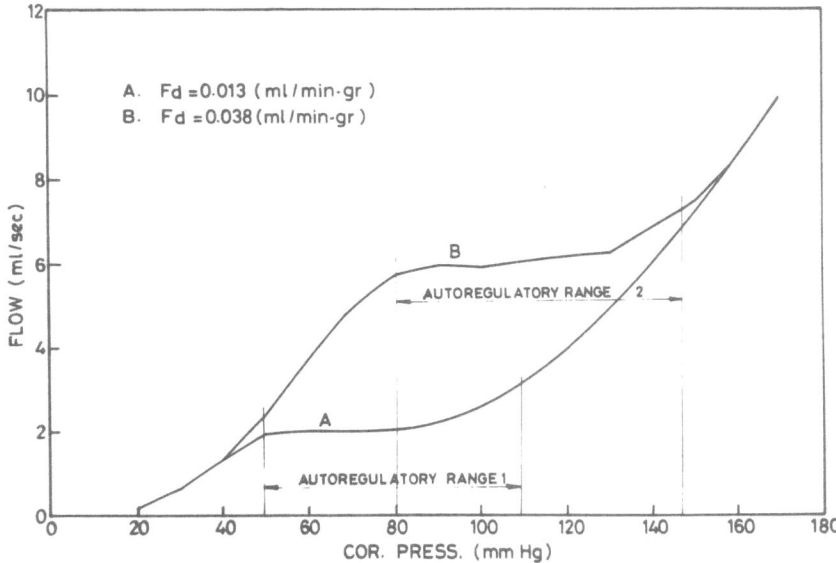

Figure 9. Total coronary flow versus coronary pressure at different flow demands (Fd) calculated from Beyar and Sideman's (1984c) model.

The spatial approach to the energy demand of the cardiac muscle is based on our mechanical, distributed-parameters, model. As outlined in Figure 10a, the distributed parameters which determine the local oxygen consumption are stress $\sigma(y, t)$, strain $\varepsilon(y, t)$ and strain rate $\dot{\varepsilon}(y, t)$. The contractility of the muscle may have a direct effect through the uncoupling of some chemical reactions, or a secondary effect, by modifying the stress or strain rates. The basal metabolic rate is another component of energy demand which is assumed to be uniform throughout the myocarium. A specific combination (either linear or nonlinear) of $\sigma(y, t)$, $\varepsilon(y, t)$, $\dot{\varepsilon}(y, t)$ and the basal metabolic rate which results in a physiological compatible forumations is to be searched. The relative contribution of the contractility, stress, external work and basal metabolism should be reflected in the desired combination. Such a combination may be developed on the basis of a theory or may be searched for by experimental parameters estimation. In general, unrelated to the specific model selected, such an approach will result in an intramural distribution of the energy demand. A theory-based formula for the description of the myocardial energy demand was related to the cross bridge theory of the sarcomere. (Beyar and Sideman, 1984d). An example of the local energy demand vs. preload, based on the results of Beyar and Sideman's (1984b) distributed mechanical model, is shown in Figure 10b.

The model shows that the endocardial oxygen demand is higher than the epicardial demand within the LV wall at normal and high preloads. This is

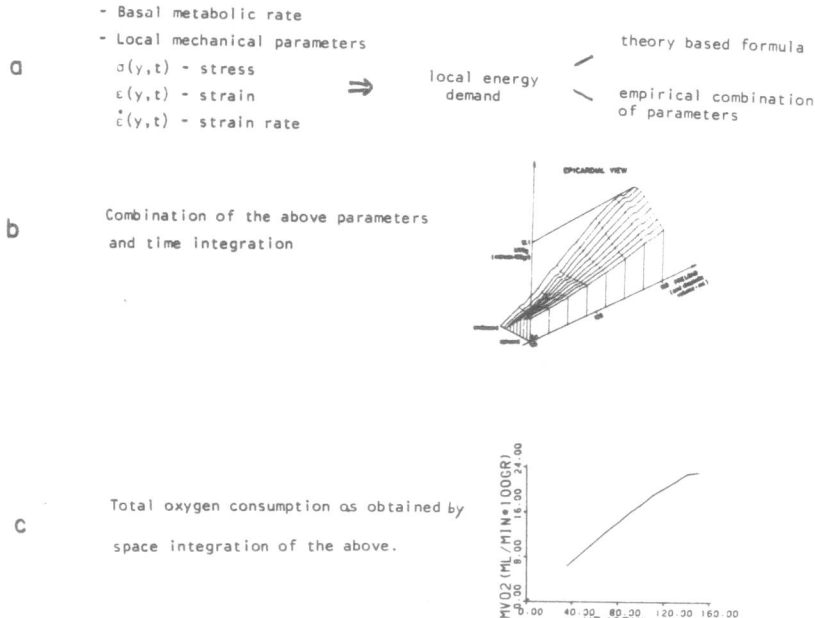

Figure 10. A spatial approach for interrelating the local energy demand to the local mechanical parameter (*a*). Oxygen demand distribution as a function of the end distolic volume (*b*) and the total oxygen demand vs. heart rate (based on Beyar and Sideman's, 1984d).

consistent with experimental data and can be explained qualitatively by the increased extensions and shortening which are attributed to the subendocardial fibers. Space integration of the spatial oxygen demand yields the global energy demand of the LV, Figure 10c. The average oxygen demand is shown here as a function of the heart rate. As most of the experimental data relates to the global energy parameters, rather than the local parameters, the adjustment of the system parameters should relate to the global average results. Thus a first approximation of the local phenomena is obtained from the global approach.

An approach to a 3-D geometric model

The above relationships which describe the distributed properties of the mechanical parameters, as well as coronary perfusion and energy demand laws, are the physiological cornerstones for the development of a global 3-D geometrical model. The local properties of the cardiac muscle can be approximated by symmetrical models which utilize distributed properties as a function of y, the radial distance from the endocard. This results in the evaluation of the constants which relate the local phenomena of the cardiac muscle to local structure, stress, strain and strain rate of the muscle.

The analysis of the nonisotropic nonhomogeneous asymmetric mechanical 3-D problem is an important step to be accomplished. Independent of the precise method which will be selected for the solution of the mechanical problem, a time dependent field of mechanical parameters $\varepsilon(y, \varphi, \theta, t)$, $\dot{\varepsilon}(y, \varphi, \theta, t)$, $P_w(y, \varphi, \theta, t)$, $\sigma(y, \varphi, \theta, t)$, will eventually be obtained. Based on the above data, the local energy demand will be related to the local coronary perfusion, autoregulated by local metabolic autoregulatory functions as well as by general control systems.

The above 3-D model will be able to relate to common diseases of the heart, i.e. myocardial infarction, aneurism, disturbances in the electrical activation, etc. Local perturbation may then be studied, i.e. the regional coronary flow may be interrupted in order to study the time development of the nonsymmetric effects on cardiac mechanics.

Summary

The important physiological laws which interrelate the different cardiac functions were presented and discussed. The mechanical aspects of the cardiac cycle are the 'heart' of the problem. Simple approaches, interrelating overall parameters like pressure, flow, volume, can be used to describe cardiac activity. However, spatial distribution within the wall requires knowledge of the cardiac structure as well as distributed mechanical characteristics.

The function of the contractile segment – the sarcomere – determines the global cardiac function. This is the combined effect of the sarcomeres through the entire myocardium, activated in a well-defined sequence by the activation function. The spatial mechanical parameters in the myocardium, i.e. the stress, strain and strain rate, determine the energy metabolism and the coronary perfusion. The triangle set by the mechanical perfusion, and energetic interactions is the cornerstone for a global description of the cardiac function.

References

Archie JP (1978) Transmural distribution of intrinsic and transmitted left ventricular diastolic intramyocardial pressures in dogs. Cardiovasc Res 12:255–262

Bellamy RF (1978) Diastolic coronary artery pressure flow relationship in the dogs. Circ Res 43;92—101

Bellamy RF (1980) Calculation of coronary vascular resistance. Cardiovas Res 14: 261–269

Berne RM, Rubio R (1979) Coronary circulations. In: Berne RM, Sperlakis M, Geiger SR (eds), Handbook of Physiology. The Cardiovascular System: The Heart. An Physiol Soc Bethesda Maryland, pp 873–952

Beyar R, Sideman S (1984a) A model for left ventricular contraction combining the force length velocity relationship with the time varying elastance theory. Biophys J 45:1167–1177

Beyar R, Sideman S (1984b) A computer study of the left ventricular performance based on the fiber structure, sarcomere dynamics and transmural electrical propagation valocity. Circ Res 55:358–375.

Beyar R, Sideman S (1984c) Time dependent coronary blood flow distributed in the left ventricular wall. Submitted for publication

Beyar R, Sideman S (1984d) Spatial energy balance within a structural model of the left ventricle. Submitted for publication

Diamond G, Forrester JS, Hargis J, Parmley WW, Danzig R, Swan HJC (1971) Diastolic pressure volume relationship in the canine left ventricle. Circ Res 29:267–275

Feigl EO (1983) Coronary physiology. Physiol Rev 63:1–202

Gibss CF (1977) Cardiac energetics. Physiol Rev 58:1,174–254

Hill AV (1938) The heat of shortening and dynamic constants of muscle. Proc R Soc London, Ser B, 126–136

Hoffman JIE (1978) Determinants and prediction of transmural myocardial perfusion. Circulation 58(3):281–391

Johnson EA (1979) Force interval relationship of cardiac muscle. In: Berne RM, Sperelakis N, Geiger SR (eds.) Handbook of Physiology, Sect 2. Am Physiol Soc Bethesda Maryland pp. 475–496

Mirsky I, Ghista DN, Sandler H (1974) Cardiac mechanics physiological clinical and mathematical considerations. John Wiley & Sons Inc New York p 45

Pollack GH, Krueger JW (1978) Myocardial sarcomere mechanics: Some parallels with skelatal muscle. In: Baan Y, Noordegraaf A, Raines J (eds.) Cardiovascular System Dynamics Cambridge, pp 3–10

Sherman IA, Grayson AJ, Bayliss CE (1980) Critical closing and critical opening phenomena in the coronary vasculature of the dog. Am J Physiol (Heart Circ Physiol 7) 238:H533–H538

Streeter DD, Ramesh RN, Patel DJ, Spotnitz HM, Ross J, Sonnenblick EH (1970) Stress distribution in the canine left ventricle during diastole and systole. Biophys J 10:345–363

Streeter DD, Vaisnav RN, Patel DJ, Ross Jr, Sonnenblick EH (1969) Fiber orientation in the canine left ventricle during diastole and systole. Circ Res 24:339–247

Suga H, Sagawa K, Shoukas A (1973) Load independence of the instantaneous pressure volume ratio of the canine left ventricle and effects of epinephrine and heart rate on the ratio. Circ Res 32:314–322

Suga H, Sagawa K, Koustuik DP (1976) Controls of ventricular contractility assessed by pressure-volume ratio Emax. Cardiovasc Res 10:582–592

DISCUSSION

RITMAN: What assumption did you use to convert the compressing forces to calculate the intra-myocardial blood flow?

ANS: This point is further extended in the paper by Beyar and Sideman to be presented later in this workshop. We assume that the coronary perfusion pressure is equal to the aortic pressure. We also assume that no flow occurs when the coronary pressure is less than the intramural pressure at a certain location and time. We further assume that the critical closing pressure (as it is known for general microvascular bed) is not subjected to compressive effects. We combine these effects to yield the zero flow parameter, both locally and for the global LV. The coronary resistance, Rcor(y), depends on the basal coronary resistance, which is also a function of the location within the LV wall. This relates to the distributed nature of the density of capillaries within the LV wall which is highest for the endocardial layers. Knowing the coronary resistance, we inversely relate it to wall compression, i.e., an increase in the vessel's transmural pressure causes a decrease in the coronary resistance. A regulatory function Twf(y) modifies the basal coronary resistance which affects the oxygen delivery to the tissues until the oxygen demand of the myocardium equals the oxygen supply. We use this function to adjust the time average flow distribution to the distributed metabolic demand, which is assumed here to be constant for the myocardium.

HEINTZEN: The main problem in the cooperation between physicians and bioengineers is to avoid being confused by theoretical models. We have to improve the techniques for measuring the things on which the calculations are based. It is easy to assume things and, with a computer, make 3-dimensional models of everything . . . However, we need better instruments to measure the original input data. We can make any assumption we want about these things and make 3-dimensional models, but I just want to stress the danger of modelling if your model parameters are not based on actual measurements. Just a general statement.

ANS: I agree with your statement regarding the need for measurement but I believe that models help in understanding the general behaviour of highly complicated systems. Obviously, models have to be supported by experimental data which provide us with the actual judgement of our assumptions. Neither of the two approaches stand on its own and the combined approach, relating theory to measurements, and vice versa, is the preferred one.

MIRSKY: I want to comment about the recent models that have been coming out, trying to put forth tortional effects may be very important in rearranging the distributions of properties within the wall. There is going to be an abstract presented at the April meeting of FASEB coming out from Dr. Fon's group and he seems to show that the shear stresses are very small in the epicardial layers and maybe 10–15% of the the endocardial layers. It might be that the stress distribution is the same as it was without the tortional effects. But obviously there's a lot more to done in this area. The fact is also that there must be quite a variation in the shear stresses going from apex to base. Are your calculated stress distribution limited only to the equator?

ANS: We didn't try to evaluate stress distribution along the longitudinal axis and concentrated only on equatorial stresses.

MIRSKY: I want to comment on Dr. Heintzen's remark. About ten years ago I developed a model which I thought was the worst model I ever developed, yet I came up with the same stress distribution as Dr. Streeter got with different assumptions. So we have to be careful. We may end up with the same results with different assumptions.

SIDEMAN: I want to relate to the comment made by Prof. Heintzen regarding models, model assumptions and reality. He knows the answer himself but I will amplify it. What we are trying to do here is an example of the checks and balances that we need, and must have, between modelling and reality, assumptions and experimental verification. One does not go without the other. The difficulty arises when we intermix theoreticians and clinicians, people who come from very varied backgrounds. The hard thing is to believe that the other guy really knows what he's doing . . . The aim of models is obviously to define the parameters which must be experimentally checked. Otherwise we will make numerous experiments and then try to correlate the results. The best way is to know what you are trying to do. This is the name of the game. I'm sure this is what Prof. Heintzen meant but I couldn't avoid relating to it because it is important in this gathering of people of different disciplines.

The role of mathematical models in an assessment of myocardial function

ISRAEL MIRSKY

Department of Medicine, Harvard Medical School and Brigham and Women's Hospital, Boston, Mass 92115 USA

Abstract

This review demonstrates the importance of mathematical modelling in an assessment of myocardial function, and addresses the following questions:
(1) What is the effect of shape on the diastolic LV pressure-volume relationship and on the quantitation of myocardial stiffness-stress relations?
(2) What are the important determinants of chamber stiffness and what are the mechanisms involved in the shifts of the P-V curves following certain drug interventions?
(3) How do infarcts affect diastolic and systolic function? and
(4) How may contractile reserve be assessed?
   Employing the theory of elasticity, these models demonstrate that; (a) in the absence of segmental disease, diastolic P-V and stiffness-stress relations are little affected by LV shape, (b) intrinsic chamber stiffness is complexly related to myocardial elasticity, cavity size, volume/mass ratio and the coronary blood volume, and external pressures are the dominant factors causing dramatic shifts in the P-V relations following certain drug interventions, (c) normal myocardium is restrained by neighbouring infarcts which disrupt border zone contraction patterns. Furthermore, there is a progressive degradation of cardiac performance with increasing infarct size, (d) end systolic P-V relations and end diastolic P-V relations determine the critical EDV at which maximum stroke volume occurs.

Introduction

The past two decades have seen a proliferation of mathematical models which have been developed for the purpose of assessing myocardial function. Most of these models have focused on the quantitation of ventricular wall stresses and deformations which take place during diastole.

The first generation of models were based on idealized geometries (sphere, ellipsoid, cylinder) for the left ventricle (LV) and the myocardium assumed to behave as an isotropic, homogeneous elastic medium. In addition, deformations were assumed small so that the classical linear theory of elasticity could be applied. This generation of models was later to be followed by one based on the finite element technique (Zienkiewicz, 1971), a method developed some 25 years ago for the analysis of stresses and deformations in complex structures. The application of this technique enabled one to employ more realistic ventricular geometry, assume large deformation theory (generally encountered with biological tissue) and to incorporate other factors such as nonhomogeneity and anisotropy.

Streeter et al. (1970) were the first to incorporate fiber orientation into a model for the quantitation of both fiber and wall stresses. In recent years fiber orientation has been reintroduced into the models assuming a cylindrical geometry for the LV (Feit, 1979; Arts, 1979; Chadwick, 1982; Tozeren, 1983). With these models it is possible to examine the effects of torsional deformations on fiber stress distribution and also quantitate the intramyocardial pressure distribution.

While most models of wall stress developed thus far, either on the basis of small or large deformation theory, have their limitations, each provide some useful information. However, until we obtain more reliable experimental information on the mechanical properties of the myocardium, the simpler type models are adequate for many qualitative type studies except in the cases of coronary artery disease.

Since the subject of wall stress evaluation has been discussed in detail in the review articles by Mirsky, 1974, 1979; Huisman et al, 1980 and Yin, 1981, this article will focus on several models which may be applied in the assessment of myocardial function. Particular attention will be given to those models which assess diastolic function since there is growing evidence from both clinical (Bonow et al., 1981; Soufer et al., 1983) and animal studies (Mirsky et al., 1983) that diastolic abnormalities in myocardial function precede abnormalities in systolic pump performance.

Specifically this presentation with the aid of mathematical models, will address the following questions:

(1) What is the effect of ventricular shape on the diastolic LV pressure-volume relations and on the quantitation of myocardial stiffness-stress relations?

(2) What are the dominant factors affecting the diastolic P-V relations during certain drug interventions?

(3) What are the effects of infarcts on the diastolic and systolic function of the LV?

(4) How can the end systolic pressure-volume relations (ESP-ESV) be employed in an assessment of myocardial contractile reserve?

Effect of shape on the diastolic pressure-volume relations

Janz *et al.* (1980) developed a mathematical model for the finite deformation of a prolate spheroidal membrane subjected to a hydrostatic pressure and unconstrained with respect to eccentricity. Figure 1 displays the deformed and undeformed geometry of this membrane model. This deformed geometry is determined by solving a system of differential equations for the stretch ratios λ_θ, λ_φ and angle φ in terms of the polar angle Φ.

Constitutive equations

Assuming the membrane material to be isotropic and homogeneous, the stress-stretch (σ–λ) relations are expressed in the form

$$\sigma_i = N_i/t = \sum_{j=1}^{2} A_j \, \lambda_i^{\alpha j} + Q \quad i = \theta, \varphi, n.$$

where A_j, α_j are the 'elasticity constants', Q is a hydrostatic pressure due to

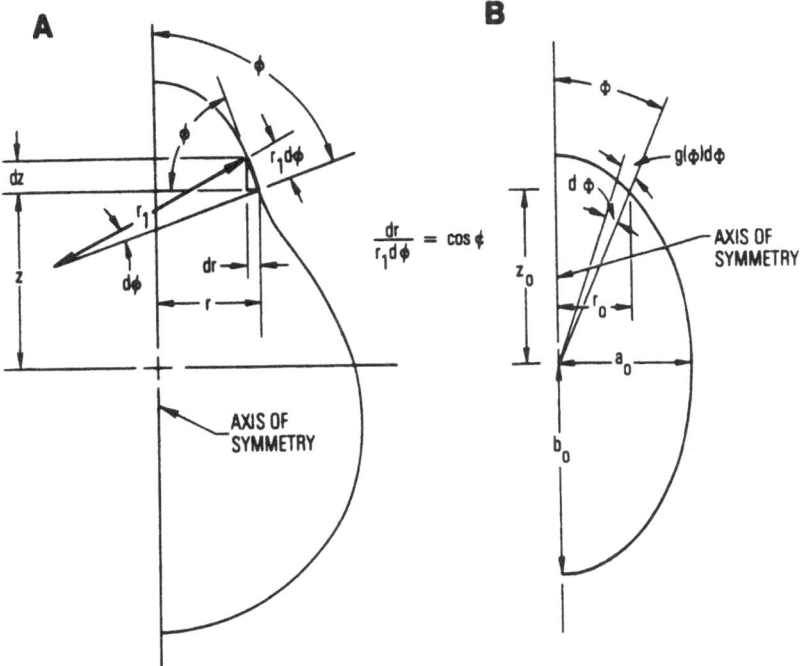

Figure 1. A. Deformed geometry of membrane model. B. Undeformed geometry which is assumed to be that of an ellipsoid. The independent variable is the polar angle Φ. (Reproduced from Janz *et al.*, Amer J Physiol 238: H917, 1980 with permission of the American Physiological Society.)

incompressibility and N_θ, N_φ are, respectively, the membrane stresses in the circumferential and meridional directions.

In membrane theory, one assumes that the radial stress component (σ_n) is small compared to the other two components and from the incompressibility condition $\lambda_\theta \lambda_\varphi \lambda_n = 1$, one obtains finally

$$\sigma_i = \sum_{j=1}^{2} A_j \left[\lambda_i^{\alpha j} - (\lambda_\theta \, \lambda_\theta)^{-\alpha j} \right] \quad (i = \theta, \varphi).$$

Evaluation of the elasticity constants

Based on human data from the studies of Fester *et al.* (1974) and assuming a spherical membrane, the resulting P-V relation in terms of the constants A, α is given in the form

$$P = (2At_0/\varrho_0) \left[(V/V_0)^{(\alpha-3)/3} - (V/V_0)^{-(2\alpha+3)/3} \right]$$

where t_0, ϱ_0 and V_0 are respectively the wall thickness, radius and cavity volume at zero pressure. The values for A, α obtained by curve-fitting the above expression to the known pressure-volume data, are $A = 0.293\,\text{mmHg}$ and $\alpha = 12.66$.

Pressure-volume curves for ellipsoidal shells

Assuming the same undeformed cavity volume V_0, wall volume and elasticity constants, and solving the system of differential equations, pressure-volume curves for various eccentricities (including the sphere) are determined and these are displayed in Figure 2. Note that the curve corresponding to the Fester data (major/minor axis ratio $= b_0/a_0 = 1.927$) coincides with that for the sphere. Similar results were obtained by Janz *et al.* (1980) employing a thick-walled finite element model.

The results from these studies therefore imply that a thick-walled sphere is adequate for the determination of the elasticity constants and that pressure-volume relations are essentially unaffected by the eccentricity of the ellipsoid.

Effect of ventricular shape on the myocardial stiffness-stress relations

The model just described is in general not suitable for clinical applications since it is difficult to obtain V_0 (cavity volume at zero pressure) with sufficient accuracy. Therefore an alternative method is described here and is based on the concept of an incremental elastic modulus (Mirsky and Rankin, 1979).

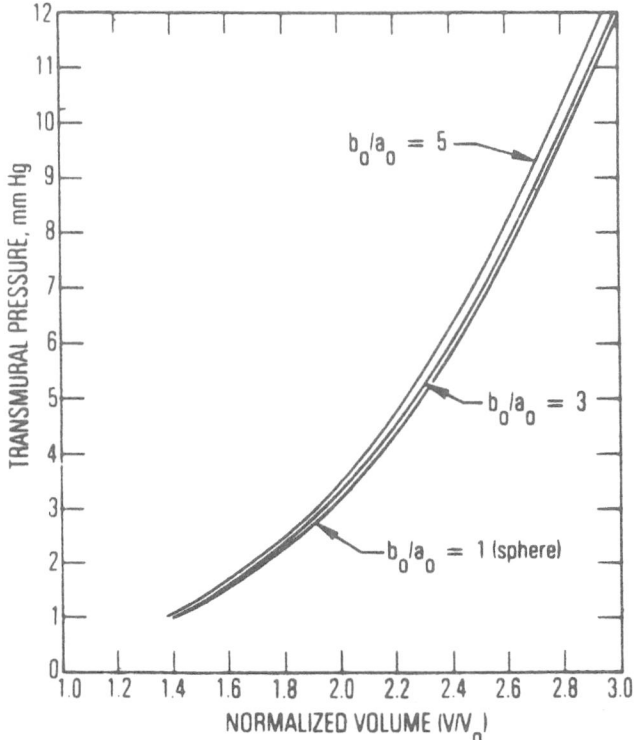

Figure 2. Pressure-volume curves for 4 ellipsoids (including sphere). The curve corresponding to undeformed major/minor axis ratio $b_0/a_0 = 1.927$ coincides with that for the sphere. (Reproduced from Janz *et al.*, Am J Physiol 238: H917, 1980 with permission from the American Physiological Society.)

Assuming an ellipsoidal geometry for the LV, the myocardial stiffness or incremental modulus (E_e) at the equator of the ellipsoid may be approximated by the expression (Mirsky, 1984)

$$E_e \sim (3/2)d\sigma_e/(db/b)/(2 + b^2/a^2)_{ave} = (3/2)(2 + \gamma)(Vd\sigma_e/dV)/(2 + b^2/a^2)_{ave},$$

where σ_e = difference of the circumferential and radial stress components at the endocardium, a, b are respectively the semi-major and semi-minor axes, V = cavity volume and γ is defined by the relation $\log a = \gamma \log b + \delta$.

For the special case of the sphere, an analysis based on the classical linear theory of elasticity (Lame formulae) yields the following expression for the incremental modulus (E_s) namely $E_s = (3/2)Vd\,\sigma_s/dV$. This same result is obtained from the expression for E_e on setting $a = b$, and $\gamma = 1$.

There are several reasons for employing endocardial stresses: (1) the modulus E and stress σ are expressed in terms of directly measured parameters; (2) recent studies by Gallagher *et al.* (1983) have demonstrated marked thickness changes in the subendocardial layers during systole. Thus one may expect also in diastole, that the same fiber is not being observed at the midwall at each instant of time; (3)

endocardial layers are more susceptible to ischemia (as may occur in aortic stenosis) than midwall layers and (4) comparisons of theoretical results with biopsy data may be more meaningful since most samples during biopsy are taken from the endocardium.

Pressure-volume relations in normal and hypertrophied LV

Figure 3 displays the diastolic P-V data obtained angiographically from 4 controls and from a patient with left ventricular hypertrophy pre- and post administration of nifedipine. The administration of appropriate drugs enables one to obtain additional P-V data in diseased ventricles which overlap data in normal ventricles. However, caution must be exercised in the use of drugs that may cause parallel shifts in the pressure-volume relations.

Myocardial stiffness-stress relations based on ellipsoidal and spherical geometries

Employing the expressions for E_e, E_s and stresses σ_e, σ_s (Mirsky, 1984) and P-V data shown in Figure 3, myocardial stiffness-stress relations are obtained for both ellipsoidal and spherical geometries. The results are displayed in Figure 4 where it is observed in the left panel for the control group, that there are no significant

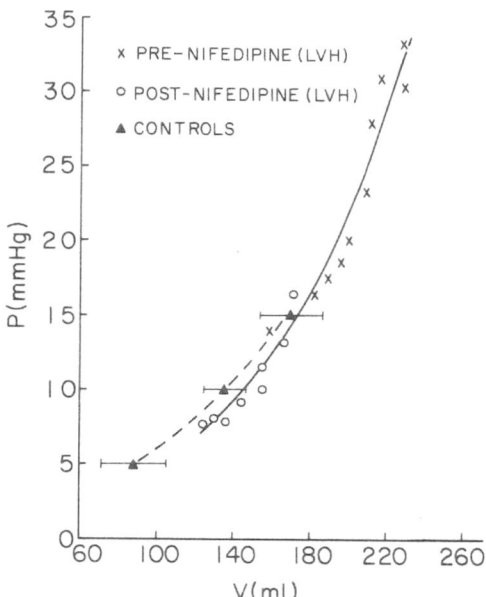

Figure 3. Pressure-volume relations for 4 controls (▲) and for a patient with LVH pre (×) and post nifedipine (○).

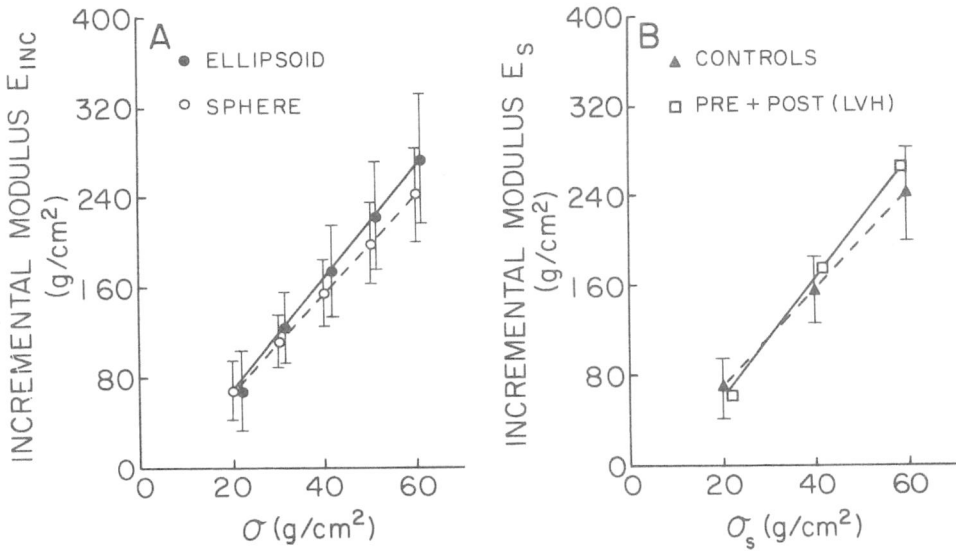

Figure 4. Left. Myocardial stiffness-stress relations for controls based on ellipsoidal and spherical models. At common levels of stress there are no significant differences in myocardial stiffness. *Right.* Stiffness-stress relations for control and patient with LVH. There is no marked difference in stiffness levels at common stress values.

differences in myocardial stiffness at common levels of stress for both geometries. This result is essentially equivalent to the one obtained by Janz *et al.* (1980). On the right panel, we observe that the stiffness-stress relation for the hypertrophied ventricle is not markedly different from that for the controls.

Validation of the incremental modulus concept in the clinical setting

As yet there is no experimental evidence validating current mathematical models which quantitate myocardial stress distributions. However, it will be shown in the following sections that validation in a qualitative sense can be obtained for models which assess myocardial stiffness, employing clinical data obtained from patients with valvular disease.

Expressions for myocardial stiffness and stress based on combined pressure and echocardiographic measurements

If we assume that at the site of measurement, the section of the left ventricle may be approximated by a cylindrical annulus, the resulting expressions for myocardial stiffness (E_c) and stress (σ_c) are:

$$E_c = (3/4)(d\sigma_c/d\varepsilon_c) = (3/4)d\sigma_c/(dD/D) \text{ and}$$
$$\sigma_c = \sigma_{\varphi c} - \sigma_r = P(D + 2h)^2/2h(D + h)$$

where P is the left ventricular pressure, D = internal diameter, h = wall thickness and σ_c is the difference of the circumferential ($\sigma_{\varphi c}$) and radial stress (σ_r) components at the endocardial surface, and $d\varepsilon_c$ is the incremental strain at the endocardium.

Myocardial stiffness-stress relationships in valvular heart disease pre and post aortic valve replacement

Employing data taken from patients (Hess *et al.*, 1984) with aortic stenosis (AS), aortic insufficiency (AI) and with mixed lesions (AI + AS) pre-operatively and following successful valve replacement (ave. 17.5 yr), the myocardial stiffness-stress relations are evaluated for each group and compared with that for the group of controls (Figure 5).

At common levels of stress, the stiffness-stress relations pre-operatively were not significantly different in valve disease patients compared to controls. Following surgery, intrinsic myocardial stiffness was significantly increased in the AS group ($p<.04$, paired t-test). These results are in qualitative agreement with those obtained by Hess *et al.* (1984) who employed a more complex model.

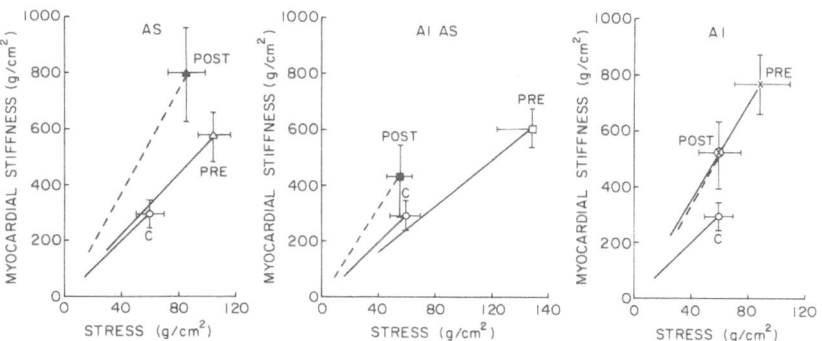

Figure 5. Myocardial stiffness-stress relations for groups of patients with AS, AIAS and AI pre- and post valve replacement compared with controls (C). Pre-operatively, there were no significant differences compared with controls. In AS and AIAS there were increases in the intrinsic stiffness following surgery and the increase was significant in the AS group ($p<.04$, paired t-test). Mean values ± SEM are given at end diastole.

Relationship between myocardial stiffness and interstitial fibrosis

Figure 6 displays the pre- and post-op values for the myocardial stiffness constant k ($E_c = k\sigma_c$) and interstitial fibrosis (IF %) for each individual patient in the 3 groups AS, AI, and AIAS. The quantity IF was obtained by morphometric analysis of biopsy data (Hess *et al.*, 1984). Although interstitial fibrosis tended to increase post-operatively, paired *t*-tests indicated that these increases were significant in the AS group only. Furthermore, the results for the stiffness constant k paralleled those of IF, i.e., k increased in AS but was unaltered in AI and AIAS. These studies and those by Hess *et al.* (1984) provide the first clinical validation for these models.

Factors affecting the diastolic pressure-volume relations following drug interventions

The problem concerning the mechanisms involved in the dramatic shifts of the diastolic P-V relations following drug interventions appears to have been resolved in recent years.

Various factors have been hypothesized by different investigators and these include changes in the external pressures (in particular pericardial pressures), incomplete relaxation and the erectile effect due to increased coronary perfusion (Alderman *et al.*, 1976; Brodie *et al.*, 1977; Mirsky and Rankin, 1979).

In earlier studies (Mirsky and Rankin, 1979), a mathematical model was developed to examine individually and collectively the effects of these various factors. This model has been modified (without altering the original conclusions) in order to express the diastolic pressure directly in terms of LV volume rather than midwall radius. The resulting P-V relation is expressed in the form $P = G(\alpha + \beta V^\delta) + G_0 P_0$ where G, G_0 are geometric factors, α, β, δ are curve-fitting

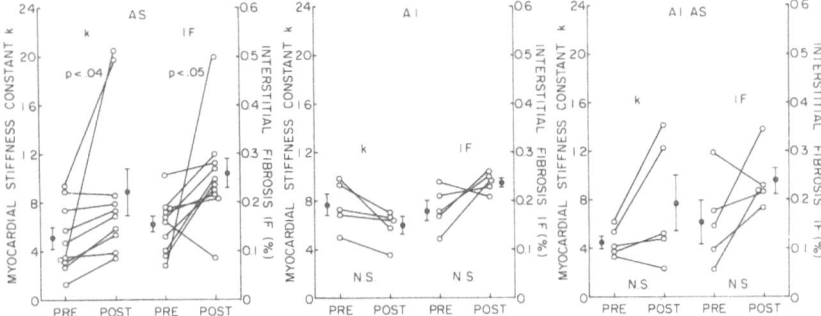

Figure 6. Pre- and post-operative values of the myocardial stiffness constant (k) and percentage interstitial fibrosis (IF) for valvular heart disease patients. Post-op, IF increased in all groups, but was significant in AS only. The qualitative behavior for k and IF was similar in the three groups.

parameters for the stress-volume relation and P_0 is a uniform external pressure which is a weighted average of RV and pericardial/pleural pressures.

Effects of elasticity, geometry and wall mass on the diastolic P-V relations following methoxamine infusion

Figure 7 displays the diastolic P-V relations in the control state and following methoxamine infusion. Note the dramatic parallel shift in these relations following the infusion. Also shown are the computed pressure-volume curves resulting from variations in the various factors namely (a) an increase in elasticity constants by 30%, (b) assuming a spherical geometry for the LV and (c) an increase of 30% in the LV wall mass to simulate the 'erectile effect' due to increased coronary perfusion. In these computations, external pressure was assumed to be zero. It is

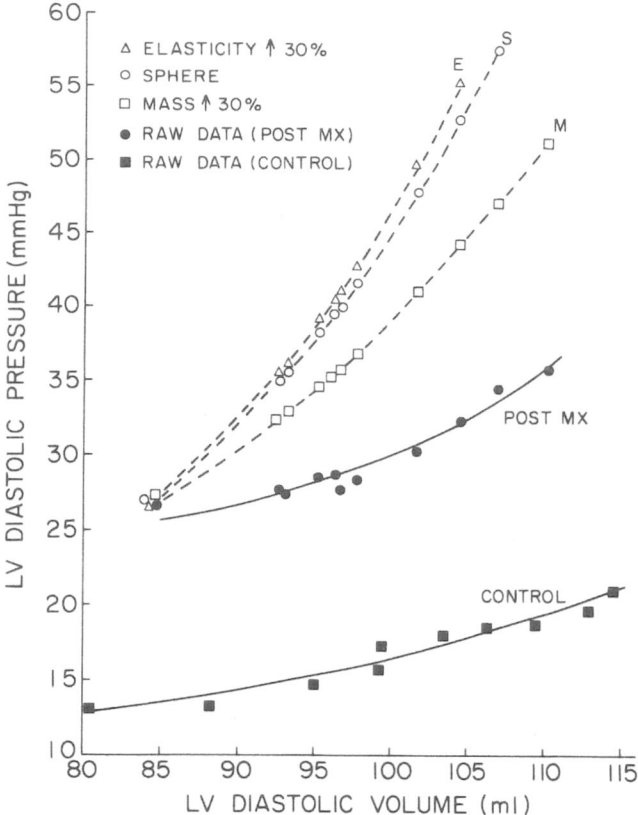

Figure 7. Pressure-volume relations in a patient in control state (■) and following methoxamine infusion (●). Note the dramatic parallel shift upward following the drug infusion. Altering the factors elasticity, geometry, and LV wall mass individually did not reproduce the methoxamine curve.

quite apparent that alterations of these factors individually do not result in a P-V relation that closely approximates the post methoxamine curve.

Effects of external pressures on the P-V relations following methoxamine infusion

In Figure 8 external pressure-volume relations (P_0-V), required to produce the post methoxamine curve, are shown for two cases namely; (1) when LV mass, geometry and elasticity are unaltered and (2) when mass and geometry are unaltered and elasticity is increased by 30%. The results indicate that in either case, substantial external pressures must be present in order to produce the dramatic shift following methoxamine infusion.

Experimental validation of the theoretical model

Animal studies conducted by Shirato *et al.* (1978) provide a partial validation of the results obtained from the model just described. These investigators demon-

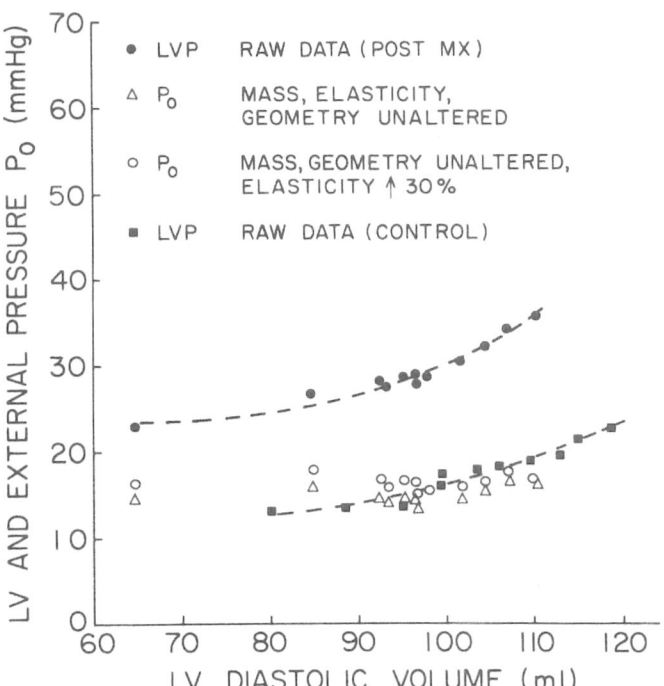

Figure 8. External pressure-volume relations (P_0-V) simulating the post methoxamine P-V relations. It is apparent that substantial external pressures must be present in order to reproduce the methoxamine curve regardless of alterations in the other factors.

strated that the pericardium contributed significantly to the increased diastolic pressure in acute dilatation and to the shifts following sodium nitroprusside infusion.

Pressure-segment length relations for two dogs are shown in Figure 9 for the control state, acute volume loading and following nitroprusside infusion. With the pericardium intact, the curves were shifted upward during acute volume loading and following nitroprusside infusion, the curves shifted downward towards control. Without the pericardium, each condition resulted in a single curve.

Further evidence that external pressures are dominant factors during drug interventions, is provided by the clinical studies of Ludbrook *et al.* (1979). In these studies, the effects of nitroglycerin on the P-V relations in 13 patients, suspected of having coronary artery disease, were examined. In all patients, the diastolic P-V curves were significantly displaced downward and leftward. These shifts were associated with a 36% decrease in the RV systolic and 41% decrease in the RV end diastolic pressures. Furthermore, the time constants of isovolumic relaxation were unchanged after the drug infusion. On the other hand, amyl nitrite infused in 13 patients resulted in single P-V relations (i.e. no shifts) and there were no significant reductions in LVEDP, RVEDP or RV systolic pressures.

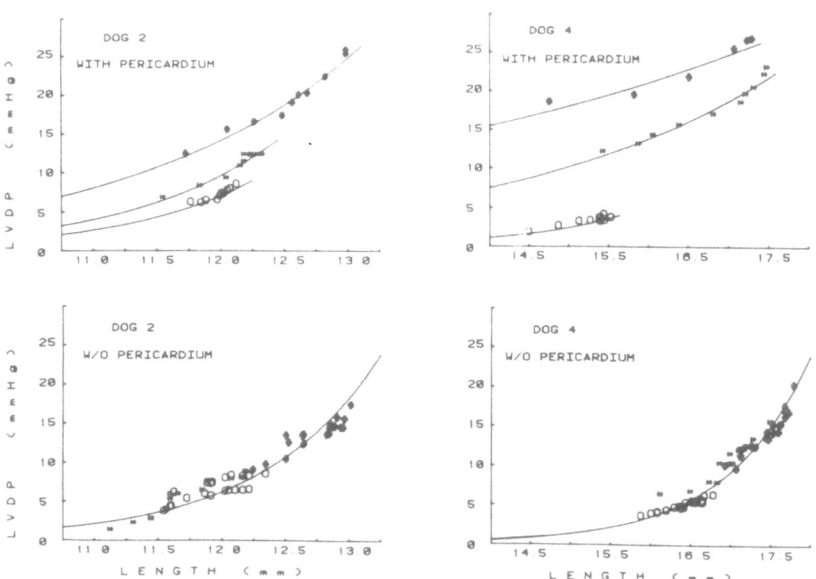

Figure 9. Left ventricular diastolic pressure-segment length relations before and after removal of the pericardium in two dogs. With intact pericardium, the curves were shifted upward during acute volume loading (#) and sodium nitroprusside (*) infusion lowered these curves towards control (0). Without the pericardium, each condition fitted a single curve. (Reproduced from Shirato *et al.*: Alteration of the left ventricular diastolic pressure-segment length relation produced by the pericardium: Effects of cardiac distension and afterload reduction in conscious dogs, Circulation 57: 1191, 1978 with permission of the American Heart Association.)

Thus both animal and clinical studies support the hypothesis that external pressures are the dominant factors involved when dramatic shifts take place in the diastolic P-V relations following certain drug interventions.

Relationship between ventricular stiffness, cavity size, wall mass, coronary blood volume and myocardial stiffness

The confusion surrounding the terms ventricular or chamber stiffness (dP/dV), myocardial stiffness E_{INC} ($d\sigma/d\varepsilon$) and factors affecting the diastolic P-V relation are best explained by a simple mathematical model which is based on the classical linear theory of elasticity.

Assuming a spherical geometry for the LV which is subjected to a cavity pressure P and external pressure P_0, the chamber stiffness (dP_T/dV) is expressed in the form (Appendix 1)

$$dP_T/dV \sim (4/9)E_{INC} (1 - \frac{V \Delta V_B}{V_w \Delta V})/V(1 + V/V_w),$$

where $P_T = P - P_0$ is the transmural pressure, V = cavity size or volume, E_{INC} = myocardial stiffness based on transmural pressures, V/V_w is the volume/wall volume ratio and V_B is the coronary blood volume. It is the interplay between all these various factors that enables one to explain what may appear to be conflicting results namely, that a stiff chamber may be associated with normal myocardial stiffness constants and vice versa.

The mechanical and hemodynamic behavior of the infarcted left ventricle

In the previous sections, we discussed mathematical models based on idealized LV geometries, in relation to an assessment of diastolic function. These 'simpler models' are inappropriate in the case of coronary artery disease and one must resort to more sophisticated techniques such as the finite element approach. In this section two such models developed by Janz et al. (1978) and Bogen et al. (1980), will be discussed.

Effect of aneurysms on the mechanical behavior of the LV

Janz et al. (1978) attempted to describe the effects of various types of aneurysms on the local fiber elongation and also obtain a relationship between ventricular stiffness and aneurysm size.

48

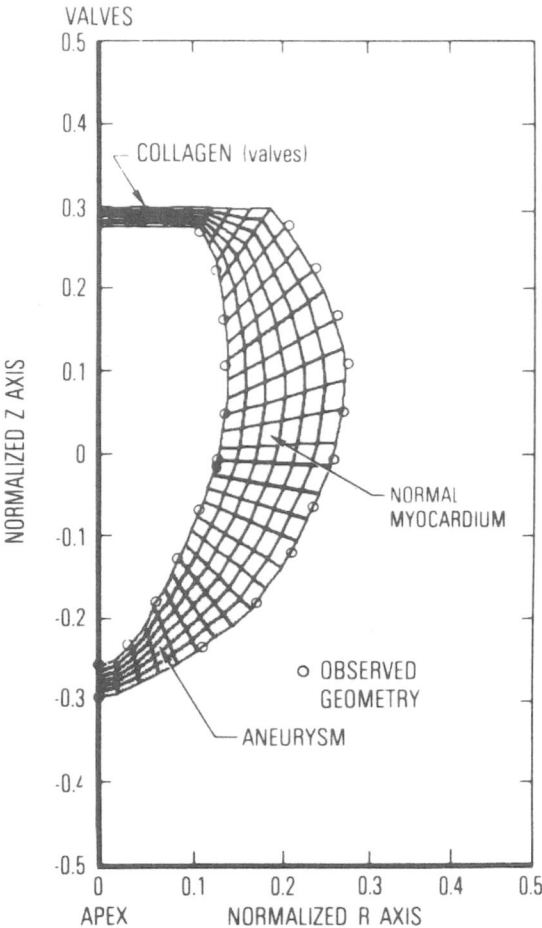

Figure 10. Undeformed shape of the free wall of a normal rat left ventricle. The network superimposed on the wall geometry illustrates the finite-element substructure in the mathematical model. (Reproduced from Janz and Waldron: Predicted effect of chronic apical aneurysms on the passive stiffness of the human left ventricle, Circ Res 42: 255, 1978 with permission from the American Heart Association.)

Figure 10 shows the undeformed shape of the free wall of a normal rat LV and the network superimposed on the wall geometry illustrates the finite element substructure in the model. Uniaxial passive stress-stretch data for fibrous and fibrous muscular aneurysms, obtained from the studies of Parmley *et al.* (1973), are displayed in Figure 11. For comparison purposes, normal human data are also shown. These data were used to determine the elastic constants.

In Figure 12 (left panel), the predicted free wall geometry of the human LV with an apical transmural fibrous-muscular aneurysm encompassing approximately 10% of the wall volume, is displayed. The right panel shows the predicted

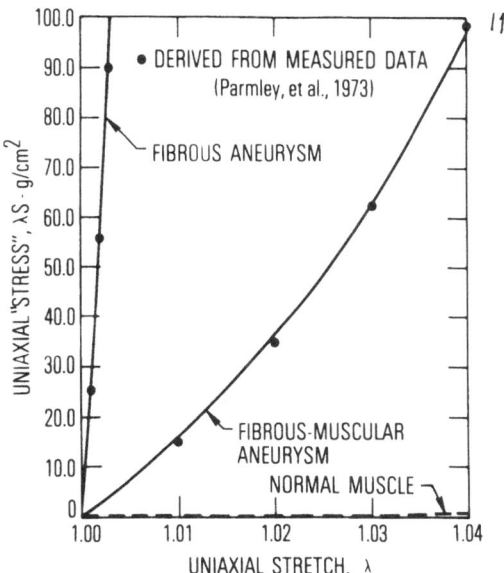

Figure 11. Uniaxial stress-stretch ($\sigma-\lambda$) data for fibrous and fibrous muscular aneurysms taken from the studies of Parmley *et al.* (1973). (Reproduced from Janz and Waldron: Predicted effect of chronic apical aneurysms on the passive stiffness of the human left ventricle, Circ Res 42: 255, 1978 with permission of the American Heart Association.)

variation of midwall circumferential stretch with position in the wall at a pressure of 12 mmHg. It is apparent that the aneurysm severely limits the fiber elongation in the normal myocardium adjacent to the aneurysm. As a result of this restraining influence on deformation, the predicted cavity volumes of the aneurysmal LV at a given pressure, are always less than those of the normal LV as seen in Figure 13 (left). In Figure 13 (right), the relationship between α and aneurysm size is shown to be linear up to an aneurysm size of 20%. Here α is the slope of the relation $dP/(dV/V_0) = \alpha P + \gamma$ (V_0 = cavity volume at zero pressure). The utility of α as an index of aneurysm size will require further study.

Diastolic and systolic P-V relations in infarcted LV

In their theoretical studies, Bogen *et al.* (1980) assumed an initially spherical membrane model for the infarcted LV. Employing a finite element method, it was possible to obtain end diastolic and end systolic pressure-volume curves. From these P-V curves, the effects of infarct size and infarct stiffness on the

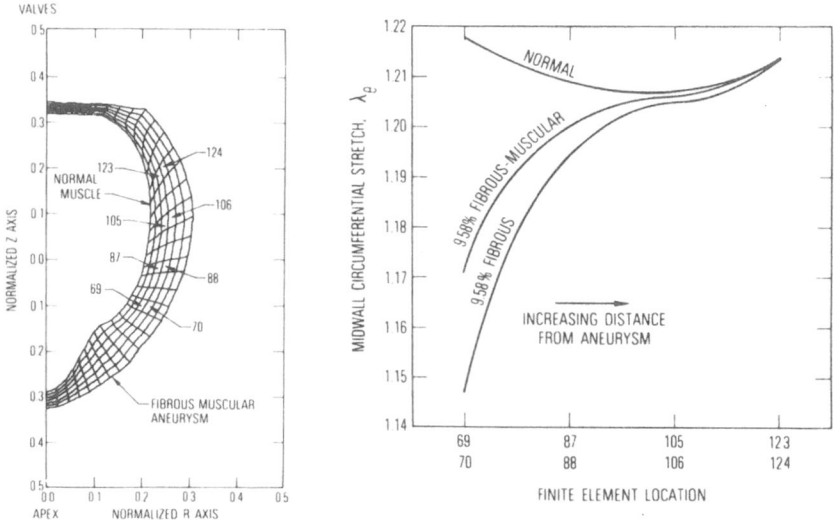

Figure 12. Left. Predicted free wall geometry in a human LV with an apical fibrous muscular aneurysm. *Right.* Variation of midwall circumferential fiber stretch with position. Note that adjacent to the aneurysm, elongation of the normal myocardium is severely limited. (Reproduced from Janz and Waldron: Predicted effect of chronic apical aneurysms on the passive stiffness of the human left ventricle, Circ Res 42: 255, 1978 with permission from the American Heart Association.)

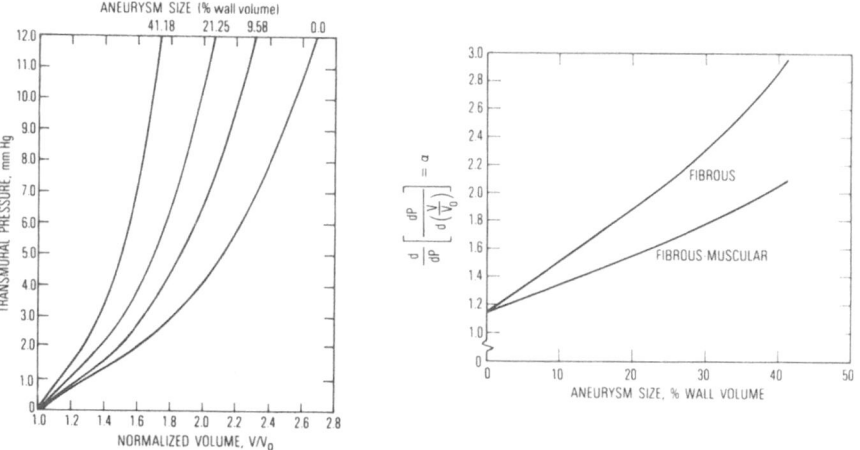

Figure 13. Left. Comparison of predicted pressure-volume curves for the normal ventricle and ventricles with fibrous aneurysms. *Right.* Variation of the parameter α with aneurysm size. For aneurysms encompassing less than 20% of wall volume, the curves are linear. (Reproduced from Janz and Waldron: Predicted effect of chronic apical aneurysms on the passive stiffness of the human left ventricle, Circ Res 42: 255, 1978 with permission of the American Heart Association.)

pumping performance of the ventricle were determined. A brief summary of their results is given in this section.

Based on a strain energy function developed by Ogden (1972), one can show that the diastolic pressure-stretch relation for a spherical membrane is given in the form

$$P_d = A(\lambda^{k-3} - \lambda^{-2k-3}) \sim A(V/V_0)^{(k-3)/3}$$

since k is generally large. Here A, k are elastic constants, λ is the stretch ratio, V = cavity volume and V_0 = cavity volume at zero diastolic pressure.

Assuming developed tension is essentially linear with extension over a certain range during peak isometric contraction, and $k = 2$ during systole, end systolic pressure-extension relations are given by P_s, total

$$= 0.82(v^{13/3} - v^{-35/3}) + 246(1.39v^{-1/3} - 0.52v^{-7/3}) \text{ for } \lambda \geqslant 1$$
$$246(1.39v^{-1/3} - 0.52v^{-7/3}) \text{ for } \lambda < 1$$

where $v = V/V_0$. Note that $P_d = 0$ for $\lambda < 1$ since resting tension and developed tension do not both fall to zero at the same length.

Ventricular function and infarct size relationships

Figure 14 displays the relationships between stroke volume (relative to the stroke volume in the normal ventricle) and infarct size for various values of infarct stiffness. For EDP = 12 mmHg, the percentage decrease in stroke volume exceeds the percentage of myocardial infarction e.g. a 41% infarct reduces function to levels of 48% and 28% of normal depending on the infarct stiffness.

Extension and stress distributions in large acute infarcted hearts

The extension and stress distributions based on the model by Bogen *et al.* (1980) are shown in Figure 15 for the infarcted region and border zone. In panel A the systolic extensions are shown. Due to the forces imposed by the bulging aneurysm, circumferential extensions in the border zone adjacent to the infarct, are larger than normal. As a consequence, the circumferential stresses at 80° (edge of infarct) are approximately 3.7 times those at 180° (panel B). Away from the border zone, extensions and stresses are approximately uniform.

In summary, these studies demonstrate that; (i) there is a progressive degradation of cardiac performance with increasing infarct size such that normal cardiac outputs cannot be maintained for infarct sizes >41% of surface area, (ii) the relationship between infarct stiffness and cardiac function is complex and is

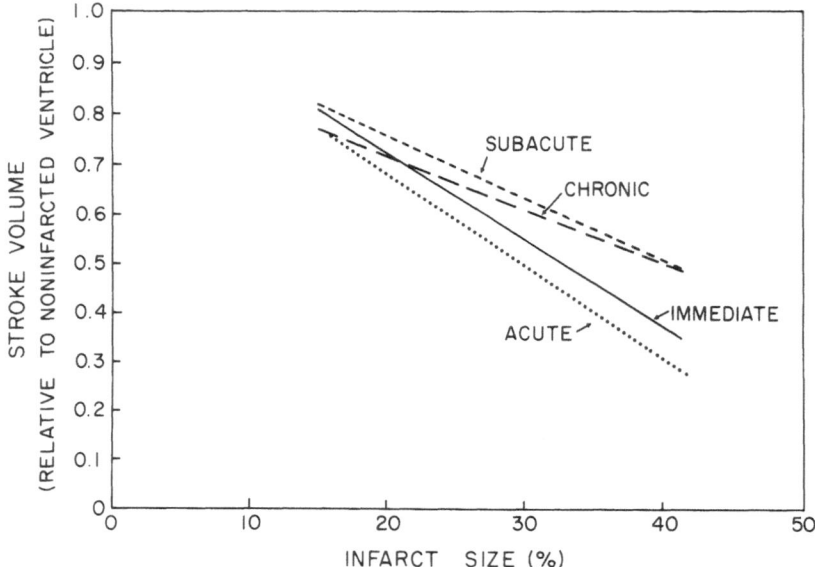

Figure 14. Stroke volume versus infarct size relationships for various infarct stiffnesses. The percentage decrease in stroke volume exceeds the percentage of myocardial infarction. (Reproduced from Bogen *et al.*: An analysis of the mechanical disadvantage of myocardial infarction in the canine left ventricle, Circ Res 47: 728, 1980 with permission of the American Heart Association.)

dependent on both infarct size and end diastolic pressure. However, function is better with moderately stiff subacute infarcts than in the presence of extensible acute infarcts and (iii) there is a considerable disruption of the border zone contraction patterns as well as an elevation of border zone systolic stress.

An approximate assessment of myocardial contractile reserve

In the past few years there has been an increased interest in the application of the end systolic pressure-end systolic volume concept (Suga and Sagawa, 1974), to the clinical setting. While this concept is useful for assessing changes in the contractile state, its limitation at present lies in the fact that the slope of this end systolic pressure-volume relation (ESP-ESV) cannot be employed as an index of contractility when making patient to patient comparisons. Sagawa (1981) has touched on this problem of normalization of the slope, however, cardiologists have yet to address this problem.

This final section explores in a preliminary manner, an approximate method for assessing the contractile state and myocardial contractile reserve in terms of ejection fraction-afterload-preload relationships. The analysis is based on the concept of developed stress defined here to be the difference of end systolic stress and end diastolic stress.

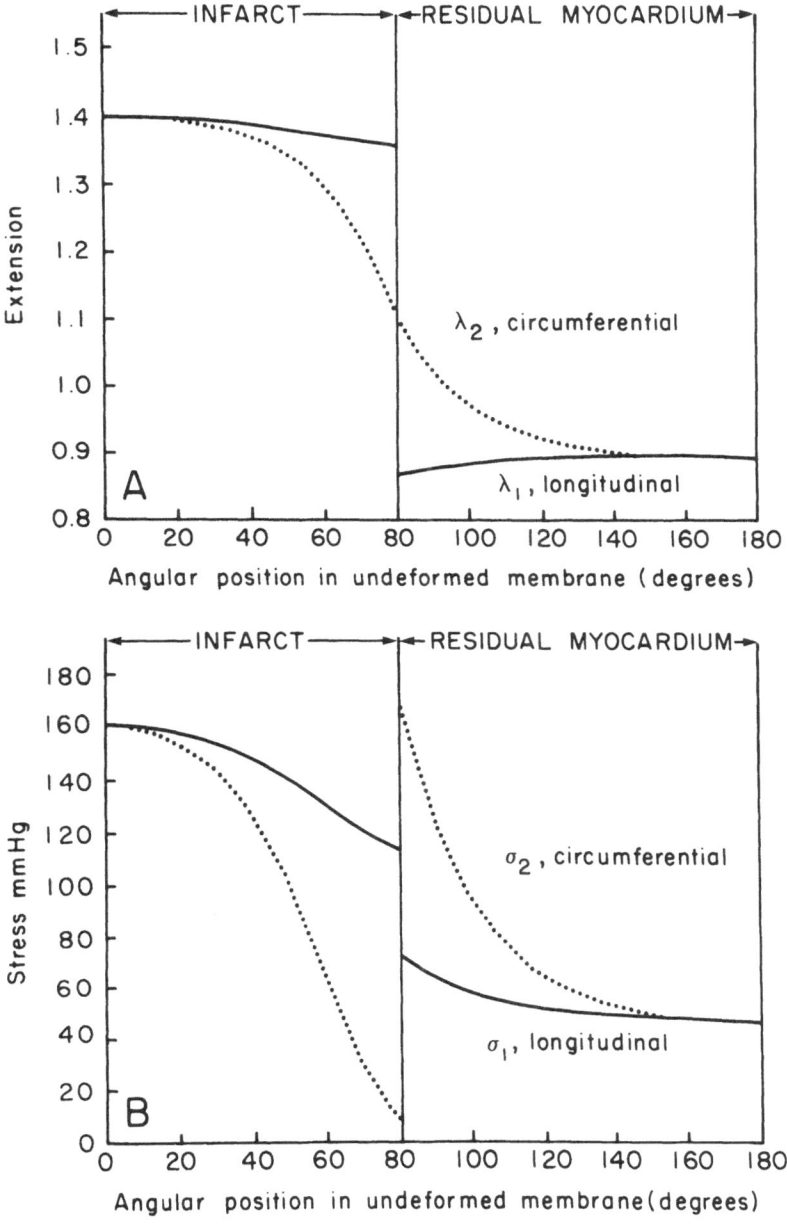

Figure 15. Extension and stress distributions in infarcted heart. A. Systolic circumferential extensions in the border zone are larger than normal. B. Circumferential stresses at the edge of the infarct are 3.7 times greater than those at 180°. (Reproduced from Bogen *et al.*: An analysis of the mechanical disdvantage of myocardial infarction in the canine left ventricle, Circ Res 47, 728, 1980 with permission from the American Heart Association.)

Expressions for end systolic, end diastolic and developed stresses

Assuming a spherical geometry for the LV, the global average end systolic and end diastolic stresses are given by

$$\sigma_{thho3ee\ 533eew10.0} = P_S \, / [(1 + V_w/V_{es})^{2/3} - 1]$$

and

$$\sigma_{ed} = P_{ed}/[(1 + V_w/V_{ed})^{2/3} - 1],$$

where V_w = LV wall volume, V_{es} and V_{ed} are respectively the end systolic and end diastolic volumes. The end systolic pressure (P_{es}) is expressed in the linear form $P_{es} = AV_{es} + B$ (Suga and Sagawa, 1974) and the end diastolic pressure (P_{ed}) is assumed in the exponential form $P_{ed} = Ce^{aVed}$. Hence the developed stress (σ_{DEV}) is defined by $\sigma_{DEV} = \sigma_{es} - \sigma_{ed}$ and may be expressed as a function of end diastolic and end systolic volumes.

Stroke volume versus end diastolic volume relationship

Writing $s = V_{ed} - V_{es}$ = stroke volume, the expression for the developed stress becomes (on substitution for P_{es} and P_{ed}),

$$\sigma_{DEV} = \sigma_{es} - \sigma_{ed}$$

$$= (AV_{ed} - As + B)/[(1 + (V_w/V_{ed} - s))^{2/3} - 1] - Ce^a V_{ed}/[(1 + V_w/V_{ed})^{2/3} - 1]$$

It is this relation that enables one to determine the critical end diastolic volume (V_{cr}) at which maximum stroke volume occurs for constant levels of developed stress.

Ejection fraction versus afterload relationships

The term afterload has taken on several meanings in the literature and these include mean systolic stress, peak systolic stress, stress at aortic valve opening, mean aortic pressure and more recently, end systolic pressure and end systolic stress. The variety of definitions is simply due to the fact that afterload varies continuously throughout ejection.

For the purposes of the present discussion, afterload will be defined in terms of both end systolic and developed stress. The rationale for the choice of developed stress as a definition of afterload stems from the studies of Monroe *et al.* (1970) who demonstrated in isolated dog hearts that actively developed pressure or stress attain maximum values at physiological pressures. As a consequence, myocardial performance and contractile reserve may be better assessed in terms of developed stress in many clinical situations.

Since $V_{es} = V_{ed} - s = V_{ed}(1 - EF)$, one can readily obtain ejection fraction (EF) versus afterload relations at constant end diastolic volumes employing the previous expressions.

Figure 16 displays the stroke volume vs. V_{ed} relationships at constant levels of developed stress, employing the dog data from the early studies of Suga and Sagawa (1974). It is observed that at each level of developed stress, there is a critical end diastolic volume at which peak stroke volume occurs. The optimal developed stress occurs when peak stroke volume is a minimum namely zero and provides the basis for determining the optimal EF-afterload and EF-preload relationships shown in Figures 17, 18. Comparisons of the contractile state between different ventricles may thus be made with the aid of these relationships.

Conclusions and discussion

While the concept of myocardial stiffness is a difficult one for cardiologists and physiologists to grasp, they must become more familiar with sophisticated methods for assessing diastolic function. For many qualitative type studies not involv-

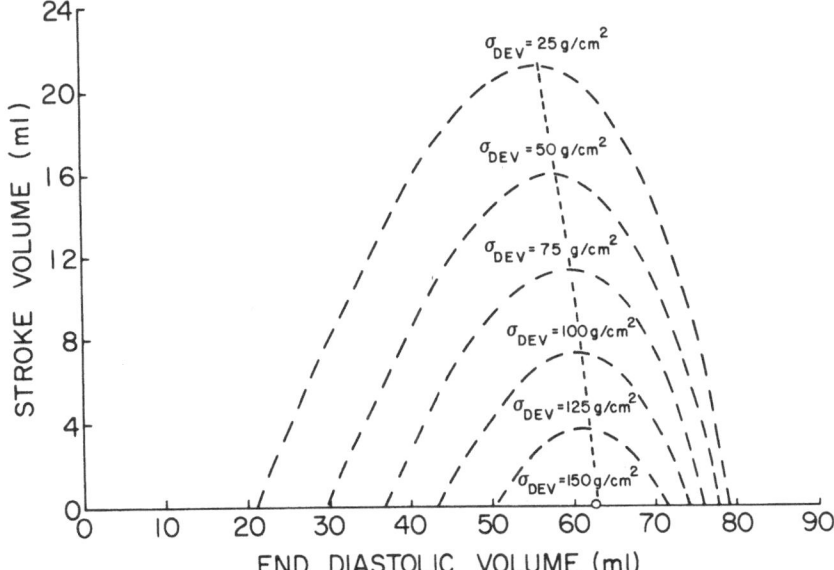

Figure 16. Stroke volume versus end diastolic volume relationships at constant levels of developed stress. At each level of developed stress there is a critical volume at which the stroke volume is a maximum. Data taken from the studies of Suga and Sagawa (1974).

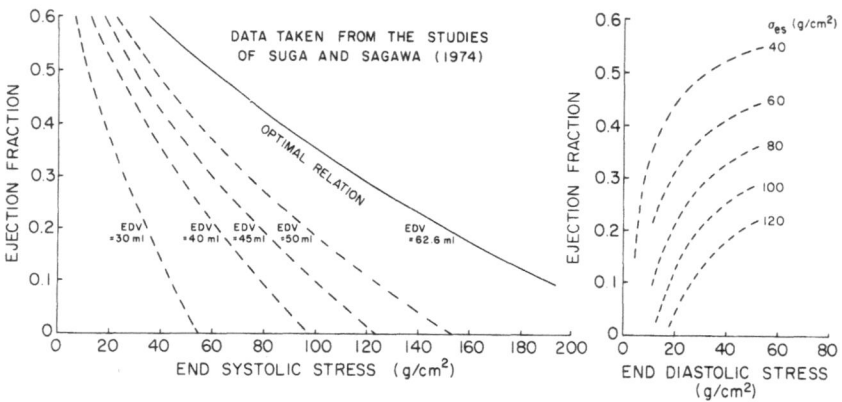

Figure 17. Ejection fraction versus afterload and preload relationships. *Left.* Ejection fraction-end systolic stress relations at constant levels of end diastolic volume. The optimal relation corresponds to the absolute maximum value of developed stress. *Right.* Ejection fraction – end diastolic stress relations at constant levels of afterload. These relationships enable one to compare the contractile states between different ventricles.

ing coronary artery disease, there are relatively simple methods for quantitating myocardial stiffness. The studies described here indicate that the effects of LV shape on the diastolic P-V and myocardial stiffness-stress relations are of secondary importance and a simple spherical model may be employed for such assessments. These models have been partially validated in clinical studies by Hess *et al.* (1984) with the aid of endocardial biopsy data.

The result that diastolic P-V relations are little affected by the eccentricity of an ellipsoid (the generally assumed shape of the LV) can be explained in part by the expression for chamber stiffness derived in Appendix 1. Although the sphere as a structure is stiffer than that of an ellipsoid having the same volume and mass, the

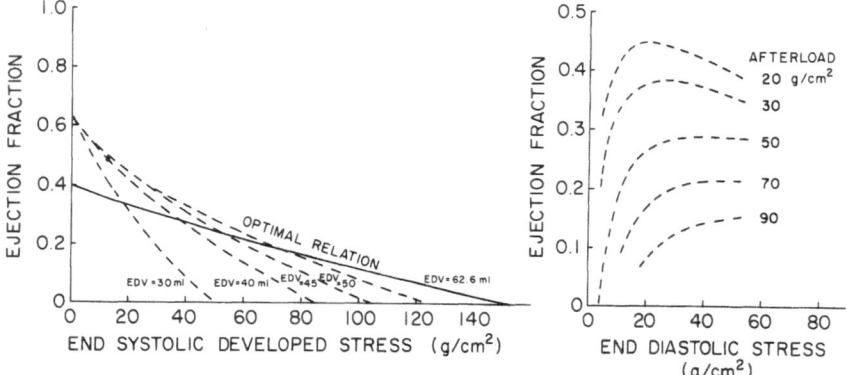

Figure 18. Ejection fraction versus afterload and preload relationships. *Left.* Ejection fraction – developed stress relations at constant levels of end diastolic volume. The optimal relation corresponds to the absolute maximum value of developed stress. *Right.* Ejection fraction-end diastolic stress relations at constant levels of developed stress.

wall stress at a given level of pressure is smaller in the sphere and hence the operating level of myocardial stiffness is reduced. Hence the interplay between chamber stiffness and myocardial stiffness results in comparable P-V relations for both geometries. This same mathematical expression also explains how it is possible for hypertrophied ventricles to display elevated levels of chamber stiffness in the presence of normal intrinsic myocardial stiffness and vice versa. In particular, the recent studies in the spontaneously hypertensive rat (Mirsky et al., 1983) have shown that intrinsic myocardial stiffness is elevated in heart failure however, the ventricle is compliant. Furthermore, these studies also demonstrated that increases in myocardial stiffness occurred before marked depression of the ejection fraction, and that the increased myocardial stiffness was associated with a depressed myocardial contractile state.

With the increased use of drug therapy in heart disease, it is important to understand the mechanisms involved that result in dramatic shifts of the diastolic P-V relations following certain drug interventions. By means of a mathematical model, it was possible to quantitate the effects of various factors and to conclude that external pressures play the dominant role. These conclusions have also been validated by animal and clinical studies (Shirato et al., 1978; Ludbrook et al., 1979).

For problems involving the mechanical and hemodynamic behavior of ventricles in patients with coronary artery disease, it is inappropriate to employ simple geometric models and one must resort to the more sophisticated methods such as the finite element approach. However, we should not fall into the trap of developing models so complicated that sorting out the important parameters in a particular situation becomes very difficult. The particular models developed by Janz et al. (1978) and Bogen et al. (1980) have yielded results that are in qualitative agreement with the rat studies by Pfeffer et al. (1979) and Fletcher et al. (1981), and appear to be manageable from the computational point of view. Obviously these sophisticated finite element models have little clinical utility, but they do provide explanations for complex phenomena taking place and aid in guiding the course of future animal experimentation.

The development of practical methods for the assessment of myocardial contractility continues and while the ESP-ESV concept provides one approach for quantitating changes in the contractile state, it requires further modification in order that it may be employed for patient to patient comparison. The preliminary studies described here on the basis of the developed stress concept shows some promise, however, further studies are required to examine the relationships between peak systolic pressure and end diastolic volume in order to explore an alternative definition for developed stress.

Areas requiring further research

There are a number of areas requiring further study and where mathematical models could play important roles in guiding the course of future experimentation. These may be outlined as follows:

(1) One of the most difficult experimental studies in cardiac mechanics is the determination of the mechanical properties of the myocardium and the associated wall stress distributions. In light of this fact it would appear more important to focus on the experimental aspects of this problem rather than pursuing the development of more complex models. However, in recent years the incorporation of fiber angle distribution into models have yielded some interesting results (Arts, 1979; Feit, 1979; Chadwick, 1982; Tozeren, 1983) and their approach should be further explored.

(2) The question of intramyocardial pressure distributions has been a controversial one for over 40 years. Most models developed thus far demonstrate that these distributions are qualitatively similar to those of radial stress i.e. decreasing from the cavity pressure at the endocardium to lower pressures at the epicardium. These distributions are often obtained experimentally. A recent model by Pierce (1981) however, indicates the possibility of intramyocardial pressures in the subendocardial layers being higher than the cavity pressures, a result that has also been observed experimentally.

(3) It is important to quantitate regional stresses in the border zones of infarcts, particularly at times early after the infarct. While such problems generally require the application of the finite-element technique, Janz (1982) has developed an analytical model which may have more clinical value and these studies should be extended.

(4) The factors affecting the diastolic P-V relations following pacing-induced angina, remain controversial. Different investigators have hypothesized different factors as being important, namely, myocardial elasticity, incomplete relaxation, coronary perfusion pressure etc. One approach might be to examine the shape changes of these P-V curves and examine the possible correlations with these various factors. With drug interventions, the shifts are usually parallel, however, with angina this is not the case.

(5) In the past few years cardiologists have focused on the quantitation of a time constant in attempts to develop 'an index of isovolumic relaxation'. However, the resulting controversies have stemmed mainly from the different computational methods employed. What has been lacking, is the development of mathematical models which may provide insights into the various mechanisms involved in these processes of relaxation. Brower *et al.* (1983) have made a beginning in this direction and their model could provide a basis for future studies. Furthermore, an added stimulus for further studies in this area is provided by the recent editorial by Brutsaert *et al.* (1984) who propose a redefinition of systole and diastole.

Finally, it should be emphasized that in the development of mathematical models, several basic points need to be adhered to namely (i) the assumptions made should be reasonable and wherever appropriate, based on previous experimental or clinical evidence (ii) where feasible, the model should be tested in the physiological setting either in a quantitative or qualitative manner and (iii) always consider their possible applications to the clinical setting.

Acknowledgements

The study was supported by U.S. Public Health Service Grant HL 12711 National Heart, Lung and Blood Institute.

The author is indebted to Drs PA Ludbrook, HP Krayenbuehl and OM Hess for providing the clinical data. He is also grateful to Dr Eugene Braunwald for his stimulating discussions associated with the question of the stroke volume-end diastolic volume relations.

Appendix 1

Relationship between ventricular stiffness, myocardial elasticity, coronary blood volume, cavity size and the volume mass ratio

For a sphere subjected to internal pressure P and external pressure P_0, Love (1944) has shown that the radial displacement $u(r)$ at any radius r is given by

$$u(r) = (3/4) \ P_T a^3 b^3 / E r^2 (b^3 - a^3),$$

where a, b are respectively the internal and external radii, E is the Young's modulus which is identified here with the incremental modulus E_{INC}, and $P_T = P - P_0$ is the transmural pressure. Hence the radial displacements at the endocardial and epicardial surfaces are respectively

$$u_a = (3/4) P_T a b^3 / E_{INC} (b^3 - a^3) \text{ and } u_b = (3/4) P_T a^3 b / E_{INC} (b^3 - a^3).$$

Now $V = (4/3)\pi a^3$ and $V + V_w = V + V_B + V_M = (4/3)\pi b^3$, where V = cavity volume, V_M = muscle volume, V_B = coronary blood volume and V_w = LV wall volume. Thus

$$\Delta V = 4\pi a^2 \Delta a,$$
$$\Delta V + \Delta V_w = \Delta V + \Delta V_B = 4\pi b^2 \Delta b \text{ assuming incompressibility of}$$
cardiac muscle.
Therefore,

$$\Delta V / V - (\Delta V + V_B)/(V + V_w)$$
$$= [\Delta V - (V/V_w)\Delta v_B]/V(1 + V/V_w)$$
$$= 3\Delta a / a - 3\Delta b / b.$$

Furthermore, an increment ΔP_T in the transmural pressure results in incremental displacements in the endocardial and epicardial surfaces given by $\Delta u_a = \Delta a = (3/4)\Delta P_T a b^3 / E_{INC} (b^3 - a^3)$
$$\Delta u_b = \Delta b = (3/4)\Delta P_T a^3 b / E_{INC} (b^3 - a^3)$$

60

Hence $[\Delta V - (V/V_w)\Delta V_B]/V(1 + V/V_w) = (9/4)\Delta P_T/E_{INC}$
or

$$\Delta P_T/\Delta V = (4/9)E_{INC} (1 - \frac{V \, \Delta \, V_B}{V_w \, \Delta \, V})/V(1 + V/V_w)$$

Note that for a cylindrical geometry, the factor 4/9 is replaced by a factor 1/3, a result obtained by Moskowitz (1980).

References

Alderman EL, Glantz SA (1976) Acute interventions shift the diastolic pressure-volume curve in man. Circulation 54:662–671

Arts T, Reneman RS, Veenstra PC (1979) A model of the mechanics of the left ventricle. Ann Biomed Eng 7:299–318

Bogen DK, Rabinowitz SA, Needleman A, McMahon TA, Abelmann WH (1980) An analysis of the mechanical disadvantage of myocardial infarction in the canine left ventricle. Circ Res 47:728–741

Bonow RO, Bacharach SL, Green MV, Kent KM, Rosing DR, Lipson LC, Leon MB, Epstein SE (1981) Impaired left ventricular diastolic filling in patients with coronary artery disease: Assessment with radionuclide angiography. Circulation 64:315–323

Brodie BR, Grossman W, Mann T, McLaurin LP (1977) Effects of sodium nitroprusside on left ventricular diastolic pressurevolume relations. J Clin Invest 59:59–68

Brower RW, Meij S, Serruys PW (1983) A model of asynchronous left ventricular relaxation predicting the bi-exponential pressure decay. Cardiovasc Res 17:482–488

Brutsaert DL, Rademakers FE, Sys SU (1984) Editorial: Triple control of relaxation: implications in cardiac disease. Circulation 69:190–196

Chadwick RS (1982) Mechanics of the left ventricle. Biophysical J 39:279–288

Feit TS (1979) Diastolic pressure-volume relations and distribution of pressure and fiber extension across the wall of a model left ventricle. Biophysical J 28:143–166

Fester A, Samet P (1974) Passive elasticity of human left ventricle: The 'parallel elastic element.' Circulation 50:609–618

Fletcher PJ, Pfeffer JM, Pfeffer MA, Braunwald E (1981) Left ventricular diastolic pressure-volume relations in rats with healed myocardial infarction. Circ Res 49:618–626

Gallagher KP, Matsuzaki M, Kemper WS, Ross J Jr (1983) Inner wall thickening during coronary stenosis in conscious dogs. Circulation 68 (Suppl 111) 156

Hess OM, Ritter M, Schneider J, Grimm J, Turina M, Krayenbuehl HP (1984) Diastolic stiffness and myocardial structure in aortic valve disease before and after valve replacement. Circulation 69:855–865

Huisman RM, Sipkema P, Westerhof N, Elzinga G (1980) Comparison of models used to calculate left ventricular wall force. Med & Biol Eng & Comput 18:133–144

Janz RF, Waldron RJ (1978) Predicted effect of chronic apical aneurysms on the passive stiffness of the human left ventricle. Circ Res 42:255–263

Janz RF, Kubert BR, Pate EF, Moriarty TF (1980) Effect of shape on pressure-volume relationships of ellipsoidal shells. Am J Physiol 238:H917–H926

Janz RF (1982) Estimation of local myocardial stress. Am J Physiol 242:H875–881

Love AEH (1944) A Treatise on the Mathematical Theory of Elasticity ed 4. New York: Dover Publications, pp 142

Ludbrook PA, Byrne JD, McKnight RC (1979) Influence of right ventricular hemodynamics on left ventricular diastolic pressure-volume relations in man. Circulation 59:21–29

Mirsky I (1974) Review of various theories for the evaluation of left ventricular wall stresses. In: I Mirsky, DN Ghista, and H Sandler (eds) Cardiac mechanics: Physiological, Clinical, and Mathematical Considerations. New York: Wiley

Mirsky I (1979) Elastic properties of the myocardium: a quantitative approach with physiological and clinical applications. In: R Berne, N Sperelakis (eds) Handbook of Physiology – The Cardiovascular System 1, chap 14. Washington D.C.: American Physiological Society, pp 497–531

Mirsky I, Rankin JS (1979) Special Article: The effects of geometry, elasticity, and external pressures on the diastolic pressure-volume and stiffness-stress relations. How important is the pericardium? Circ Res 44:601–611

Mirsky I, Pfeffer JM, Pfeffer MA, Braunwald E (1983) The contractile state as the major determinant in the evolution of left ventricular dysfunction in the spontaneously hypertensive rat. Circ Res 53:767–778

Mirsky I (1984) Perspectives Article: Assessment of diastolic function: Suggested methods and future considerations. Circulation 69:836–841

Monroe RG, Gamble WJ, LaFarge CC, Kumar AE, Manasek FJ (1970) Left ventricular performance at high end diastolic pressures in isolated perfused dog hearts. Circ Res 26:85–99

Moskowitz SE (1980) On the mechanics of left ventricular diastole. J Biomechanics 13:301–311

Ogden RW (1972) Large deformation isotropic elasticity: On the correlation of theory and experiment for incompressible rubber-like solids. Proc R Soc Lond A326:565–584

Parmley WW, Chuck L, Kivowitz C, Matloff JM, Swan HJC (1973) In vitro length-tension relations of human ventricular aneurysms: Relation of stiffness to mechanical disadvantage. Am J Cardiol 32:889–894

Pierce WH (1981) Body forces and pressures in elastic models of the myocardium. Biophysical J 34: 35–59

Pfeffer MA, Pfeffer JM, Fishbein MC, Fletcher PJ, Spadaro J, Kloner RA, Braunwald E (1979) Myocardial infarct size and ventricular function in rats. Circ Res 44:503–512

Sagawa K (1981) Editorial: The end systolic pressure-volume relation of the ventricle. Definition, modifications and clinical use. Circulation 63:1223–1227

Shirato K, Shabetai R, Bhargava V, Franklin D, Ross J Jr (1978) Alteration of the left ventricular diastolic pressure-segment length relation produced by the pericardium: Effects of cardiac distension and afterload reduction in conscious dogs. Circulation 57:1191–1198

Soufer R, Wohlgelernter D, Vita N, Amuchastegui M, Sostman D, Berger HJ, Zaret BL (1983) Normal systolic left ventricular function in patients with congestive heart failure. Frequent diastolic dysfunction. Circulation 68 (Suppl 111) 101

Streeter DD, Vaishnav RN, Patel DJ, Spotnitz HM, Ross J Jr, Sonnenblick EH (1970). Stress distribution in the canine left ventricle during diastole and systole. Biophysical J 10:345–363

Suga H, Sagawa K (1974) Instantaneous pressure-volume relationships and their ratio in the excised, supported canine left ventricle. Circ Res 35:117–126

Tozeren A (1983) Static analysis of the left ventricle. J Biomech Eng 105:39–46

Yin FCP (1981) Ventricular wall stress. Circ Res 49:829–842

Zienkiewicz OC (1971) The Finite Element Method in Engineering Science. London: McGraw Hill

DISCUSSION

JANICKI: I want to address the dramatic shifts in the pressure-volume relationship with drugs. I've looked at the literature and I wonder how dramatic these shifts are. These observations are based on a diameter measurement to yield the diameter-pressure relationship. The data that was obtained was primarily from the end of the rapid filling phase to end diastole. Now, you are focusing on the end diastolic pressure-volume relationship, which I think is different. In our isolated heart preparation we looked at the end diastolic pressure-volume relationship and the shift occured when the volume in the other ventricle was varied. It wasn't a big shift and it occured only when we varied the volume in the other ventricle over a pressure range of 0–20 mm of mercury, which is a lot of external force.

ANS: The model presented in the manuscript stems from my early studies. It has human patient data and methoxamine was used. The pressure-volume data was measured from, approximately, minimum diastolic pressure to end diastole and there were shifts of roughly 15–16 mmHg. If you look at the studies by Shirato et al. (1978), you'll also see these shifts in the pressure-segment length relations (pericardium absent), following certain drug interventions.

JANICKI: If you look at Shirato's data and if you look at the end diastolic point, they, more or less, fall on the exponential curve, even though the curves he gives, which are from the end of rapid filling to end diastole, are shifted. But they still end up on what looks like the end diastolic pressure-volume relationship.

ANS: You mean the end diastolic points are similar in the control as in the intervention state?

JANICKI: Yes.

ANS: Well, this did not occur in the methoxamine study. They were really parallel shifts and I think that you'll find that, with drugs, the shifts are invariably parallel. What you are saying may be true in the case of pacing induced angina, where you may get both a parallel shift and a shape change in the pressure-volume relation.

JANICKI: The point I'm trying to make is that these shifts aren't at end diastole. They are just shifts you see during filling. The end diastolic curve has not shifted itself. It may shift a little bit but not directly the way the data would indicate.

MIRSKY: Maybe more studies are needed to settle this point but the evidence at present appears to validate my result.

SAGAWA: Dr. Mirsky's conclusion that the major factor is the external pressure is the answer to the question. Dr. Janicki mostly studied the excised heart and we see exactly the same thing. The small effect of those factors mentioned in the literature are on the excised heart. In the in vivo chest, a lot of interaction occurs from the right side to the left side, through the pericardium and the myocardium, and because of that the external pressure is much more amplified, which we can't see in the excised heart. I have no objection to calculating and regarding end systolic developed stress as an afterload for muscle.

DINNAR: Relating to Figure 18. You plotted ejection fraction as a function of developed stress for various preload values, Ved, and there was a crossing of the optimal curve with those at lower values of Ved. What is it in your model that gives a better ejection fraction with less stress?

ANS: I thought about this for a long time. Maybe one has to disregard the region of those very early afterloads. I don't know what physiological meaning they have. The crossing may be an artifact and may be a consequence of the assumption of the linear end systolic pressure volume relationship which probably doesn't hold in that range. If you look at the whole range of end systolic pressure-volume relations, you'll find non linearity at both extremes. This could be a reason for (the apparent optimization) the crossing of the solid line. I don't really have a good answer.

DINNAR: You can see it on the right panel too where ejection fraction is plotted versus preload (end diastolic stress).

ANS: It's on the right side that you get the peaks; you don't get the sort of descending limbs with the higher afterload, though.

SKORTON: I am confused by your result that both fibrosis and elasticity were increased post operatively in aortic stenosis patients. What is your interpretation of that? I would think it would be the other way around.

ANS: The answer is very simple: once fibrosis, always fibrosis and there is a regression of LV mass. As these ventricles regress in mass the fibrosis content remains the same but the masses come down and the fibrosis percentage obviously has to go up. The concerns I have relate to the endocardial biopsy measurements. One may be overestimating fibrosis in, say, aortic stenosis and in aortic insufficiency, fibrosis may be more diffuse so obviously one really needs to do transmural biopsies and not too many investigators do that. My colleagues, Drs. Krayenbuehi and Hess, also got the same results with a much more complicated model, and I didn't believe it at first. However, when you think about it, it is really an obvious result. That is the best way to validate a model.

SKORTON: How long after surgery were the second measurements taken?

ANS: The average was 17.5 months. That's quite a while. It would be no good to study even within 6 months. Probably, you wouldn't find the regression of mass by that period.

SKORTON: In Janz's finite element model that you showed there were 4, 5, or 6 elements distributed across the wall. Was the assumption made throughout the cardiac cycle, or the portion that was studied, that those elements maintained the same relative sizes throughout the cycle?

ANS: I don't think you need to asusme this. I remember that the shape of the LV was calculated at one pressure measurement, namely 12 mmHg. Dr. Janz's model is an interesting model and one explanation that shape may have little effect on the pressure-volume relationship might be as follows. For the same volume and mass, the sphere as a structure is much stiffer than an ellipsoid of equivalent volume and mass. But on the other hand, at a given pressure level, the wall stresses in the sphere will be lower, and therefore the operating myocardial stiffness will be lower. So you have this interplay between chamber stiffness, myocardial stiffness and cavity size which could possibly produce similar pressure-volume relations

Left ventricular performance and its systolic mechanical properties

JOSEPH S. JANICKI, SANJEEV G. SHROFF and KARL T. WEBER
Cardiovascular Research Institute, Department of Medicine, Michael Reese Hospital and Medical Center, Chicago, IL 60616, U.S.A.

Abstract

The myocardium is a viscoelastic material whose mechanical properties are reflected in the pumping behavior of the ventricular chamber. Hence, the relationships between left ventricular (LV) pressure, volume, and flow may be characterized in terms of the chamber mechanical properties, elastance and resistance which are phenomenological descriptors of the observed behavior between pressure and volume and pressure and flow, respectively. For example, during the isovolumic phase of systole, the ability of the ventricle to generate pressure is expressed by the degree to which elastance increases, while during the ejection phase instantaneous LV pressure depends on both instantaneous volume (elastic behavior) and flow (resistive behavior). From the onset of systole to the end of ejection the following observations have been made; (a) ventricular elastance can be represented by a third order polynomial in time, (b) elastance is only sensitive to variations in contractile state and (c) ventricular resistance can be uniquely quantified as a linear function of LV pressure. Accordingly, a mathematical model which equates the pressure generated within the LV to the sum of the resistive and elastic components has been found to adequately describe ventricular dynamics. Using this model, it is possible to calculate the intrinsic mechanical properties of the LV from measurements of LV pressure, flow and volume obtained over a single cardiac cycle. These properties may prove useful in quantifying the functional state of the LV.

Introduction

The heart is a muscular pump that provides energy to circulate blood to and from the metabolizing tissues. The pumping characteristic of each ventricle, or the relation between its pressure, volume and flow is a complex function of the contractile state of the myocardium and the mechanical interaction that takes place between the ventricles and the venous and arterial circulations. For example, two of the primary determinants of ventricular function namely the filling volume of the ventricle and the pressure against which it ejects blood are the results of the external loads imposed by the vasculature. Because of this interplay betweeen ventricle and external load, it is difficult to assess the contractile state simply from the measurement of pressure, volume and flow. By definition the contractile state must reflect the intrinsic ability of the ventricle to pump blood independently of the extrinsic determinants of function. Hence the measure of contractile state must be invariant to changes in either the filling volume or the level of ejection pressure.

Recently, the relationship between pressure-volume or force-length at the end of systole has attracted a great deal of interest as a descriptor of the contractile state of the heart. This interest stems from a series of studies in isolated, canine left ventricular preparations (Taylor *et al.* 1969; Suga *et al.*, 1973; Suga and Sagawa, 1974; Weber *et al.*, 1976; Weber and Janicki, 1977), which demonstrated the end-systolic pressure-volume relation to be quite sensitive to variations in contractile state and relatively insensitive to variations in load. In addition, the relation is linear over a wide range of volumes so that its slope can be used to quantitate the contractile state.

While the slope of the end-systolic pressure-volume relation does provide a measure of the contractile state, this relation is difficult to obtain in the intact animal and in man. For example, the definition of end systole is not straightforward (Sagawa, 1981; Shroff *et al.*, 1984), and the loading conditions must be varied without invoking a reflexive regulation of the contractile state in order to obtain multiple end-systolic points. In addition, valuable information regarding ventricular dynamics is lost by focusing on just one instant in the cardiac cycle where flow is essentially zero. An alternative approach, which overcomes these problems and shortcomings has recently been described (Shroff *et al.*, 1983b). This approach utilizes a mathematical model to calculate ventricular elastance and resistance from measurements of ventricular pressure, volume and flow obtained over one cardiac cycle; the peak elastance is equivalent to the slope of the end-systolic pressure-volume relation. It will be the purpose of the present review to briefly discuss both approaches with respect to their ability to describe the intrinsic properties of the ventricle.

Peak isovolumetric pressure-volume relation

The maximal pressure which can be developed for any level of filling volume and contractile state is obtained when the contraction of the myocardium does not result in a change in chamber volume (i.e. isovolumetric contraction). The only way this peak isovolumetric pressure could be changed is via a change in filling volume or a change in contractile state. When the contractile state is held constant and the filling volume increased, there is an associated augmentation in the peak isovolumetric pressure. Over the physiologic range of filling pressure, the relationship between maximal developed pressure and filling volume can be considered linear (Figure 1).

Ventricular elasticity describes the relation between chamber pressure and volume. During ventricular contraction this stiffness increases steadily (Hunter *et al.*, 1979; Suga and Sagawa, 1974). Conceptually, this behavior at different instants of systole can be represented by a family of lines in the pressure-volume (P-V) plane. Increasing ventricular stiffness during systole appears as the increasing slope of these P-V lines for times progressively later in systole. The slope of the peak isovolumetric pressure-volume relation would therefore represent the maximal elasticity the ventricle can achieve. Alterations (pharmacological or intrinsic) in the contractile state of the myocardium create nonparallel shifts in the relation (Figure 1); positive and negative inotropic interventions raise or reduce the slope or maximally achieved elasticity, respectively, (Suga *et al.*, 1973; Suga and Sagawa, 1974; Weber *et al.*, 1976). Thus since the slope of the relation is sensitive to inotropic interventions and is independent of the filling volume, it can be used to quantitate the contractile state of the ventricle.

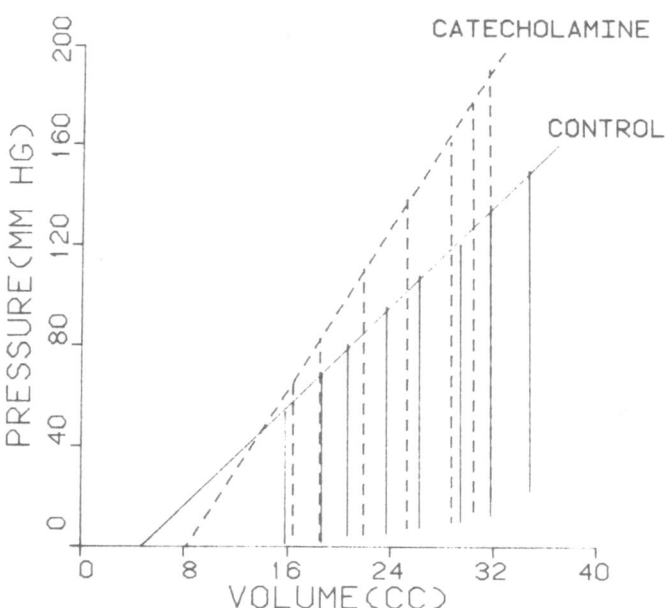

Figure 1. Steady state isovolumetric pressure-volume loops (vertical lines) are plotted for various ventricular volumes. Two contractile states are presented: control (solid lines) and enhanced (broken lines, 6 μg/min Dobutamine). The linear regression lines for the peak isovolumetric pressure-volume points are also illustrated.

End-systolic pressure-volume relation

When the contractile state is held constant and loading conditions are varied, a characteristic set of pressure-volume loops are obtained. For example, from a given filling volume, the loops obtained at increasing levels of ejection pressure become narrower with the end systolic pressure-volume point moving upward and to the right (Figure 2). On the other hand, when ejection pressure is fixed, and filling volume is increased, the loops widen but the end systolic pressure-volume point is invariant. These loops are related to one another via the end-systolic pressure-volume relation which can be considered to be linear over the physiological range of filling pressure (Figure 2). That is, for a given contractile state, the ejecting portion of the pressure-volume loops will terminate on the linear end-systolic pressure-volume relation regardless of the loading condition. There is one notable exception when the flow at the end of systole is non-zero (*vide infra*).

When the end systolic and peak isovolumic pressure-volume relations are compared, they are found to be equivalent. This equivalency has been verified for

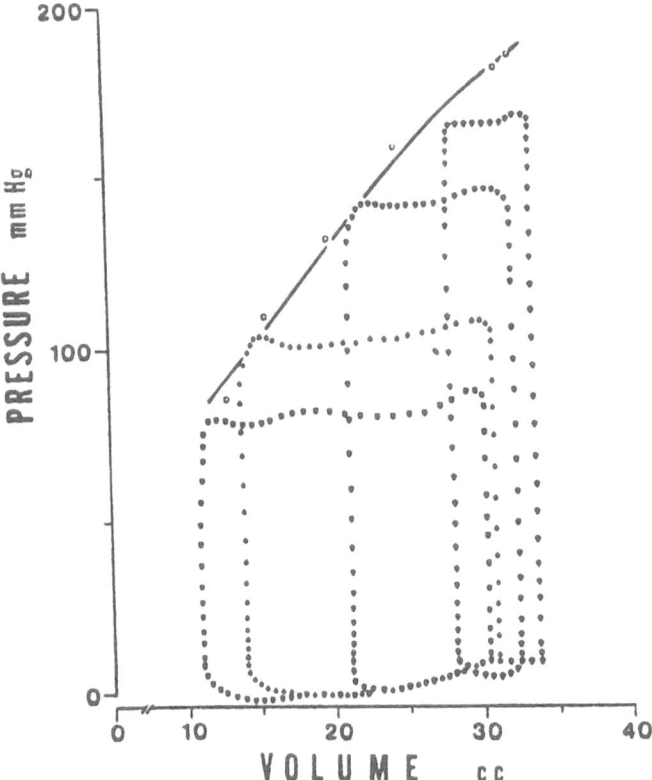

Figure 2. Superimposed pressure-volume data for a series of variably afterloaded, ejecting (solid symbols) contractions and isovolumic (open circles) state.

positive and negative variations in contractile state (Weber *et al.*, 1976). Thus the slope of the end-systolic pressure-volume relation, is a measure of the maximum elastance and the contractile state of the ventricle.

Unlike the peak isovolumetric pressure-volume relation, the end-systolic pressure-volume relation can be obtained in man (Grossman *et al.*, 1977; Mehmel *et al.*, 1981; Carabello *et al.*, 1981) and its usefulness in the evaluation of the diseased ventricle is actively being investigated. Obtaining this relation, however, is not without difficulty. As discussed in two recent reviews (Sagawa, 1981; Shroff *et al.*, 1984), the definition of end-systole is not straightforward, particularly in cardiac cycles where systolic pressure is declining during ejection or when the dichrotic notch pressure or the end-ejection pressure is used in place of end systolic pressure. It is also difficult to obtain multiple end systolic points over a wide range of loading conditions without invoking a reflexive regulation of contractile state unless of course complete pharmacologic blockade is induced. Finally, the slope of the end-systolic pressure-volume relation may overestimate that of the peak isovolumetric pressure-volume relation if the resistive effects are significantly elevated or substantial flow is occurring at end-systole (Shroff *et al.*, 1983a). Here it should be noted that the end of systole is not necessarily the same as end of ejection and it is therefore quite possible to have a flow at the end of systole.

Systolic mechanical properties

As an alternative to focusing on just the end-systolic pressure-volume relation or equivalently maximum elasticity to describe the contractile state, a mathematical model of ventricular dynamics has been developed recently (Shroff *et al.*, 1983b). This model utilizes the following information: end diastolic volume and all of the systolic pressure-flow data from a single cardiac cycle to calculate the time varying mechanical properties, elastance and resistance. The basis of the mathematical model is an assumption that the dynamic behavior of the left ventricle may be characterized in terms of the global chamber properties of elastance and resistance; inertance has been found to be negligible (Shroff *et al.*, 1983b). The elastance and resistance functions were shown, via the flow pulse technique (Hunter *et al.*, 1978), to be a independent of filling volume and ejection pressure. Elastance (E) was a function of both systolic time (t) and contractile state; its variation with time during systole could be approximated by a third order polynomial. Resistance (R) was found to be linearly related to instantaneous pressure and this linear relationship was independent of the contractile state.

The equation for the model is as follows:

$$R(P) \cdot \dot{V}(t) + E(t) [V(t) - V_d] = P(t), \tag{1}$$

where

$$R(P) = A1 + A2P(t) \tag{2}$$

and

$$E(t) = A3 + A4t + A5t^2 + A6t^3. \tag{3}$$

Here $P(t)$, $V(t)$ and $\dot{V}(t)$ are the instantaneous ventricular pressure, volume and flow and Vd is the absolute residual volume that is associated with zero end-systolic pressure. Thus from end-diastolic volume and ventricular pressure and flow data or, equivalently, ventricular pressure and volume data one can use a least squares minimization technique to obtain $A1$ through $A6$ and V_d such that the sum of the squared residuals between calculated and measured pressure is minimized. Maximum elastance could then be obtained from the elastance function.

This model can also be used to predict the isovolumetric pressure $P_{ISO}(t)$. Thus during an isovolumetric contraction the flow is zero, the volume remains constant at its end-diastolic value (EDV), and the model reduces to the following form:

$$E(t) [EDV - V_d] = P_{ISO}(t). \tag{4}$$

If the elastance function is replaced by the maximum elastance (E_{max}), peak isovolumetric pressure (P_{max}) is obtained. That is:

$$E_{max} [EDV - V_d] = P_{max}. \tag{5}$$

Results and discussion

The accuracy of the model was tested using a servocontrolled isolated heart preparation (Janicki *et al.*, 1974) whereby it was possible to have controlled ejecting and isovolumetric contractions. The model parameters (i.e., $A1$–$A6$ and V_d) were calculated from the ejecting pressure-volume data and the model was then used to predict the peak isovolumetric pressure. When the predicted and measured peak isovolumetric pressure from 10 experiments were compared a correlation coefficient of 0.97 was found (Figure 3). Similar results have been obtained in open chest experiments with the heart intact.

The advantage of this approach is obvious. Maximum elastance that has been corrected for resistive effects can easily be obtained from the elastance function without having; (1) to perturb the system and (2) to identify the end of systole. In addition, information concerning the resistive behavior of the ventricle is obtained. Because the myocardium is a viscoelastic material, the pressure generated by the ejecting left ventricle will not solely reflect its elastic properties. Instead, a

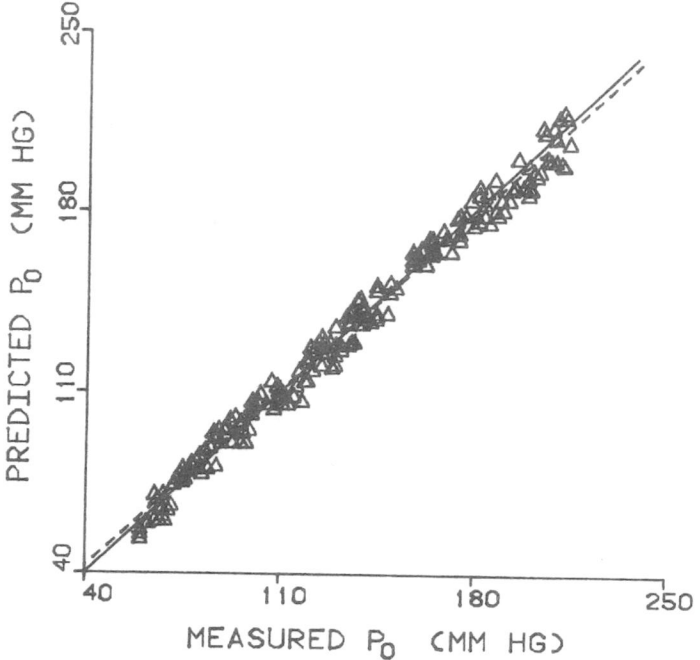

Figure 3. Predicted peak isovolumetric pressures (P_O) are plotted against measured P_Os ($n = 225$). Solid line represents line of identity; dashed line is linear regression line (slope = 0.97 ± 0.13, intercept = 4.4 ± 8.6 mmHg and correlation coefficient = 0.97).

portion of the pressure-generating capacity is spent to overcome the internal viscous resistance to motion. As a result, the actual pressure within the ventricle will be less than that which would have been expected if the ventricle were purely elastic. Hence the above model includes a resistive component.

The importance of the resistive component in comparision to the elastic can be seen in the following example. In 10 experiments (dogs) the average slope of the linear resistance-pressure relationship was found to be 0.0015 s/ml and the intercept was statistically equal to zero (Shroff *et al.*, 1983b). If we take aortic flow and pressure to be 150 ml/s and 100 mmHg, respectively, then the resistive component (resistance at 100 mmHg × flow) amounts to 22.5 mmHg. Accordingly if there are no resistive effects (i.e., a purely elastic ventricle), the corresponding pressure would have been 122.5 mmHg. Thus in this example the resistive component is 18.4% of the elastic component, which certainly cannot be ignored.

Physical significance of ventricular resistance is not yet completely clear. Phenomenologically, it represents a loss in ventricular pressure whenever the ventricle attemps to eject blood as the muscle fibers are allowed to shorten. However, ventricular resistance does not solely originate from the 'viscous like' behavior of the myocardial material which resists motion. In addition, the origin of ventricular resistance is associated with the contractile process itself. This is supported by our results that resistance is uniquely proportional to pressure and this relationship is independent of time, end diastolic volume, ejection pressure, and contractile state (Shroff, 1983b). Thus, resistance represents some fundamental rate limiting process of the contractile machinery itself. Results from preliminary experiments with 26 week old spontaneously hypertensive (SH) and Wistar-Kyoto (WKY) rats indicate the SH rats to have a 2–3 fold higher resistance than the WKY rats. It is known that SH rats possess a significantly higher proportion of the V3 type of isomyosin which is the slow acting type. Therefore, it is conceivable that ventricular resistance, as measured by our technique, may correlate with the relative proportion of myosin isoforms. It should be emphasized that the contribution of purely extra cellular components (e.g., collagen) and geometric factors to ventricular resistance can not be completely ignored. It is conceivable that excess collagen may hinder the contraction of muscle fibers (increasing resistance) while not altering the ability to generate isovolumetric pressure. The collagen concentration has been reported to be significantly increased from 2.5% to 3.8% (Pearlman et al., 1982) in hypertrophied, pressure overloaded human myocardium. Thus, a knowledge of ventricular resistance may provide valuable additional information regarding the structure-function of the myocardium in normal and diseased states.

The role of ventricular resistance in the coupling of the ventricle to its arterial load was also investigated. For this purpose, a computer simulation study was performed where the LV was represented by the above model and the arterial load by a modified Windkessel (i.e., peripheral resistance, lumped arterial compliance and a characteristic impedance). It was observed that inclusion of a ventricular resistance slightly decreased mean arterial pressure (3 to 10%) and stroke volume (3 to 7%). In contrast, the pulsatile nature of the flow was markedly altered suggesting that ventricular resistance may play an important role in minimizing the external pulsatile power and in optimally coupling the ventricle to its arterial load (Shroff et al., 1983a).

Summary

The LV systolic dynamics can be adequately represented by a time varying elastance in series with a pressure dependent resistance. Using a model such as the one presented above, it is possible to calculate the functional forms of these mechanical properties from the measurements of the LV pressure, end diastolic volume and flow over a single cardiac cycle. From the elastance function a measure of intrinsic pressure generating capacity (without shortening) is obtained while from the resistance function an idea of the loss in the pressure generating capacity due to shortening can be estimated. Furthermore, resistance characterization may be correlated to the proportion of myosin isoforms and collagen content.

72

References

Carabello BA, Nolan SP, McGuire LA (1981) Assessment of preoperative left ventricular function in patients with mitral regurgitation: Value of the end-systolic stress-end-systolic volume ratio. Circulation 64:1212–1217

Grossman W, Braunwald E, Mann T, McLaurin LP, Green LH (1977) Contractile state of the left ventricle in man as evaluated from end-systolic pressure-volume relations. Circulation 56:845–852

Hunter WC, Janicki JS, Weber KT, Noordergraaf A (1979) Flow-pulse response: A new method for the characterization of ventricular mechanics. Am J Physiol 237:H282–H292

Janicki JS, Reeves RC, Weber KT, Donald TC, Walker AA (1974) Application of a pressure servo system developed to study ventricular dynamics. J Appl Physiol 37: 736–741

Mehmel HC, Stockins B, Ruffman K, Olshausen K, Schuler G, Kubler W (1981) The linearity of the end-systolic pressure-volume relation in man and its sensitivity for the assessment of left ventricular function. Circulation 63:1216–1222

Pearlman ES, Weber KT, Janicki JS, Pietra G, Fishman AP (1982) Muscle fiber orientation and connective tissue content in the hypertrophied human heart. Lab Invest 46: 158–164

Sagawa K (1981) The end-systolic pressure-volume relation of the ventricle: Definitions, modifications and clinical use. Circulation 63:1223–1227

Shroff SG, Janicki JS, Weber KT (1983a) The importance of internal resistance in the description of ventricular mechanics. Bull Philadelphia Phys Soc 2:32–43

Shroff SG, Janicki JS, Weber KT (1983b) Left ventricular systolic dynamics in terms of its chamber mechanical properties. Am J Physiol 245:H110–H124

Shroff SG, Weber KT, Janicki JS (1984) End systolic relations: Their usefulness and limitations in assessing left ventricular contractile state. Int J Cardiol 5:253–259

Suga H, Sagawa K, Shoukas AA (1973) Load independence of the instantaneous pressure-volume ratio of the canine left ventricle and effects of epinephrine and heart rate on the ratio. Circ Res 32:314–322

Suga H, Sagawa K (1974) Instantaneous pressure-volume relationships and their ratio in the excised, supported canine left ventricle. Circ Res 35:117–126

Taylor RR, Covell JW, Ross J Jr (1969) Volume-tension diagrams of ejecting and isovolumic contractions in left ventricle. Am J Physiol 216:1097–1102

Weber KT, Janicki JS, Hefner LL (1976) Left ventricular force-length relations of isovolumic and ejecting contractions. Am J Physiol 231:337–343

Weber KT, Janicki JS (1977) Instantaneous force-velocity-length relations in isolated dog heart. Am J Physiol 232:H241–H249

DISCUSSION

GESELOWITZ: As a bioelectrician I tread in here with some trepidation, but let me try. It is certainly attractive when looking at the pressure-volume-flow relations of the heart to consider the heart as a pressure source or flow source with some internal impedance. Apparently that is the approach you are taking now. This is something that I looked at casually a number of years ago but have not followed. I think that Drs. Elzinga and Westerhof have looked at the heart in this fashion and found that they could represent the resistance as being rather linear. That is, using a Fourier series analysis they concluded that the heart can be discribed by a driving pressure and a source impedance. Your model which describes ventricular dynamics in a different fashion seems to lead to a different result. Incidentally, I assume that this model is independent of valve resistance.

ANS: Yes. Our model is independent of valve resistance as well as filling volume and level of ejection pressure.

GESELOWITZ: Does the resistance that you are measuring include the valve resistance?

ANS: As I indicated earlier, our resistance is a phenomenological descriptor of the relationship between ventricular pressure and flow. That is, ventricular flow, along with volume and time, is an independent determinant of pressure. As a result, the actual pressure within the ejecting ventricle will be less than that which would have been expected if the ventricle was purely elastic. Therefore, phenomenologically, resistance represents a loss in ventricular pressure whenever the ventricle attempts to eject blood or, equivalently, the muscle fibers are allowed to shorten. Our resistance has nothing to do with blood flow across the valve.

GESELOWITZ: One can conceptualize a pressure source with an internal resistance and that is the kind of resistance you are talking about. The group of Elzinga and Westerhof also developed a representation independent of load.

ANS: I am familiar with their work but I am not sure how successful they were in applying it to the intact heart. Moreover, one of the basic differences between their approach and ours is that they completely removed the pulsatile nature of pressure and flow when calculating the source impedance. Thus, their approach represents an uncomplicated method to express the net, integrated ability of the ventricle to pump blood. However, it is important to recognize that such an averaging process sacrifices considerable discriminating information regarding pulsatile hemodynamics and the cyclic variation of the mechanical properties. This average internal impedance incorporates all of the ventricular mechanical properties and their variations during contraction into a single value and it is not possible to distinguish between elastance and resistance. Consequently, mean internal or source impedance may not be a sensitive indicator of changes in ventricular performance. One thing we found attractive in our model is that it provides us with information regarding the contracility of the ventricle independent of the loading conditions. When applied to the intact heart with the valves in place, etc., we were able to demonstrate that the model gave us good results. That is, we again compared the measured and predicted isovolumetric peak pressures and found excellent agreement.

GESELOWITZ: They put a lot of emphasis on the DC term but I think they also used the pulsatile data and did a Fourier analysis.

DINNAR: A comment. They did a Fourier series on the results but Hunter and Noordergraf subsequently published an article claiming that such a series analysis cannot be used for the heart and leads to a misinterpretation. That is, the Fourier series is not appropriate for the ventricle in which the mechanical properties vary widely over the course of one heart cycle.

GESELOWITZ: We also have used this approach. That is, a pressure source with an impedance source together with a Fourier analysis. We showed that analytically, if the time variation is pulsatile, even though it is essentially a non uniform kind of situation, you can use Fourier analysis. In fact, it is fairly common in other electric engineering applications with non linear and non uniform behavior. If you have an essentially uniform time variation, you can use Fourier analysis and get valid information. So despite the claims of Hunter et al., we feel it is a reasonably good approximation to use the Fourier analysis on ventricular pressure and flow. I'll show you some of the results in my forthcoming presentation.

FEIGL: I have a little trouble with your terms 'elastance' and 'resistance'. It seems to me that elastance is similar to what cardiac muscle mechanics people might be tempted to call the length-strength relationship, since you've derived it from isovolumic contractions. Similarly, resistance would be called the force-velocity relationship. What is your reason for choosing the terms elastence and resistance?

ANS: The resistance and elastance we are using give us, essentially, the same information you would obtain if you were looking at isolated papillary muscle. Elastance is describing the relation between ventricular pressure and volume. The major difference is that these terms are a measure of chamber or global properties. In the strictest sense, if you were to measure the material properties and you were to get elasticity, it should be independent of the shape of that material. Our elastance and resistance are global or apparent properties, not material properties. For example, the maximum elastance for dogs is typically 4 mm Hg/ml, while for the rat, which has a smaller left ventricule, the maximum elastance is approximately 600 mm Hg/ml. That is, for a smaller chamber, the same pressure is generated but with lower volume changes. Therefore, what we are measuring here is not the material property but rather a description of pressure as a function of volume.

FEIGL: I don't want to quibble about terminology, but elastance or elastic properties are passive properties to me and you are describing something which is active in the muscle. There has been nearly a 100 years work on trying to describe active muscle and the length-tension relationship, sometimes called Starling Law. Therefore, while it is true that the variables can be the same (pressure-volume and tension-length), I wouldn't choose these terms to describe the active behavior of muscle.

ANS: I would disagree with your statement that elastance cannot be used to describe both the passive and active relationship between pressure and volume. If it were possible to examine the ventricle at a specific time in systole and measure the mechanical properties, you will find that that elastance has increased from its diastolic value. We could show this using our flow pulse technique where within 30 ms we were able to withdraw 1–2 ml of volume. We typically observe a large decrease in pressure, more so than we would see during diastole. That is, it is a stiffer appearing ventricle.

FEIGL: The point is that you now perturb the ventricle, you add a stress and you watch the strain. But this has been going on a long time and A.V. Hill described the new elastic body as a way of describing active muscle a long time ago. There is no question that there is a difference in diastole and systole between the elastic and the viscuous properties.

SAGAWA: I also disagree with Dr. Feigl. I don't see any reason why the word elastance should be used strictly as a passive property. Even the so-called passive property of muscle is quite active. It is very difficult to draw a sharp line between passive and active muscle. In addition, in engineering, the suffix 'ance' is not used to represent a material property. Instead it represents a systems property. For example, the elastance of the balloon at a given volume is not a measure of the elasticity of the balloon material. Instead, the term elasticity, or modulus of volume elasticity, is used to describe the material property. So I think it's right to use the term elastance for the ventricular chamber regardless of its state of activation.

GESEWOLITZ: I am also going to defend Dr. Janicki's use of the terms elastance and resistance. I think that it is very useful to talk about the ventricle as a compliance or capacitance. The pressure-volume relation of the heart is related to the muscle properties in, of couse, a complex way. The models of the cardiovascular system in terms of representing the heart as a time varying elastance have been very successful. As someone who has worked with artificial hearts, I'm intrigued by the fact that the pneumatic artificial heart is a pressure source, and the motor-driven artificial heart is a flow source while the natural heart is a time-varying elastance.

ANS: One of the major points here is that we also have to include some resistance. That is something that we have overlooked in the past.

GESELOWITZ: Incidentially, I published a paper, that was buried in some Proceedings a number of years ago, which showed that if you took the model of Suga and Sagawa, you could show that it is consistent with the resistance.

ANS: Yes, the time varying behavior of elastance will mathematically result in an inverse force-velocity relationship of muscle. However, as I have just shown there is an additional dependence of pressure on flow that is independent of volume and it is this additional pressure loss that must be accounted for by a resistance term. Furthermore, Dr. Suga recently published the results of a study which indicated a correction term had to be added to his time varying elastance model in order for the isovolumetric and ejecting pressure-volume relationships to coincide. This correction term was of the same magnitude as our resistance term. So you cannot just use a time-varying elastance to describe the dynamics of the left ventricle.

GESELOWITZ: We are talking about details of fitting data but my point is if you take that relationship, you can convert it, let's say at least for the mean values, into a pressure source with a resistance.

ANS: No, we are not simply talking about details of fitting data. Resistance is significant and must be accounted for when mathematically describing ventricular dynamics *throughout* systole as opposed to one instant in systole such as the end of systole, where flow is essentially zero. Moreover, as I indicated earlier, our resistance appears to have physical significance in that it represents some fundamental rate limiting process of the contractile machinery.

Three-dimensional models of the heart: advantages and limitations

Y.C. PAO
Department of Engineering Mechanics, University of Nebraska,
Lincoln, NA 68588, U.S.A.

Abstract

The three-dimensional models of the heart that have been hitherto proposed are critically reviewed. Finite element analysis of the stress distributions in the cardiac walls and valves, and the developed methods for inverse estimation of myocardial elasticity and contractility during cardiac cycles are especially examined to assess their advantages and limitations. Future finite element cardiac researches are projected and regional myocardial studies are advocated. A blood-myocardium composite model which can simulate the measured ventricular wall volume changes during cardic cycles is proposed. A methodology is described for calculating the myocardial fiber contraction during systolic phase based on the proposed model and by use of the measured regional wall thickness and blood volume data. These data are to be collected with a high spatial and temporal resolution scanning device such as the dynamic spatial reconstructor (DSR) available at the Mayo Clinic.

Introduction

The first model proposed for approximated analysis of the left ventricle of the heart was a spherical shell (Pao, 1980a and Mirsky, 1974) which was adopted by Woods in 1892 so that the Laplace law could be applied for calculation of the wall stresses. When the biplane silhouettes can be obtained by the X-ray technique, the left ventricle has since been analyzed as axisymmetric thick-walled shells. The advances in computer-aided tomography in recent years make it possible to image and reconstruct the cross-sectional shapes of the heart (Ritman, 1983). As a result of this development, the true three-dimensional structural shape of the heart can be accurately formed by stacking of the reconstructed cross sections together. Various finite element models have been proposed (Figure 1) for the analyses of the ventricles as well as for the cardiac valves both natural and prothetic (Pao,

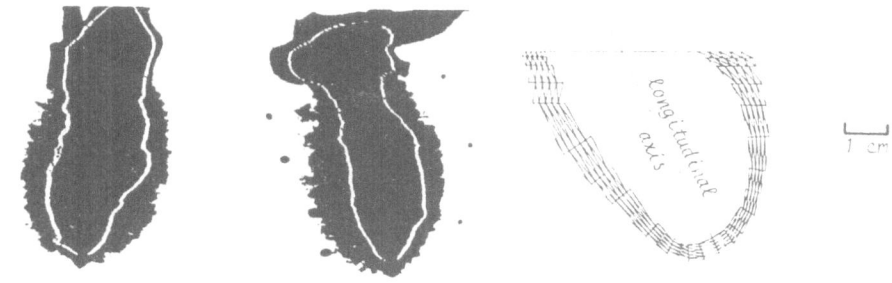

(a) Left ventricular silhouettes and axisymmetric finite-element model

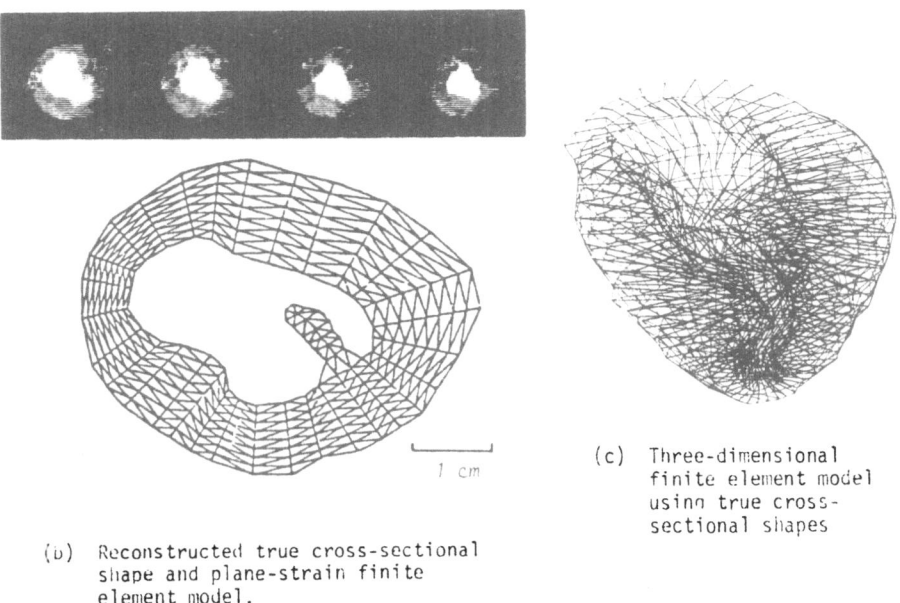

(b) Reconstructed true cross-sectional shape and plane-strain finite element model.

(c) Three-dimensional finite element model using true cross-sectional shapes

Figure 1.

1982a). This paper presents an up-to-date review of the three-dimensional models of the heart and assesses their advantages and limitations, and projects on future finite element cardiac researches.

Idealized and finite element models

To evaluate the pumping performance of the heart, to calculate the myocardial and valvular sresses and strains, and to quantify the blood flow in the circulation system undoubtedly are among the major objectives for most cardiac studies. In cardiac studies, there are two distinct groups of parameters involved, *global* and

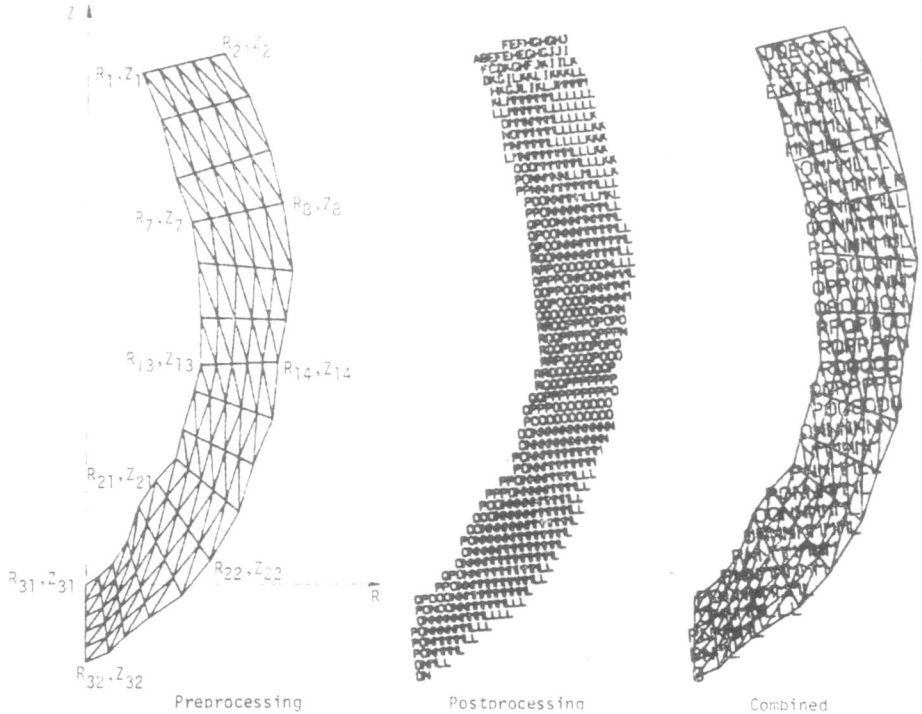

Figure 2. Axisymmetric finite-element analysis.

local. Stroke volume and left ventricular chamber pressure are examples of the former and left ventricular wall thickness and transmural pressure are examples of the latter. The global analysis estimates the *average* value of the performance and chaacteristic variables. Idealized geometries of the heart which use spherical, ellisoidal, cylindrical and nested shells are quite adequate in evaluation of the parameters such as the stroke volume, average wall thickness change, average diatsolic and systolic muscle strength, mechanical work and other. In such global analysis, it is also adequate to assume the myocardial properties as hetero-geneously isotropic, transversely isotropic, or, orthotropic. And, if necessary, these properties can be considered as time-dependent, or, stress- or strain-dependent (Pao and Ritman, 1977a; Pao *et al.*, 1980). The space-dependence of the myocardial properties are greatly simplified or completely ignored in using the idealized models of the heart.

Figures 2 to 4 illustrate the applications of the axisymmetric (Pao *et al.*, 1974), plane-strain (Pao *et al.*, 1976), and three-dimensional (Pao 1980a) finite element models, respectively, for calculations of the stress destributions in the left ven-tricular, or, in the connected left and right ventricular walls. The axisymmetric and plane-strain models assume that there are no variations in deformations and

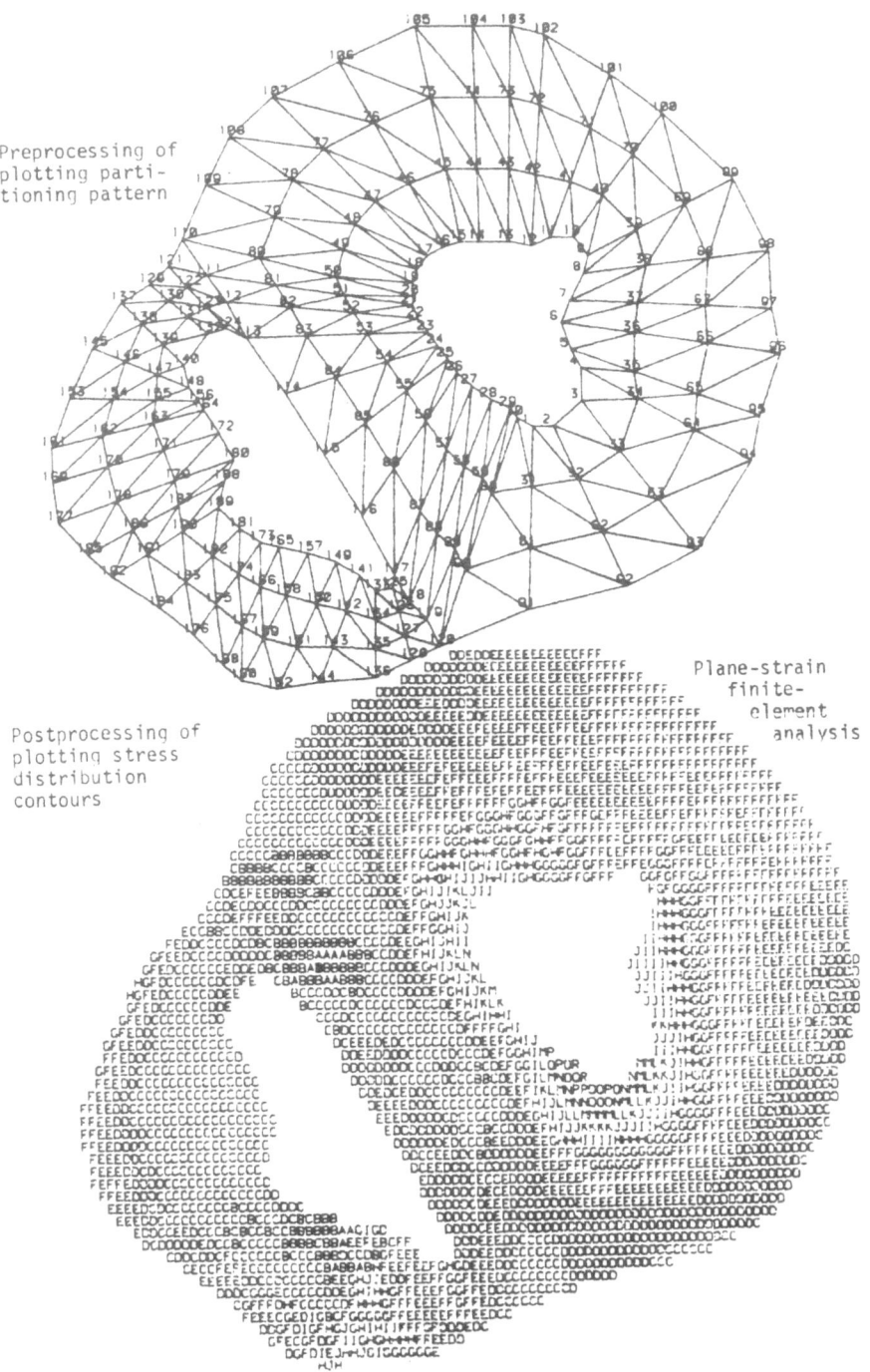

Preprocessing of plotting partitioning pattern

Plane-strain finite-element analysis

Postprocessing of plotting stress distribution contours

Figure 3.

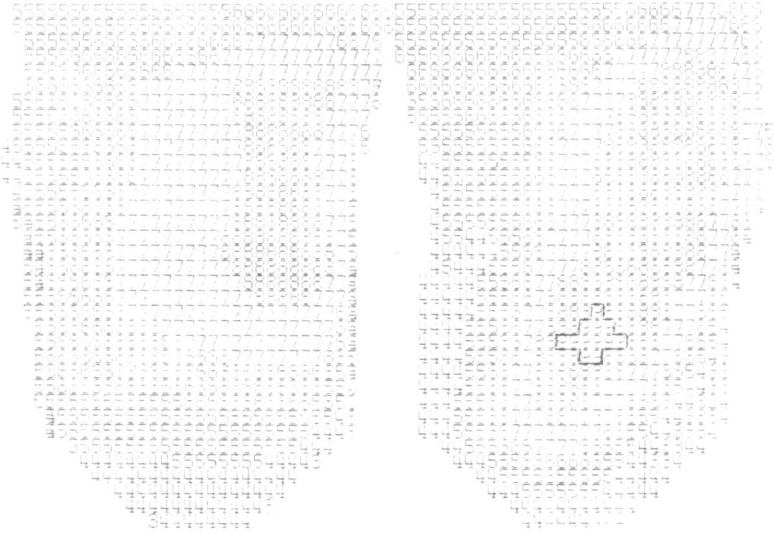

Figure 4. Stress distribution contour on endocardial surface of an isolated left ventricle calculated by three-dimensional finite element analysis.

hence no variations in strains and stresses, in the circumferential direction and in the direction normal to the cross section, respectively. The three-dimensional model is most general and considers all variations.

Admittedly, the finite element methods predict the same order of magnitude as by use of the idealized models (Mirsky, 1974; Streeter, 1979). However, the finite element analyses can give detailed spatial variations of the deformations, strains and sresses, and can therefore map out the precise locations where the maximum stresses and strains occur because the true shapes and dimensions of the ventricular silhouette or cross sections are utilized in the analyses. In Figures 2 to 4, the modern graphics technique of contour plotting (Pao, 1984a) has helped delineate the stress distributions and pin-point the locations of the maximum stresses. Such information is essential in study of the local deterioration of myocardial strength. In a later section, regional investigation by application of the finite element analyses will be elaborated.

Calculation of myocardial passive and active characteristics

Finite element models also have the advantage of providing more precise simulated studies of the myocardial passive and active properties. Using either the left ventricular silhouettes or cross-sectional geometries at three critical instants of a cardiac cycle, as sketched in Figure 5 for a cross-sectional study, computer simulation can be conducted to estimate the diastolic Young's modulus and

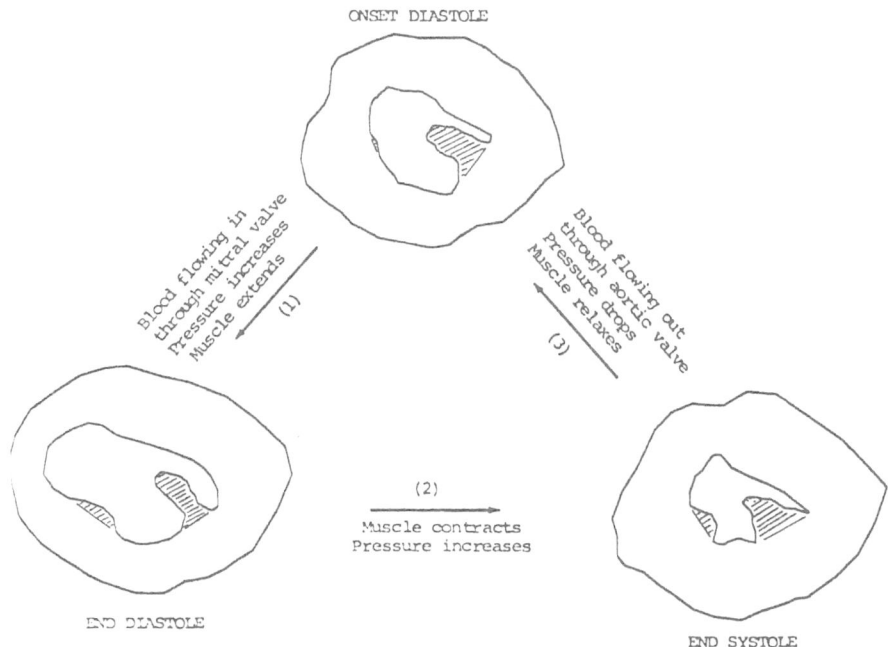

Figure 5. Three critical cross-sectional shapes required for estimation of the average passive stiffness and active contraction of the myocardial fiber during a cardiac cycle, by application of plane-strain finite element analysis.

systolic contraction (Pao and Ritman, 1976; Pao *et al.*, 1976; Pao, 1981a). Due to large deformation, incremental-loading finite element analysis needs to be implemented (Pao and Ritman 1977b). The incremental-loading approach also allows adjustments to be made during the step-by-step increments to take into account the viscoelastic(Pao and Ritman, 1977a), or, strain-dependent characteristics of the myocardium. An axisymmetric finite-element model (Pao and Ritman, 1976) has generated a parabolic equation for relating the diastolic Young's modulus, E in dyne/cm^2, in terms of the left ventricular chamber pressure, P in mmHg, as

$$E = 1660 - 139P + 320P^2. \tag{1}$$

A plane-strain finite-element method was employed in (Pao *et al.*, 1976) for deriving the E and P relationship

$$E = 24.9P - 33\,000 \tag{2}$$

except that here E and P are both in dyne/cm^2. Based on Eq (2) and by extrapolation of the E values at systolic pressures, the myocardial contractions during systolic phase of the same cardiac cycle were also calculated in (Pao *et al.*,

1976). Instantaneous fiber shortening ranging from 4% to 14% were obtained. In arriving at these fiber contraction data, the fibers were assumed to be circumferentially oriented. This leads to the discussion of another advantage of using the finite element models, in that the fibrous properties of the myocardium and its changes of orientation across the ventricular wall thickness can be easily incorporated.

Fibrous studies of the heart

In (Pao et al., 1980), the stretching tests of the strips circumferentially cut and longitudinally cut from the left ventricular wall were reported. The calculated instantaneous stress and strain data revealed that significant differences in the wall muscle properties existed between these two groups of strips because of the different directions along which they were cut. It points out the fact that the myocardial fibrous characteristics should be incorporated into cardiodynamics studies. When the stress and strain data were treated in (Pao et al., 1980) by application of the theory for laminated composites, the following stess-dependent stiffness equations for the circumferentially cut strips were obtained:

$$E_f = 23.2\sigma_f + 3.09 \quad \text{(3-layer)}, \tag{3}$$
$$E_f = 23.7\sigma_f - 2.92 \quad \text{(5-layer)}, \tag{4}$$
$$E_f = 22.7\sigma_f + 2.26 \quad \text{(10-layer)}, \tag{5}$$

where E_f and σ_f are the instantaneous tangent modulus and stress, respectively, along the fiber direction and are both in gm/mm². The fiber orientations for the 10-layer study followed closest to those values which were published by Streeter (1979), but the insignificant difference in Eqs. (3) through (5) suggested that the 3-layer analysis of using fiber angles $60°/0°/-60°$ is accurate enough as far as the derivation of the stress-dependent stiffness equation is concerned (Pao et al., 1979; Pao et al., 1981).

In (Pao and Ritman, 1978), the 3-layer analysis was adopted in the investigation of the transmural pressure distributions in the left ventricular wall before and after the coronary artery ligation. The stress-dependent E equation such as Eq. (3) enables the fiber stiffness to be adjusted from one element to another in accordance with the instantaneous stress level in each element calculated during the incremental-loading finite element analysis.

Since $E_f = d\sigma_f/d\varepsilon_f$ where ε_f is the instantaneous strain, the instantaneous stress-strain relationship can be easily obtained to be

$$\sigma_f = K[exp(C\varepsilon_f)-1], \tag{6}$$

where K and C are constants. Horowitz et al. (1984) have recently employed a stress-strain relationship in the form of Eq. (6) for investigation of an idealized geometry of the left ventricle composed of nested toroidal shells. The nested-shell approach resembles that of the Streeter's investigation (1979) where ellipsoidal shells were adopted. In Horowitz *et al.* (1984), it is shown that geodesically oriented myocardial fibers result in minimal energy spent during systolic contraction.

Limitations of finite element models

For analyzing *real* heart geometry, the finite element models are definitely the best tools. The accuracy of the computed results by the finite element analysis is only limited by; (1) the geometric description of the heart, (2) the loading and boundary conditions, (3) material properties of the cardiac components, and (4) the available computer hardware and software for finite element calculations.

Geometric shape

Regarding the accurate description of the heart geometry, the availability of high spatial (1 mm) ad temporal resolutions (60 images per second) provided by the advanced scanners (Ritman *et al.*, 1980) is more than adequate. This solution is far better than that for the problem of describing accurate loading and boundary conditions.

Loading and boundary conditions

Most of the finite element analysis hitherto conducted only consider *uniform* chamber pressure loading of the ventricles; the shear and turbulent effects of the blood flow in the ventricular chambers are not dealt with. As far as the boundary conditions are concerned, isolated left ventricles and connected left and right ventricles have mostly been treated as radially deformable at the sites of the cardiac valves.

The valvular analysis, such as (Chrisic and Medland, 1981), could be easily combined with the ventricular analysis. In fact, the substructuring technique treating the valve and the ventricle each as a substructure has been well developed in finite element analysis. This combined analysis is yet to be tried.

The incorporation of the blood flow effects to provide refined loading conditions for the ventricular finite element analysis has not been fully developed. More basic research is needed for defining the flow and loading relationships. Currently, analytical studies on the microscopic blood flow are being intensively conducted by Professor Richard Skalak and his associates (1981) at Columbia

University; experimental works are being conducted on blood flows in tapered, branched arteries by Dr. Paul Stein's group (1981) in Detroit, on mitral valve by Dr. Ned Hwang's group (1981) in Houston, on pulsatile flow by Dr. D. Young's group (1981) and in aorta by Dr. C.J. Chen's group (Khalighi *et al.*, 1983) both in Iowa. The present author has edited a section on application to 'Biomechanics' in a finite element handbook (Pao, 1984b), in which more pertinent references are given on the subject of fluid cardiodynamics.

Material properties

Whether or not the *in vitro* test results of the myocardial properties are applicable for the *in vivo* cardiac analyses remains as a heated debate topic. As has already been discussed earlier, the finite element models enable te myocardial passive and active characteristics to be estimated *in vivo*. It is an *inverse* problem of knowing the loading and the consequent deformation and of continuously guessing the material properties until the simulated and measured deformations are approximately matched.

So far, only the methods for estimating the global or average values of the myocardial fiber properties for a silhouette or a cross section of the ventricle have been proposed. In a later section, a method based on a blood-myocardium composite model will be discussed for the *in vivo* estimate of the regional myocardial properties.

Computer hardware and software requirements

It is evident from the above discussion that the finite element analysis can be continuously improved by providing further refined data to define the problem more accurately. All refinements, however, are to be gained at the expense of additional computer storage and time requirements. The cost effectiveness hence becomes a matter of concern. Mathematically, the finite element analysis leads to the solution of matrix equations. For a three-dimensional analysis of the isolated left ventricle shown in Figure 1c, a matrix equation involing 3 600 unknowns has to be solved. Unless a large mainframe computer is available for solution of such a large matrix system, special software must be developed (Pao, 1978; 1980b; 1981b) for solution of the problem on a minicomputer or microcomputer. Even if a supercomputer such as Cray-1 (Russel, 1978) is available, the expense is formidable because the solution for one cardiac instant requires hours of computer time.

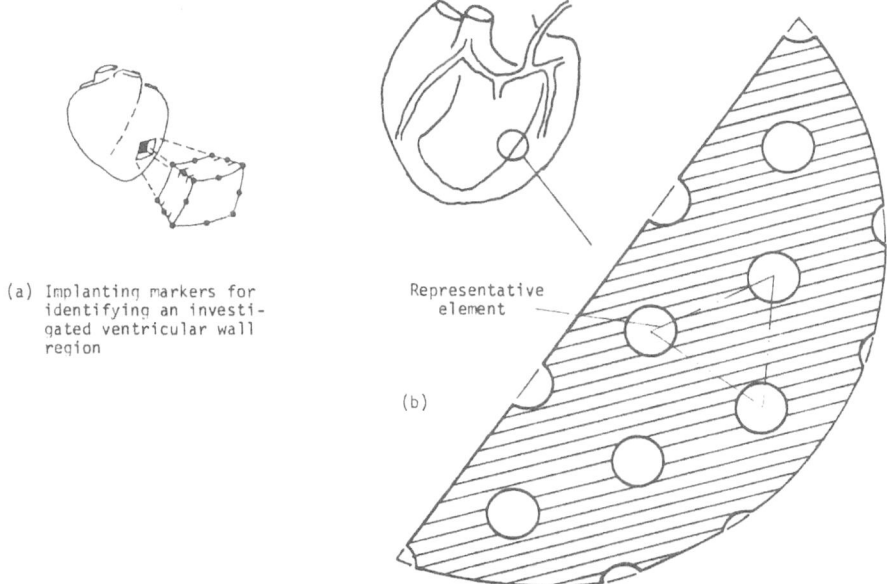

(a) Implanting markers for
identifying an investi-
gated ventricular wall
region

Representative
element

(b)

Figure 6. A blood-myocardium composite model.

Prospect: regional finite element analysis

As has been asserted earlier, the idealized heart models are effective tools for global estimates of cardiac performance and functional status. Finite element models for the *whole* heart or ventricle with refined loading and boundary conditions wil produce more accurate results but *impractical* because of the computational cost. The real future of finite element cardiac models is for *regional* analyses, particularly for the inverse, *in vivo* quatification of the regional myocardial properties. From the viewpoint of clinical applications, local muscle dysfunction which initiates various cardiac problems should be investigated with highest priority than for the whole heart. Especially, the increased availability of the imaging devices now permits easy scrutiny of the regional cardiac activities.

The author has developed a blood-myocardium composite model (Pao, 1982b; 1982c) for the heart wall muscle. It enables the regional wall volume changes during different phases of cardiac cycles to be taken into account in the stress and strain analyses of the heart. Using this model, the regional wall-muscle volume changes can be attributed to the changes in transmural blood perfusion (Hoffman, 1978) when the myocardium remains to be assumed as incompressible. Figure 6 illustrates that an investigated cardiac region is to be identified by implanting markers and the wall muscle is to be considered as composed of small fibrous masses. The cross-sectional shape of the fiber bundles is idealized as comprising with the blood vessels located at the vertices of the equilateral-

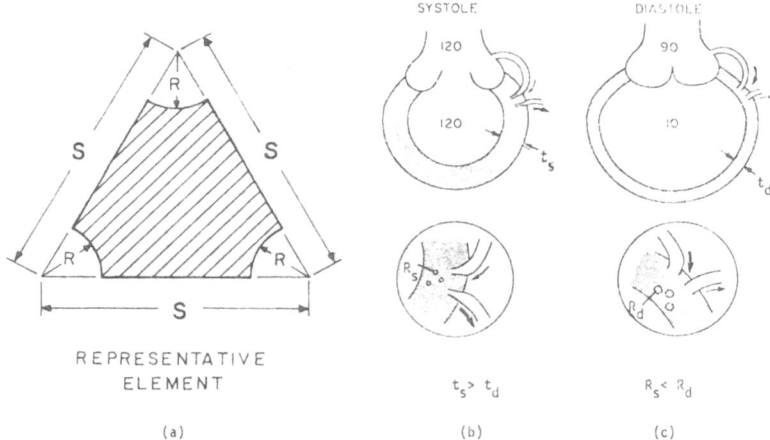

Figure 7. Use of the representative element of the proposed blood-myocardium model explaining the myocardial fiber relaxation and contraction, and the corresponding transmural perfusion patterns. (Adapted from (Hoffman, 1978), Courtesy of Professor J.I.E. Hoffman.)

triangle representative element representing the myocardium. The number of markers that needed for identifying the region depends on the number of transmural layers, of which the *in vivo* muscle properties are to be evaluated. For example, the 20 markers shown in Figure 6a enable the differential in material properties in two, subendo- and subepicardial, layers to be quantified.

By tracing the three-dimensional displacements of the markers along with recording of the transmural perfusion during cardiac cycles, the wall thickness, t, of the muscle layer and the blood volume fraction, f, can be calculated. It is easy to show that the dimensions R and S for the representative element shown in Figure 7a are related to f by the equation

$$f = 2\pi R^2/\sqrt{3}S^2. \tag{7}$$

Equation (7) is derived based on the fact that the blood volume fraction f is equal to the three cut-out area at the vertices divided by the total area of the equilateral triangle. The cut-out and shaded areas shown in **Figure** 7a represent the spaces occupied by the blood and the incompressible myocradium, respectively.

While Eq. (7) indicates that the blood volume fraction f is related to the R/S ratio, the thickness t can be shown to be related to the overall size S of the representative element. This blood-myocardium composite model also help explain the observations made by Hoffman (1978) regarding the transmural perfusion which are illustrated in Figure 7b and 7c. At end of systole of a cardiac cycle, the myocardial fiber contracts but its cross section expands because of incompressibility. The spaces between fibers hence become narrower. At end of diastole of a cardiac cycle, the myocardial fiber relaxes and extends, its cross-sectional area decreases. The spaces between fibers hence become larger. The explanation above leads to the results of $t_s > t_d$ and $R_s < R_d$ where the subscripts s and d denote systole and diastole, respectively.

For calculations of *in vivo* diastolic and systolic myocardial strains, denoted as ε_d and ε_s respectively, the following equations expressed in terms of the wall muscle thickness t and the blood volume fraction f have been derived:

$$\varepsilon_d = [(t_r/t_d)^2(1 - f_r)/(1 - f_d)] - 1 \tag{8}$$
$$\varepsilon_s = [(t_r/t_s)^2(1 - f_r)/(1 - f_s)] - 1 \tag{9}$$

where the subscript r is for a reference state, for that the early diastolic instant of the cardiac cycle is a reasonable choice.

Thus, a methodology has been proposed for the *in vivo* quantification of the myocardial fiber's diastolic extension and systolic contraction during cardiac cycles. The traditional evaluation of the myocardial force-length relationship is only of pasing interest for achieving the ultimate goal of quantifying the real-time myocardial fiber contraction during cardiac cycles. Now, the proposed method makes it possible to directly measure the *in vivo* myocardial contraction of the heart during cardiac cycles, the force-length relationship study may no longer be needed.

The proposed model follows the theme of finite element analysis, in that the number of transmural layers can be increased by implanting more markers so that more layer elements can be investigated to account for the tansmural fiber direction changes.

Concluding remarks

In summary, the author advocates that the finite element models for cardiac analyses should be applied for regional studies while the idealized models should remain as effective tools for global assessments of the cardiac performance and functional reserves.

The proposed blood-myocardium composite model enables the regional analysis to be realistically implemented by application of the finite element method at reasonable computer cost. It permits not only regional stress and strain calculations but more importantly the *in vivo* quantification of myocardial fiber contraction of the heart during cardiac cycles. The diastolic and systolic fiber strains can be easily computed at any instant of a cardiac cycle by use of Eqs. (8) and (9) if the myocardial layer thickness t and the blood volume fraction f in that layer are known. Presently, the layer thickness t can be calculated using the three-dimensional displacement data of the implanted markers which can be monitored by the biplane or computer-aided tomographic technique, and the blood volume

88

fraction f is to be determined using high-spatial-resolution scanning (such as the 1 mm resolution of the Dynamic Spatial Reconstructor (Ritman et al., 1980) of the transmural perfusion.

Both the implantation of the markers and the prevailing ways of injecting constrasting fluid or microspheres into the blood stream for measurement of blood volum fraction are not truly non-invasive methods. There are a few anatomically easily identifiable sites of the heart which can be readily adopted in place of the markers, but certainly are not sufficient for providing in-depth study of the differential in myocardial material properties across the wall thickness and at different regions. So, it is evident that the proposed method is yet to be perfected.

Acknowledgements

This work was supported in part by the National Institutes of Health and the Engineering Research Center, the University of Nebraska-Lincoln.

References

Christie GW, Medland IC (1981) The effects of tissue anisotropy on the mechanics of bioprothetic heart valves. Biomechanics Symposium: 11–14

Hoffman JIE (1978) Transmural myocardial perfusion, George E Brown Memorial Lecture. Circ Res 58:381–391

Horowitz A, Perl M, Sideman S (1984) Geodesics as a mechanically optimal fiber geometry for the left ventricle. Technion – Israel Institute of Technology, Haifa, Israel, submitted for publication.

Hwang NHC Jussain AK, Hui PW, Striplng T, Weiting TW Turbulent flow through a natural human mitral valves. Biomech 13: 1007–1022

Khalighi B, Chandran KB, Chen CJ (1983) Steady flow development past valve protheses in a model human aorta – I. Centrally occluding valves and II. Tilting disc valves. Biomech 16: 1003–1018

Mirsky I, Ghista DN, Sandler H (1974) Cardiac Mechanics: Physiological, Clinical and Mathematical. New Hork: John-Wiley

Pao YC, Ritman EL, Wood EH (1974) Finite element analysis of left ventricular stresses. Proceedings of the Seventh US National Congress of Applied Mechanics 170–171 (abstr), J Biomech 7:469–477

Pao YC, Ritman EL (1976) An energy method for evaluating the effective global stiffness of the left ventricle in the passive state. Proc Fourth New Eng Bioeng Conf 209–212; Biotelemetry (1975) 2:77–79

Pao YC, Wang HC, Ritman EL, Robb RA, Wood EH (1976) Computer simulation of the cross-sectional shape change of a beating heart. In: Dekker J (ed.) Simulation of Systems. North-Holland Company, pp 609–615

Pao YC, Robb RA, Ritman EL (1976) Plane-strain finite element analysis of reconstructed diastolic left ventricular cross section. Ann Biomed Eng 4:232–249

Pao YC, Ritman EL (1977a) Viscoelastic, fibrous, finite-element, dynamic analysis of beating heart. Proc Symp on Application of Computer Methods in Engineering, Los Angeles: Univ South Cal Press, pp 477–486

Pao YC, Ritman EL (1977b) Iterative evaluation of left ventricular cross-sectional contraction by incremental-loading finite-element analysis. Proc Sixth Can Appl Mech 911–912

Pao YC, Ritman EL (1978) Quantitative analysis of the change of transmural pressure distribution in the left ventricular wall following coronary artery ligation. Proc San Diego Biomedical Symp 17:109–117

Pao YC (1978) Algorithms for direct-access gaussian solution of structural stiffness matrix equation. Numer Methods Eng 12:751–764

Pao YC, Nagendra CK, Padiyar R, Ritman EL (1979) Analysis of heart wall muscle as a three-layer laminated composite. Proc Can Cong Appl Mechanics:817–818

Pao YC (1980a) Discussion on geometric modelling of the human left ventricle. J Biomech Eng 102:274–275

Pao YC (1980b) On triangular decomposition of nonpositive definite matrices using complex FORTRAN programming. Int J Numer Methods Eng 15:611–616

Pao YC, Nagendra GK, Padiyar R, Ritman EL (1980) Derivation of myocardial fiber stiffness equation based on theory of laminated composite. J Biomech Eng 102:252–257

Pao YC, Ritman EL (1980) Stress analysis of connected right and left ventricles by idealized geometry and finite element models. In: Mow VC (ed), Advances in Bioengineering, Publ G00176, Am Soc Mech Eng, pp 49–52

Pao YC (1981a) Modelling the heart wall muscle contraction by application of spline curve-fit with tension. Third Int Conf on Math. Modelling. Univ of Missouri-Rolla Press, p 63

Pao YC (1981b) Solving large structural stiffness matrix equations by resumable segments. Computers and Structures Int J 14: 247–254

Pao YC, Nagendra GK, Ritman EL (1981) Isoparametric finite-element analysis of heart wall muscle as layered composite. In: Viano DC (ed), Advances in Bioengineering, Publ H00199 Am Soc Mech Eng pp 139–142

Pao YC (1982a) Finite elements in stress analysis and estimation of mechanical properties of working heart. In: Finite Elements in Biomechanics. New York: John-Wiley, Chapter 8, pp 127–142

Pao YC (1982b) Recent developments in finite-element cardiovascular analysis. Proc 4th Annual IEEE/EMBS Conf, IEEE Publ #82CH1729-3:253–257

Pao YC (1982c) A myocardium-blood composite model for in vivo strain measurement of ventricular wall muscle. 9th US Cong Appl Mechanics (abstr), 141–142

Pao YC (1984a) Elements of computer-aided design/manufacturing. CAD/CAM, New York: John-Wiley

Pao YC (1984b) Biomechanics In: Kardestuncer H (ed), Finite Element Handbook. New York: McGraw-ill, in press

Ritman EL, Kinsey JH, Robb RA, Gilbert BK, Harris LD, Wood EH (1980) Three-dimensional imaging of heart, lung and circulation. Science 210: 273–280

Russel RM (1978) The Cray-1 computer system. Commun ACM 21:63–72

Skalak R, Keller SR, Secomb TW (1981) Mechanics of blood flow. J Biomech Eng 103: 102–115

Stein PD (1981) Relation of fluid dynamics to cardiovascular pathophysiology. In: Viano DC (ed) Advances in Bioengineering Publ. H00199 ASME pp. 71–76

Streeter DD (1979) Gross morphology and fiber geometry of the heart. In: RM Berne et al. (eds), Handbook of Physiology, section 2: The Cardiovascular System. Volume I – The Heart,Baltimore, Maryland: Williams & Wilkins

Young DF, Rogge TR, Gray TA, Rooz E (1981) Indiret evaluation of system parameters of pulsatile flow in flexible tubes. J Biomech 14: 339–347

A cardiac model convenient for vascular load coupling

KIICHI SAGAWA, LOWELL MAUGHAN and KENJI SUNAGAWA
Department of Biomedical Engineering, The Johns Hopkins Medical School, Baltimore, MD 21205, U.S.A.

Abstract

To answer the question of optimal matching between the ventricle and arterial load, we developed a framework of analysis which uses simplified models of ventricular contraction and arterial input impedance. The ventricular model consists only of a single volume (or chamber) elastance which increases to an endsystolic value E_{es} with each heart beat. With this elastance, stroke volume SV is represented as a linearly decreasing function of ventricular endsystolic pressure. Arterial input impedance is represented by a 3-element Windkessel model which is in turn approximated to describe arterial end systolic pressure as a linearly increasing function of stroke volume injected per heart beat. The slope of this relationship is E_a. Superposition of the ventricular and arterial endsystolic pressure-stroke volume relationships yields stroke volume and stroke work expected when the ventricle and the arterial load are coupled. From theoretical consideration, a maximum energy transfer should occur from the contracting ventricle to the arterial load under the condition $E_{es} = E_a$. Experimental data on the external work that a ventricle performed on extensively varied arterial impedance loads supported the validity of this matched condition. The matched condition also dictated that the ventricular ejection fraction should be nearly 50%, a well-known fact under normal condition. We conclude that the ventricular contractile property, as represented by E_{es}, is matched to the arterial impedance property, represented by a three-element windkessel model, under normal conditions.

Introduction

The circulatory system contributes to the homeostasis of an organism by transporting and exchanging substances and information via blood. The heart of course provides the mechanical energy needed to circulate blood through the vascular system. Therefore a cardiac model which cannot be readily coupled with the vascular load is a pie in the sky. Since the heart periodically pumps blood from the vein into the artery, matching between the dynamic characteristics of myocardial contraction and vascular impedance has been discussed by the physiologist and biomedical engineer (Noordegraaf, 1969).

Two kinds of cardiovascular impedance matching have been studied. One kind of optimal matching is a condition in which there is no wave reflection from the peripheral part of the arterial tree back to the heart (O'Rouke, 1982). The second kind of matching has been studied with reference to the general engineering discipline that a maximum energy transfer occurs from the energy source to its load when the load impedance is matched to the source (internal) impedance. Applied to the question of ventriculo-arterial impedance matching, the discipline directs us toward a comparison between the outflow port (internal) impedance of the ventricle as a chamber with the input impedance of the arterial system.

'Matching' is a teleological notion; there should be something good associated with the matched condition. So let us examine what is good about the first kind of matched condition, i.e., absence of wave reflection. If a large reflected pressure wave arrives at the heart during the ejection period, it will certainly impede the ejection of blood and, therefore, absence of pressure wave reflection will be generally good. If, however, the wave arrives at the heart in the diastolic phase it can enhance coronary blood flow without doing any harm to ejection. In fact, an extensive review by 0'Rouke (1982) indicates that, in most large mammals, the impedance is favorably matched to allow the heart to operate at the pressure node and at the flow antinode. This is not the case, however, with the human elderly who has dilated, tortuous and stiffened arteries.

How about the notion of a maximum energy transfer from the heart to the arterial tree? Some physiologists may be rather skeptic about the physiological meaning of this concept. For, at the tissue level (exchange vascular bed) what really matters is perhaps not the amount of energy delivered by blood flow but whether enough oxygen is delivered and metabolic wastes are adequately washed out. Both functions depend on flow rather than energy. At the ventriculo-arterial junction, however, a maximum energy transfer is obviously beneficial because for a given impedance load, the flow generated by the source will be proportional to the energy transferred from the source. Therefore, under a given constant preload (i.e., end-diastolic volume), a maximum transfer of myocardial mechanical energy to the arterial system is certainly a desirable condition for efficient use of myocardial energy to transport blood.

In the evolution of the homeostasis served by blood circulation, it is reasonable to consider that tissues (the user of the transport service) dictated the extent and nature of the vascular network and the heart evolved in an adaptation to this given vascular load system. Then, a relevant question to ask will be 'Is the internal impedance of the ventricle matched to the input impedance of the arterial tree?', rather than if the latter is matched to the former.

We present here the results of two sequential studies from our laboratory. First, we tested the afterload insensitivity of the endsystolic P-V relationship (volume-elastance model) of the left ventricle (Maughan et al, 1984; Sunagawa et al., 1983a). We then studied whether a maximum amount of energy is extracted from a ventricle beating at a constant end-diastolic volume and under a given contractile state (i.e., if it does a maximal external work) when the ventricle is coupled with an arterial input impedance which is matched in magnitude to the internal impedance of the ventricle (Sunagawa et al., 1983b).

Ventricular pressure-volume relationship

Over the past decade, we (Sagawa, 1978) have measured the ventricular pressure (P)-volume (V) relationship in an isolated and blood perfused canine heart preparation and came to consider that the ventricular *end-systolic* P-V relationship (ESPVR) is; (a) linear as opposed to the highly nonlinear P-V relationship of the frog's ventricle reported by Otto Frank a century ago, (b) rather insensitive to the preload and afterload and (c) changes its slope (E_{es}) sensitively with inotropic interventions without a significant shift in the volume intercept (V_0). This is to say that our model of the ventricle merely consists of a linear volume elastance E which varies with each heart beat from a smaller end-diastolic value E_{ed} to a larger end-systolic value E_{es}. Thus E is time-varying, and so is V_0 (Suga and Sagawa, 1974). For the present discussion, however, we would deal only with the end-systolic volume elastance E_{es} and the end-systolic volume axis intercept V_0 of the ESPVR (left panel in the 2nd row of Figure 1). With this model of unique ESPVR, end-systolic pressure P_{es} and end-systolic volume V_{es} are related to each other by

$$P_{es} = E_{es} (V_{es} - V_0). \tag{1}$$

Substitution of $V_{es} = V_{ed} - SV$ (stroke volume) in Eq. (1) yields

$$SV = (V_{ed} - V_0) - \frac{P_{es}}{E_{es}}. \tag{2}$$

Equation (2) states that, given an end-diastolic volume V_{ed}, SV is inversely proportional to P_{es} (the line coursing from the lower left to upper right corner of the bottom panel of Figure 1). This rectilinear relation is denoted the '*ventricular end-systolic pressure-stroke volume relationship (VPSVR)*'.

Now, in order to facilitate the coupling of the arterial input impedance load to the elastance model of the left ventricle, it is also necesary to convert arterial input impedance into an effective (nonphysical) elastance E_a such that the rela-

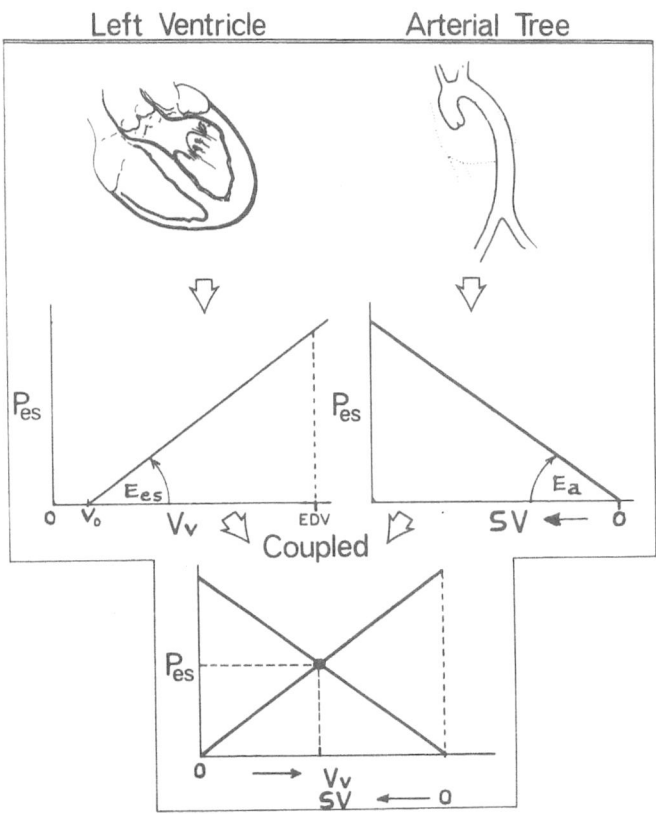

Figure 1. Schematic explanation of coupling the left ventricular contraction with the systemic arterial tree. In the middle left panels, left ventricular contraction is represented by its end-systolic pressure-volume relationship. Given a particular end diastolic volume (EDV), this relationship can be converted into ventricular end-systolic pressure P_{es} stroke volume *(SV) relationship, which is shown by the rectilinear curve coursing from the lower left to upper right corner in the graph at the bottom. In the right middle panel, the aortic input impedance property is represented by a rectilinear arterial end-systolic pressure (P_{es})-stroke volume (SV) relationship* curve (Eq. (5)). See the text for the explanation of this representation. This arterial P_{es}-SV relationship is transcribed in the bottom panel in superposition with the ventricular P_{es}-SV relationship. The intersection of the two P_{es}-SV relationship curves indicates the end-systolic pressure and stroke volume which should result from coupling a left ventricle with the given EDV and the slope parameter E_{es} with a systemic arterial tree with the slope parameter E_a.

tionship between *arterial* end-systolic pressure and stroke volume injected in the arterial system (APSVR),

$$P_{es}' = E_a \, SV, \tag{3}$$

can be plotted in the same graphical co-ordinate (as shown in the right panel of the 2nd row of Figure 1). The stroke volume and external stroke work of the ventricle resultant from its coupling with a given arterial input impedance can then be found graphically by superimposing the VPSVR and APSVR lines, as shown in the bottom panel at the bottom of Figure 1.

The conversion of the arterial impedance property into an effective elastance can be done by first representing the arterial impedance by a three-element Windkessel model (consisting of R_c, C, and R) and then by manipulating the model equations to arrive at an approximation of arterial end-systolic pressure P_{es}' as

$$P_{es}' \simeq \frac{R_c + R}{t_s + \tau[1 - \exp(-t_d/\tau)]} SV, \tag{4}$$

in which t_s and t_d are the durations of the systolic and diastolic phases of aortic pressure wave, respectively, and τ is RC (4). Comparison of Eqs. (3) and (4) indicates that

$$E_a = \frac{R_c + R}{T_s + \tau[1 - \exp(-t_d/\tau)]}. \tag{5}$$

Note that use of a lumped parameter model of the arterial tree neglects the wave reflection phenomenon which exists more or less in reality and thus artificially achieves the first kind of matching mentioned at the beginning.

Substituting Eq. (4) into Eq. (2), we obtain

$$SV = \frac{V_{ed} - V_0}{1 + E_a/E_{es}}, \tag{6}$$

which indicates that, given V_{ed} and E_a, there is no optimal E_{es} which maximizes SV. Simply, the greater E_{es}, the greater will be SV. The inotropic effect on SV will quickly saturate in a hyperbolic fashion, however.

The framework for experimental testing of the validity of the ventricular model is complete now. To make the afterload imposed on the canine ventricle in the experiment the same as the 3-element arterial impedance model used in the above analysis, we set up the identical model in a digital computer and let it generate the volume command signal for the servo-volume control pump connected to the excised ventricle (Sunagawa et al, 1983a). Thus, when canine ventricular pressure exceeds the arterial pressure in the arterial model, the computer calculates in real time (at every 5 ms interval) how much ejection should occur under the existing ventricular pressure into the model arterial system. The time integral of ejected volume from the onset of systole is subtracted from the end-diastolic volume and the difference is given to the ventricular volume control pump as the command signal.

The test proceeded as follows (Figure 2). We chose from the literature a set of R_c, C and R values as the normal canine arterial impedance parameters, imposed this control afterload on a given left ventricle at 4 end-diastolic volumes, and identified the E_{es} and V_0 parameter values of the ESPVR of this ventricle. The E_{es} and V_0 values were incorporated in the ventricular model (Eq. 1), which was then used to predict stroke volumes that the real ventricle will produce under 8 noncontrol sets of arterial impedances parameters. The prediction was performed by specifying the APSVR line with the R_c, C and R value of each of the noncontrol afterloads and substituting t_s and t_d values averaged from the 4 control beats into Eq. (5), and then equilibrating this APSVR with the VPSVR determined from the control beats.

A total of 32 stroke volumes were thus predicted in each ventricle and the predicted stroke volumes SV_p were compared against the actual stroke volumes SV_m measured in the ventricle under the 8 identical noncontrol afterload sets (Sunagawa *et al.*, 1983a). The regression analysis of SV_p on SV_m yielded a regression equation which had the following mean coefficient and intercept values averaged from 8 ventricles:

$$SV_p = 1.00 \ (\pm \ 0.04) \ SV_m + 1.0 \ (\pm \ 0.2) \ \text{ml}. \tag{7}$$

The mean correlation coefficient was 0.985 ± 0.004 (SE). The result demonstrates that, as far as prediction of SV is concerned, our linear end-systolic volume-elastance model is reasonably accurate despite its neglection of a slight afterload dependence (a small sift of V_0 with changes in afterload resistance and characteristic impedance) (Maughan *et al.*, 1984).

Piene (1980) reached the same conclusion using a similar ventricular model (ventricular instantaneous pressure-volume surface) and by experiments in a cat right ventricular preparation. He compared, however, not just stroke volume but instantaneous ventricular pressure and aortic pressure and flow curve configurations reconstructed from the time-domain models of the ventricle and arterial load by using a flow impulse technique. The agreement of predicted configurations with measured configurations does not seem to be as good as the agreement of predicted and actual stroke volumes presented here. This is expected because many studies including ours (Suga *et al.*, 1980; Hunter *et al.*, 1979) suggested that the single elastance model produces significant errors in predicting *instantaneous* systolic pressure-volume relationship. As Dr. Janicki pointed out, addition of a force-dependent internal resistance greatly improves the prediction (Demoment and Hinglais, 1981; Campbell *et al.*, 1982; Shroff *et al.*, 1983).

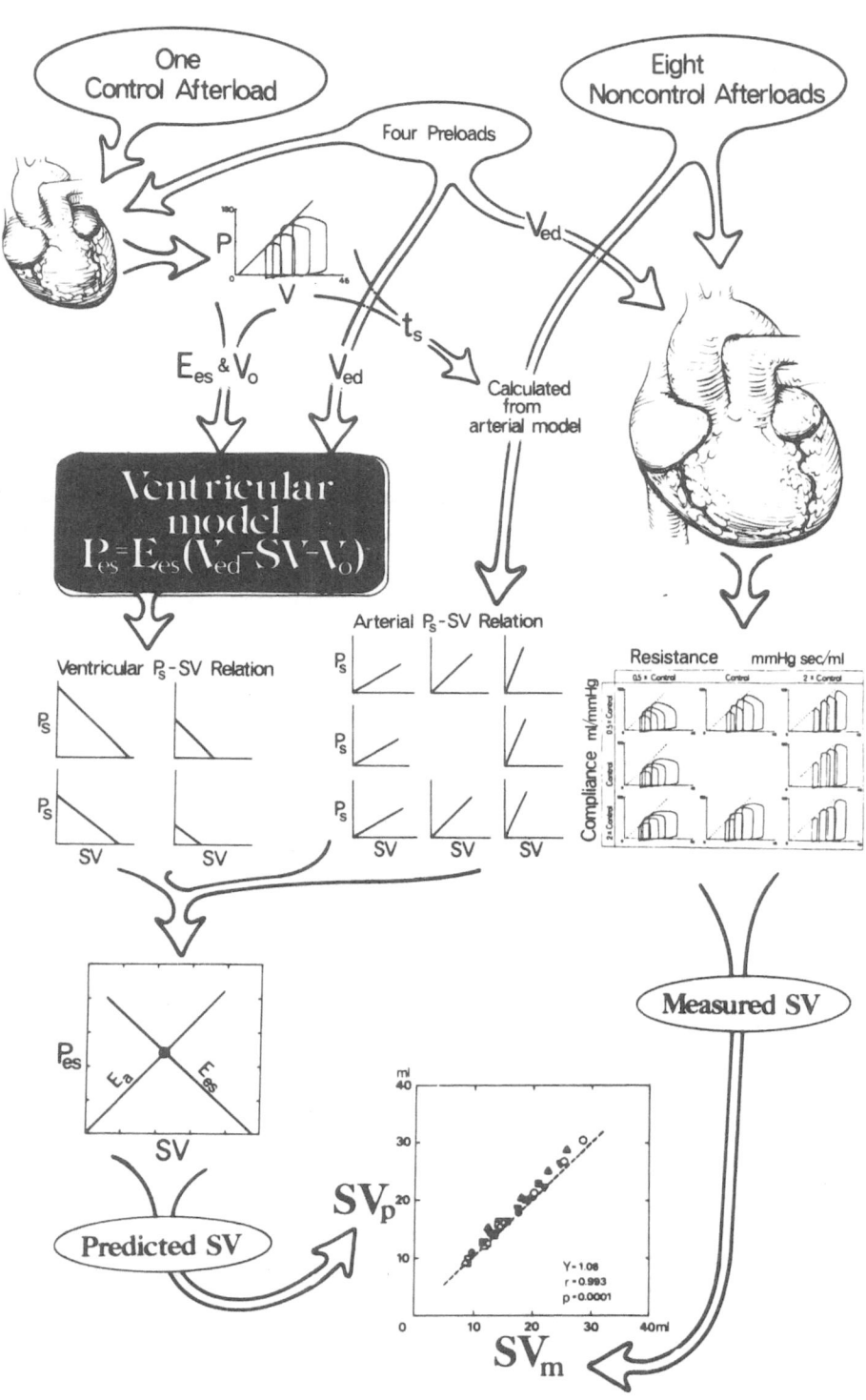

←
Figure 2. Flow chart of the procedures to test the ventricular model (in terms of end-systolic pressure-volume relationship) and the arterial model by end-systolic pressure-stroke volume relationship using one control set of loads (4 preloads and 1 afterload) and 8 noncontrol load sets (4 preloads and 8 afterloads).

Analysis of ventriculo-arterial impedance matching

Let us now move to the second phase of our study, i.e., analysis of ventriculo-arterial impedance matching. The key point is to examine whether a maximum external work is performed when the source impedance of the ventricular model is made equal to the afterloaded arterial impedance. What is the source impedance of our ventricular model? Since the model consists only of a volume elastance which becomes E_{es} at end-systole, the source impedance is E_{es} itself (reciprocal of capacitance). Because of impedance refers to opposition to flow, however, it is probably better to refer to E_{es} as the source stiffness. Then the matched condition becomes $E_{es} = E_a$. Although we argued above that the heart probably adapted to the arterial load rather than vice versa, the real ventricular E_{es} is difficult to manipulate experimentally whereas arterial model E_a can be easily and accurately varied as we like through the computer terminal. Therefore, we searched an optimal E_a which maximizes the external work of a given ventricle and examined how close the existing ventricular E_{es} is to the optimal E_a thus identified. Since E_a is a function of several parameters such as heart rate (HR), R_c, C and R, we chose R as the main variable while setting one of the other parameters (R_c, C, or HR) at 50%, 100% and 200% of its normal value and keeping the remaining parameters at their normal values. The external work under each impedance afterload was determined as the P-V loop area constructed from the $P(t)$ and $V(t)$ information.

The results indicated that the optimal E_a value thus found was very close to the ventricular E_{es} of the given heart (5). That is, the external work became maximum when the slopes of VPSVR and APSVR were equal as shown in the schematic diagram of Figure 3. Further, it is obvious in the diagram that the stroke volume under this matched condition is one half of the maximum possible stroke volume ($V_{ed}-V_0$). In other words, the ejection fraction EF is about 50% when the ventricular elastance is matched to the afterloaded arterial elastance. This is an interesting finding in view of the well known fact that the EF of the normal left ventricle in a resting subject is only slightly greater than 50%.

When a subject is mentally stressed, a mild increase in the sympathetic drive of cardiac contractility, heart rate and vasomotor tone occurs. As a result both E_a and E_{es} will increase but the matched condition for a nearly maximal external work may be maintained, as illustrated by the shift of the intersection point from 1 to 2 in the equilibrium diagram of Figure 4.

98

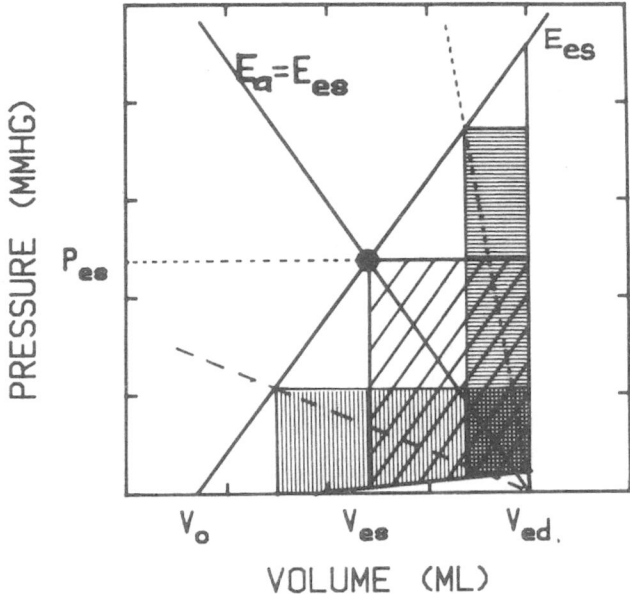

Figure 3. Schematic illustration of the dependence of the amount of the external mechanical work (shown by shaded area) that a ventricle performs at a constant preload and under a constant contractility (i.e., a fixed slope (E_{es}) of end-systolic pressure-volume relationship) on afterloaded arterial elastance E_a. Note that the shaded area becomes maximum when E_{es} equals E_a.

When a person physically exercises and requires a large increase in cardiac output, the ventricular contractility and thereby E_{es} will significantly increase. However, E_a is unlikely to change due to the balancing effect of large reduction in R on the one hand and a large decrease in heart period on the other (note that Eq. (4) can further be approximated as $P_{es}/SV \simeq (R + R_c)/T$ where $T = T_s + T_d$). Thus stroke volume increases mildly (at a high heart rate) with a mild increase in the ejection fraction and a slight deviation of the ventriculo-aortic coupling from the matched condition. This is illustrated in Figure 4 by the shift of the intersection point from 1 to 3. In contrast, when a patient suffers from an acute cardiomyopathy, the ventricular contractility is low (with a small E_{es}) while arterial impedance is rather augmented (with a high E_a). Use of the afterload reduction therapy will bring the equilibrium point from the mismatched Point 4 to Point 5 in the diagram in Figure 4.

Summary

We have presented here a rather simple framework for analysis of ventriculo-arterial interaction, using an equilibrium diagram in which the LV contraction is

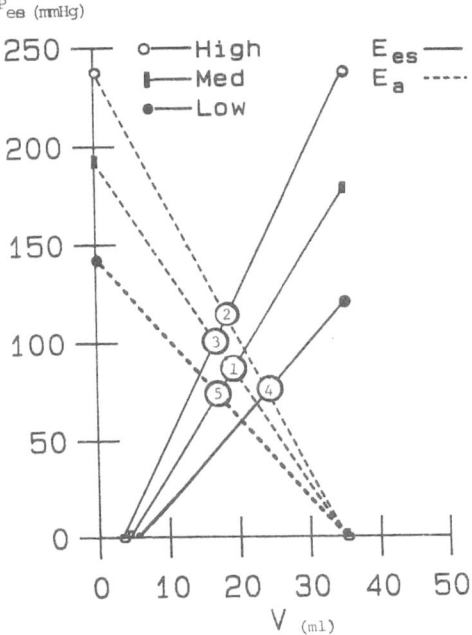

Figure 4. Equilibrium diagram for ventriculo-arterial coupling. See Figure 3 legend for explanation of the E_{es} and E_a curves. Points 1 to 5 indicate equilibria between the ventricular pump performance and arterial impedance property under various conditions discussed in text. The ventricule is assumed to contract at a fixed end-diastolic volume of 35 ml

represented by its endsystolic pressure-stroke volume relationship and aortic input impedance by the arterial endsystolic pressure-stroke volume relationship. It shows that, from the energetics point of view, the ventricle is matched to the arterial load in the physiological conditions transferring a maximum fraction (50%) of the total mechanical energy liberated per contraction under a given contractility and an end-diastolic volume. The concept of matching is well supported by the experimental data from isolated canine ventricle. Thus it seems worthwhile to extend the experimental study to the heart *in vivo* on the one hand and to examine on the other if coupling more detailed and isomorphic models of the LV to the arterial system model leads us to the similar basic findings on the optimal matching condition.

Acknowledgement

This study was supported in part by US National Heart Lung Blood Institute Research Grant HL 14903 and Ischemic Disease SCOR HL-17655.

References

Campbell KB, Ringo JA, Wakao Y, Klavano PA, Alexander JE (1982) Internal capacitance and resistance allow prediction of right ventricle outflow. Am J Physiol 243 (Heart Circ Physiol 12):H99–H112

Demomont G, Hinglais J (1981) Global parametric search and left ventricular identification: Evaluation of cardiac contractility through computed maximal isovolumic elastance. Ann Biomed Eng 9:59–74

Hunter WC, Janicki JS, Weber KT, Noordergraaf A (1979) Flow-pulse response: a new method for the characterization of ventricular mechanics. Am J Physiol 237 (Heart Circ Physiol 6):H282–H292

Maughan WL, Sunagawa K, Burkhoff D, Sagawa K (1984) Effect of afterload impedance changes on end-systolic pressure-volume relationship. Circ Res 54:595–602

Noordergraaf A (1969) Hemodynamics In 'Biological Engineering' edited by HP Schwan. New York: McGraw-Hill: 391–545

Piene H (1980) Interaction between the right heart ventricle and its arterial load: a quantitative solution. Am J Physiol 238 (Heart Circ Physiol 7): H932–H937

O'Rouke MF (1982) Vascular impedance in studies of arterial and cardiac function. Physiol Rev 62:570–623

Sagawa K (1978) The ventricular pressure-volume diagram revisited. (Brief Review) Circ Res 43:677–687

Shroff SG, Janicki JS, Weber KT (1983) Left ventricular systolic dynamics in terms of its chamber mechanical properties. Am J Physiol 245 (Heart Circ Physiol 14): H110–H124

Suga H, Sagawa K (1974) Instantaneous pressure-volume relationship and their ratio in the excised, supported canine left ventricle. Circ Res 35:117–125

Suga H, Sagawa K, Demer L (1980) Determinants of instantaneous pressure in canine left ventricle: time and volume specification. Circ Res 46:256–263

Sunagawa K, Maughan WL, Burkhoff D, Sagawa K (1983a) Left ventricular interaction with arterial load studied in isolated canine ventricle. Am J Physiol 245 (Heart Circ Physiol 14): H773–H780

Sunagawa K, Maughan WL, Sagawa K (1983b) Optimal condition for maximum left ventricular external work on arterial load. (abstr.) Circulation 68:I11–I34

DISCUSSION

BEYAR: I would like to ask about the relationship of the maximum elastance to the heart rate. It is known from physiologic measurements that in isovolumic contractions the pressure which the left ventricle develops is higher with the increase in rate; that means, a higher elastance value is induced by accelerating the heart rate. In one of your papers you report the effect of the heart rate on the elastance value, saying that the elastance function shortens in duration but is quite steady in magnitude. That means it doesn't increase with the heart rate. Would you like to comment about these two discrepancies?

SAGAWA: In the earlier study the excised preparation showed a heart rate between 120 and 140 and we really couldn't see any clear-cut effect of the heart rate on the maximum elastance value when we paced the heart at faster rates. Recently it has become possible to study the heart rate effect between 60 and 120 cpm, and yes, there was a clear-cut effect there; roughly a 20–30% increase in end systolic elastance. Above 120 cpm the increase became very small all the way to 180 cpm, probably an extra 10% increase. Above 180 cpm, statistical analysis shows an increase, although it is very small.

For a more accurate detailed modelling, therefore the heart rate should be taken into consideration. About the time to peak elastance Tmax, it decreased with increase in heart rate.

DINNAR: You presented an analysis between the left ventricle and the aorta, across the aortic valve, and eliminated the time scale very nicely from the picture. The build up of pressure in the aorta, depends also on the velocity and the time of contraction, coming back to the same problem of heart rate. Where is the velocity in your presentation? And what is the effect of velocity across the valve, or a stenotic valve?

SAGAWA: We put all these difficult problems under the carpet. And the reason we did so, as initially shown, is that when you look at the end systolic pressure stroke volume relationships, things suddenly simplify very much. If you try to describe instantaneous pressure-volume relationships during systole, as Dr. Janicki showed, you find that there are additional number of details to which you must pay attention. I'm sure that Dr. Janicki is convinced that including this pressure-dependent nonlinear resistance solves the major problems. Dr. Piene of Trondheim thinks it is unnecessary to include anything but compliance. These differences of opinion come from the extent of precision you want to quantify and predict. If you go to the precise prediction, then the reproducibility of the experimental data should also be taken into consideration. Predicting some particular data obtained at one moment may not fit at all to the data obtained 3 min later, because we know things tend to fluctuate, not tremendously, but enough to make people wonder how much precision we should really seek in modelling. This depends, of course, on the use of models. You must define the purpose of your modelling. The purpose of our studies presented today was to analyze the determinants of stroke volume and stroke work, not instantaneous pressure-volume-flow dynamics in the ventricle and aorta.

FEIGL: The maximization of work seems like a very intriguing point and particularly appealing for engineering. Could you expand on what is happening to cardiac output or stroke volume?

SAGAWA: In reference to Figure 3, given an end-diastolic volume the stroke volume depends upon end-systolic pressure. When the end-diastolic volume is between 30 and 40 ml and arterial impedance is normal, the stroke volume is something like 15 ml, which is pretty close to half of the end-diastolic volume. Thus, the ejection fraction seems to become 50% under the matched condition of $E_a = E_{es}$, which you can observe in normal dogs and patients.

FEIGL: My feeling is that an optimum work scheme, as far as energetics goes, may not serve the rest of the organism very well because the task of the heart in physiological circumstances is usually to increase cardiac output. Cardiac output increases in heavy exercise, perhaps fivefold, blood pressure changes 20%, so that optimizing work may not be the design parameter the designer had in mind.

SAGAWA: Your point is very well taken and that is exactly what we think. There is no reason why the design of our system should be working uniformly all the time. There can be different policies depending upon what the status of the organism is. When that organism must run away from an enemy and must use a lot of oxygen, it may not have time to care about the matching between the pump and the conduit system and it might fulfill the requirements at the expense of less efficient performance of the heart. However, there is a limitation to reduction of arterial pressure for maintenance of perfusion of those visceral beds in which the capillaries are connected in series.

GESELOWITZ: This is a simplistic argument that indicates that there is not necessarily an inconsistency. I think that this analysis is basically for systole and if you argue that the increased cardiac output during exercise is coming from increased heart rate, then there is some modification in stroke volume. It can still be at the optimum. Each stroke is close to the optimum and you get the increased cardiac output from an increased rate.

FEIGL: Your answer is quite right in that the increased cardiac output during exercise is done almost entirely by an increase in heart rate. The confusing part is that blood pressure goes up, not down, during exercise. As a matter of fact, any patient whose blood pressure goes down during exercise manifests cardiac disease. Yet, this kind of analysis would predict that it ought to go down and Dr. Sagawa's answer to my question was: the way to optimize this parameter is in fact to make it fall, but portal circulations and other things are a constraint on the system. Physiologically, in hundreds of measurements, the blood pressure goes up. Why? And what does this have to do with cardiac aortic impedance matching?

SAGAWA: Everybody knows that increasing heart rate is quite costly from energetic point of view. I must point out, however, that when people exercise the heart rate goes up markedly and resistance decreases consequently. This Ea curve may not change very much, because, as seen in Eq. (5), the increased heart rate effect cancels out the decreased resistance effect on E_a by reducing T_d and T_s in the denominator. Therefore, as Dr. Gezelowitz pointed out, the shift of this matching point, in terms of stroke volume or stroke work, may not be so great thanks to this increase in heart rate.

Models of ventricular dynamics

WALTER WELKOWITZ
Department of Electrical Engineering, Rutgers State University,
Piscataway, NJ 08854, U.S.A.

Abstract

A number of models of ventricular dynamics are discussed from the point of view of understanding the function of the heart and possible methods of diagnosis and treatment. In particular, work at Rutgers University, including studies of a variety of models, has been presented. These models include an hydraulic pressure source model, an ellipsoided shell model and a segmented shell model. Some of these models are interacted with each other to provide further insight into the use of models in understanding the physiology of the heart.

Introduction

One can study the physiology and the mechanics of cardiac function on many levels. These include details of muscle contractions from the anatomical, physiological, and model based descriptions as well as the gross functioning of the various heart chambers such as the left ventricle. Study of the chamber performance can again be carried out at the anatomical, physiological, and model based levels. This paper deals with some model based descriptions of the functioning of the left ventricle and of necessity includes some model based descriptions of muscle contraction.

Some of the applicable muscle models include the Maxwell, Voigt, Hill and Carlson models (Figure 1). In particular, the Carlson (1957) equation is used in much of this work to describe the stress-velocity relationship of cardiac muscle over the entire cardiac cycle. Min *et al.* (1978) found very little difference in analyzing ventricular dynamics when he alternately used Carlson's equation only during isotonic contraction and Hill's equation during isovolumic contraction.

There are many models that have been used to describe ventricular dynamics. One of the most popular is the description of the left ventricle as a time varying hydraulic capacitor as proposed by Suga and Sagawa (1974). This paper will

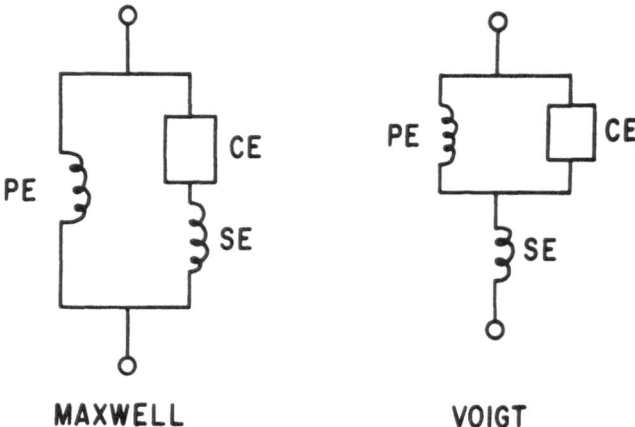

Figure 1. Muscle contraction models.

discuss alternatives to this approach, including an equivalent hydraulic pressure source model, a dynamic vibrating mechanical shell model, and a segmented shell model. The first and last of these can be cast as equivalent electrical networks – an approach that greatly simplifies manipulations of the models.

Detailed description of models

Hydraulic pressure source model

There have been a number of models described which represent the ventricle as a pressure source with an internal hydraulic impedance (Westerhof *et al.*, 1977; Abel, 1966; Fish *et al.*, 1973; Shastri, 1969; Buonochristiani, 1973; Elzinga and Westerhof, 1973). Such an approach lumps all the spatially distributed characteristics and all the diverse physical entities such as contractile strength, wall stress, elasticity and size into a Thevenin source equivalent. While this approach may appear to be a simplisitic way of describing something as complex as the heart it is certainly not unique and in fact it is the most common approach used in describing electrical generators when analyzing electrical systems. Extending this description, a simplified lumped network representation of the systemic circulation is shown in Figure 2. In this figure P_g, P_v and P_a correspond to the source pressure, left ventricular pressure and aortic pressure, respectively, while Z_g, Z_v and Z_a correspond to the source impedance, aortic valve impedance and aorta input impedance. These six parameters are generally time-varying functions. An examination of Figure 2 indicates that $P_g(t)$ represents the isovolumic equivalent pressure of the left ventricle throughout the cardiac cycle of the intact heart. The left ventricular pressure for an infinite load can be measured by cross-clamping the aorta prior to ejection. Figure 3 demonstrates the agreement between this

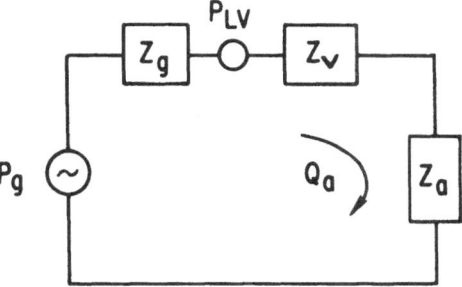

Figure 2. Equivalent source representation of the left ventricle.

measured value and the analytically derived $P_g(t)$ from Figure 2. If the time variation of the parameters is of a steady-state pulsatile nature, Min (1972) has shown that this network can be treated like a linear network with the quantities P_g, P_v, P_a and Q_a (aortic flow) resolvable into their Fourier components and representable by phasors.

Using a balloon pump to produce variable loading, a typical calculated discrete frequency spectrum of source pressure phasors from measurements made on a dog before and after induced heart failure is shown in Figure 4.

A pressure source time function reconstructed from these phasors is shown in Figure 5. The corresponding source impedances as a function of frequency are shown in Figure 6.

Ellipsoidal shell model

The left ventricle can be diagrammed approximately as shown in Figure 7. Because of this a number of investigators have modeled the left ventricle as a vibrating shell in the shape of a truncated ellipsoid of revolution with a circular cross section. Both thin and thick walled versions of the ellipsoid model have

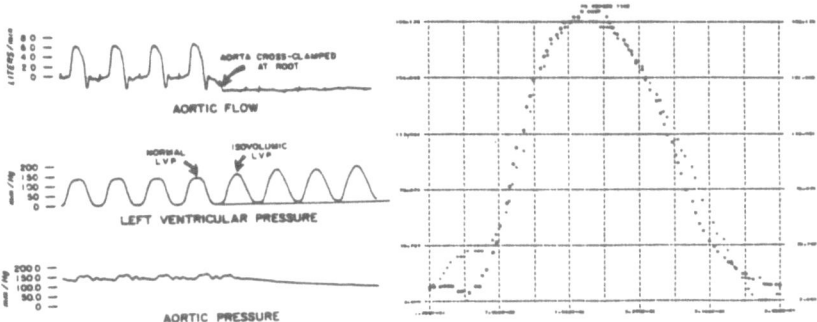

Figure 3. Comparison of measured and computed isovolumic left ventricular pressure.

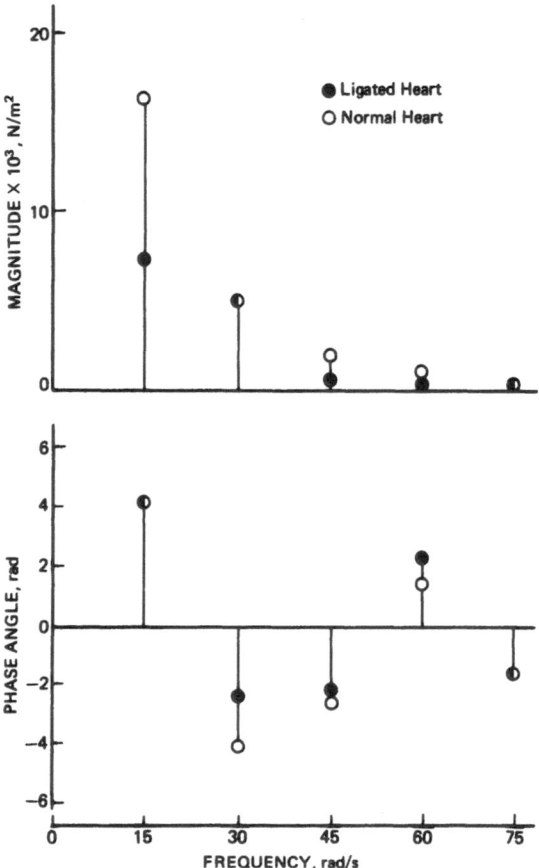

Figure 4. Calculated spectrum of equivalent source pressure before and after induced failure.

been analyzed by Hood (1969) who demonstrated good correlation between midwall stress predicted by the thick walled model and the average stress calculated from the thin walled model. Eggleton *et al.* (1970) observed that during contraction infolding occurs at the inner layers of the ventricle with most of the stress concentrated in a thin layer. Given these observations and calculations it appears reasonable to analyze the ventricle as a thin walled shell.

When the heart contracts, the apex is displaced to a new position due to the spiral nature of the muscle fibers. During ventricular motions the septum separating the right and left ventricle is essentially in a fixed position. Therefore, the base to apex length of the left ventricle changes only slightly. In this analysis the base to apex length will be assumed constant as will the wall thickness during the cardiac cycle.

Using the Carlson (1957) equation to describe the stress-velocity relationship of cardiac muscle

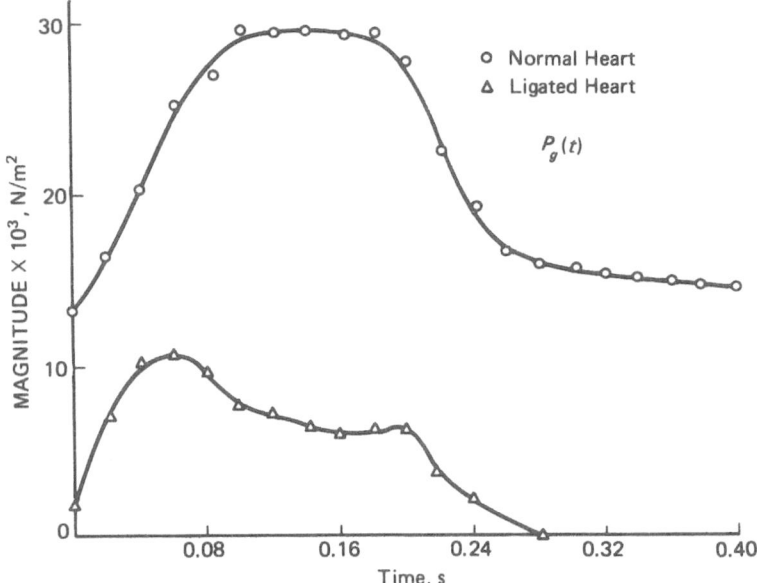

Figure 5. Time-domain representation of equivalent source pressure before and after induced failure.

$$\sigma\,(t) = \sigma_s - m\,\frac{dL(t)}{dt}, \tag{1}$$

where $\sigma(t)$ = active stress as a function of time,

$\quad\quad\sigma_s$ = isometric stress (which can vary under physiological control and is a function of muscle length),

$\quad\quad m$ = a constant,

$\quad\quad L(t)$ = muscle segment length as a function of time.

Incorporating the previously stated assumptions the volume of the semi-ellipsoid model as a function of time can be expressed as

$$V_v(t) = B\,L^2(T), \tag{2}$$

where B = a constant,

$\quad\quad L(t)$ = the greatest circumference of the ellipsoid.

The relationship between the wall stress and the internal pressure in the ellipsoid can be expressed by the appropriate Laplace equation as

$$\left(\frac{\sigma_{R1}}{R_1} + \frac{\sigma_{R2}}{R_2}\right) = \frac{P_v}{h}, \tag{3}$$

108

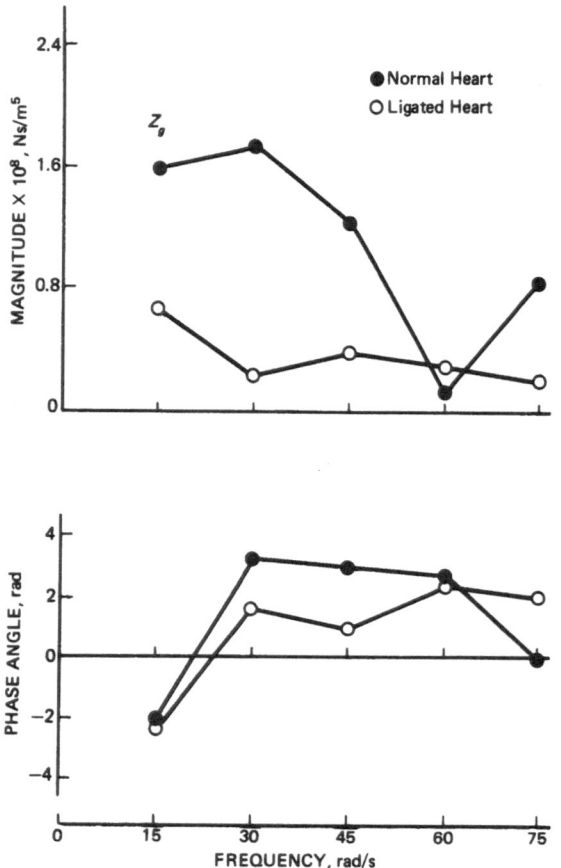

Figure 6. Calculated source impedance before and after induced failure.

where: σ_{R_1}, σ_{R_2} = wall stresses,

     R_1, R_2 = radii of curvature at locations σ_{R_1} and σ_{R_2},

     h = left ventricle wall thickness (assumed constant).

Measurements by Sandler and Dodge (1963) suggest that

$$R_1 > 4R_2 \tag{4}$$

and

$$\sigma_{R_2} > 2\sigma_{R_1} \tag{5}$$

or approximately,

$$\sigma_{R_2} = \frac{bP_v}{h}, \tag{6}$$

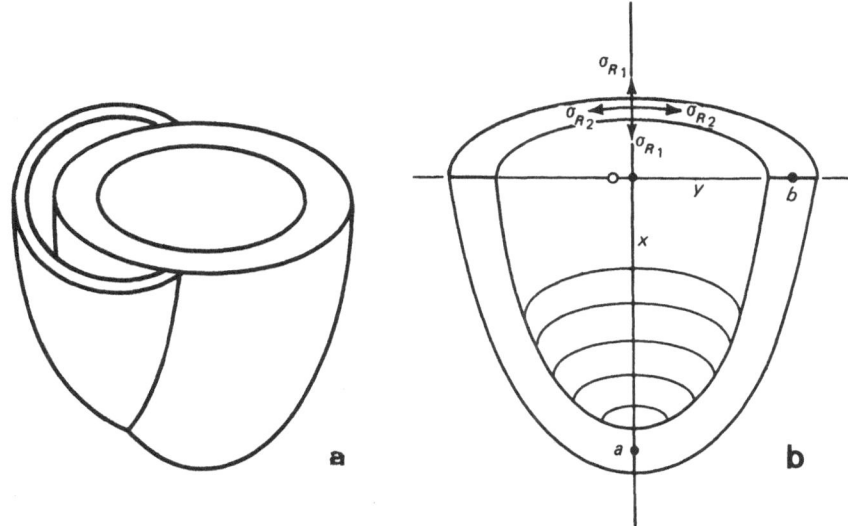

Figure 7. Ellipsoid model of left ventricle.

where: b = minor semiaxis of ellipsoid.

Averaging the circumferential stress over the entire semiellipsoid and defining the average stress as

$$\sigma_a = \frac{1}{a} \int_0^a \sigma(x) \, dx \tag{7}$$

then

$$\sigma_a(t) = \frac{1}{8h} L(t) P_v(t). \tag{8}$$

Substituting this equation into Carlson's equation and introducing Eq. (2) for volume, a pressure-volume equation for this model of the left ventricle results.

$$P_v(t) = 8h\sqrt{B} \frac{\sigma_s}{\sqrt{V_v(t)}} - \frac{4h \, m}{V_v(t)} \left[\frac{dV_v(t)}{dt} \right]. \tag{9}$$

Using the hydraulic pressure source model of Figure 2 and the usual network equations, it is apparent that the hydraulic pressure source model yields a pressure-volume equation

$$P_v(t) = P_g(t) - Z_g(t) \left[\frac{dV_v(t)}{dt} \right], \tag{10}$$

since
$$Q_a(t) = \frac{dV_v(t)}{dt}.$$

These two equations are clearly of the same form – as they should be since they represent the same phenomenon described by two different models. The two Eqs. (9) and (10) can be related term by term to express physical quantities such as volume and stress in terms of the measurable parameters $P_g(t)$ and $Z_g(t)$.

Segmented shell model

It has been pointed out (Beyar and Sideman, 1984) that it would be convenient to have a model which can contain variations of structure from epicardium to endocardium and which can permit variations in timing of the electrically induced contractions as the electrical wave moves over the myocardium. Such a model should also permit the description of localized abnormalities (such as infarcts) which is not permitted in a uniform shell model. A segmented shell model as discussed by Watts (1974) and by Welkowitz (1977) satisfies these needs.

For comparison purposes the segmented shell model can be analyzed using the same basic physiological assumptions that were used in the uniform semi-ellipsoid shell model. These are:
   (1) contraction is circumferential,
   (2) left ventricle is a thin walled shell,
   (3) the wall thickness is constant is a plane orthogonal to the major axis,
   (4) variations of wall thickness during systole are neglected, and
   (5) Carlson's equation describes muscle contraction.
In addition to these assumptions, it will be assumed that:
   (1) rings of muscle tissue contract independently.

In comparison to the uniform shell model, the segmented shell model consists of the uniform structure cut up into rings as shown in Figure 8. The number of rings can be varied depending upon the fineness specified for the geometric variations in anatomy or electrical excitation. Each of the rings can be considered a uniform cylinder with input flow and pressure, output flow and pressure, and dimensions shown in Figure 9. During contraction, the force-flow equations for each cylinder can be expressed approximately as

$$\Delta F = \left[\frac{8\pi v}{A_{ji}} Q + \rho \frac{\partial Q}{\partial t} \right] \Delta z \tag{11}$$

$$\Delta Q = - \frac{\partial A_j}{\partial t} \Delta z. \tag{12}$$

In terms of circumferential tension, Carlson's equation can be expressed as

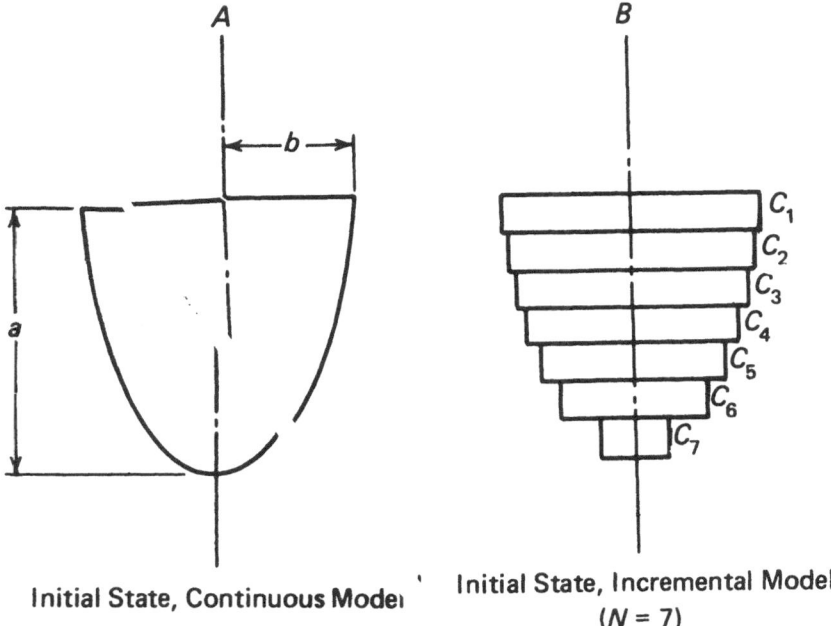

Figure 8. Segmented ventricle model.

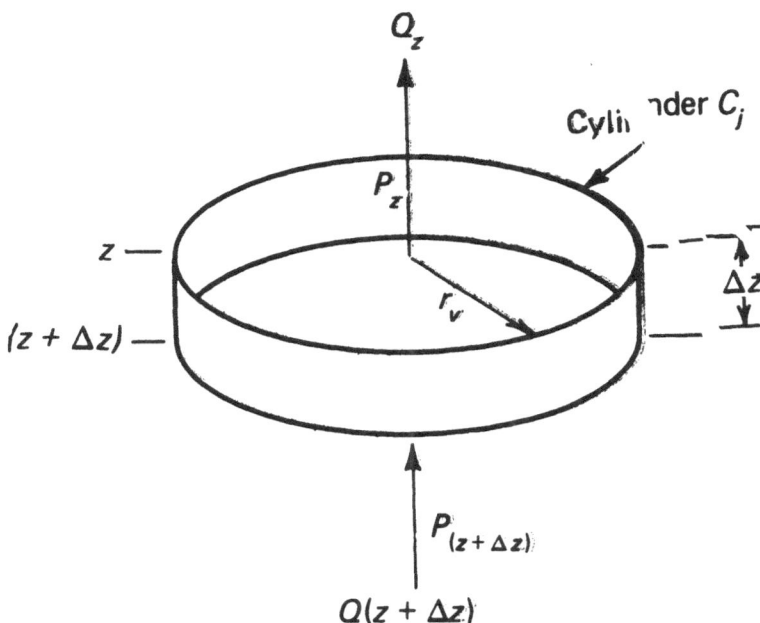

Figure 9. Pressures and flows at incremental cylindrical section.

$$T_\theta = T_s + m_1 \frac{dL_j(t)}{dt},$$ (13)

where: T_s = isometric tension (which can vary under physiological control and as a function of muscle length),

m_1 = a constant,

L_j = circumference of jth cylinder.

Laplace's equation for a thin walled circular cylinder becomes

$$P = \frac{T_\theta}{r_j},$$ (14)

where P = pressure inside of cylinder.

Force is then given by

$$F = \pi r_j^2 P.$$ (15)

Substituting for area

$$\Delta Q = - 2\pi r_j \frac{dr_j(t)}{dt} \Delta z$$ (16)

and

$$P = \frac{T_s}{r_j} + \frac{2\pi m_1}{r_j} \frac{dr_j(t)}{dt} \Delta z.$$ (17)

Combining these two equations

$$P = \frac{T_s}{r_j} - \frac{m_1}{r_j^2} \Delta Q$$ (18)

or

$$F = \pi r_j^2 P = \pi r_j T_s - \pi m \Delta Q$$ (19)

The equivalent circuit for each cylindrical segment of the ventricle is shown in Figure 10

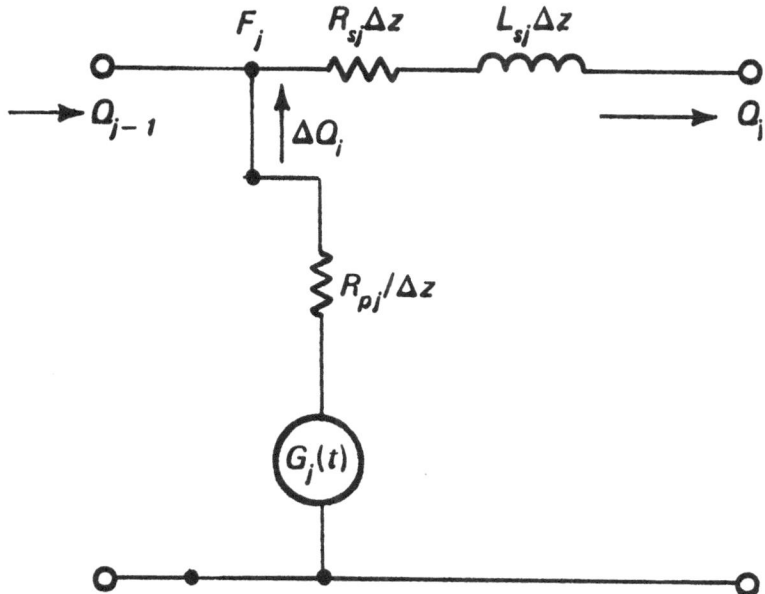

Figure 10. Network analog model for incremental cylindrical section.

where: $L_{gj} \quad = \varrho$

$$R_{sj} = \frac{8\pi v}{A_j}$$

$$G_j(t) = \pi r_j T_s$$

Since $G_j(t)$ can vary in timing and magnitude for each cylinder it can represent variations in the electrically induced contractions as the electrical wave moves over the myocardium. Figure 11 shows a complete netwerk model for the entire left ventricle. Exercising this model for various structural differences or excitation timing arrangements just consists of solving for various forces and flows (especially the output force and flow) using standard computer network analysis programs.

In the event that there is a localized infarct, the effected cylinders can be represented by a segment of normal contractile tissue (obeying Carlson's equation) and a segment of abnormal (non-contractile) tissue with only elastic properties. Using this description, Watts (1976) has shown that the individual cylinder equivalent cricuit is modified as illustrated in Figure 12

where:

114

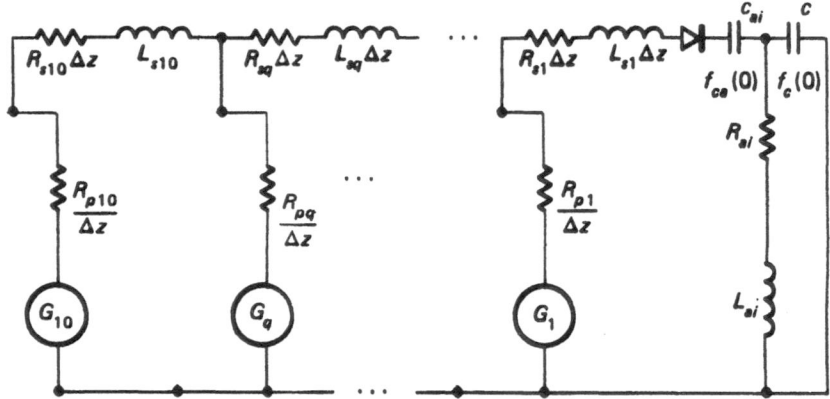

Figure 11. Network analog for segmented shell model of left ventricle.

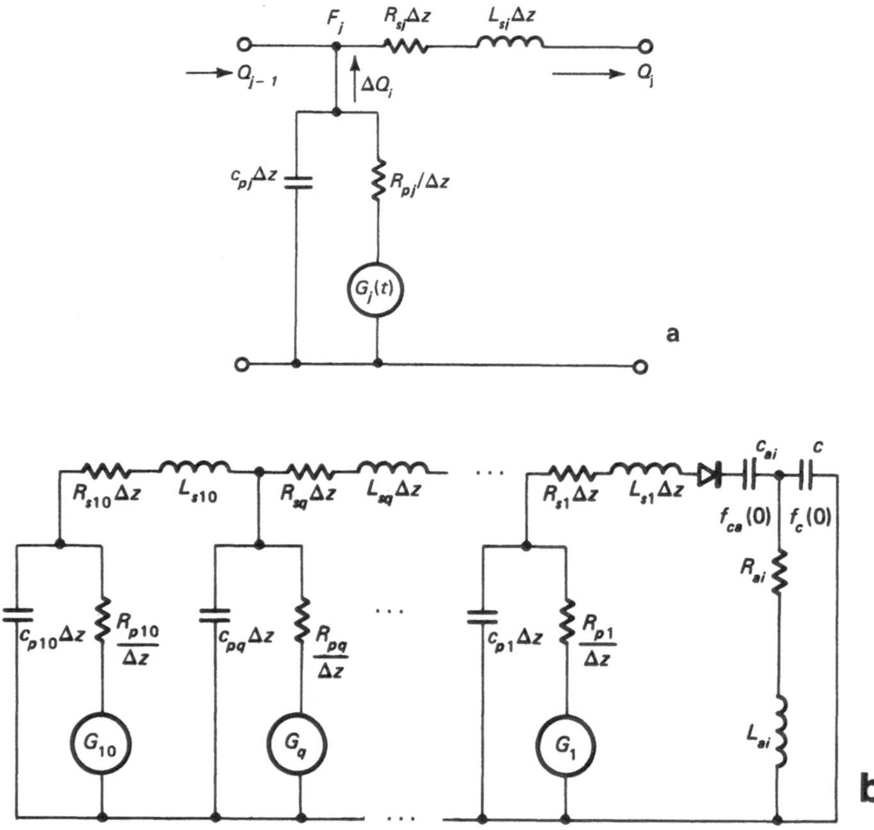

Figure 12. Network analog model for incremental cylindrical section including effect of infarcted tissue.

$$C_{pj} = \frac{l2j}{\pi E_{2j} h}$$

l_{2j} = circumferential length of cylinder that is normal tissue,
E_{2j} = Young's modulus for this tissue section,
h = wall thickness of cylinder.

This transition from a resistive-inertial reactance for the internal source impedance to a resistive-compliant reactance has been demonstrated experimentally by Kresh *et al.* (1976) in a series of animal experiments where infarcts were induced by tying off portions of the coronary artery.

Conclusion

In conclusion, it has been shown that a variety of models can be developed which can help clarify the understanding of the anatomy and physiology of the left ventricle and which may have utility in diagnosing cardiac disorders or in establishing parameters for appropriate mechanical assistance for the failing heart. By combining the hydraulic pressure source model and the ellipsoidal shell model, Welkowitz (1981) has developed indices which can characterize cardiac status. Using the segmented shell model, Watts (1974) has been able to develop some differential characteristics for a ventricle with localized infarcts. This has been confirmed experimentally by Kresh *et al.* (1976). Finally, by using the pressure source model Welkowitz *et al.* (1972) has developed a system description which can be used in the automatic computer control of heart assist devices.

References

Abel FL (1966) An analysis of the left ventricle as a pressure and flow generator in the intact systematic circulation. IEEE Trans Biomed Eng BME-13:182–188

Beyar R, Sideman S (1984) A computer study of the left ventricle performance based on fiber structure, sarcomere dynamics and transmural electrical propagation velocity. Circ Res, in press

Buonocristiani JF, Liedtke AJ, Strong RM, Urschel CW (1973) Parameter estimates of a left ventricular model during ejection. IEEE Trans Biomed Eng BME-29:110–114

Carlson FD (1957) Kinematic studies of mechanical properties of muscles. In: JW Remington (ed) Tissue Elasticity, Am Physiol Soc Washington, D.C

Eggleton RC, Townsend C, Herrick J, Templeton G, Mitchell JH (1970) Ultrasonic visualization of left ventricular dynamics. IEEE Trans on Sonics and Ultrasonics 17:143–153

Elzinga G, Westerhof N (1973) Pressure and flow generated by the left ventricle against different impedances. Circ Res 32:178–186

Fich S, Welkowitz W, Shastri S (1973) An equivalent pressure source for the heart. Int J Eng Sci 11:601–611

Hood WP (1969) Comparison of calculation of left ventricular wall stress in man from thin-walled and thick-walled ellipsoidal models. Circ Res 24:576

Kresh JM, Min BG, Welkowitz W, Kulikowski A, Kostis JB (1976) Source impedance and internal reactive power in the impaired left ventricle. Proc. 29th Ann Conf Eng. in Biol and Med:215

116

Min BG (1972) Analysis and optimization of cardiac assistance by intraaortic balloon pumping. Ph D Thesis, New Brunswick, NJ:Rutgers Univ

Min BG, Kresh JM, Fich S, Kostis JB, Welkowitz W (1978) Relation between computed zero-load aortic flow and cardiac muscle mechanics. J. Biomech 80:227–235

Sandler J, Dodge HT (1963) Left ventricular tension and stress in man. Circ Res 13:91

Shastri SJ (1969) A thevenin equivalent model of the left ventricle derived from hemodynamic measurements obtained by use of a ventricular assist pump. Ph D Thesis, New Brunswick, NJ:Rutgers Univ

Suga H, Sagawa K (1974) Instantaneous pressure-volume relationships and their ratio in the exercised supported canine left ventricle. Circ Res 32: 314–322

Watts RN (1974) A mathematical model for studying the mechanical properties of the impaired left ventricle. Ph D Thesis, New Brunswick, NJ:Rutgers Univ

Welkowitz W (1977) Engineering Hemodynamics: Application to Cardiac Devices. Boston, MA:Lexington Books

Welkowitz W (1981) Indices of cardiac status. IEEE Trans Biomed Eng BME-28:553–567

Welkowitz W, Fich S, Min B, Jaron D, Kantrowitz A (1972) Analysis of assisted circulation. Bibl Cardiol 29:14–27

Westerhof N, Elzinga G, Sipkema P, vanDen Bos GC (1977) Quantitative analysis of the arterial system by means of pressure-flow relations. In: Hwang NHC and Norman NA (eds) Cardiovascular Flow Dynamics and Measurements, Baltimore, MD:Univ Press

Material and structural limitations in a 3-D finite element model of the left ventricle

MORDECHAI PERL and ARIE HOROWITZ
Departments of Mechanical and Biomedical Engineering, Technion – Israel Institute of Technology, Haifa 32 000 Israel

Abstract

A short chronological review of the diverse available mechanical models of the LV precedes a critical reassessment of the various main factors involved in a finite element analysis of the ventricle. These factors constitute the three-dimensional geometry of the LV and its kinematical boundary conditions; the extent of the deformation the ventricle undergoes; the pressure distribution on the endocardium; the myocardial constitutive law as well as its anisotropy, and the activation mechanism of the muscle. A rationale for developing an improved finite element model, gradually incorporating these factors, concludes the presentation.

Introduction

During the past two decades a major effort to model the mechanical structural behaviour of the human left ventricle (LV) has been made. In the early stages of this effort the LV was modeled as a sphere or an ellipsoid of revolution subjected to uniform internal pressure. The myocardial wall was assumed to be made of an isotropic linear elastic material, and no active role was attributed to the muscle during the systolic phase of the cardiac cycle (Wong and Rautaharju, 1968; Ghista and Sandler, 1968; Mirsky, 1969; Streeter *et al.*, 1970). These models have been constantly improved to account for a more realistic geometry of the LV (Gould *et al.*, 1972; Pao *et al.*, 1974; Heethaar *et al.*, 1977; Neckyfarow and Perlman, 1976; Panda and Natarajan, 1977; Ghista and Hamid, 1977; Ghista *et al.*, 1980; Yettram *et al.*, 1983), for the anisotropy of the fibrous structure (Streeter *et al.*, 1970; Ross, 1972; Wong, 1973; Neckyfarow and Perlman, 1976; Panda and Natarajan, 1977; Feit, 1979; Arts *et al.*, 1979; Chen *et al.*, 1980; Chadwick, 1982; Yettram *et al.*, 1983), for the nonlinearity of the muscle constitutive law (Ross, 1972; Wong, 1973; Janz *et al.*, 1974; Feit, 1979; Arts *et al.*, 1979; Ghista *et al.*, 1980) and for the active role of the contraction mechanism during the systolic phase (Chen *et al.*,

1980). A chronological representation of the various proposed models of the LV, though incomplete, is given in Table 1. The main improvements, already achieved, are mainly due to the application of the finite element (FE) method in solving this problem (Gould et al., 1972; Ross, 1972; Pao et al., 1974; Janz et al., 1974; Pao et al., 1976; Heethaar et al., 1977; Neckyfarow and Perlman, 1976; Panda and Natarajan, 1977; Ghista and Hamid, 1977; Ghista et al., 1980; Chen et al., 1980; Yettram et al., 1983). The relative flexibility of this method to deal with irregular complex geometries, its potential ability to handle material and geometrical nonlinearity, and the availability of and easy access to standard codes have considerably contributed to the increasing implementation of the finite element method in trying to solve the LV mechanics. Nevertheless, there are still many limitations to the existing finite element models of the LV. It is the purpose of this presentation to reassess the various factors involved in a finite element analysis of the LV, and to propose a rationale for constructing an improved and more realistic mechanical model for simulating the cardiac cycle.

Basic factors concerning the LV FE analysis

Several basic factors are involved in the process of modelling the mechanical behaviour of the LV by the FE method. These factors are: the geometry of the ventricle including its kinematic boundary conditions, the extent of the deformation that the LV undergoes, the pressure distribution on the endocardium, the myocardial constitutive law as well as its anisotropy and the activation mechanism of the muscle, mainly manifested in the systolic phase. Furthermore, computer resources such as storage and computation time requirements should also be considered.

The LV geometry

The geometry of the LV appears to be the most important factor in carrying out a stress analysis of the myocardium during the diastole (Yettram et al., 1983) and probably of no lesser importance in analysing the systolic phase. Until a few years ago the trend was to model the ventricular geometry by assuming ellipsoids of either circular of elliptical cross sections. It is only since the late seventies that improved techniques such as biplane angiocardiograms (Yettram and Vinson, 1979) and computer-aided tomography (Ritman et al., 1980) have been introduced, yielding better imaging and threedimensional (3-D) reconstructions of the true ventricular shape. Presently, an effort to improve the ultrasound technique for obtaining better 3-D reconstruction of LV is being carried out at the Technion.

Tabel 1.

Parameters	L.V. Geometry	Model Dimensional-ity	Type of Deformation	Type of Loading (Pressure)	Material Law	Material Anisotropy	Active Passive	Method of Analysis
Wong and Rautaharju (1968)	Ellipsoid of Revolution. Uniform Thickness	2-D	Small	Uniform Pressure	Linear	Isotropic	Passive: Systole	Analytical
Ghista and Sandler (1969)	Ellipsoid of Revolution. Varying Thickness	2-D	Small	Uniform Pressure	Linear	Isotropic	Passive: Systole + Diastole	Analytical
Mirsky (1969)	Ellipsoid of Revolution. Uniform Thickness	2-D	Small	Uniform Pressure	Linear	Isotropic	Passive: Systole + Diastole	Analytical
Streeter et al. (1969)	Truncated Ellipsoid of Revolution. Varying Thickness	2-D	Small No Strain Calculation	Uniform Pressure	Linear No Strain Calculation	Anisotropic (Fibrous Structure, $-60° \div +60°$)	Passive: Systole + Diastole	Analytical
Gould et al. (1972)	Axisymmeric Body Obtained by A-P Contour	2-D	Small	Uniform Pressure	Linear	Isotropic	Passive: Diastole	Finite-Element

Tabel 1.

Parameters	L.V. Geometry	Model Dimensionality	Type of Deformation	Type of Loading (Pressure)	Material Law	Material Anisotropy	Active Passive	Method of Analysis
Ross (1972)	Ellipsoid of Revolution. Uniform Thickness	2-D	Small	Uniform Pressure	Nonlinear	Anisotropic (Fibrous)	Passive: Diastole	Finite-Element
Wong (1973)	Truncated Ellipsoid of Revolution. Varying Thickness	3-D	Small	Uniform Pressure	Nonlinear Exponential	Anisotropic (Fibrous Structure, $-60° \div +60°$)	Active: Systole + Diastole	Analytical
Pao et al. (1974)	Axisymmetric Body Obtained by A-P Contour	2-D	Small (Plane Strain)	Uniform Pressure	Linear	Isotropic	Passive: Diastole	Finite-Element
Janz et al. (1974)	Truncated Ellipsoid of Revolution. Varying Thickness	2-D	Large	Uniform Pressure	Nonlinear Exponential	Isotropic, Two Layers	Passive: Diastole	Finite-Element
Pao. et al. (1976)	True Cross Sectional Shape	2-D	Small (Plane Strain)	Uniform Pressure	Linear	Isotropic	Passive: Diastole	Finite-Element
Heethaar et al. (1977)	True 3-D Shape	3-D	Small	Uniform Pressure	Linear	Isotropic	Passive: Diastole	Finite-Element

Tabel 1.

Parameters	L.V. Geometry	Model Dimensionality	Type of Deformation	Type of Loading (Pressure)	Material Law	Material Anisotropy	Active Passive	Method of Analysis
Pao and Ritman (1977)	True Cross Sectional Shape	2-D	Small (Plane Strain)	Uniform Pressure	Linear	Isotropic	Passive: Diastole	Finite-Element
Neckyfarow and Perlman (1976)	A-P Contour, Circular Cross Sections	2-D	Small	Uniform Pressure	Linear	Orthotropic (Circumferential & Longitudinal Directions)	Passive: Diastole	Finite-Element
Panda and Natarajan (1977)	Axisymmetric Body Obtained by A-P Contour	2-D	Small	Uniform Pressure	Linear	Orthotropic (3 layers)	Passive: Diastole	Finite-Element
Ghista and Hamid (1977)	A-P Contour, Elliptic Cross Sections	3-D	Small	Uniform Pressure	Linear	Isotropic	Passive: Systole	Finite-Element
Arts et al. (1979)	Finite Circular Cylinder	3-D	Large	Uniform Pressure	Nonlinear	Anisotropic (8 layers)	Active: Systole	Analytical
Feit (1979)	Finite Circular Cylinder	3-D	Large	Uniform Pressure	Nonlinear Exponential	Anisotropic (Fibrous Structure $-80° \div +60°$)	Passive: Diastole	Analytical

Tabel 1.

Parameters	L.V. Geometry	Model Dimensionality	Type of Deformation	Type of Loading (Pressure)	Material Law	Material Anisotropy	Active Passive	Method of Analysis
Ghista et al. (1980)	A-P Contour, Elliptic Cross Sections	3-D	Small	Uniform Pressure	Nonlinear Exponential	Isotropic	Passive: Diastole	Finite-Element
Chen et al. (1980)	Finite Circular Cylinder	3-D	Large	Uniform Pressure, 6 increments	Linear	Orthotropic (2 Layers)	Active: Systole	Finite-Element
Chadwick (1982)	Finite Circular Cylinder	3-D	Small	Uniform Pressure	Linear	Anisotropic (Fibrous Structure, Linear Distribution, $-80° \div +80°$)	Passive Systole + Diastole	Analytical
Yettram et al. (1983)	Irregular 3-D Shape Obtained by 2 Normal Longitudinal Contours	3-D	Small	Uniform Pressure	Linear	Anisotropic (Varying $-60° \div +60°$)	Passive: Diastole	Finite-Element
Hadingham (1983)	A-P Contour Circular Cross Sections	2-D	No Strain Calculation	Uniform Pressure	No Strain Calculation	Anisotropic	Passive: Systole + Diastole	Analytical
Tozeren (1983)	Finite Circular Cylinder	3-D	Large	Uniform Pressure	Nonlinear Exponential	Anisotropic (Fibrous Structure $-60° \div +60°$)	Passive: Systole + Diastole	Analytical

At present it seems that the sequence of geometries of the LV obtained at various stages of the cardiac cycle by tomography (via the DSR – Dynamic Spatial Reconstructor) at the Mayo Clinic (Ritman *et al.*, 1980) are the best available 3-D reconstructions of the ventricle. Though this technique is not yet widely spread, it would be recommended to use the DSR geometries in the FE analysis in view of the importance of the exact configuration of the LV.

The LV kinematical boundary conditions

In order to perform a FE analysis it is necessary to constraint the model so as to prevent rigid body displacements and rotations. Anatomically, the LV movement is restrained by the right ventricle and the atria, by the pericardial sac, and by the aorta, none of which constitutes an absolute clamp. The common approach is to hinge the model at the base constraining it from vertical movement. This approach, due to the St. Venant principle, seems to have only a local effect and thus it will not affect the stress distribution in most of the LV.

The LV deformation

During the cardiac cycle the LV undergoes large deformations with sarcomere elongations of up to 15% (Sonnenblick *et al.*, 1963). Although this value is far beyond the limits of infinitesimal strain, most of the existing models (see Table 1) perform a small deformation analysis. It seems that the future FE analysis can be much improved by accounting for the large deformation of the LV. This can be achieved by an incremental updated lagrangian scheme which will be combined with a load incrementation procedure. It is expected that the finite deformation analysis will yield more accurate displacements, strains and stresses. This information is also valuable for trying to assess the optimal structural design of the LV (Horowitz *et al.*).

The pressure distribution on the endocardium

All the models herein presented (Table 1) considered only uniform internal pressure loading in the LV. Nevertheless, it is quite evident that pressure gradients as well as fluid shear stress are present at the endocardium. A first attempt to calculate the pressure distribution in the LV during systole was recently made by the authors. The analysis was performed by the Pheonics code (Gunton *et al.*, 1983). Preliminary results do indicate the presence of pressure gradients in the LV during systole. Further research, both experimental and numerical, is needed in order to quantify the exact normal and shearing stresses prevailing in the ventricle during both phases of the cardiac cycle.

The myocardial material law

When considering the myocardial material law one refers mainly to the stress-strain relation obtained from a uniaxial tensile test of an isolated heart muscle bundle, such as the pappilary muscle (Pinto and Fung, 1973), or a wall muscle strip (Pao *et al.*, 1980). The experimental results indicated a nonlinear stress-strain relation of the form

$$\sigma = c(e^{k\varepsilon} - 1), \tag{1}$$

where c and k are material constants.

Nonetheless, most of the existing models assume a linear material for the ventricle. Since the material is considerably nonlinear and since large strains are present, it would be most advantageous to perform a nonliner material analysis. This improvement can be implemented in the FE analysis by employing an incremental approach and by assuming a piece-wise linear material. It seems that the large deformation and the material nonlinear analyses can be incorporated into the algorithm. Although the relative importance of these two nonlinearities has not yet been determined, it is preferable to treat the geometrical nonlinearity first because of the large variability in the experimentally measured material constants which might produce ambiguous results.

The anisotropic structure of the LV

The myocardium exhibits an anisotropic response during its loading and unloading stages due to its complex fiber structure. Several attempts have been made to incorporate this anisotropy (or orthotropy) in the mechanical modelling of the LV (Streeter *et al.*, 1970; Wong, 1973; Neckyfarow and Perlman, 1976; Panda and Natarajan, 1977; Feit, 1979; Arts *et al.*, 1979; Chen *et al.*, 1980; Chadwick, 1982; Yettram *et al.*, 1983; Tozeren, 1983). Anatomical studies by Streeter (1979) suggested a helical arrangement of the fibers with an angle varying with respect to the ventricle circumferencial direction. This angle was reported to vary linearly from about $-80°$ at the epicardium to $+80°$ at the endocardium. It was also suggested by Peskin (1975) that the fibers should follow geodesic paths. Recently Greenbaum *et al.* (1981), following clinical studies, suggested a more complex configuration of the fiber angle. Yettram *et al.* (1983) have implemented these findings in a FE analysis of the LV. Performing a parametric study of the influence of the fiber orientation on the LV stres analysis during diastole, they concluded that the analysis 'is not critically dependent on variation in fiber architecture'. Nevertheless, it is probably in the systolic phase that the fiber configuration importance is more apparent.

The passive and the active LV

During the diastolic phase of the cardiac cycle the ventricle is usually considered to be a passive material deforming under the increasing blood pressure pumped into it. Contrary to this, during the systolic phase the myocardium actively contracts. The active properties of the muscle fibers have been implemented only in one model of the LV (Chen *et al.*, 1980). It would therefore be important in future FE simulations of the LV to incorporate the active characteristics of the myocardial fibers.

Computer resourses

The present FE models such as that of Yettram *et al.* (1983) employ a spatial discretization of the LV of about 72 20-nodes brick elements, representing about 1200° of freedom. The computational time for solving such a model is a few hundreds of CPU sec on a CDC 7600 computer. Future improved mechanical analyses of both the active and passive phases of the cardiac cycle, employing a more accurate and detailed geometry, and allowing for geometrical and material nonlinearities will thus lead to excessive exploitation of computer resources. The increased storage and CPU-time requirements will necessitate the use of a mainframe, or a supermini, solely dedicated to this project, and virtually equipped with an array processor. Hardware developments presently underway may result in the very near future in substantial reduction of computer resources demanded for simulating the cardiac cycle.

A comprehensive finite element model of the LV

A comprehensive FE model of the LV, gradually accounting for the various factors described in the previous section will be hereafter presented. The geometry of the LV is probably the main factor affecting its analysis. Therefore it is proposed to employ 3-D reconstruction of the LV such as those obtained at the Mayo Clinic via computerized tomography. Once the LV shape is determined it is necessary to discretisize it prior to the FE analysis. A tentative break-down of elements is presented in Figure 1, consisting of two types of isotropic elements: the 3-D solid and the truss elements. The LV is divided into two layers of 3-D $9 \div 12$ node isoparametric bricks reinforced in several directions by truss elements.

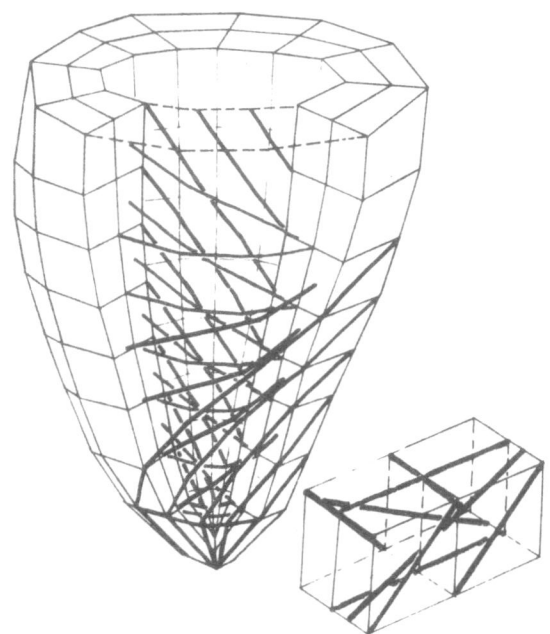

Figure 1. Tentative break-down of elements for the left ventricle

The truss elements are introduced to simulate the directional orthotropy of the muscle due to its fibrous structure and are practically oriented in the actual direction of the fibers (Greenbaum *et al.*, 1983). The fiber angle variation through the thickness of the ventricle is represented in Figure 1 by five distinct angles. The truss and the 3-D elements will be respectively assigned such material moduli so as to account for the axial and transversal fiber properties. This basic configuration which accounts for the real geometry and anisotropy of the myocardium will be applied in all forthcoming stages.

As a first approach it is suggested to perform a linear elastic, small deformation analysis of the diastolic phase assuming uniform blood pressure throughout the cavity by means of a standard FE code such as SAP 7 (1982). Once this basic concept is proved, gradual implementation of improvements in the various basic factors previously discussed is proposed.

The second stage will include the development of an incremental procedure together with an updated Lagrangian scheme to enable a large deformation analysis. Eventually the real pressure distribution on the ventricle wall, provided this information is available, will be taken into account.

A further refinement will be to implement a nonlinear material law in the simulation. At first the material can be assumed to be piece-wise linear, and thus its nonlinear characteristics can be incorporated in the incremental procedure previously described.

Once all the above improvements are put into the effect and the diastole is satisfactorily evaluated, it would be recommended to incorporate the active features of the fibers in the model so as to enable the simulation of the systolic phase. This can be done by introducing initial strains in the truss elements and so reproducing the active contraction of the fibers. The time of introduction of the initial strains can vary from element to element and follow the activation sequence of the electrophysiological excitation.

The following information will serve as input to all the above simulation:
(a) The *in vivo* measured end-systolic 3-D geometry of the ventricle.
(b) The space-time pressure variation in the LV during the cardiac cycle.
(c) The myocardial mechanical properties.
(d) The time and spatial sequences of the electrophysiological activation (only for the systole).
As output the simulation will provide us with:
(a) The time varying geometry of the LV during the cardiac cycle.
(b) The space-time distribution of stresses and strains in the ventricular wall.

The evaluation of the FE model, in its diverse variations, will be carried out as follows: Each of the simulations commences with an *in vivo* measured 3-D reconstruction of the LV: either with the end systolic or the end-diastolic one. Then the changing geometry of the ventricle during the cardiac cycle is numerically evaluated. On the other hand a similar sequence of the time varying shape of the ventricle is provided by the computerized tomography. Thus, the comparison between respective numerically evaluated geometries and experimentally measured ones can serve to assess the accuracy of the model.

Concluding remarks

In this paper the main parameters affecting a finite element simulation of the LV cardiac cycle have been reviewed. As a result, a step-by-step procedure towards developing a more comprehensive model is proposed based on the combination of 3-D brick and truss elements. Though the task of performing a realistic simulation of the cardiac cycle still seems enormously difficult, it is hoped that the gradual sophistication of the model will enable its materialization.

Acknowledgements

This work was supported by a generous grant endowed by Mr. M. Kennedy-Leigh. The advice and continuous interest of Professors S. Sideman, Technion-IIT, and Y.C. Pao, University of Nebraska, Lincoln, is highly appreciated.

References

Arts T, Reneman RS, Veenstra PC (1979) A model of the mechanics of the left ventricle. Ann Biomed Eng 7:299–318

Chadwick RS (1982) Mechanics of the left ventricle. Biophys J 39:279–288

Chen CJ, Kwak BM, Rim K, Falsetti HL (1980) A model for an active left ventricle deformation – formulation of a nonlinear quasi-steady finite-element analysis for orthotropic, three-dimensional myocardium. Int Conf Finite Elements in Biomechanics 2:639–655

Feit TS (1979) Diastolic pressure-volume relations and distribution of pressure and fiber extension across the wall of a model left ventricle. Biophys J 28:143–166

Ghista ND, Sandler HD (1968) An elastic viscoelastic model for the shape and the forces in the left ventricle. J Biomechanics 2:35–47

Ghista DN, Hamid MS (1977) Finite-element stress analysis of the human left ventricle whose irregular shape is developed from single plane cineangiocardiogram. Comp Prog Biomed 7:219–231

Ghista DN, Ray G, Sandler H (1980) Cardiac assessment mechanics: 1. Left ventricular mechanomycardiography, a new approach to the detection of diseased myocardial elements and states. Med Biol Eng and Comp 18:271–280

Gould P, Ghista D, Brombolich L, Mirsky J (1972) In-vivo stresses in the human left ventricular wall: analysis accounting for the irregular 3-dimensional geometry and comparison with idealised geometry analyses. J Biomechanics 5:521–539

Greenbaum RA, Ho SY, Gibson DG, Becker AE, Anderson RH (1981) Left ventricular fiber architecture in man. B Heart J 45:248–263

Gunton MC, Rosten HJ, Spalding DB, Tatchell DG (1983) Phoenics, an instruction manual. CHAM TR/75

Hadingham PT (1983) The stress state in the human left ventricle. Adv Cardiovascular Phys 5:88–105

Heethaar RM, Pao YC, Ritman EL (1977) Computer aspects of three-dimensional finite-element: analysis of stresses and strains in the intact heart. Comp and Biomed Res 10:291–295

Horowitz A, Perl M, Sideman S: Minimization of fiber length changes and mechanical work in the heart muscle. Submitted for publication

Janz RF, Kubert BR, Moriarty TF, Grimm AF (1974) Deformation of the diastolic left ventricle – II. Nonlinear Geometric Effects. J Biomechanics 7:509–516

Mirsky I (1969) Left ventricular stresses in the intact human heart. Biophys J 9:189–208

Neckyfarow CW, Perlman AB (1976) Deformation of the human left ventricle: material and geometric effects. Proc 4th New-England Bioeng Conf, 169–172

Panda SC, Natarajan R (1977) Finite-element method of stress analysis in the human left ventricular layered wall structure. Med Biol Eng Comp 15:67–71

Pao YC, Ritman EL, Wood EH (1974) Finite-element analysis of left ventricular myocardial stresses. J Biomechanics 7:469–477

Pao YC, Robb RA, Ritman EL (1976) Plane-strain finite-element analysis of reconstructed diastolic left ventricular cross section. Ann Biomed Eng 4:232–249

Pao YC, Ritman EL (1977) Viscoelastic, fibrous, finite-element, dynamic analysis of beating heart. Proc Symp Appl Comp Meth, 477–486

Pao YC, Nagendra GK, Padiyar R, Ritman EL (1980) Derivation of myocardial stiffness equation based on theory of laminated composites. J Biomech Eng 102:252–257

Peskin CS (1975) Mathematical aspects of heart physiology. Courant Institute of Mathematical Sciences, New York

Pinto JG, Fung YC (1973) Mechanical properties of the heart muscle in the passive state. J Biomechanics 6:597–616

Ritman EL, Kinsey JH, Robb RA, Gilbert BK, Harris LD, Wood EH (1980) Three-dimensional imaging of heart, lung and circulation. Science 210:273–280

Ross AL (1972) A finite element computer program for the nonlinear structural analysis of the heart. General Electric Report No. 72SD213

SAP7, User Manual, 1982 Structural mechanics computer laboratory, University of Southern California

Sonnenblick EH, Skelton CL, Spotnitz WD, Feldman D (1963) Redefinition of the Ultrastructural basis of cardiac length-tension relations. Circ 48

Streeter DD, Ramesh N, Vaishnav DJP, Spotnitz HM, Ross J, Sonnenblick EH (1970) Stress distribution in the canine left ventricle during diastole and systole. Biophys J 10:345–363

Streeter DD (1979) Gross morphology and fiber geometry of the heart. In: RM Berne et al. (eds) Handbook of Physiology, Section 2: The Cardiovascular System, Vol. 1, The Heart, Bethesda Md, American Physiological Society

Tozeren A (1983) Static Analysis of the Left Ventricle. J Biomech Eng 105:39–46

Yettram AL, Vinson CA (1979) Geometric Modelling of the human left ventricle. J Biomech Eng 101:1221–1223

Yettram AL, Vinson CA, Gibson DG (1983) Effect of myocardial fiber architecture on the behaviour of the human left ventricle in diastole. J Biomed Eng 5:321–328

Wong YK, Rautaharju PM (1968) Stress distribution within the left ventricle wall approximated as a thick ellipsoidal shell. Am Heart J 75:649–662

Wong YK (1973) Myocardial mechanics: application of sliding-filament theory to isovolumic contraction of the left ventricle. J Biomechanics 6:565–581

DISCUSSION

JANICKI: I realize your problem is very complicated, but I noticed you overlooked the role of external forces, such as thoracic pressure, for example. I wonder if you just overlooked it, or if you think it is not important in your modelling?

ANS: Once you specify the forces, i can put them into the model. That's the easiest part of the program. the problem is to identify the forces. As with the many other parameters that I have mentioned, the problem is to know exactly the physiology and not how to introduce them into the model.

FEIGL: If you are interested in an engineering solution, one that contains coronary blood flow, then dividing the ventricle into inner and outer halves puts you at a big disadvantage because there are literally hundreds of papers which divide the ventricle in 3 or 4 or sometimes more layers and measure coronary blood flow with microspheres and so forth. Those data are tabulated and one can have them.

ANS: I presented only a tentative picture because if I had put 10 layers into the picture, nobody would have seen anything. I don't really mean to put 2 layers. The number of layers will depend upon the capacity of the computer we shall be employing. I am not quite sure if we can handle 10 layers with our present capacity, but I think we can have 3 or 4 layers, at least. You can have fewer layers in the peripheral direction at the expense of more layers in the thickness.

BEYAR: There are 2 brick elements in this model which actually represents 5 layers, and thus one can specify stresses, strains and any other parameter at 5 points through the LV wall thickness.

ANS: Indeed, in the same way that we can put 5 layers of truss elements, one can put 5 layers of whatever you wish. But this is not the point. The number 2 is not a magic number. It is only a matter of means. If we get a bigger computer, we can have 6 layers or more.

RITMAN: You mentioned that you fixed the base in space. Certainly all our information in the intact dog seems to indicate that the apex stays fixed. If that is the case, then the myocardium might, in a manner of speech, be pulled over the blood, as a sleeve might be, so you don't really have to postulate a pressure gradient within the ventricular chamber for the blood to move out into the aorta.

ANS: I thank you for this information. It wouldn't be difficult to choose clamping or fixation or hinging or any other boundary condition as long as it can prevent rigid body movements. We need to have more than one point fixed in space in order to prevent rigid body movement and I don't know at this moment exactly how to do it at the apex, but it is probably possible. What we do know, and Dr. Sagawa may correct me, is that hinged base, can prevent rigid body movement.

SKORTON: My comment about the finite elements has to do with Dr. Feigl's request to have more than 2 layers. We have been doing an analysis somewhat similar to this and I find it always an act of faith as to where the nodal coordinates of any nodes are inside the wall, even if you only have 2 layers and you're finding the nodal coordinates of the separation between those layers by always dividing the wall in half throughout the cycle. We know, of course, that the endocardial and epicardial layers don't thicken the same amount. And if you have 5 or 6 layers across the wall, how do you decide where the nodal coordinates are in those layers? The only way you can do it is either to assume an even distribution across the wall or to put in intracardial markers which is a big task and probably changes the parameters.

ANS: I am not going to do this. I would like to comment that if you assume a linear distribution for the fibers, then, probably, an equal thickness for the inner and outer layers will be normal. There is a dispute today about the fiber distribution through the wall, and if someone is really able to give us the real distribution, we'll use this information in order to decide about the thickness of the layers. The better information we have, anatomically speaking, the better the model.

SAGAWA: You wanted somebody to give you the information as to how the thickening from layers and layers proceeds. I think we can. We are investigating one method, i.e. by implanting a large number of beads, some 40 beads, in various layers and locations of the ventricle and taking biplane X-rays. We have been successful in identifying the spatial position of these beads in the ventricular wall with an accuracy of something like 0.1 mm, which is pretty good.

General discussion on cardiac mechanics

DINNAR: I want to direct may questions to Dr. Perl, Prof. Pao, and maybe Prof. Skorton. We saw the complexity in tackling this problem, especially in the idea of adding markers and changing the description from a shape into a vector displacement which is actually the real picture at a time. Can a mathematical model, like the one suggested here by Dr. Sagawa, or by others, be of any help? Can they reduce the complexity of the problem? Can we use the knowledge from 1-D models to help solve the 3-D actual models?

PAO: We are lacking the knowledge as to how to measure regional effects. There are difficulties involved, but Dr. Sagawa advised us that there's already been some work done by implanting of beads and I know that Dr. Ritman has done the Rentgen opacity. So there's a hope. We may be able to estimate the intramyocardial blood volume relative to the entire wall during every instant and that would help to estimate the local material property. You expect this property to change from region to region. I don't think I have an answer to your question because you tried to lump the 3-D problem into a 1-D problem.

BASSINGTHWAIGHTE: I'm concerned with priorities. What is to be done first; simplification of the model for convenience, or reduction of the model after gaining specific knowledge. We are facing the problem of not having enough data but at the same time wanting to develop models that work. Therefore there is a basis for *a priori* simplification. The problem is that the parameters you derive from much oversimplified models are probably wrong and then the question is, what can you do instead? If you follow Dr. Perl's scheme, you would spend many years evolving a scheme wherein you put in the correct data, integrate them appropriately and after that you would be in a position to do model reduction. That is a desirable but lengthy state of affairs. Of this afternoon's presentations, the one that appealed to me the most in one sense was Dr. Welkowitz's. He actually showed the fitting of an isovolumic pressure time curve. That was a step in the right direction. Dr. Sagawa gave a presentation that was beautiful from the didactic point of view, but it did not give me an understanding of how the ventricle could be constructed in order to produce the result. What I would have liked him to have done was to fit the pressure-volume curves with his model, at each of the different pre-conditions, volume or length, and then to show that the behaviour of the complex model could be well represented by the simplified state that he ended up with. Instead, he seemed to jump from the concept to the simplified state and showed that it made general sense. It surely does, but it is a nice teaching exercise rather than a means of understanding what goes on in the tissue. That is my problem today and that is why I ask whether Dinnar's question is appropriate. Can we reduce the model without understanding it in the complex, more realistic, form. Reduction without comprehension gives simplification, to be sure, but with the risk of serious error.

GESELOWITZ: I was going to come along the same lines to a slightly different conclusion. We've has a number of discussions about models, and their role. An important aspect of models is elegance.

Any cursory review of the history of physics indicates the importance of beauty in models. Dr. Welkowitz's presentation started out by talking about a system where pressure, impedances, etc. is time varying. If you're starting out with a system with time varying impedences, you have, I think, an elegant model. Dr. Sagawa and co-workers used a single capacitance that varies with time. All these models have limitations. I'm not sure exactly what limitations Dr. Sagawa's model has. I'm sure it doesn't have any limitations worse than others. It contains everything that Dr. Welkowitz's model has. Furthermore, I can see in that model what is going on in the heart muscle in terms of the active processes and so forth.

BASSINGTHWAIGHTE: This is a very good point. Simplifying features allow understanding. The question is whether the parameters of the simplified model give you correct information with respect to cellular events. In a way we have two goals: one is to understand the physiology from the cellular level all the way to the dynamics of the myocardium; the other is to obtain an appreciation of mechanical events that can be applied to be understanding of more global events, as in disease states. These are in a sense, separate, sometimes opposing, goals. The elegance lies more toward the latter understanding than the cellular end.

SAGAWA: I would like to respond to these points. First, obviously, my model is a lumped parameter model, with everything lumped into a single parameter. Dr. Welkowitz's model is also a lumped parameter model, although it has a much more components in it. Does it tell anything of the cell? I don't think either model can tell us anything directly about the cell. The purpose of the model is, certainly, to evaluate the global functions of the ventricle as a pumping chamber; we also try to characterize some pathological changes in terms of these parameters. Can a single elastance parameter, for example, represent the local, regional schemic condition of the heart? Yes. We showed that when we caused various degreess of regional ischemia, the end systolic pressure-volume curve, instead of decreasing its slope as in the case of global ischemia shifted to the right side, to a degree proportional to the size of regional ischemia. So the end systolic pressure-volume relationship can tell us of some kind of regional abnormalities, as well. I didn't understand quite clearly what Dr. Bassingthwaighte said about my not explaining ventricular dynamics and instead jumping to some didactic concept.

BASSINGTHWAIGHTE: I don't wish to appear overly critical of your masterful work, but merely to emphasize a principle. If I tried to make a model encompassing myofilament shortening within the sarcomere, force transmission through the interconnections between sarcomeres and cells, and the cells with interstitial collagen, and then take into account the fiber directions in the ventricle, I should end up with a model of the performance of the whole ventricle, as you do, and examine flow versus impedance. But it would be a hardy soul who would try to encompass all those things in one model. However, if one were to have all of those things in one model, one could make certain reductions by taking simple equations that would describe the elements that you know precisely, because then you could make descriptors out of what would be a physical-chemical model and shorten them up. That would be, formally, model reduction. My criticism of your presentation was that I couldn't see the steps from the pressure volume curve which your model probably describes, for each of those individual flow-impedance curves rather than just providing the loops. I would have enjoyed seeing the fitting of the loops to the model.

SAGAWA: I now understand your question and I think it comes back to the same question as Dr. Dinnar raised. I agree with everything you said. This is a temporary model for quick and dirty understanding and it should be replaced with a more detailed, precise and reduced kind of model. In my talk today, the whole set of pressure-volume loops has been reduced to a single volume elastance by opting to look only at their end systolic points. This is the first drastic reduction. P-V loops thus disappear. Likewise, aortic input is represented simply by another volume elastance which is non-physical. At each end systole, so much stroke volume is transferred to the aortic effective elastance (or compliance). As a result, some pressure will be generated in the arterial elastance which is very close to incisura pressure. Because no parallel resistance is coupled to the elastance, the stroke volume transference and arterial pressure built up remain unaltered. The stroke volume has to be discharged before the next transfer of stroke volume happens. Thus, arterial pressure will stepwise go down to zero and then quickly rise to the next pressure in response to the next stroke volume transferred from the ventricular elastance. It is a dynamic, pulsatile, but discrete, quantized simulation of ventricular ejection.

JARON: I want to make one more coment about the issue of modelling. It is clear to all of us that we don't have a comprehensive model at this point in time that will describe everything in which we are interested. Consequently we are all dealing with models which are imperfect which describe only part of the phenomena. In looking at these models, one has to ask whether the models that we construct answer the specific questions in which we are interested? If we are interested in the global properties of the left ventricle, and how it is coupled to the arterial system, then we have, at least a partial handle on it through some models that were presented here. If we are interested in the biochemical aspects, then there are other ways to approach it. Obviously it would be ideal to combine all of them into one comprehensive model. We can not do that at present.

I want to make one other comment regarding the difference between Dr. Sagawa's model and Dr. Welkowitz's model. Both are lumped models. Dr. Sagawa's model, however, is appropriate for only one point in time, namely end systole. Dr. Sagawa has extended the model to represent the ventricular system in the normal state. The lumped model that Dr. Welkowitz presented represents the full cardiac cycle.

Another question is whether the models that Dr. Sagawa and Dr. Janicki have presented deal with the isolated ventricle. I would like to hear what is the applicability of the isolated case to the in situ system.

GESELOWITZ: We had a very elegant presentation from Dr. Pearl as to all the complexities of modelling of the ventricle. What we would end up with through all of this is the details of the actual shape and the pressures, stresses in the wall. As far as the heart as a pump is concerned, what we have is a volume of the ventricle, and the intraventricular pressure. This is precisely what Dr. Sagawa's model gives us. In a very simplistic way I can go from that through a spherical model, and Dr. Mirsky has said that spherical models don't vary very much from non spherical models in certain cases. And you can put in all the cardiac mechanics you want – a thin wall, a thick wall, the forcelength relations, etc – and you can see how his time varying elastance pairs with what the predictions of that are. But if we don't want to wait 5 years until an exact model really tells us what that is, I see a very direct connection between the parameters of the Sagawa model and the parameters of this complex cardiac mechanical model.

MIRSKY: A comment to Dr. Geselowitz's comment. We are missing the power of the mathematical model. First, I think that the qualitative aspects are very important. If you go through all the literature in physiology, I'm sure that you will find that 60–70% of the experiments conducted in the animal lab are of a qualitative nature. That is where the mathematical models are probably needed the most. Maybe we are overemphasizing the quantitative aspects of these models and we shouldn't. When we can't get a good model, we can fall back on the experimentalist; we just don't have the data. One of the main purposes of mathematical modeling, I think, is to help guide the course of what the next experiment should be. One can save a lot of animals, a lot of money and a lot of labour by conducting a lot of numerical experiments first. This is something that has been overlooked. I really think it is a feedback system; a two-way street. We don't just model ad infinitum and we shouldn't be conducting experiments ad infinitum. Unfortunately, that's what we do, and a lot of experiments are just wasted. If some of the experimentalists took time out to acquaint themselves with some of the models that are being developed and formed relationships with some of these investigators, maybe they would not have conducted some of the experiments in the first place.

JANICKI: I want to reply to the comment about the isolated heart preparation. First of all, I don't want to be in the position where I have to defend any model, but we did check out our models in the intact open chest dog where we could cross clamp it and were able to produce the isovolumetric relationships as well as the measured peak isovolumetric pressure. I think that the model does apply equally well to the open chest intact heart.

JARON: There is a very close relationship between the models that were presented by Drs. Janicki and Sagawa and Welkowitz, and the finite element models that we are talking about. The important thing to remember is that the differences of concern are the differences between the global behaviour of the left ventricle and the behaviour that deals with regional differences. Obviously, the global model will never be able to represent these regional issues.

FEIGL: I'd like to reply to Dr. Mirsky. As one of the few experimentalists in the room, I think it goes both ways. It's difficult for the experimentalist to keep up with the mathematics and the sophisticated techniques that you use. Your papers are hard for us to read so we don't design our experiments to answer exactly the questions that you would like answered. On the other hand, you often present us with models which don't relate to a whole generation's worth of experimental work that's been done in cardiac muscle mechanics. There is a lot of muscle mechanics that's been done and Dr. Mirsky's particularly aware of this. The potential beauty of the Haifa Model is that the linear papillary muscle type cardiac muscle mechanics may be incorporated into a global model. It can be tested at these two levels: global perfomance and fiber cardiac mechanics. That gives us to two points to test and compare and that has a nice potential. It remains to be seen how much fruit it bears.

Quantitative 3-D imaging of the heart: myocardium and chambers

ERIK L. RITMAN, ERIC A. HOFFMAN, TSUTOMU IWASAKI,
ROBERT S. SCHWARTZ, and LAWRENCE J. SINAK
Department of Physiology and Biophysics and Division of Cardiovascular Diseases and Internal Medicine Mayo Foundation Rochester, MN 55905, U.S.A.

Abstract

Accurate quantitation of the shape and dimensions of all cardiac chambers and myocardium is possible with the Dynamic Spatial Reconstructor (DSR). Generally a single bolus injection of approximately 2 ml/kg roentgen contrast agent in the right atrium will provide information of the chamber volumes and myocardial mass within 5% of the actual value. The detailed shape of the chambers and myocardium facilitates evaluation of heart deformed by complex congenital heart disease or myocardial infarction (aneurysm).

Introduction

Form and motion combine, in a proportion depending on the organ in question, to generate function. For the heart, motion is particularly important, the anatomy itself would not allow one to confidently predict its function. Although we need to measure both form and motion, in the heart a major limitation to analysis has been the inability to measure form precisely and without ambiguity.

Methods

The dynamic spatial reconstructor system

In response to this problem we built the Dynamic Spatial Reconstructor (DSR) which is illustrated in Figure 1 (Kinsey *et al.*, 1980; Ritman *et al.*, 1980). This artist's rendition of the machine shows a subject lying horizontally along the axis of rotation of a circular drum. To one half of the perimeter of this drum are attached 14 television cameras and on the opposite half of the drum are attached 14 X-ray tubes. By rapid sequential electronic actuation of these X-ray tubes and

136

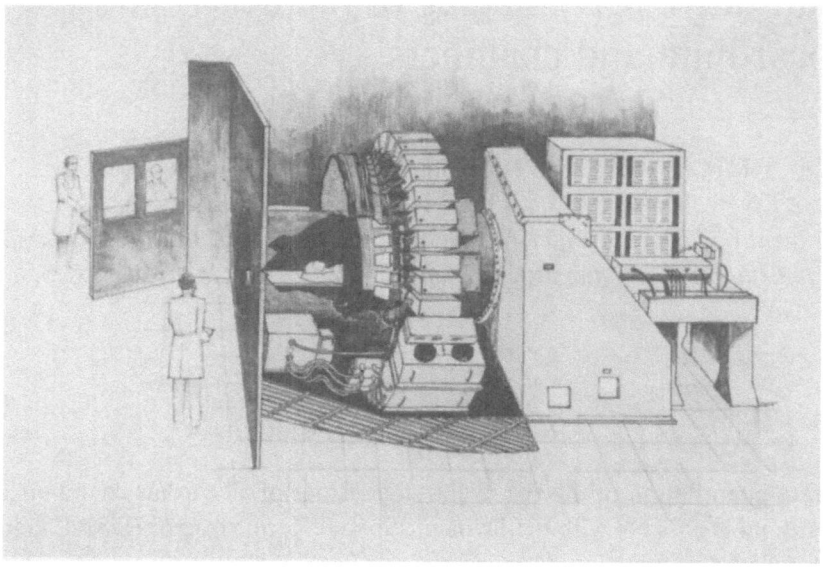

Figure 1. Artist's concept of Dynamic Spatial Reconstructor. Cutaway diagram shows a patient lying on a table that is surrounded by a semicircular array of 14 X-ray tubes (lower half) and television cameras (upper half). At the patient's feet is a large bearing that enables the gantry to be rotated continuously around the patient (Schwartz *et al.*, 1983b).

their corresponding opposite TV cameras, we obtain a complete scan in 1/100th of a second. Because the system is television based, the scans can be repeated 60 times per second.

The four major features of the DSR scanner that we believe to be important for the accurate measurement of structure to function relationship in the cardiovascular system are; (1) It scans a volume, (2) it does so synchronously, (3) it does this in stop-action so that the blurring due to motion is less than one pixel (generally less than 1 mm on a side) and (4) it can repeat this scan at 60 times per second. This latter feature is important for evaluation of the motion part of the structure-to-function relationship.

Figure 2 is a schematic representation of how the DSR works. A TV camera scans many cross sections of the heart over its entire apex to base extent. The TV image is an electronic analog signal with its amplitude proportional to the brightness in the image which in turn is proportional to the amount of x-ray impinging on the fluorescent screen. A computer uses this image information from many angles of view in order to calculate the cross section image using computed tomographic principles.

The entire DSR system is conveniently divided into the DSR scanner section, the reconstruction section, and the data analysis section. The reconstruction system utilizes a filtered back-projection fan beam reconstruction system based on a floating point array processor (Robb *et al.*, 1980). Most important to the

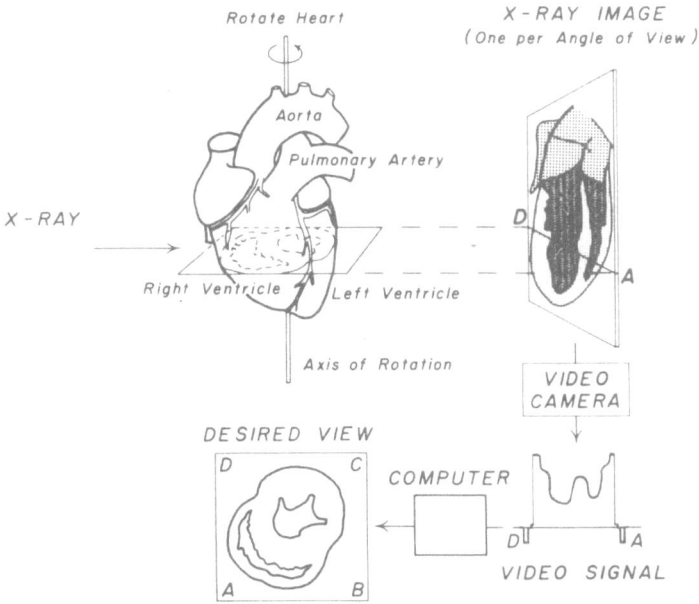

Figure 2. Illustration of geometry and data pathways for reconstructing cross section of canine heart from multiplanar roentgen projections. Three-dimensional X-ray absorption images of the heart can be constructed at 1/60 s intervals throughout the cardiac cycle in the form of a sequence of up to 120 parallel adjacent two-dimensional X-ray attenuation cross-sectional images covering the full anatomic extent of the heart (Robb *et al.*, 1974).

presentation in hand is the data analysis system where the operator interacts with the 3-dimensional image set (Harris, 1981). First, the DSR generates a cubic array of picture elements. This array can be sectioned into coronal, sagittal and transverse sections, as well as oblique sections. Various 3-D imaging techniques can also be used. A key feature of the DSR is that each of the multiple slices is 0.9 mm thick. This is of critical importance if the 3-D resolution of the DSR is to be equal in all directions. This feature is readily illustrated in Figure 3. We used the resolution phantom shown and scanned it with its resolution elements at the three orientations relative to the scanning plane. It is quite clear that the resolution, in all three directions, is comparable.

DSR image data analysis

Figure 4 is an artist's concept of the three major techniques for display of 3-D image information. The upper row indicates what we can *projection dissolution*, a method by which 3-D image information is displayed on a 2-D screen as though projected like a conventional X-ray. Unlike a conventional X-ray we can selectively 'dissolve' our tissues at various contrast levels. The middle row shows that

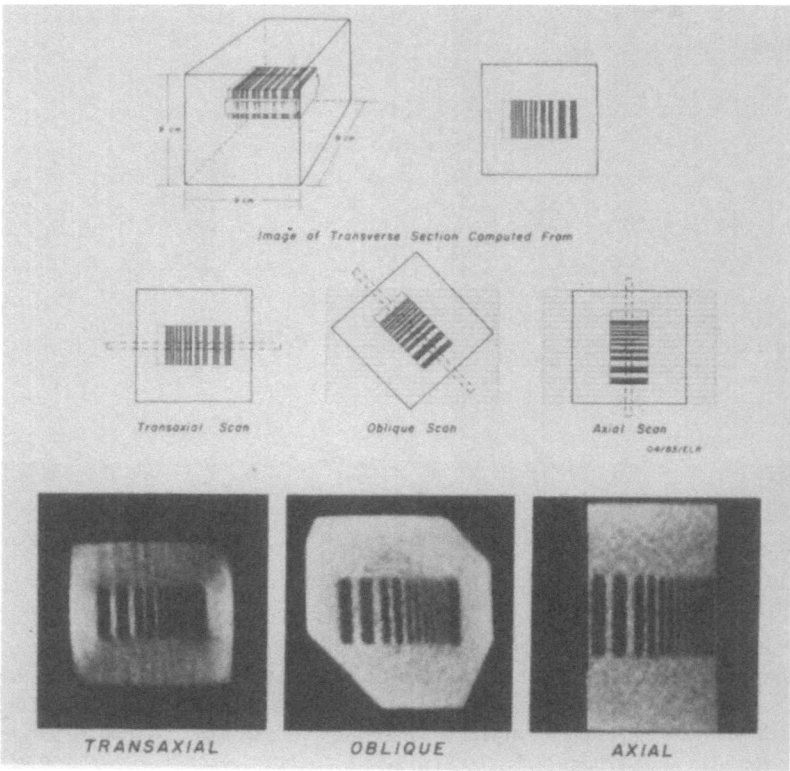

Figure 3. (Upper panel) Plexiglas Phantom was scanned with the plane containing the resolution elements held parallel, oblique, and at right angles to the DSR scan plane. The reconstructed transverse sections were used to compute images of slices in the plane containing the resolution elements. (Lower panel) DSR tomographic images of 3.6 mm thick slices of the radiologic phantom. The corners in the oblique image and the truncation of the left and right sides of the axial scan image are due to restriction of the volume reconstructed to the region of interest in the original scan data. The spatial resolution in all images is essentially identical. (*Upper panel* – Ritman *et al.,* in press 1984;

we can *rotate* the image information in the computer prior to display and provide angles of view not available in conventional *X-rays*. The bottom row shows the ability to do *numerical 'surgery'* on these images. This technique is useful for facilitating comprehension of complex anatomic relationships as might occur inside the heart.

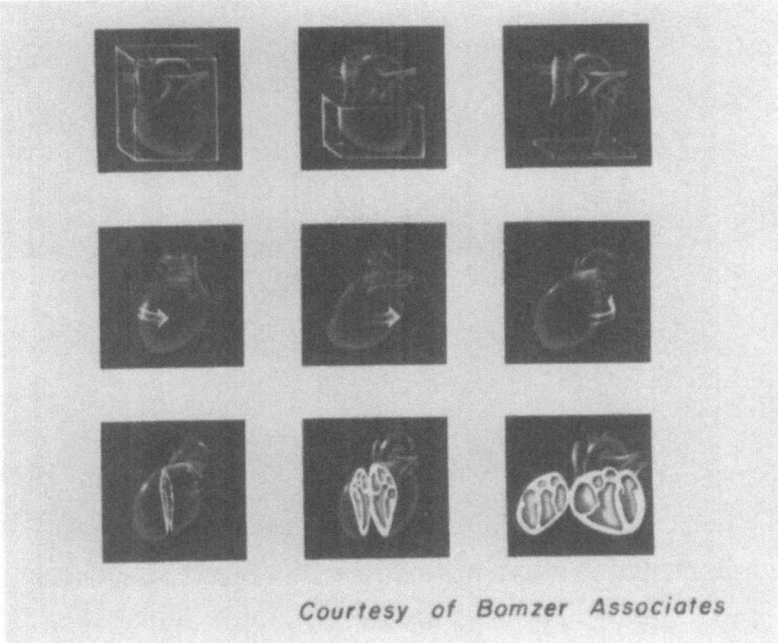

Courtesy of Bomzer Associates

Figure 4. Artist's description of three methods of 3-D image display. *Upper row* – projection 'dissolution' applied progressively so as to leave only the dye-filled vessels. *Middle row* – surface display with rotation of entire heart. *Lower row* – numerical 'dissection' of the surface display.

Results

Cardiac chambers

In the lower three panels of Figure 5 is a display of a plastic cast of the right and left cardiac chambers and the corresponding major vessels. This cast was scanned *in situ* in a dead dog using a scan aperture of 0.06 s which would allow for stopaction imaging of end diastole and end systole of a beating heart (Hoffman *et al.*, 1984a). The animal was scanned and the DSR data were used to compute a 3-D type image surface display as shown in the upper row. This cast and the 3-D image data were later broken down into the right and left side chambers. The real and DSR-based shapes correspond closely and the volumes computed from the DSR image corresponds very closely to that measured by water displacement. In Figure 6 we see that the volume of the ventricular chambers measured by water displacement and by DSR image analysis is very close to a one-to-one relationship over a considerable range of volumes. This display analysis method has been applied to some preliminary physiological experiments (Hoffman *et al.*, 1983,

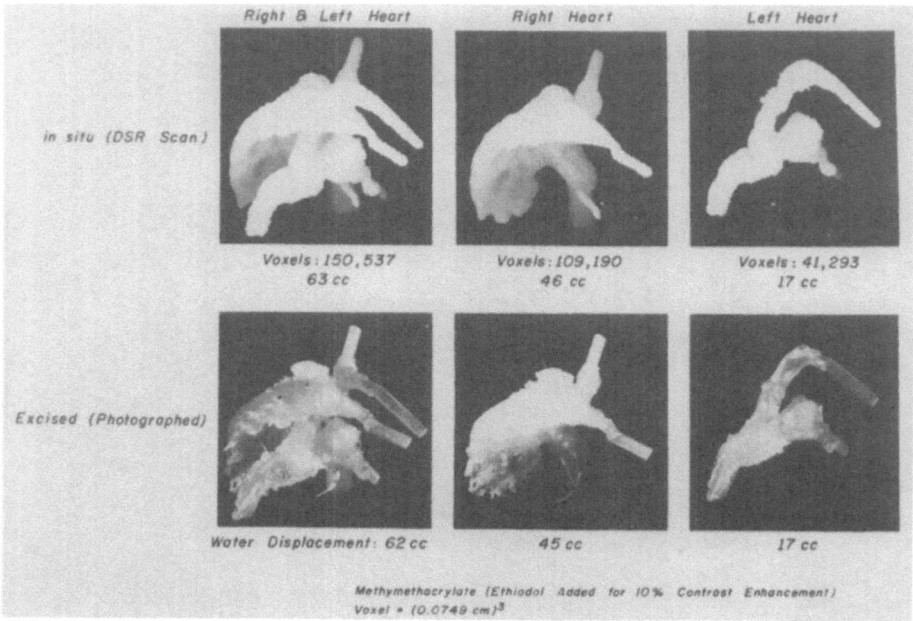

Figure 5. Upper row – Surface displays of the contrast agent in the right and left cardiac chambers. Dog's heart chambers were filled with methyl methacrylate so as to form a fixed cast in the in situ heart. Ethiodol was added to increase roentgen contrast to that expected following intravenous injection of 2 ml/kg contrast agent. *Lower row* – the casts removed from the dog following the scan. (Hoffman and Ritman, submitted 1984a.)

1984b). As shown in Figure 7 the change in shape and size of the cardiac chambers from end diastole to end systole is as expected. Consequently we are confident that the dynamic 3-D shape of the cardiac chambers can be accurately measured with the DSR.

The same display approach was applied to the DSR data acquired in a patient with congenital heart disease (Sinak *et al.,* 1984a and Sinak *et al.,* 1984b). In the patients we have little chance of accurately validating what we see with the DSR, but in view of the accuracy demonstrated in the dog studies we are very confident that the DSR image is a realistic representation of the true chambers.

In another application of this type of image analysis is in a patient as shown in Figure 8 (Schwartz *et al.,* 1983a). An aneurysm of the left ventricle chamber is shown in a conventional view in the upper two panels. In the lower two panels the ventricle is shown from the diaphragmatic aspect. The active part of the ventricle, as well as the large apical bulbous aneurysmal region, is clearly defined and the extent of the normal myocardium is also clearly visible. This sort of information can also be analyzed quantitatively as shown in Figure 9 which shows that the

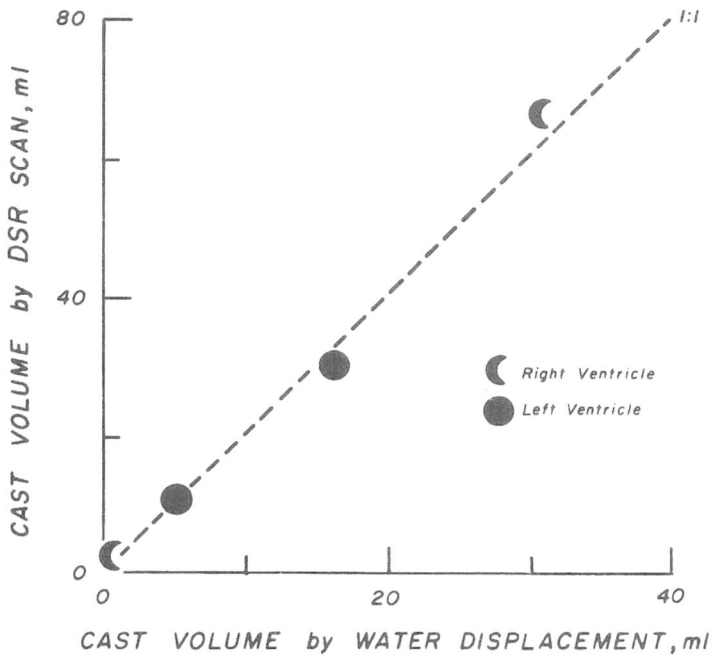

Figure 6. Accuracy of DSR based estimates of ventricular chambers compared with direct water displacement of the plastic casts of the chambers. Data from (Hoffman and Ritman, submitted 1984a).

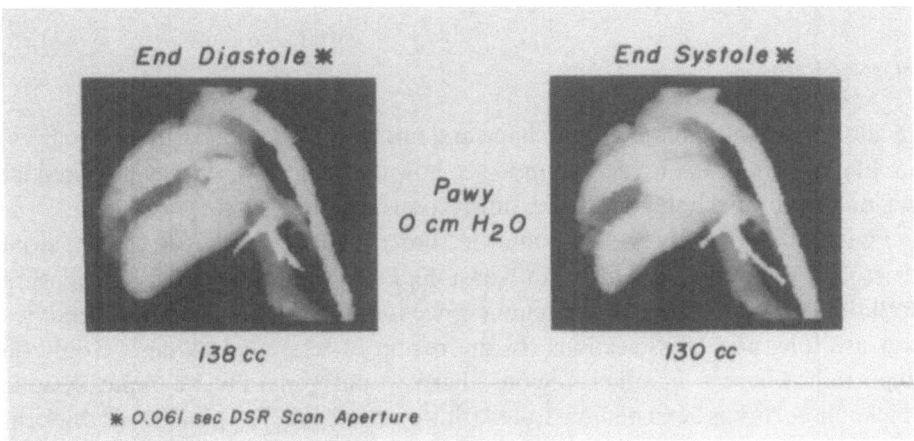

Figure 7. 3-D surface displays of cardiac chambers at end systole and end diastole with airway open to atmosphere. Note appropriate change in size of chambers and major vessels with phase of cardiac cycle (Hoffman and Ritman, 1984a).

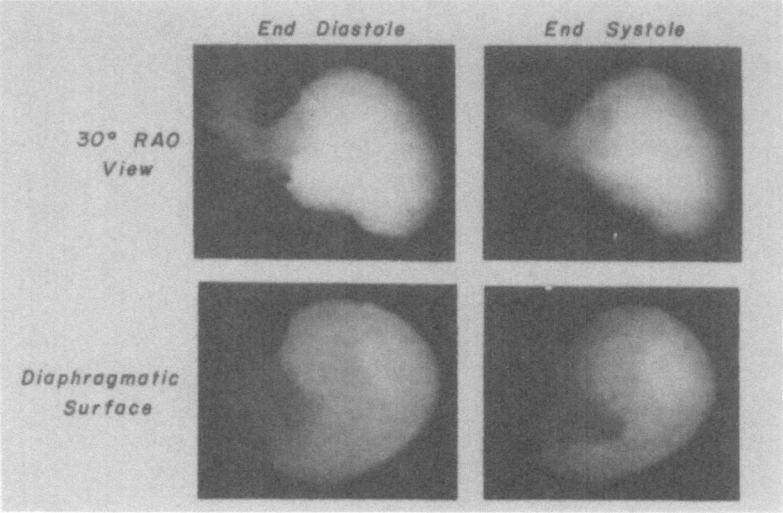

Figure 8. Surface display of human (62 year old male) left ventricle with apical aneurysm. Scan performed during levo phase of bolus injection of renografin into pulmonary trunk (Sinak *et al.*, 1984d).

volume of just the aneurysm region does not change whereas the volume of the normally functioning region changes appropriately. It is to be hoped, and we plan to look at this, that by correlating the absolute volume of the normal part of the heart to the patient's size, that we can predict quantitatively the cardiac function after aneurysmectomy.

Myocardium

In addition to these more global shape and function aspects of cardiac chambers, we like to look at the myocardium to see how it functions. One way is to look at regional wall thickening following intravenous injection of contrast agent.

Figure 10 is of a section through the short axis of the heart of a dog, from diastole through systole and back to diastole. From these images we can measure wall thickness over the entire circumference for all cross sections. If desired, we can use long axis cross sections. In the region of infarction akinesis would be expected, whereas in other regions there would generally be rapid systolic thickening. As has been demonstrated (Sutton *et al.*, 1982), regional wall thickening during systole seems to correlate quite well with myocardial blood supply. The rate of thickening as well as the rate of thinning during diastole seem to be closely related. Another approach to extend this type of approach we need to look at the entire wall and display this in some manner as shown in Figure 11. The

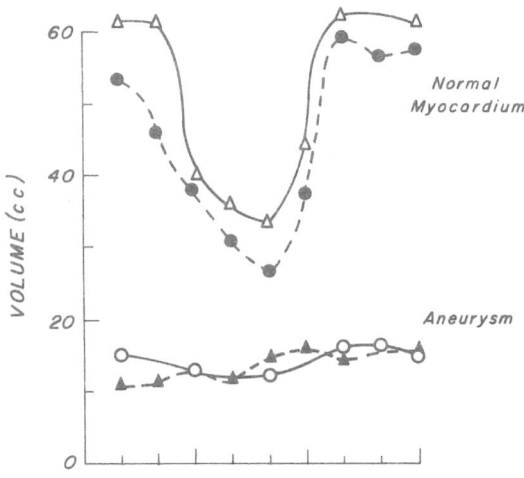

Figure 9. Volume of functional part of left ventricle chamber and of aneurysmal part in a 20.5 kg dog six weeks after occlusion of left anterior descending coronary artery. Data from (Schwartz *et al.*, submitted 1984).

magnitude of regional wall thickening at many circumferential points for all cross sections can be plotted as a square array as shown. Instead of a square array a geometrically transformed array, which retains some of the geometry of the myocardium, is shown in Figure 12. If the rate of wall thickening is plotted as an intensity at each wall location a functional surface display results. Note the aortic

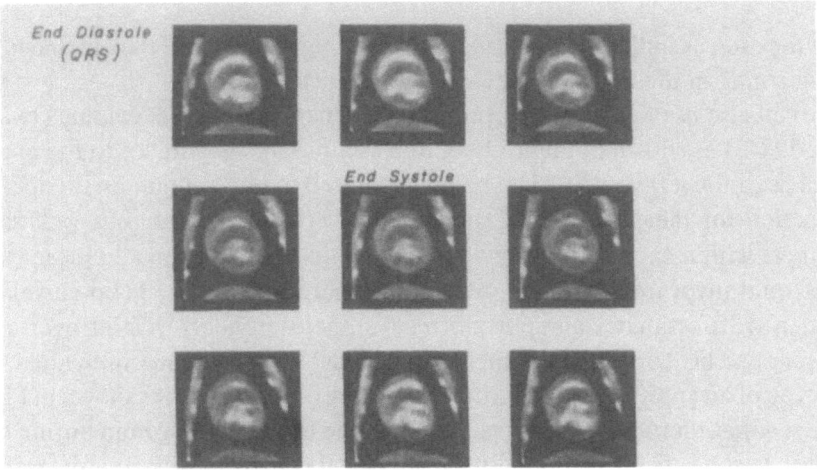

Figure 10. Sequential images of sections through the short axis of the left ventricle generated after weighted subtraction processing of volume images. Each slice is 7.8 mm thick and 0.06 s scan duration (Sinak *et al.*, 1984c).

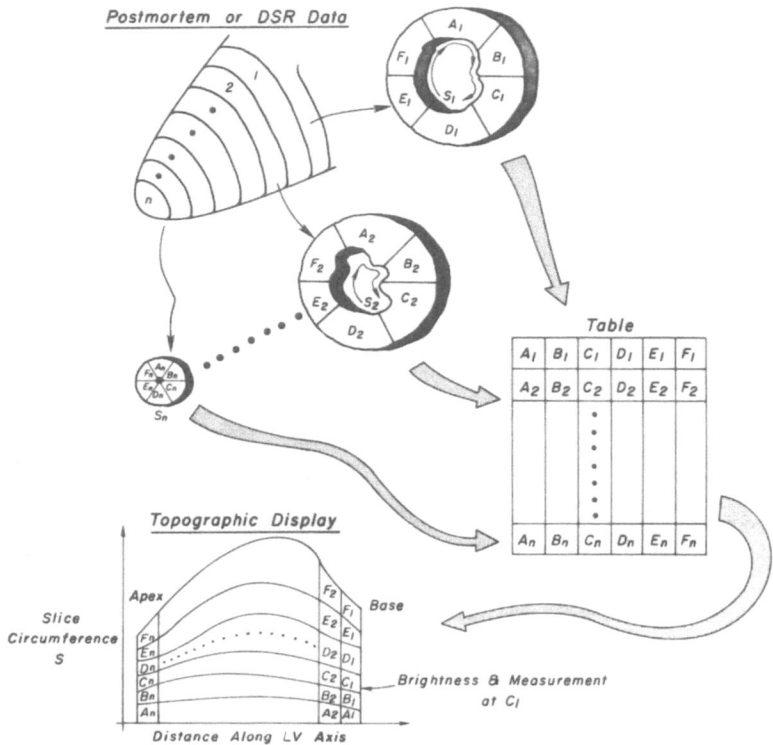

Figure 11. Schematic of analysis sequence and display of regional LV wall thickening magnitude over the entire myocardium of a dog. The resulting square array is plotted over topographic display in which brightness is proportional to regional rate of wall thickening.

valve location as indicated by a reduced rate of thickening and the enhanced rate of thickening in the apical half of the left ventricle.

We can also use this type of approach to estimate myocardial volume (Iwasaki *et al.*, 1984a) as shown in Figure 13. Cross sections at right angles to the apex to base axis of the left ventricle can be planimetered in the computer with operator interaction for measurement of the volume of the myocardium as well as the chambers within each slice. Knowing the slice thickness we can add these values to get total myocardial volume. Shown in Figure 14 is a very good correlation between DSR estimates and postmortem estimates of heart weights over a ten-fold range. This correlation is highly reproducible for any one individual dog. This type of an analysis has lead to an interesting observation. As shown in Figure 15 we see that there is phasic increase in volume of the myocardium during early systole. This has been suspected from statistical considerations in large populations but never have been observed consistently in any one animal using conventional imaging techniques. This is almost certainly due to the change in blood volume within the myocardium during the cardiac cycle (Iwasaki *et al.*, 1984b).

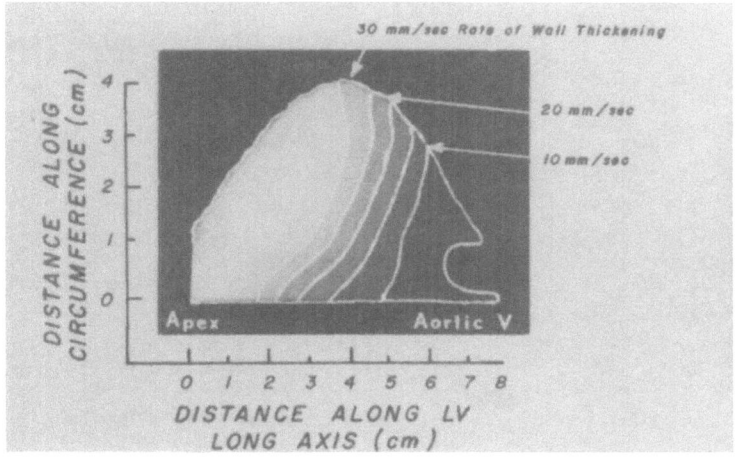

Figure 12. Contoured wall thickening map ($T_{ED} - T_{ES}$) derived from circumferential wall measurement in the images of Figure 13. The difference in wall thickness between end diastole and end systole is related to the contractile state of a region of heart muscle. The horizontal axis is distance along the left ventricular long axis from apex to base. The ordinate is circumferential dimension of the left ventricle. Intensity is the scaled rate of wall thickening (maximum = 40 mm/s; minimum = 4 mm/s) (Schwartz *et al.*, 1983a).

Occasionally we like to look at the entire myocardium, especially when we are interested in the possible surgical implications of a complex defect such as shown here. When we 'cut' the myocardium in the computer the chambers are exposed so that the integrity of the septum can be evaluated. Hopefully from this sort of display the surgeon might be able to determine the suitability of possible surgical correction procedures.

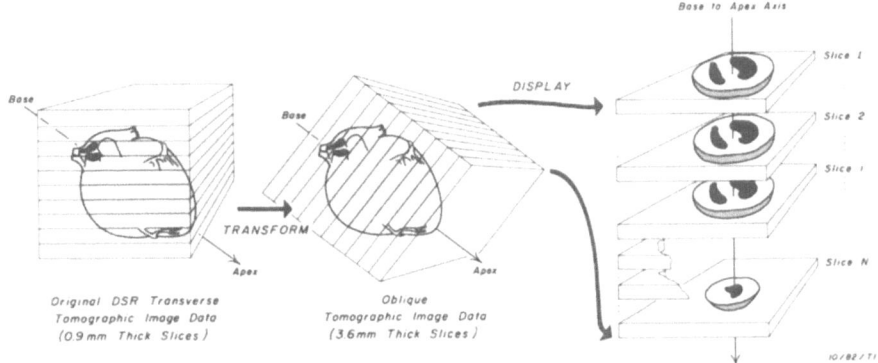

Figure 13. Schematic describing how oblique slices perpendicular to aortoapical axis are generated from original transverse slices to measure volume of left ventricular myocardial and chamber. Original volume (i.e., 3-D) image is made up of transverse slices scanned by DSR (*left panel*); volume image is retrospectively organized into oblique slices (*center*); oblique slices, from apex to base, are then ready for outlining to measure chamber and myocardial area in each slice (*right*) (Iwasaki *et al.*, 1984a).

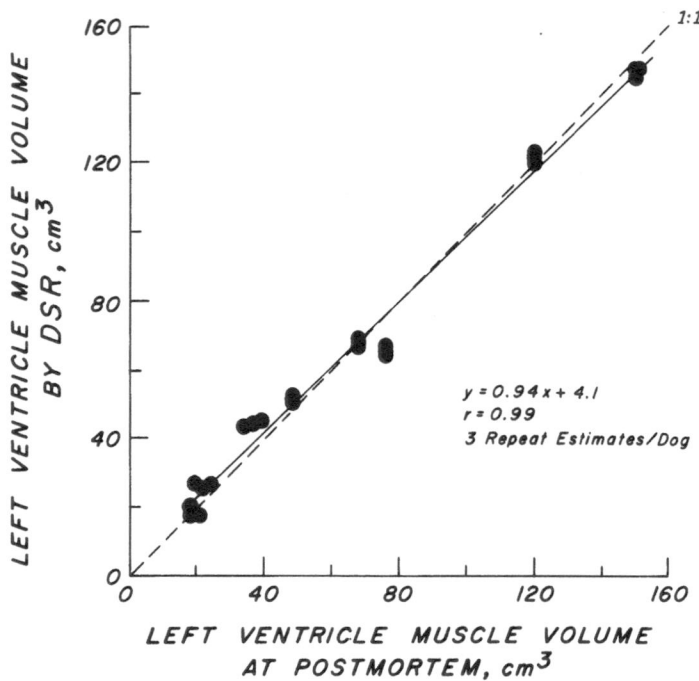

Figure 14. Correlation between left ventricular muscle volume estimated by Dynamic Spatial Recon-structor (DSR) (ordinate) and by postmortem measurements (abscissa). Volume of myocardium estimated by DSR is plotted for three separate measurements for each dog. Regression line was calculated using average of the three measurements by DSR and volume by postmortem study. The eight dogs used (2.5–32.5 kg) had morphine-pentobarbital anesthesia, end diastole, 0.06 s aperture, and superior vena cava injection of 1 ml/kg Iohexol (Iwasaki *et al.*, 1984a).

Conclusion

Using the DSR there are many aspects of cardiac shape and function, both at the global and regional level, for the chamber and myocardial geometry that can be analyzed from a single ventriculogram, often requiring only an intravenous injection of roentgen contrast agent.

Acknowledgments

The authors thank Messrs Steven Richardson and James Hanson for the original art work.

This work was supported in part by the National Institutes of Health Grants HL-04664 and RR-00007.

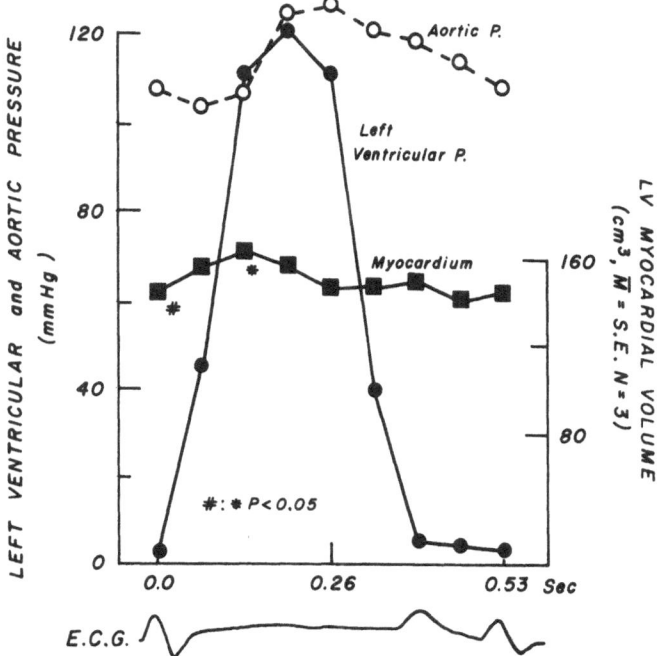

Figure 15. Change of volume of left ventricular myocardium during cardiac cycle in a 32.5-kg dog morphine-pentobarbital anesthesia, heart rate 116 beats/min, 1 ml/kg contrast into superior vena cava, scan aperture 0.061 s. Computed volume at end-diastole is significantly less ($P<0.05$) than peak volume during systole based on results from three sequential heart cycles. This reproducible pattern suggests that blood content of myocardium varies if the muscle itself is assumed to be isovolumic. Electrocardiographic, left ventricular, and aortic pressure signals were recorded in synchrony with video recordings and hence the phasic relationship between computed myocardial volume and physiological signals can be accurately established (Iwasaki *et al.,* 1984a).

References

Behrenbeck T, Kinsey JH, Harris LD, Robb RA, Ritman EL (1982) Three-dimensional spatial, density, and temporal resolution of the Dynamic Spatial Reconstructor. J Comput Assist Tomogr 6:1138–1147

Harris LD (1981) Identification of the optimal orientation of oblique sections through multiple parallel CT images. J Comput Assist Tomogr 5:881–887

Hoffman EA, Ritman EL, Wood EH (1983) Interserosal forces: the pressure environment of the central circulations and nature's internal 'G suits', part II. The Physiologist 26:S165–S168 (Suppl)

Hoffman EA, Ritman EL (Submitted 1984a) Shape and dimensions of cardiac chambers: assessment of a quantitative tomographic imaging technique. Radiology

Hoffman EA, Ritman EL (1984b) Constancy of total heart volume throughout cardiac cycle and role of lung inflation: a computer tomographic measurement with DSR (abstr). Fed Proc 43: 509

Iwasaki T, Sinak LJ, Hoffman EA, Robb RA, Harris LD, Bahn RC, Ritman EL (1984a) Mass of left ventricle myocardium estimated with the Dynamic Spatial Reconstructor. Am J Physiol: Heart and Circulatory Physiol 15:H138–H142

Iwasaki T, Ritman EL (1984b) Intramyocardial blood volume dynamics in the cardiac cycle (abstr). Fed Proc 43(3):442

Kinsey JH, Robb RA, Ritman EL, Wood EH (1980) The DSR – a high temporal resolution volumetric roentgenographic CT scanner. Herz 5:177–188

Ritman EL, Kinsey JH, Robb RA, Gilbert BK, Harris LD, Wood EH (1980) Three-dimensional imaging of the heart, lungs, and circulation. Sci 210: 273–280

Ritman EL, Robb RA, Harris LD (1984) Imaging physiological functions: experience with the DSR. Pennsylvania: Praeger, in press

Robb RA, Wood EH, Ritman EL, Johnson SA, Sturn RE, Greenleaf JF, Gilbert BK, Chevalier PA (1974) Three-dimensional reconstruction and display of the working canine heart and lungs by multiplanar X-ray scanning videodensitometry. Comput Cardiol IEEE Catalog number 74CH0879–7C:151–163

Robb RA, Lent AH, Gilbert BK, Chu A (1980) The Dynamic Spatial Reconstructor: a computer tomography system for high-speed simultaneous scanning of multiple cross sections of the heart. J Med Sys 4:253–288

Schwartz RS, Bove AA, Ritman EL (1983a) Quantitative analysis of three-dimensional images of the left ventricle generated with the DSR. Proc The Seventh Annual Symposium on Computer Applications in Medical Care IEEE Catalog Number 83CH1934–9:804–807

Schwartz RS, Ritman EL (1983b) Computed tomography in cardiac imaging. Practical Cardiol 9:224–238

Schwartz RS, Bove AA, Bahn RC, Ritman EL (Submitted 1984) Three-dimensional regional myocardial function following coronary arterial occlusion-quantitation with the DSR. Annals of Bimedical Engineering

Sinak LJ, Hoffman EA, Julsrud PR, Mair DD, Seward JB, Hagler DJ, Harris LD, Robb RA, Ritman EL (1984a) The Dynamic Spatial Reconstructor: investigating congenital heart disease in four dimensions. Cardiovasc Intervention Radiol 7:124–137

Sinak LJ, Liu YH, Block M, Mair DD, Julsrud PR, Hoffman EA, Hagler DJ, Seward JB, Ritman EL (in press 1984b) Anatomy and function of the heart and intrasthoracic vessels in congenital heart disease-evaluation with the DSR. J Am Coll Cardiol

Sinak LJ, Hoffman EA, Ritman EL (1984c) Subtraction gated computed tomography with Dynamic Spatial Reconstructor: simultaneous evaluation of left and right heart from single right-sided bolus contrast medium injection. J Comput Assist Tomogr 8:1–9

Sinak LJ, Hoffman EA, Ritman EL (1984d) Three-dimensional cardiac anatomy and function in adult heart disease: initial results with the Dynamic Spatial Reconstructor. Mayo Clin Proc, in press

Sutton MG St.J, Ritman EL, (1982) Effects of progressive reduction in coronary blood flow on regional and global left ventricular contraction and relaxation during normal and increased after load: a roentgen videometric study. Cardiovasc Res 16:535–545

DISCUSSION

QUESTION: I was curious about your slide (not shown here) where you showed relationship between coronary flow and wall thickening. Many people have shown that there is a more complicated relationship than just a linear one between those two, and wall thickening seems to be preserved over a wide range of perfusion, as studied by microspheres, for example. There's an exponential or otherwise non linear relation. Over what range of flow measurements were the wall thickning measurements made over?

ANS: Under our conditions the far right of the curve is at about 75% of the control flow and then it starts decreasing as you move to the left. That's quite a consistent finding. If you change the hemodynamic conditions, there may be something different.

SAGAWA: I just happened to notice that your diastolic pressure is rather high in the dog slide.

ANS: The scans are 0.06 s in duration and these pressures are the average over that time. In this particular dog there may already be some systolic pressure included. This dog had a big aneurysm and I'd have to check it out but I think that basically it was a failing heart.

JANICKI: Is it possible to exercise patients in this system and get another scan?

ANS: It is possible. We have not done that, but we could. Patients would have to be supine and work a bicycle. We plan to do that at some stage.

JANICKI: Can you perceive twisting or rotating type motion with this system?

ANS: You get the 3-d picture of the myocardium, but in order to notice rotation you could use the papillary muscle, in patients, or you might put in endocardial screws, in dogs, to watch twisting. You have to have some sort of a marker.

BEYAR: You showed a nice picture of the blood distribution in the myocardium in a certain phase. Do you have details as to how thick is the portion of the endocardium being compressed during systole?

ANS: Dr. Iwasaki in our group is working on it now. From a pulmonary artery injection of contrast agent, he finds the endocardial surface as the blood first comes into the LV and then as it goes around the coronary circulation into the myocardium. He can measure the distribution of the contrast agent, and hence the blood in the myocardium and then relate its concentration to that of the blood in the chamber. And there is a transmural gradient in opacity, presumably blood volume.

QUESTION: On Figure 15, showing myocardial volume and the LV pressure, it looks as if the myocardial volume peaks in early systole and that seems backward to me.

ANS: As to Figure 15 which shows an increase in myocardial volume during early systolic phase, I have the following comments. At first blush this observation does appear to be a paradox in that published data indicate a surge of flow in the coronary sinus and a concurrent cessation of flow in the coronary arteries in the systolic phase. Indeed, it would be easiest if I withdrew that figure for publication at this time. Nonetheless, I wish to keep it in for several reasons.

(1) We have a good reason to believe our measurements. We observed this phenomenon (at least measurements consistent with the phenomenon) by three different modes of image analysis.
(a) Via planimetric evaluation – this is a 'direct' measure of myocardial volume. This method is somewhat open to question because it involves a person outlining the epi and endocardium by 'hand'. On the other hand, there is no reason to believe that the epicardial vessels play a major role in this measurement.
(b) Via 'automated' recognition of the myocardium, this method involves much less operator judgement than does method (a).
(c) Via the 'brightness area product' method which measures the distribution of contrast medium in the intramyocardial blood. This method is attractive because it does not require recognition of the epi or endocardial surfaces. On the other hand, it is possible that epicardial vessels are included in this measurement.
(2) It should be noted that our measurements were performed at 0.06 s intervals – perhaps if we made measurements at more frequent intervals the peak volume may, in fact, have occurred a little earlier.
(3) There is reason to believe that some published data are consistent with our observations. Of special note is the study by Stein et al. using a catheter tip electromagnetic flow meter placed inside the coronary sinus of intact dogs. They demonstrate the maximum outflow to occur in late systole or even early diastole in some dogs. If nothing else, these data suggest that there is considerable variability from dog to dog.
(4) Most published demonstrations of early systolic outflow in the coronary sinus and cessation of

flow in the coronary arteries was performed in open chest dogs or dogs that had had their chests opened (and pericardium left open). It may well be that in the intact (i.e. never opened) chest dogs that the transient transmural pressure changes during systole are quite different in magnitude and phase from the opened chest preparations.

In summary, our observation may be controversial but not totally inconsistent with prevailing wisdom.

Three-dimensional analysis of the cardiovascular system*

PAUL H. HEINTZEN, RÜDIGER BRENNECKE, JOACHIM H. BÜRSCH,
HANS J. HAHNE, DIETRICH W.G. ONNASCH AND
KLAUS MOLDENHAUER
*Department of Pediatric Cardiology and Biomedical Engineering, University of
Kiel, West-Germany*

Abstract

Angiocardiographic methods for quantitative analysis of the dynamic geometry of the heart are described. 3D spatial 'reconstruction' of the left or right ventricle from their traced and digitized contours after contrast injection allow the generation of simplified, but clinically useful 3D models of the ventricles which form the basis for left and right ventricular volume determination and contraction pattern analysis. These models can be improved by combining the biplane density profiles of the projection images with some a priori knowledge.

For many practical purposes a '3-D' dynamic analysis of the cardiovascular system – considering the *time* as the third dimension – has been proved to be extremely useful. From digitized time series of 2-D projection images, on- and off-line processing procedures like subtraction of the background is possible, allowing contrast enhancement and intravenous, or selective angiocardiography, with reduced amounts of contrast material. The most promising applications of dynamic digital processing techniques are the so-called functional or parametric imaging procedures. Since the whole image series represents a matrix of pixel densograms, various time and volume parameters can be obtained. Using this approach, regional flow and perfusion patterns can be obtain from different parts of the circulation and central as well as regional arterial blood flow can be determined quantitatively.

Introduction

The cardiovascular system has three spatial dimensions, characterizing its *anatomy*. It changes its size, shape and blood content, due to rhythmic contraction and relaxation of the central muscle pump *with time* – as an expression of its

* This work has been supported by the Deutsche Forschungsgemeinschaft.

function. Thus for a complete geometric analysis of the anatomy and function we have to deal with four dimensions. Ideally one could try to process always the full 4D data to create the most complete model of the beating heart. From such a model one could select those parameters, or aspects, which represent the clinically relevant information in a given patient. But, provided we would have a clinically applicable method for this type of 4D reconstruction and analysis of the cardiovascular system, this procedure would be in many cases too expensive and time consuming.

Thus, even with the ideal 4-D method, the question would remain:
(1) when do we need how many dimensions? and
(2) what can be achieved by further developping the conventional radiological methods with the use of digital processing techniques applied to 2D projection image-time-series.

Quantitative video angiocardiography

When we became interested in the analysis of the dynamic geometry of the heart and the resulting blood flow we started like others (Wood *et al.*, 1964; Heintzen, 1971; Ritman *et al.*, 1971; Heintzen *et al.*, 1971a) with the attempt to quantitative biplane angiocardiographic image series both by cine- and videodensitometry as well as by videometry. With the first approach it was possible to record at a given location, or area, or at a few videodensitometric windows the temporal changes of densities caused by contrast material. Thereby we obtained clinically relevant information of the cardiovascular *function* at selected regions by a 2-D approach. Using this technique, essential parameters such as ejection fraction, stroke volume, EDV, ESV and in particular the regurgitant fraction (RF) in valvular incompetence could be determined quantitatively (Bürsch, 1971, 1974, 1978; Simon *et al.*, 1973).

With biplane *videometry* (Ritman *et al.*, 1971; Heintzen *et al.*, 1971a, 1971b) one can attack the third dimension. However the limitations in reconstructing a 3-D structure from 2 biplane projections are obvious and well recognized (Figure 1). Instead of 'real cross sections' of the heart only a rectangular area can be determined from each pair of video lines at a given level. One needs further assumptions for volume determination which have to be derived from experimental data and cast studies.

Extensive studies and clinical application could demonstrate that this type of left and right ventricular volume analysis is very usefull and provides the clinically relevant degree of accuracy (Heintzen *et al*, 1982; Lange *et al.*, 1976, 1978a, 1978b, 1978c). It should be stated that no radiological approach using contrast material as indicator will give 'absolute accurate' values. There remains at least the need and problem of border definition which depends on contrast material distribution in a trabeculated ventricle and density as well as spatial resolution in the recon-

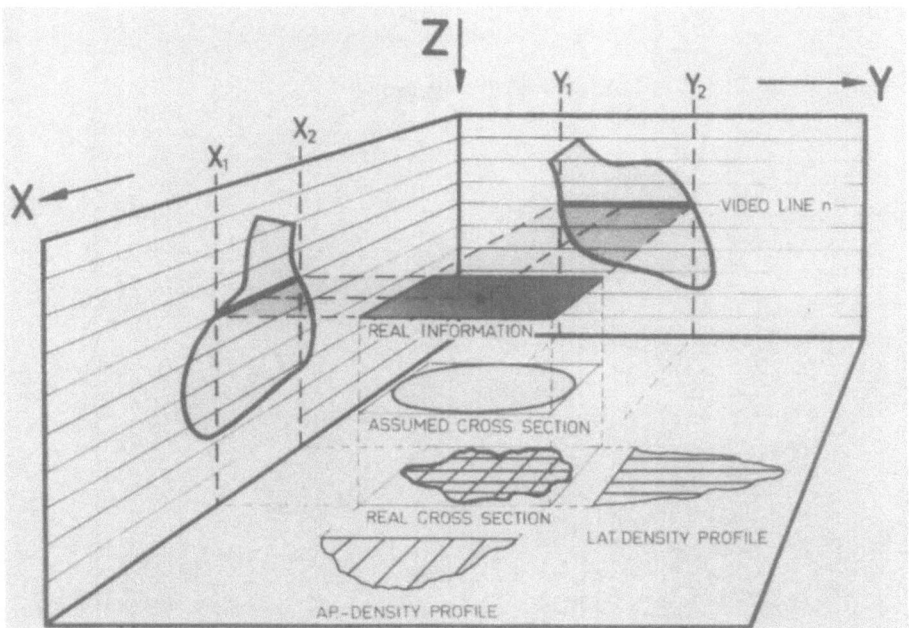

Figure 1. Schematic diagram of an ap and a lateral angiocardiographic projection. The videoline *n* is taken as an example to demonstrate the information to be gained from a biplane angiocardiogram by videometry and videodensitometry. The true area and shape of the real cross-section remain unknown unless e.g. a cast is taken and sliced mechanically, or by using tomographic reconstruction methods.

structed cross sections. (In a 100 cc sphere an error in the border of about 1 mm makes a 10% error in volume!).

Analysing the changes of size and contour-shape of the dye filled ventricles from single or biplane angiocardiograms is presently still the most commonly used approach to study the dynamic geometry of the ventricles in routine clinical cardiology. However 2-D Echocardiography is another promising way and Cine-CT as well as the DSR may become clinically available but have still to prove their superiority in daily routine.

Contraction pattern analysis

So called 3-D contraction pattern or wall motion analysis from one or two ventricular contours needs similar assumptions as for volume determination (Heintzen, Bürsch, 1978). The computer models – which can be derived for further analysis – are assuming multiple elliptical cross sections for the left ventricle. The methodology we use has been described earlier (Heintzen *et al.*, 1974). For normalization purposes in regional contraction and relaxation studies

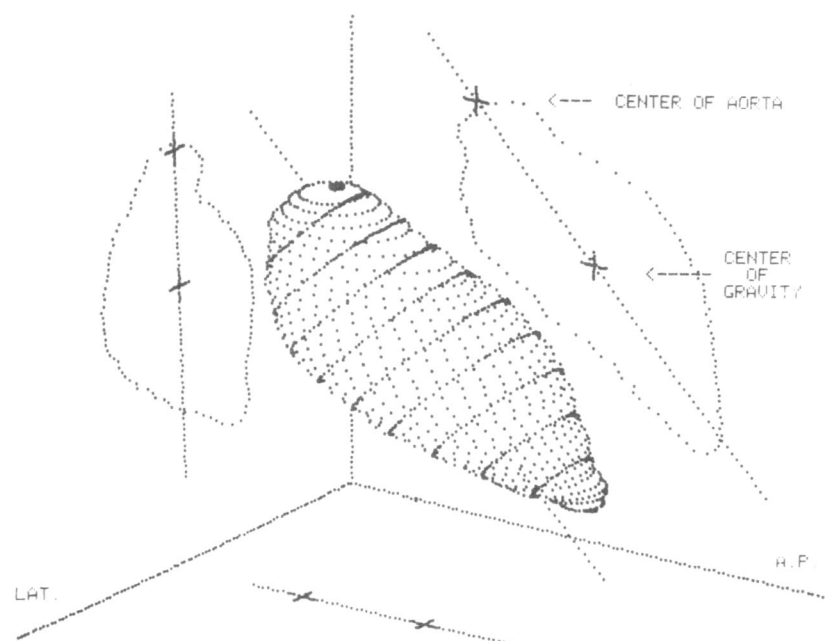

Figure 2. 3-D model of the left ventricle generated from biplane projection angiocardiogram and sliced into 9 parts, perpendicular to a line connecting the center of the aortic valve with the center of gravity.

we found the most consistent way to slice the LV in directions perpendicular to the long axis or to a line connecting the center of gravity with the center of the aortic valve plane or the apex (see Figure 2). However the best reference system may be different for specific pathological entities and has still to be worked out. Examples of the display mode for regional contraction and relaxation velocities are given in Figure 3a and b.

These 3-D models however can at the best be an approximation to the reality if the analysis is based on the contours taken from biplane projection angiocardiograms. Some improvements are possible if not only the contours but also the biplane density profiles are taken into consideration. In addition, a model cross section and subsequently the previous and adjacent cross sections can be used as a priori information to improve the reconstruction procedure (Onnasch and Heintzen, 1976; Onnasch, 1978). The philosophy of this program for reconstructing a binary array is demonstrated in Figure 4 and the corresponding flow chart (Figure 5). From the biplane density profiles first the probability of each element of the array of being inside or outside the ventricle is calculated. Than the binary array is filled by looking for the largest value of the probability array in each column and line.

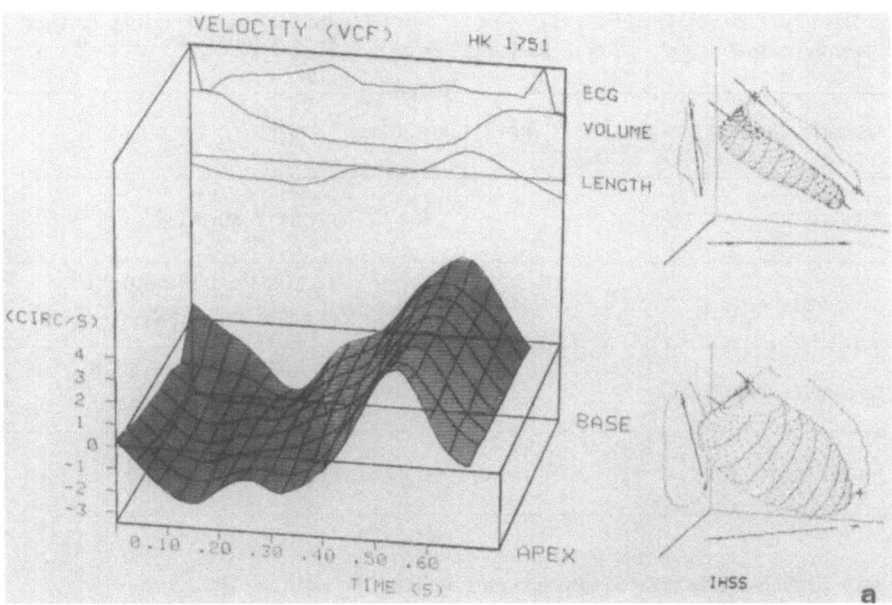

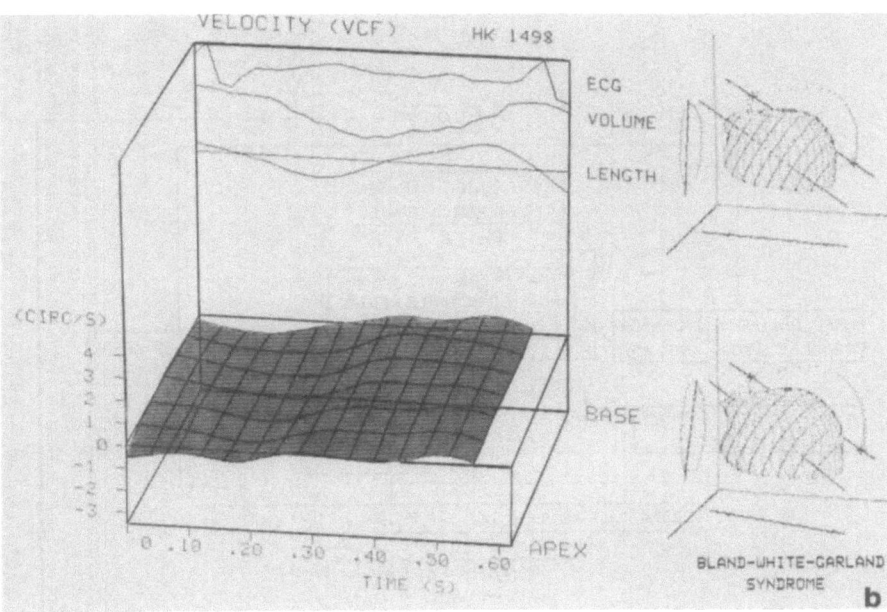

Figure 3a, b. At right, three-dimensional representation of the left ventricle derived from biplane angiocardiograms together with the antero-posterior and lateral projections in the end-systolic (above) and end-diastolic (below) phases. Computer-generated cross sections perpendicular to the long axis can be seen on the surface of the models. At left, circumferential fiber shortening velocities of eight circumferences of such ventricular slices are depicted as velocity-time plotspatial coordinates from apex to base given in the third dimension. In the case of hypertrophic cardiomyopathy (IHSS), the extreme transverse shortening compared with the longitudinal shortening is obvious from the end-systolic and end-diastolic left ventricles (A). In the Bland-White-Garland syndrome, there is a homogeneous reduction of contraction in all regions of the globular-shaped ventricle (B).

BINARY ARRAY	BA [t,s]	=	1	FOR THE LARGEST VALUES OF W(I,K) IN EACH COLUMN AND LINE OF SLICE s AT TIME t
			0	ELSE
DENSITY PROFILES	KDX (I) , KDY(K)		$\sum$ KDX(I) = $\sum$ KDY(K)	
FUNDAMENTAL PROBABILITY	F(I,K)	=	KDX(I) x KDY(K)	
SIMILARITY IN TIME	T(I,K)	=	2 D NORMAL DISTRIBUTION DERIVED FROM BA [t-1,s]	
SIMILARITY IN SPACE	S(I,K)	=	2 D NORMAL DISTRIBUTION DERIVED FROM BA [t,s-1]	
PROBABILITY ARRAY	W(I,K)	=	F(I,K) x T(I,K) x S(I,K)	

Figure 4. Definitions for the reconstruction program BASE.

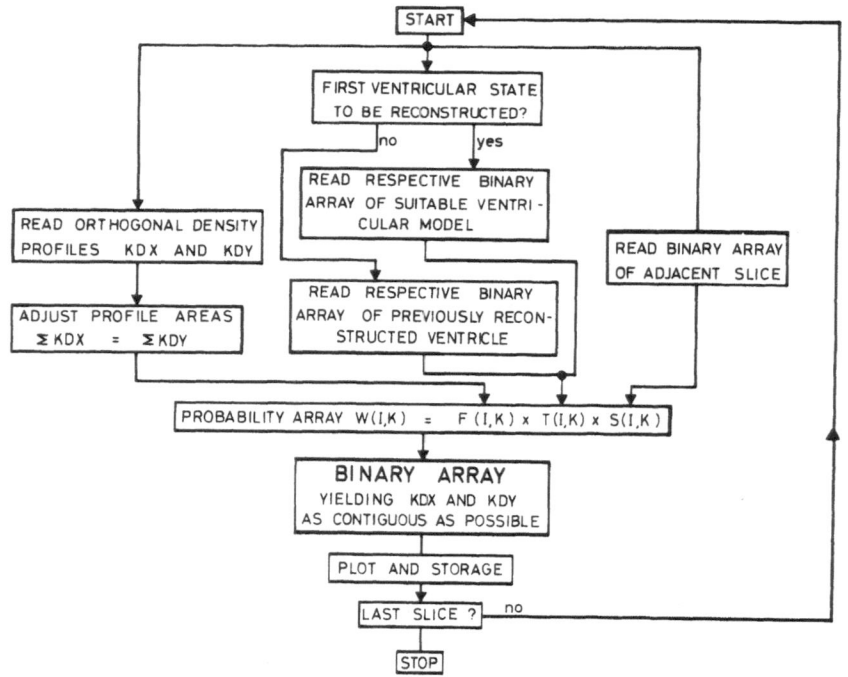

Figure 5. Flow chart of the reconstruction program BASE.

The probability array is defined as a product of three factors: the fundamental probability array, which is essentially a normalized product of the two density profiles, and two probability arrays which take the similarity of the ventricular slices in space and in time into account. These arrays are approximately two-dimensional normal distribution derived from the binary arrays of those slices.

As an example, a graphic distribution of the probability array is given in the left panel of Figure 6. It can be recognized that the probability depends not only on the largeness of the density profiles, but also on the location of the cross-section to which the similarity is demanded.

The binary pattern of the cross-section is derived from the probability array in such a way that the density profiles are reproduced and the resulting array is as contiguous as possible. In Figure 6 the four programmed steps in filling the binary array are depicted. At first, the very most probable elements of each column are filled from center to periphery. In a second step the most probable elements of each line are filled, provided the column sums are not exceeded. In a third step, the threshold elements of each column are filled, provided that an adjacent element is filled. In the last step, the complete filling of the array is reached irrespective of the probability array, provided that the column sum and the line sum are not exceeded and that an adjacent element is filled. In each step the elements are filled from center to periphery in order to strengthen the contiguity

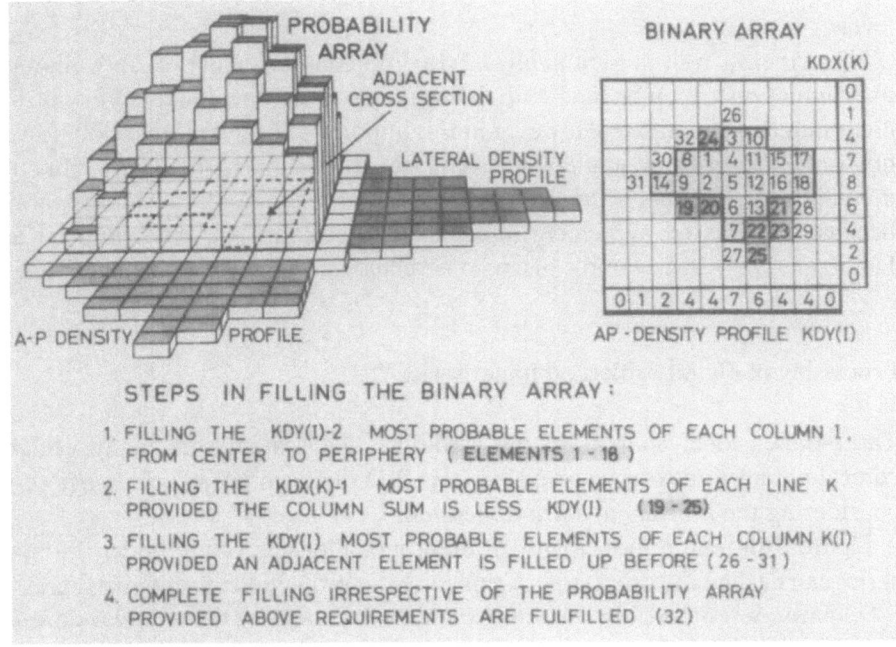

STEPS IN FILLING THE BINARY ARRAY:

1. FILLING THE KDY(I)-2 MOST PROBABLE ELEMENTS OF EACH COLUMN I, FROM CENTER TO PERIPHERY (ELEMENTS 1 - 18)

2. FILLING THE KDX(K)-1 MOST PROBABLE ELEMENTS OF EACH LINE K PROVIDED THE COLUMN SUM IS LESS KDY(I) (19 - 25)

3. FILLING THE KDY(I) MOST PROBABLE ELEMENTS OF EACH COLUMN K(I) PROVIDED AN ADJACENT ELEMENT IS FILLED UP BEFORE (26 - 31)

4. COMPLETE FILLING IRRESPECTIVE OF THE PROBABILITY ARRAY PROVIDED ABOVE REQUIREMENTS ARE FULFILLED (32)

Figure 6. The probability array (logarithmicly scaled) derived from the density profiles and an adjacent slice, and the binary array derived with the elements numbered as they are filled.

ES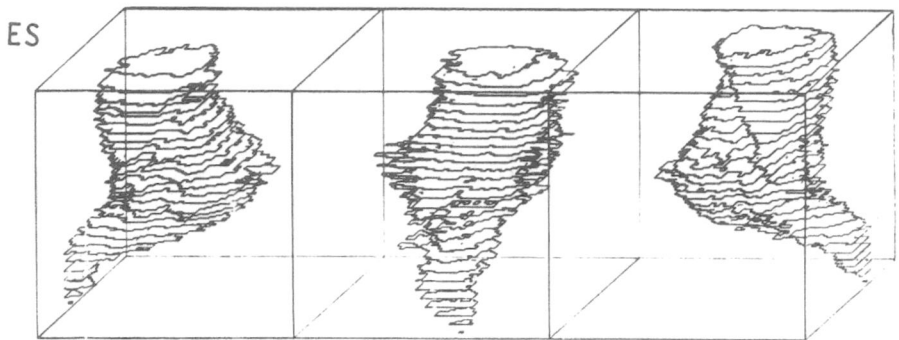

Figure 7. Examples of an improved 3-D model of the left ventricle generated by using biplane angiocardiographic contours and density profiles.

of the array. It may happen that two or three elements are not filled, even after the fourth step. As mentioned above, it is however, not necessary to demand complete agreement between the given and the derived density profiles.

More details of the method and results are given elsewhere (Onnasch and Heintzen, 1978; Onnasch, 1978). It should be clear that such a procedure can not and should not replace a complete computer tomographic reconstruction of the density distribution. At the best these results say if an element from an array belongs to a given structure (e.g. the heart) or not. There ist no gradation of gray levels.

Nevertheless wall motion analysis based on contour detection only allows to discriminate between normal and abnormal global and regional behaviour in a great number of patients. However in this important diagnostic decision process not only the instrumentation and data generation part, but even more the modeling, evaluation and analysis part creates problems and some discrepancies because there is no agreement about how to evaluate the data (Sigwart and Heintzen, 1984). An example of a reconstructed left ventricle is given in Figure 7.

Processing of digital projection image series

Three-dimensional analysis of the cardiovascular system with many valuable clinical applications can be achieved from 2-D digitized projection image series considering the *time* as the *third dimension*.

Figure 8 shows the principally different modalities according to which image series can be digitally processed. A time series of projection images gives access to 2-D anatomy *and function* whereas from a series of images taken under different angles like in CT, with a corresponding amount of data and a comparable effort only a static 3-D representation of the anatomy could be achieved – provided the image series to be processed could be taken under similar conditions (e.g. same

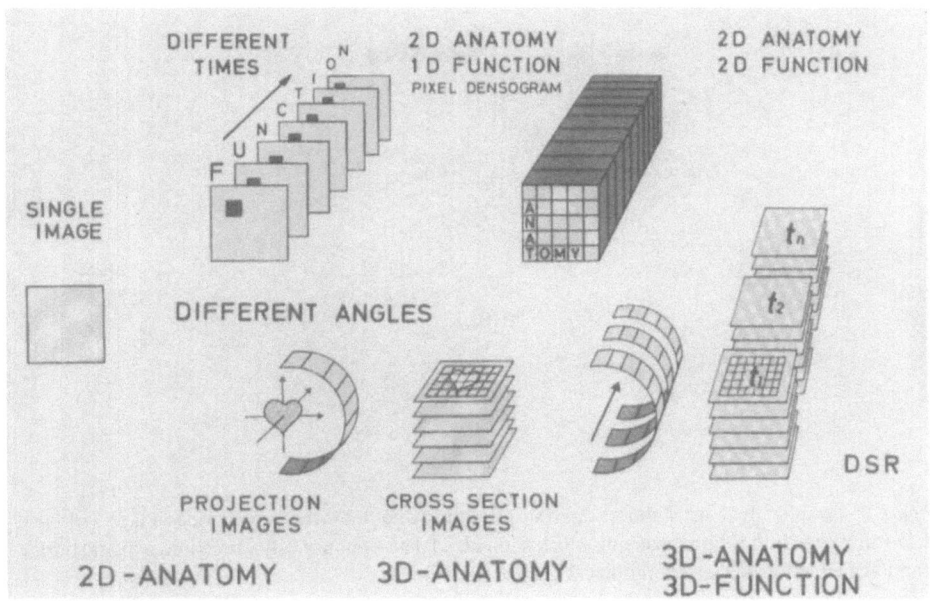

DIFFERENT TIMES — 2D ANATOMY 1D FUNCTION PIXEL DENSOGRAM — 2D ANATOMY 2D FUNCTION

SINGLE IMAGE

DIFFERENT ANGLES

PROJECTION IMAGES — CROSS SECTION IMAGES — DSR

2D-ANATOMY — 3D-ANATOMY — 3D-ANATOMY 3D-FUNCTION

Figure 8. Comparison of the different modalities for generating and evaluating image series. Upper part: images taken at different times give insight into 2-D anatomy and function. With a comparable number of pictures taken at different angles (lower part) multiple cross sections of a static 3-D object can be obtained. It requires the same number of pictures and processed data for each image if a dynamic spatial reconstruction (DSR) of the beating heart should be achieved.

heart phase). It would require an enormous additional amount of data to be perceived and processed if one would like also to obtain 3-D functional information, as with the DSR (Wood, 1977) (see also page 135–146). The principle of our method for *d*igital *v*ideo*a*ngiocardiography (DVA), for *d*igital *s*ubtraction *a*ngiocardiography (DSA) and *d*igital *f*unctional *a*ngiocardiography (DFA) will be described with some applications.

As outlined in Figure 9 the linewise structure of a video angiocardiographic image sequence is transfered by analog to digital conversion into a block of homogeneous data stored into a digital buffer which might or might not be part of the storage capacity of a digital computer. This process can be executed in real time. Each picture element ('PIXEL') represents the brightness information at a given picture site and at a given time.

By this procedure a series of subsequent pictures is transformed into a block of simultaneously available data so that the spatial and temporal information is interchangeable and can be combined or mixed, as desired! The desired or required spatial and temporal resolution may vary widely in the various fields of possible radiological applications of digital imaging techniques. In cardiovascular

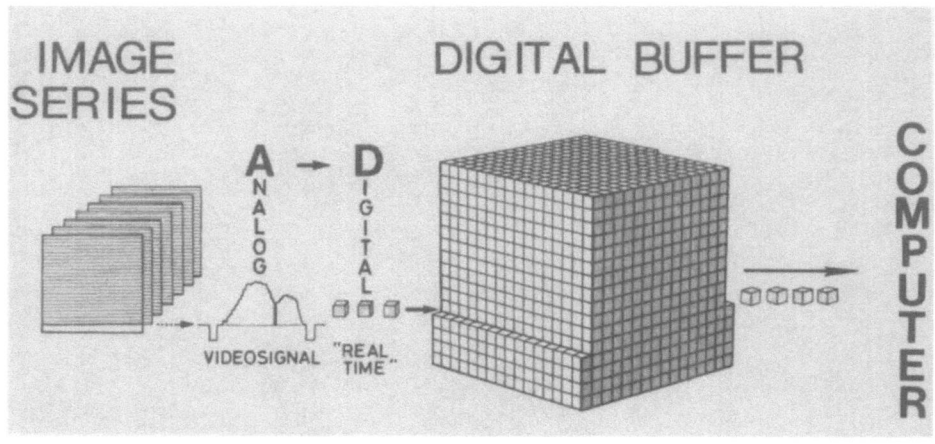

Figure 9. Graphic demonstration of the transformation of a linewise scanned videoimage series by A/D conversion into a 'homogeneous' block of digitized data – temporarily stored into a digital buffer – and available for further operations as desired.

radiology a spatial resolution of 256×256 or 512×512 and an image frequency of 1 to 50 fields per second covers most of the needs.

Figure 10 demonstrates the relationship between the various combinations of spatial and temporal resolution and the fields of useful application in cardiovascular radiology. An ideal system should have the flexibility of allowing – for a given maximum data rate – a variable choice between spatial, temporal and (possibly) density resolution, according to the clinical or experimental problem under study.

As published earlier single, 'static' images and in particular image sequences may be objected to a number of image processing techniques, such as histogram modifications, filter operations (spatial, temporal) image restorations and other kinds of 'manipulations' which can facilitate and improve the extraction of clinically relevant information by contrast enhancement, or by generating (synthetizing) new image aspects and qualities (Brennecke *et al.*, 1976, 1977, 1979, 1980, 1978a, 1978b; Brennecke, 1983; Wittmaack *et al.*, 1980).

The greatest benefit of digital image processing techniques in the field of cardiovascular radiology can be achieved not from digital processing of single, static images or just simple background subtraction operations, but from the flexible use of a whole image series due to the fact that spatial and temporal information can be combined and processed in variable modes. This however requires intelligent, experimentally elaborated and clinically relevant biological and engineering concepts.

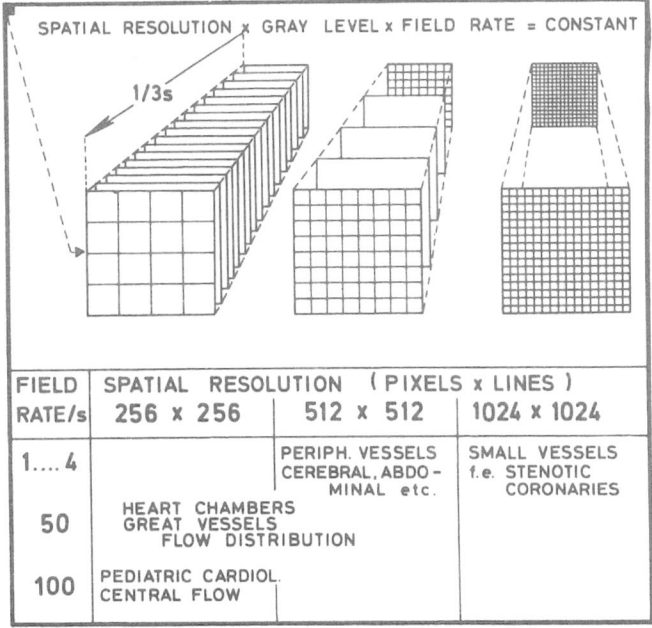

FIELD	SPATIAL RESOLUTION (PIXELS x LINES)		
RATE/s	256 x 256	512 x 512	1024 x 1024
1....4		PERIPH. VESSELS CEREBRAL, ABDO-MINAL etc.	SMALL VESSELS f.e. STENOTIC CORONARIES
50	HEART CHAMBERS GREAT VESSELS FLOW DISTRIBUTION		
100	PEDIATRIC CARDIOL. CENTRAL FLOW		

Figure 10. Demonstration of the 'interchangibility' of spatial and temporal resolution for a given data rate (as the limiting factor of a given equipment). One has the choice between low spatial and high temporal or high spatial and low temporal resolution. Possible indications for the various options are given in the lower part of the picture.

This simultaneous availability of all data characterizing the 'anatomy' of the cardiovascular system and the changes of structure and blood flow with time, i.e. 'function' is the main reason for the specific advantages of digital over conventional angiocardiographic imaging techniques.

The possibilities of contrast enhancement and thereby the revival of intravenous contrast injection techniques in angiocardiography has a number of useful clinical applications (Heintzen *et al.*, 1978; Bürsch *et al.*, 1982).

Specific imaging techniques

If the information from more than one picture of an image series (taken at different times) is combined, the result may yet only reflect anatomy. This is the case in dye filled cardiovascular structures after 'background' subtraction. There are, however, many modalities for digital image series processing – as demonstrated in Figure 11 where the information from a few or an increasing number of individual pictures is combined (subtracted, summed up, mixed etc.) whereby

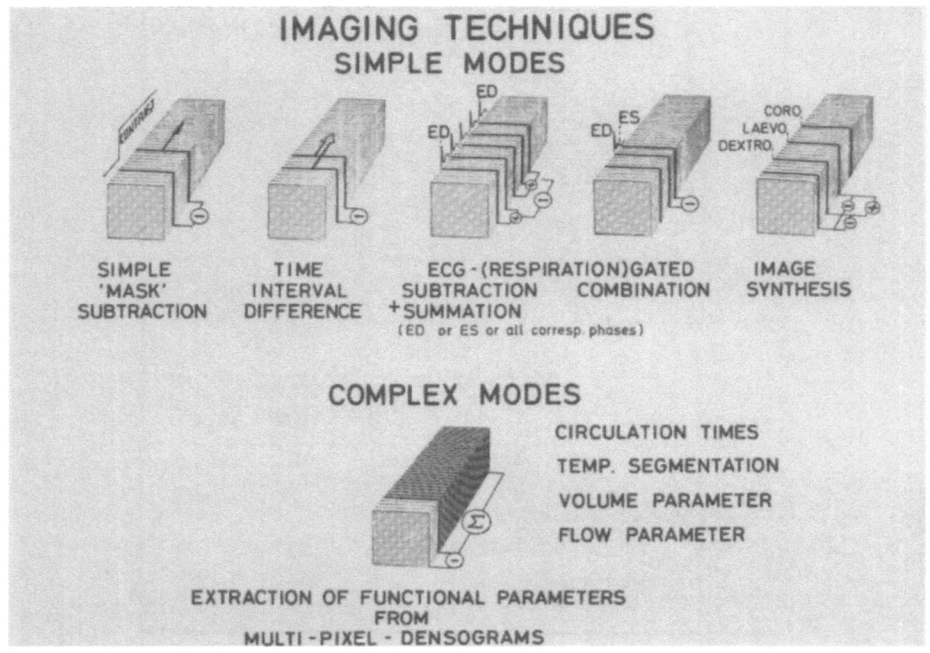

Figure 11. Survey on various techniques for extraction of clinically relevant information from angiocardiographic image series by combining in different ways the information of more than one picture from the series. The most common and simplest way is image subtraction. The most complex modes of digital image processing are using the information from the whole image series (lower part) for extraction of functional parameters from multi-pixel densograms.

these input pictures reflect the cardiovascular system at different functional states, e.g. at a given time interval (so called TID mode), or at specific instances of thec cardiac cycle (i.e. endsystolic and enddiastolic pictures). Such operation can therefore be considered already as simple types of 'functional imaging'.

Simple 'masc mode subtraction' (Figure 11), which means subtraction without considering the cardiac phase, can be performed in real time, it gives satisfying results if motional artifacts can be kept small, for example in intravenous and intraarterial subtraction angiography of the peripheral circulation.

If, however, digital subtraction techniques should be applied to the central circulation, motional artifacts are caused by the contraction of the heart and even more by the respiration. The 'slow motion' artifacts of respiration can be reduced by subtracting images which are separated by a short time interval (TID mode) thus leaving only the more rapid changes of the contrast material distribution related to the heart motion and blood flow. The contrast itself is thereby reduced, which can be compensated in part by higher amplification after background subtraction.

Based on our experience, ecg gated techniques are almost always required to give acceptable results from image subtraction if digital processing should be applied to the central circulation (Figure 11).

Respiration can cause motional artefacts, particularly in children. The method developed in our laboratory allows the selection of pictures for subtraction from a series of 'background' images taken over a whole respiratory and cardiac cycle before contrast injection in order to find those pictures by (on line) cross correlation techniques, which optimaly correspond to the actual contrast pictures. This ecg and respiratory gated subtraction is possible in real time with the Image Sequence Acquisition and Analysis Computer ('ISAAC'), developed in our laboratories (Brennecke et al., 1977, 1979, 1980, 1978a, 1978b; Brennecke, 1983). For functional studies of ventricular performance ecg gated endsystolic (ES) pictures can be subtracted from enddiastolic ones (ED) (Figure 11). The resulting subtraction images reflect the mode of contraction of the left ventricle as a 2-D correlate of stroke volume and ejection fraction (EF). From biplane pictures ventricular volumes and ejection fraction can be calculated as in conventional angiocardiography (Lange et al., 1983; Heintzen et al., 1984).

For specific studies of left or right ventricular function the radiation can also be triggered from either the computer or a microprocessor which coordinates image generation, image acquisition, digitization, processing storage and retrieval (Wittmaack et al., 1980).

In addition to the possible reduction of contrast material – which is needed for a given piece of information – the radiation dose can also be reduced in digital angiocardiography, be it intravenous or selective, depending on the diagnostic problem. Thus at least four left ventricular performance studies are possible (during rest and exercise) without increasing the patient's load.

Having the whole sequence of images stored in digital format enables any useful combination of pictures from various phases of the contrast passage to be used to synthetize composite image (Figure 11), whereby the background may be removed and the noise reduced before or parallel to image synthesis.

Combinations of dextro- and levocardiograms depicted in different gray levels or colours demonstrate the spatial relationship between the heart chambers and great vessels and thereby allow a clear delineation of the ventricular septum, in particular in the four chamber view (Bogren et al., 1981). For these studies, only a limited number of pictures from the whole series has to be processed. However, interactive search for those pictures which optimally fit to each other is required and can be done shortly after the procedure. This type of operation will probably not become a field for automatic real time digital image processing.

One particular interesting aspect of digital angiocardiography is the study of the perfusion of the cardiac muscle itself, since it allows the determination of the left ventricular muscle mass and the detection of perfusion defects (Radtke et al., 1983a, 1983b; Bürsch et al., 1983).

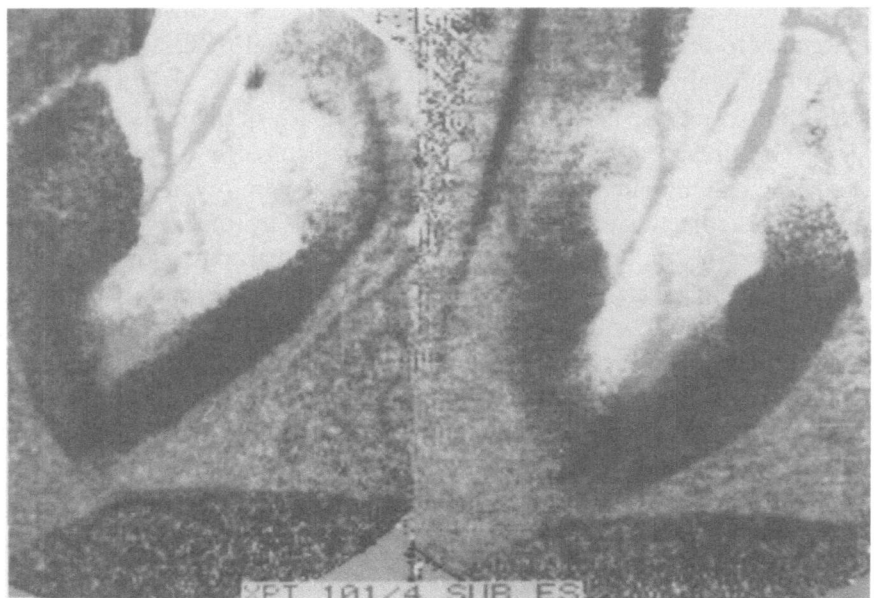

Figure 12. Opacification of the ventricular muscle mass during the capillary phase of the coronary circulation by using digital subtraction and integration techniques. End-systolic phase, ap and lateral projections.

For this purpose contrast enhancement is used by heart phase related integration and background subtraction during the capillary phase of the coronary circulation. This can be achieved by aortic, selective coronary or left ventricular dye injection. From the initial levocardiogram (LV injection) the internal surface of the left ventricular muscle wall is obtained. During the following perfusion of the heart muscle via the coronary arteries, contrast enhancement techniques allow the opacification of the myocardial wall and thereby the delineation of the epicardial surface. From this late picture the early levocardiogram is electronically subtracted, leaving only the left ventricular muscle shell opacified (Figure 12).

The left ventricular muscle mass can then be determined by subtracting the LV volume derived from the endocardial surface from the volume, obtained from the biplane epicardial contours of the left ventricle (LV), applying the established videometric methods. The calculated muscle volume correlated very well with the true LV muscle volume measured postmortem in pig hearts (Radtke *et al.,* 1983b).

In addition, animal studies with experimentally created ventricular infarctions of known size have shown that variations in the wall thickness, wall motion and myocardial perfussion become detectable by this technique.

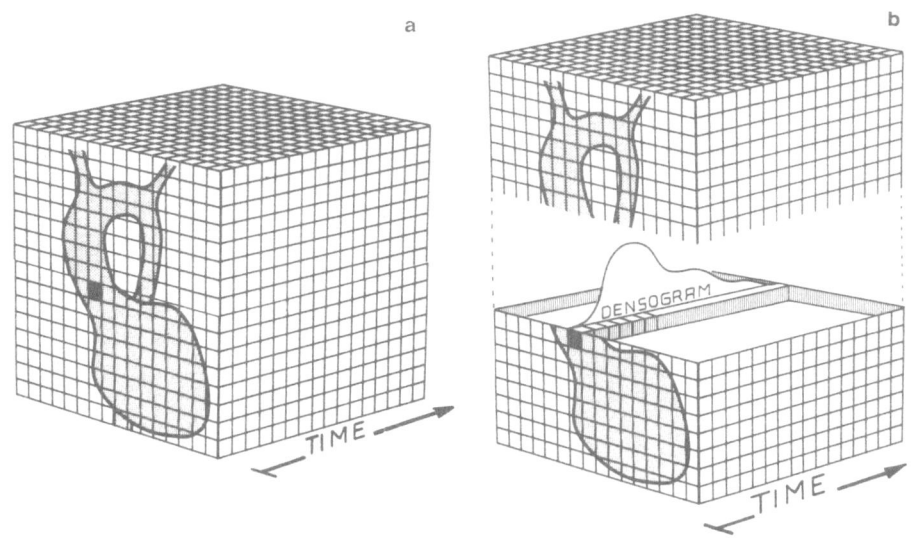

Figure 13a, b. Schematic demonstration that, in a digitized image series, each pixel can be considered as a videodensitometric window (a) so that the brightness changes with time constitute a matrix of pixeldensograms, (b) which can be evaluated in various ways applying some principles of the indicator dilution technique.

Blood flow distribution measurements

Within the block of data obtained after digitization of acomplete image series, each picture element ('pixel') can be considered as a videodensitometric window so that all kinds of indicator dilution operation can be performed in the most complete way (Figure 13a, b).

From the whole density time curves functional parameters can be derived. This is demonstrated in Figure 14a for a time parameter (maximum of densogram or arrival time). This time value can be displayed providing a new picture quality which signalizes the progress of the contrast bolus within one image. A 2-D X-ray density display is thereby converted into a 2-D time value display either in gray levels, colours or numbers.

Such time parameters can be grouped considering the underlying anatomy and the physiological problem. For flow distribution measurements in the vascular tree, programs have been developed which allow a useful 'temporal segmentation' of the contrast bolus so that its stepwise progression within a given time interval can be detected and displayed.

From the area under the same densogram (Figure 14b) another parameter can be derived representing the dephth of the cardiovascular structure within the path

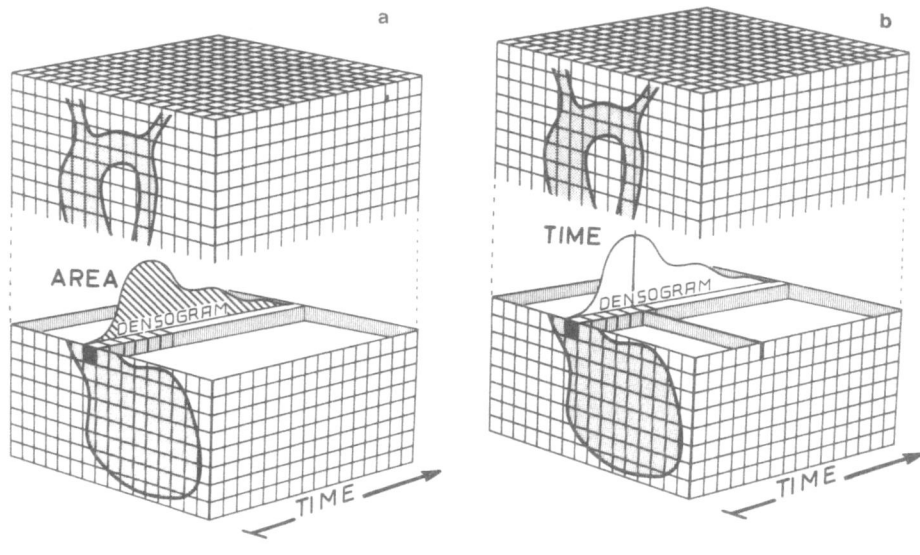

Figure 14a, b. From each pixel-densogram 'functional' (time)parameters (a) or volume parameters (area under the densogram b) can be obtained.

of radiation, and thereby a measure of the volume of the vessel in a given region or segment, of the vascular tree if all individual area-parameters are integrated.

Quantitative flow distribution measurements are possible in a branching vascular tree by a principle using time parameter extraction as described above and vascular volume parameters.

Since the isochrones obtained by temporal segmentation give a quantitative measure of the progress of the contrast bolus within a given part of the vessel, for example during a 80 ms interval, and the volume element between these isochrones is also known, the volume displacement in the vessel within a given time – i.e. the flow – at this site can be calculated. The relative flow rates in a branching vessel can be converted into absolute values, if the dimension of the vessel is determined by an independent (videometric) measurement at any site of the vessel. The calculated flow distribution can be indicated by numbers displayed with the (coloured) picture of the vascular tree.

This type of image analysis can be applied for flow pattern analysis as well as for quantitative flow measurements in other regions of the circulation. For example, to study the renal coronary, pulmonary or renal circulation or to determine the shunt volume through a aorto-pulmonary anastomosis (Figure 15, 16, 17) (Bürsch *et al.*, 1981, 1983b, 1984; Bürsch, 1982, 1983).

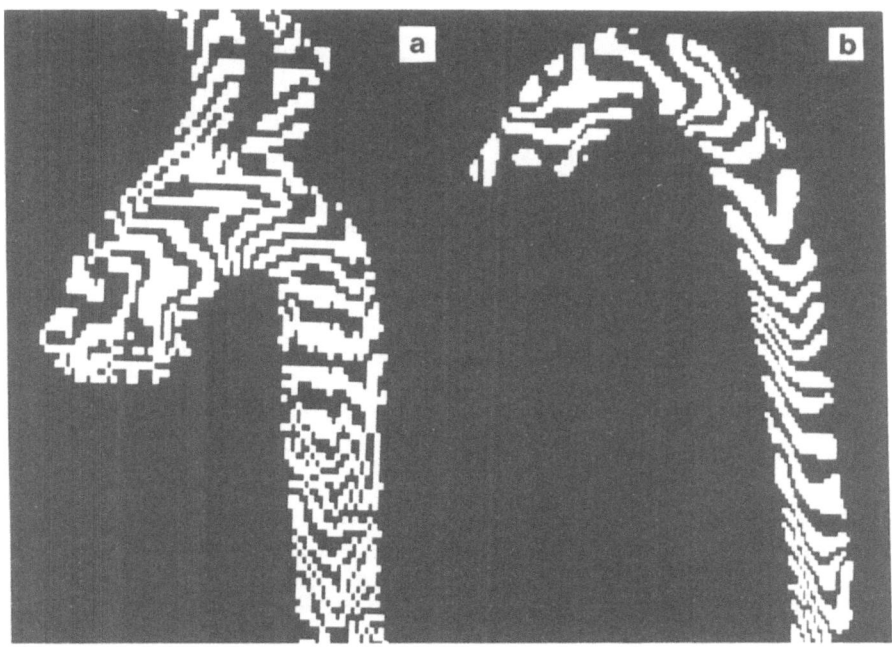

Figure 15a, b. Two examples of 'contrast flow patterns' in the aorta obtained by a display of time parameters characterizing the progress of the contrast bolus (its mean concentration time, MAZ) in steps of 20 ms.

Conclusion

The heart as a three dimensional structure with changing geometry in time can be studied by attempting to record all four dimensions as completely as possible, and also by relating to the most clinically relevant problems by selecting specific information obtained from incomplete 3D spatial 'reconstructions'. Biplane projection angiocardiograms allow a rough modeling of the left and right ventricles, respectively, for volume and contraction pattern analysis, with clinically acceptable accuracy. If, in addition to the ventricular endocardial contours, the density profiles and some a priori knowledge is applied, the correspondence between the model and reality can be improved.

Another clinically valuable way of '3D analysis' of the cardiovascular system is to consider the *time as the third dimension* and apply digital image processing techniques to 2-dimensional angiocardiographic image series. This approach is practiced in so called digital subtraction angiocardiography (DSA) and, more recently, also in qualitative and quantitative digital functional angiocardiography (DFA). This procedure represents a comparable simple expansion of conventional angiocardiographic techniques without the need for changing the whole

168

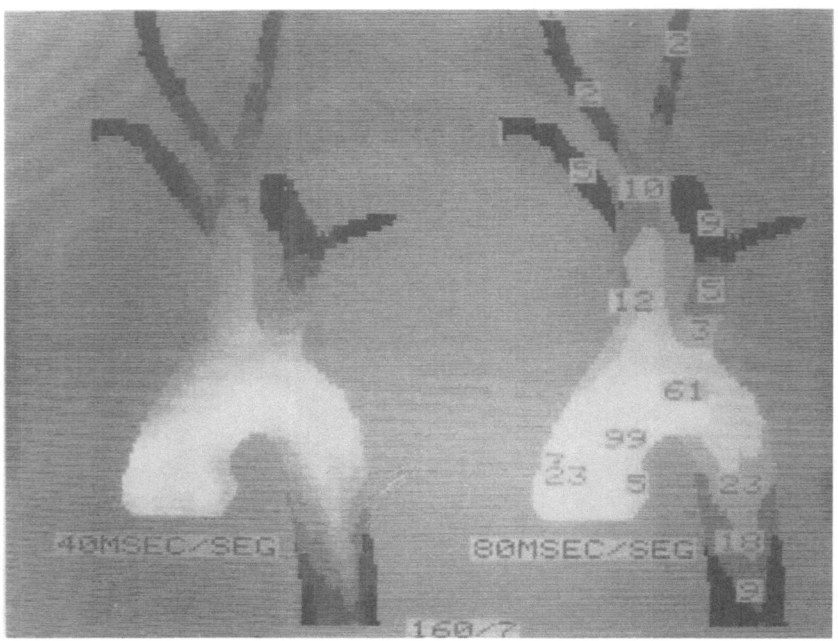

Figure 16. Contrast flow pattern in the aortic root and central arteries with temporal segmentation of 40 ms (left) and 80 ms (right). In the right pannel the flow distribution is quantitated by simultaneously time and volume parameter calculations and the percentage flow into the branching arteries is displayed. In this case the flow values are influenced by the phasic changes in blood flow velocities in the central aortic root since the temporal segmentation is not related to cycle. (Compare to Figure 8).

image generation equipment. There are many useful applications of this 2D version of dynamic and functional digital angiocardiography. They suffer less from the projection technique and superposition then the presently available dynamic 3-D reconstruction methods from limited spatial resolution.

Digital projection angiocardiography can be made in many cases less invasive (by less contrast material and radiation) than conventional techniques and can be complemented by quantitative studies of, in particular, central and regional blood flow distribution and organ perfusion.

References

Bogren HG, Bürsch JH, Brennecke R, Radtke W, Heintzen PH (1981) Intravenous angiocardiography using digital image processing: experience with axial projections in normal pigs and in pigs with experimentally generated left-to-right shunts. Conference on Digital Radiography, Stanford, USA, September 1981 Proc SPIE 314:287–293

Brennecke R, Brown TK, Bürsch JH, Heintzen PH (1976) Digital processing of videoangiographic

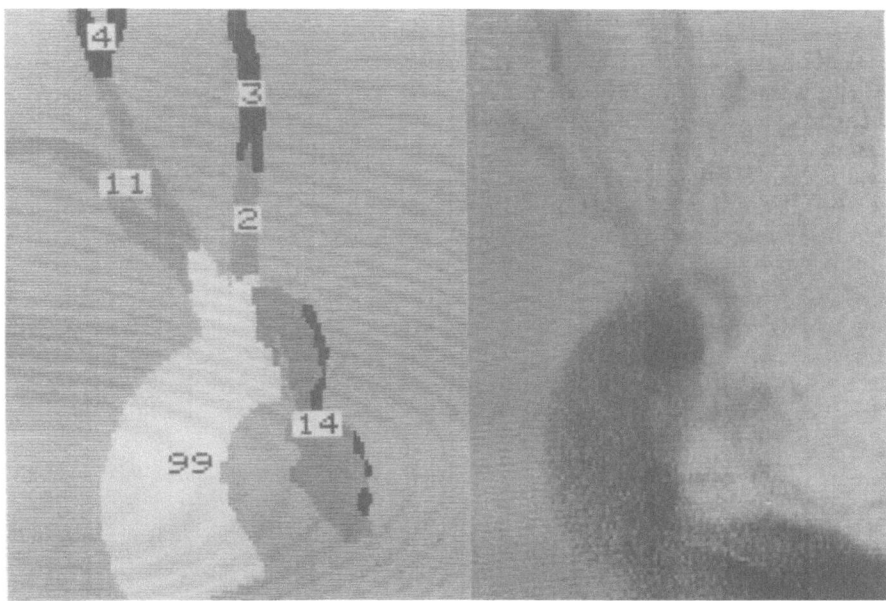

Figure 17a, b. (a) Digitized angiocardiogram from a child with a Blalock Taussig anastomosis. (b) Result of flow parameter calculation for the same patient. Progress of the bolus (temporal segmentation) is demonstrated in gray levels for time steps of one cardiac cycle length. By this method it can be shown that 14% of the cardiac output and central aortic flow is going through the Blalock Taussig anastomosis, 2% into the left carotid and 11% into the anonymous artery.

image series using a minicomputer. Proc Comp Cardiol, Long Beach. IEEE Computer Society, pp 255–260

Brennecke R, Brown TK, Bürsch JH, Heintzen PH (1977) Computerized video-image preprocessing with applications to cardio-angiographic roentgen-image series. In: Nagel HH (ed) Digital Image Processing. Berlin-Heidelberg-New York: Springer, pp 244–262

Brennecke R, Brown TK, Bürsch JH, Heintzen PH (1978a) A digital system for roentgen video image processing. In: Heintzen PH, Bürsch JH (eds) Roentgen-Video-Techniques. Stuttgart: G. Thieme, pp 150–157

Brennecke R, Hahne JH, Moldenhauer K, Bürsch JH, Heintzen PH (1978b) Improved digital real-time processing and storage techniques with applications to intravenous contrast angiography. Proc Comp Cardiol, Long Beach; IEE Computer Society, pp 191–194

Brennecke R, Hahne HJ, Moldenhauer K, Bürsch JH, Heintzen PH (1979) A special purpose processor for digital angiocardiography. Design and applications. Proc Comp Cardiol, Long Beach: IEEE Computer Society, pp 343–346

Brennecke R, Hahne HJ, Heintzen PH (1980) A multiprocessor-system for the acquisition and analysis of video image sequences. In: Pöppl SJ, Platzer H (eds) Erzeugung und Analyse von Bildern und Strukturen, Berlin-Heidelberg, New York: Springer, pp 113–122

Brennecke R (1983) Digital processing of roentgen video image sequences. In: Heintzen PH, Brennecke R (eds) Digital imaging in cardiovascular radiology. Stuttgart: Thieme, pp 24–34

Bürsch JH (1971) Quantitative Videodensitometrie. Grundlagen und Ergebnisse einer röntgenologischen Indikatormethode. Habilitationsschrift, Univ. Kiel

Bürsch JH, Heintzen PH, Simon R (1974) Videodensitometric studies by a new method of quantitating the amount of contrast medium. Europ J Cardiol 1:437–446

Bürsch JH, Ostermeyer J, Stelzer E, Heintzen PH (1978) Videodensitometric quantification of mitral insufficiency. Concepts and preliminary results. In: Heintzen PH, Bursch JH (eds) Roentgen-Video-Techniques. Stuttgart, Thieme, pp 94–100

Bürsch JH, Hahne HJ, Brennecke R, Grönemeyer D, Heintzen PH (1981) Assessment of arterial blood flow measurements by digital angiography. Radiology, 14:39–47

Bürsch JH, Brennecke R, Heintzen PH (1982) Digital angiography. Practical Cardiology 8:131–142

Bürsch JH, Seemann S, Meissner L, Hahne HJ, Brennecke R, Heintzen PH (1983a) Approaches to myocardial perfusion analysis by digital angiography. Proc Comp Cardiol, Long Beach: IEEE Computer Society, in press

Bürsch JH, Hahne HJ, Brennecke R, Eicker C, Heintzen PH (1983b) Arterial blood flow analysis by digital angiography. In: Heintzen PH, Brennecke R (eds) Digital Imaging in Cardiovascular Radiology. Stuttgart, Thieme, pp 115–123

Bürsch JH (1983) Use of digitized functional angiography to evaluate arterial blood flow. Cardiovasc Intervent Radiol 6:303–310

Bürsch JH, Radtke W, Rünger T, Moldenhauer K, Hoffmann B, Heintzen PH (1984) Endocardial and epicardial contour detection of the left ventricle by digital angiocardiography. Sigwart U, Heintzen PH (eds) Ventricular Wall Motion. Stuttgart: Georg Thieme, pp 49–57

Heintzen PH (ed) (1971) Roentgen- Cine- and Videodensitometry. Fundamentals and applications for blood flow and heart volume determination. Stuttgart: Thieme

Heintzen PH, Malerczyk V, Pilarczyk J, Scheel KW (1971a) On-line processing of the video-image for left ventricular volume determination. Comput Biomed Res 4:474–485

Heintzen PH, Malerczyk V, Pilarczyk J, Schohl HH, Vogel GW (1971b) Automatisierung der röntgenologischen Herzkammervolumenbestimmung unter Einsatz eines magnetischen Bildplattenspeichers. Fortschr Röntgenstr. 114:215–222

Heintzen PH, Moldenhauer K, Lange PE (1974) Three-dimensional computerized contraction pattern analysis. Description of methodology and its validation. Europ J Cardiol 1:229–239

Heintzen PH, Bürsch JH (eds) (1978) Roentgen video techniques for dynamic studies of structure and function of the heart and circulation. Stuttgart: Thieme

Heintzen PH, Brennecke R, Bürsch JH (1978) Computerized videoangiocardiography. In: Kaltenbach M, Lichtlen, P, Balcon R, Bussmann W-D (eds) Coronary Heart Disease. Stuttgart: G. Thieme, pp 116–121

Heintzen PH, Brennecke R, Bürsch JH, Hahne RJ, Lange PE, Moldenhauer K, Onnasch D, Radtke W (1982) Quantitative analysis of structure and function of the cardiovascular system by roentgen-video-computer techniques

Heintzen PH, Brennecke R (eds) (1983) Digital Imaging in Cardiovascular Radiology. Stuttgart: Thieme

Heintzen PH, Bürsch JH, Hahne HJ, Brennecke R, Budach W, Lange P (1984) Assessment of cardiovascular function by digital angiocardiography. J Amer Coll Cardiol (in press) and Mayo Clin Proc 57: Suppl 78–91

Lange PE, Onnasch D, Moldenhauer K, Malerczyk V, Farr F, Hüttig G, Heintzen PH (1976) The analysis of size, shape and contraction pattern of the right ventricle from angiocardiograms. Europ J Cardiol Suppl IV:153–168

Lange PE, Onnasch D, Farr F, Malerczyk V, Heintzen PH (1978a) Analysis of left and right ventricular size and shape, as determined from human casts. Description of the method and its validation. Europ J Cardiol 8:431–448

Lange PE, Onnasch D, Farr F, Heintzen PH (1978b) Angiocardiographic left ventricular volume determination. Accuracy, as determined from human casts, and clinical application. Europ J Cardiol 8:449–476

Lange PE, Onnasch D, Farr F, Heintzen PH (1978c) Angiocardiographic right ventricular volume determination. Accuracy, as determined from human casts, and clinical application. Europ J Cardiol 8:477–501

Lange PE, Budach W, Radtke W, Onnasch DGW, Heintzen PH (1983) Global and regional comparison between standard biplane and digital subtraction angiocardiography of the right ventricle. Proc 10th annual meeting computers in Cardiol, 100

Onnasch D, Heintzen PH (1976) A new approach for the reconstruction of the right or left ventricular form from biplane angiocardiographic recordings. Computers in Cardiology, IEEE Comp Soc: 67–73

Onnasch DGW (1978) A concept for the approximative reconstruction of the form of the right or left ventricle from biplane angiocardiograms. In: Heintzen PH, Bürsch JH (eds) Roentgen-Video-Techniques. Stuttgart: Thieme Verlag, pp 235–242

Radtke W, Bürsch JH, Brennecke R, Hahne HJ, Heintzen PH (1983a) Assessment of myocardial mass and infarction size by digital angiography. In: Heintzen PH, Brennecke R (eds) Digital Imaging in Cardiovascular Radiology. Stuttgart: Thieme, pp 233–240

Radtke W, Bürsch JH, Brennecke R, Hahne HJ, Heintzen PH (1983b) Assessment of left ventricular muscle volume by digital angiocardiography. Invest Radiol 18:149–154

Ritman EL, Sturm RE, Wood EH (1971) Biplane roentgen videometric system for dynamic (60/s) studies of the shape and size of circulatory structures, particularly the left ventricle. In: Heintzen PH (ed) Roentgen-, Cine- and Videodensitometry. Stuttgart: Thieme, pp 179–211

Sigwart U, Heintzen PH (eds) (1984) Ventricular Wall Motion. Stuttgart, New York: Thieme

Simon R, Callesen C, Heintzen PH (1973) Bestimmung der Regurgitationsfraktion von Pulmonalinsuffizienzen durch videodensitometrische Indikator- Mengenmessung. Basic Res Cardiol 68:509–520

Wittmaack W, Brennecke R, Heintzen PH (1980) Mikroprozessoreinsatz bei der Aufnahme von Videoangiokardiogrammen. Biomedizinische Technik, Ergänzungsband 25, pp 101–103

Wood EH, Sturm RE, Sanders (1984) Data processing in cardiovascular physiology with particular reference to roentgen videodensitometry. Mayo Clin Proc 39:849–865

Wood EH (1977) New vistas for the study of structural and functional dynamics of the heart, lungs and the circulation by noninvasive numerical tomographic vivisection. Circulation 56:506–520

DISCUSSION

MIRSKY: Were you looking at the velocity of the mid wall fibers or the endocardial fibers?

ANS: It was the velocity of the endocardium. With the digital imaging techniques, you can outline the myocardial walls, the inner and outer surface, and you can even add the left ventriculargram and the muscle shell at the same time. We conducted studies to determine the muscle volume. Then you can certainly delineate the endocardial and the epicardial surface of that ventricle in the projections which you choose.

MIRKSKY: Cardiologists have been using mid wall fiber shortening. Unfortunately if you follow the mid wall from end diastole to end systole, you are looking at a different fiber at each interval of time.

ANS: Of course, we realize that. It is possible with this technique to determine the wall thickness and add half of the wall thickness to the endocardial contours. You certainly can by no means identify and follow individual fibers.

SIDEMAN: The 3-dimensional configuration which we wish to obtain in a convenient and handy way, is probably helpful, provided we have it. From what you have said it seems that we can live without it. Indeed, we have lived without if for many centuries. You said, that instead of waiting 2 months until we get the 3-D data, we may as well use 2-D information. This is obvious. Still, please expand on your outlook as a clinician on the 3-D model and the information you can get from it. Is it really limited or is it limited because you don't have it accurately?

ANS: This is not easy to answer. I have followed the development of the DSR in the Mayo Clinic and I admire this effort which has been made there. I have always seen the danger of the discrepancy between a concept and the reality and that is one of the problems with the DSR. If, with a comparable temporal and spatial resolution, a 3-D representation of the heart would be possible, then the clinician would certainly be happy. The danger which I see is that many people say that 2-D is nothing; that the heart is a 3-D structure, hence we need a 3-D representation of everything. In fact, we don't always need that. That's my point. If we would have a good 2-D representation of the heart, be it by echo, or angio, or any other technique, it could certainly be worthwhile for a given indication. The use of the term accurate in this connection very often disturbs me because, even for the DSR, you don't get absolute volumes. You use contrast material. You have to make a delineation where the border is between the contrast material and the myocardial wall. All these problems cannot automatically be solved by the computer and, in particular, not if the spatial resolution is not as good as we hoped it to be. But nevertheless, in clinical diagnosis, in our patients, there are a few indications where we need this 3-D representation. But only if it is going to be better and cheaper, and available at the moment of the examination, then it will help the diagnosis. We should not overestimate the 3-D approach. Probably, if you have limited resources, I would suggest to use time as a third dimension with single or biplane 2-D projection images. This is more realistic until a new technology is there which really can give you what you want to have.

JARON: I am referring to your temporal analysis. How did you take care of the registration problem between your time elements. In other words: , the translation rotation?

ANS: We have 50 images per second. This is our temporal information. Each 20 milliseconds we have an outlined LV, and a cardiologist is drawing the borders. All the other calculations are based on this information obtained from the borders from biplanes taken in a time difference of 20 milliseconds.

JARON: The problem that I'm alluding to is, how do you register the different elements, from picture to picture? In other words, how do you know which part of the myocardium has moved due to the fact that the whole heart moved, or due to contraction, for example?

ANS: This is a problem which could occupy a whole symposium. I cannot answer that so easily. The point is that if you have data from a patient, you don't have markers which you can follow during contraction so you have to make some approximations. We cannot follow from time-to-time real individual points on the contours, so we cut that ventricle into a number of 10 equidistant slices and we follow these which are extending during diastole and contracting during systole. The assumption is that these cross sections are cutting somewhere in the region where they did before. Obviously we don't see any fiber. Nobody can see that. You may know of the approach of the group in the Netherlands which put markers in and believe that you can find natural markers on the contours which can be followed. I don't believe that this is real information. We have to take the most probable way to find individual points which we can follow during the contraction cycle. We can do that for the long axis and I think it is the most realistic way to do it for the LV. This gives the least deviation if you do that in a group of normal patients.

GOTTESMAN: One or two observations. Maybe we are looking at 3 completely different things. The first one is the question of the mathematician who is asking certain basic engineering questions. The second one is the physiologist who's looking at the physiological parameters in a dog model, with all its modulations which can be modelled according to your wishes. The third one is the clinician who has to look at the clinical problem. And I would agree with Dr. Heintzen on certain aspects. When one looks at pediatric cardiology, the question is whether the ventricle works or doesn't work and how badly is it impaired. When one looks at adult cardiology, one is looking at regional ventricular dysfunction and I think that the regional ventricular dysfunction in this case is extremely important. Echocardiography, and possibly the DSR may give us a lot of functional anatomy that one may not be seeing so accurately with angiography, although the angiography is extremely accurate. We've really got a lot to learn. We have to marry the 3 disciplines together – the applied mathematician who has the basic ideas of an engineer, the dog physiologist and the clinician who is asking the specific questions.

Another point is the LV aneurism which Dr. Ritman mentioned. Acute myocardial infarction, the development of the infarction, the development of the aneurism and, in the different structure of the myocardium, how much is it due to the mycardium; how much is functional and how much is it fibrous tissue.

ANS: As to aneurism, infarction or regional abnormalities, a 'cut' into the ventricle gives a rough estimation. We had a whole symposium about ventricular wall motion and it's very difficult to find any agreement among all these experts. They all detect regional abnormalities differently. It's a problem because we don't have enough landmarks and that is true for 3-D and 2-D approaches.

Three-dimensional ultrasonic cardiac reconstruction: general aspects and application to finite element analysis of the left ventricle

DAVID J. SKORTON, K.B. CHANDRAN, STEVE M. COLLINS, LAWRENCE P. PETREE, DAVID D. McPHERSON, BRIAN OLSHANSKY, MICHAEL P. NOEL and RICHARD E. KERBER. *Cardiovascular Center, Departments of Internal Medicine, Biomedical Engineering, Electrical and Computer Engineering and Radiology, University of Iowa and VA Medical Center Iowa City, IA 52242, U.S.A.*

Abstract

Two-dimensional (2-D) echocardiography is well suited to evaluate regional left ventricular dynamics because of its ability to depict wall motion and thickening in real time throughout the cardiac cycle. Recently, several investigative groups have combined the fine spatial and temporal resolution of 2-D echocardiography with a method of three-dimensional (3-D) spatial registration of individual images to produce 3-D geometric reconstructions of the intact heart. We have devised a method of finite element analysis of left ventricular myocardial elastic properties based upon 3-D echocardiographic reconstructions and simultaneous high-fidelity pressure measurements. The technique consists of predicting left ventricular cavity expansion and wall thinning during diastole, using; (1) an assumed myocardial elastic modulus, and (2) the measured change in cavitary pressure during diastole as the endocardial loading condition. The predicted cavity expansion is compared to that actually derived from echocardiographic data. An iterative algorithm is used to derive an 'optimal' elastic modulus for the myocardium- that elastic modulus which allows the closest prediction of chamber expansion during diastole. We have used this technique in preliminary studies in open-chest dogs to derive normal and abnormal regional and global left ventricular elastic modulus.

Introduction

The ultimate goal of any technique aimed at depiction of the morphology of the intact heart is a three-dimensional (3-D) representation of cardiac anatomy throughout the heart cycle. The clinical echocardiographer attempts to derive this information by mentally 'reassembling' the image data from multiple two-dimensional (2-D) echocardiographic images into a conceptualization of the 3-D geometry of the heart. Each of the individual 2-D echocardiographic images is obtained along a different plane, with a variable relationship between the planes used to obtain individual images. The goal of 3-D echocardiographic reconstruction is to replace this somewhat approximate mental reassembly with a computer-generated model of the heart, derived from the individual 2-D echocardiographic images and information concerning the spatial relationship between individual images (Skorton and Geiser, 1983). Once a 3-D model of the heart has been reconstructed, the data can be used for derivation of ventricular volume (Moritz *et al.*, 1980) and ejection fraction, ventricular mass, and for qualitative morphological analysis. In this paper, we will briefly discuss the general aspects of three-dimensional ultrasound cardiac reconstruction and then describe an application of this technique to the finite element analysis of left ventricular (LV) diastolic biomechanical properties.

Three-dimensional echocardiography: General aspects

The general requirements for producing a 3-D reconstruction of the heart from ultrasound data are; (1) several individual 2-D echocardiographic images, obtained from a variety of orientations, and encompassing as much of the cardiac anatomy as possible, (2) data concerning the position and orientation of each 2-D echocardiographic image with respect to other images, or to a common, external reference point, (3) digitized endocardial and epicardial boundaries from each of the 2-D echocardiographic images, (4) a method of reconstruction of the image data into a 3-D data structure, and (5) a method of display of the 3-D data.

2-D Echocardiographic Data Acquisition

Echocardiographic images for 3-D reconstruction have been obtained from studies performed with the transducer in the parasternal position (Geiser *et al.*, 1980), at the cardiac apex (Maurer *et al.*, 1981; Ueda *et al.*, 1980), and by a combination of these approaches (Moritz and Shreve, 1974). Various advantages and disadvantages of each approach have been reviewed previously (Skorton and Geiser, 1983). In general, the parasternal short-axis views give the most complete information on endocardial and epicardial contours, but fail to give optimal visualization of the LV apex. Apical views remedy the latter problem but give less than perfect visualization of the endocardial contours. Although each of the approaches to data acquisition has its strong advocates, it is quite likely that accurate reconstructions may be achieved using any of the techniques.

Transducer position registration

After obtaining several 2-D cross-sectional images and after digitizing the endo-cardial and epicardial borders from each image, some method is needed to relate the position and orientation of each image to all other 2-D images which will be used to generate the 3-D reconstruction. Several systems have been developed to accomplish this task including systems based on acoustic (Moritz and Shreve, 1974), mechanical (Geiser *et al.*, 1980), and laser techniques (Joskowicz *et al.*, 1982). In general, the laser and acoustic techniques will probably prove to be more accurate than the mechanical techniques, but the latter, mechanical meth-ods will be less expensive, more portable, and simpler to use. Using all of these systems, apparently accurate 3-D reconstructions have been obtained. In the data to be presented subsequently, we have utilized a mechanical system with six degrees of freedom, modified from that originally described by Geiser and coworkers (1980).

Endocardial and epicardial recognition and digitization

At the present time, digitization of the endocardial and epicardial contours is accomplished by manually tracing these borders using a digitizing tablet or light pen system. The identification of endocardial and epicardial contours in individ-ual 2-D echocardiographic images represents a significant source of error in 3-D ultrasound reconstructions (Geiser *et al.*, 1980), and considerable investigation is being devoted to automated methods of edge detection in echocardiographic imagery (Skorton *et al.*, 1981; Garcia *et al.*, 1981; Collins *et al.*, 1984). Successful completion of these investigations may facilitate this important step in 3-D echocardiographic reconstructions.

Reconstruction of image data into a 3-D data structure

The methods of reconstructing the 2-D images and transducer position and orientation data into a 3-D data structure vary somewhat, depending upon the type of spatial registration system used and the echocardiographic views em-ployed. However, all methods basically consist of superimposing the individual 2-D images (either relative to an external reference system or relative to one another) and then interpolating (connecting sections) by straight lines, calculated curves, or other mathematical approximations. Our method of reconstructing 3-D echocardiographic image data is in general representative of many other approaches, and will be described in detail later. In brief, a 3-D (x, y, z) coordinate system is constructed using three of the short-axis images. The trans-ducer position and orientation data from each individual cross-section are then used, along with the digitized positions of the endocardial and epicardial borders, to align these cross-sections within the x, y, z system (Nikravesh *et al.*, 1984). That is, each 2-D cross-sectional 'plane' has its own registered position within the x, y, z coordinate system. After proper alignment of each 2-D cross-section within the coordinate system, some method of interpolating or filling in data is desired. Some investigators have chosen not to perform this interpolation for visualization of data, but interpolation is always necessary for calculation of derived indices such as volume and mass.

Display of 3-D data

Methods for the application of 3-D computer display techniques to 3-D data structures are well-established in such engineering endeavors as computer-aided design. Thus, a large amount of experience and previously-written software can be brought to bear on displaying 3-D echocardiographic reconstructions including display of data with and without removal of hidden lines, with indication of hidden lines, with sophisticated methods of shading of the contours to achieve the impression of three dimensions, and with other computer graphic techniques (Figure 1).

In addition to the difficulty in identifying endocardial and epicardial borders, briefly mentioned above, another important shortcoming of 3-D echocardiographic reconstructions in general should be emphasized. A 3-D echocardiographic reconstruction is obtained using data from several cardiac cycles – each 2-D image from approximately the same point in a different cardiac contraction. Therefore, any cycle-to-cycle variation in heart rate or hemodynamics will cause some degradation of the final 3-D data structure. Furthermore, the technique is somewhat time consuming. Newer tomographic imaging technology such as rapid computed tomography (Ritman *et al.*, 1980) will allow the acquisition of data on the morphology of large portions of the heart within a single cardiac cycle. In the next few years, further studies should help clarify the relative roles of ultrasound and other imaging modalities in the acquisition of 3-D cardiac data.

Importance and methods of assessing diastolic function

Diastole is the period of the cardiac cycle during which ventricular filling occurs prior to ventricular ejection. The importance of diastolic function includes at least three considerations; (1) by Starling's law, adequate LV filling is required for adequate ejection of blood during systole, (2) impaired diastolic filling may contribute to the symptoms of congestive heart failure and (3) certain changes in diastolic function may occur independently of systolic abnormalities (Grossman

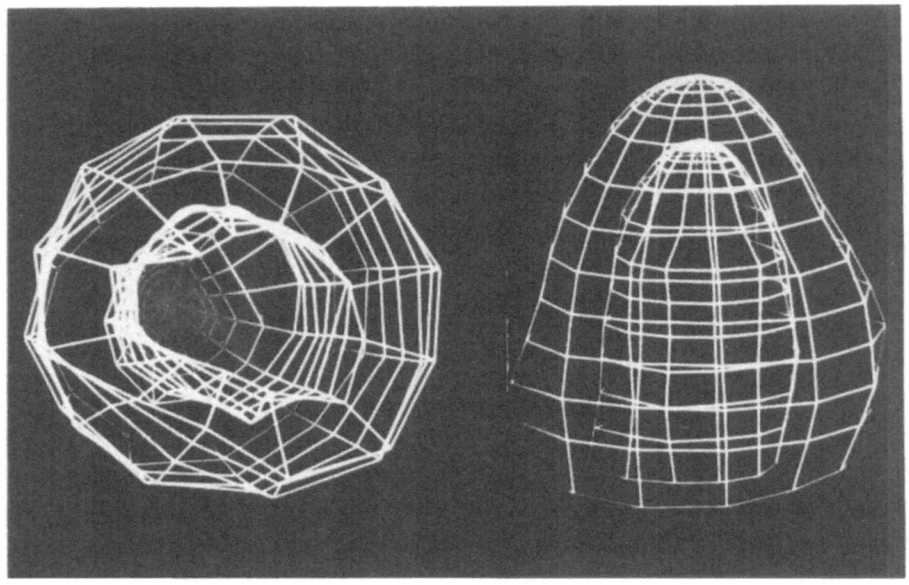

Figure 1. Three-dimensional finite element reconstruction of the intact left ventricle. These two perspective views of a finite element reconstruction of a normal human left ventricle were photographed from a vector graphics display system.

and McLaurin, 1976). Of these considerations, one that is particularly intriguing is the evidence that alterations of diastolic ventricular function may occur independently of abnormalities in systolic function (Hirota, 1980). In one clinical study of patients evaluated using radioisotope ventriculography, the time-to-peak filling rate was abnormal in patients with coronary artery disease at a time when no systolic abnormalities were noted (Bonow *et al.*, 1981). These findings suggest that the evaluation of global diastolic LV function might be a sensitive measure of early cardiac perfusion abnormalities. Since coronary artery disease is the most common cardiac disorder in Western society, and since it is by nature a regional abnormality, the study of regional LV diastolic properties might prove to be a useful technique.

The clinical evaluation of LV diastolic properties has been difficult because of technical and conceptual problems in accurately measuring LV volume and shape throughout the heart cycle. Measurements of parameters such as LV end-diastolic pressure, pulmonary artery wedge pressure, or global LV pressure/volume relationships give information on the compliance of the entire LV chamber and thus do provide some estimation of overall diastolic function (Bunnell *et al.*, 1965). However, these measurements do not delineate abnormalities in function at a regional or segmental level. Since regional myocardial dysfunction might not be reflected in overall diastolic performance, due to compensatory changes in normal regions, such a regional analysis might be important in the evaluation of diastolic abnormalities in ischemic heart disease. Attempts have been made to evaluate regional LV material properties utilizing a stress/strain analysis using hemodynamic and M-mode echocardiographic data (McLaurin *et al.*, 1973). The small sample of tissue studied and the uncertain orientation of the M-mode echocardiographic beam, however, necessitate questionable assumptions concerning LV shape and thus preclude an accurate assessment of the regional distribution of LV material properties using this approach.

The numerical method, finite element analysis, is especially well suited to the evaluation of regional biomechanical behavior. The finite element analysis of LV function has been accomplished by combining hemodynamic data with either angiographic images (Ray *et al.*, 1976) or by using computed tomographic analysis (Pao, 1980). The difficulties with the angiographic technique are well known and include; (1) the injection of angiographic contrast material which may alter some of the parameters of interest such as wall stress, (2) the fact that the volume calculations are based upon somewhat inaccurate assumptions concerning LV size and shape (LV shape does not conform to any idealized geometric model) and (3) the fact that contrast ventriculography does not allow measurement of LV wall thickness; such measurements are necessary to derive diastolic properties such as the regional elastic modulus. The use of computed tomographic scanning as another method to obtain accurate 3-D geometric data is extremely promising. However, rapid computed tomography is not widely available at this time, and at present, the time required to perform conventional CT scans (over one second) precludes the evaluation of dynamic cardiac events.

Two-dimensional echocardiography does allow evaluation of the shape of virtually the entire LV in real time, at a sampling rate of 30 frames per s. Coupled with LV pressure measurements, echocardiography may be used to determine regional and global pressure/dimension relationships. Standard 2-D echocardiography at present can give only approximate information on the 3-D shape of the LV, since the orientation of each 2-D imaging plane relative to other planes is uncertain.

It was our intention to develop a combined hemodynamic/ultrasonic method of evaluating regional diastolic LV properties based on finite element analysis of LV diastolic function. The rationale for this approach is that the relatively high spatial and temporal resolution of 2-D echocardiography, including information on the regional distribution of wall thickness, could be combined with high fidelity pressure measurements to derive a close approximation of regional LV elastic properties.

Introduction to finite element analysis

The finite element method, an approximate numerical solution procedure, was developed to solve complex problems in structural analysis where closed-form solutions to the governing equations were difficult to obtain (Cook, 1981; Desai, 1979). The method is versatile, so that problems involving complex geometries and loading conditions can be solved using high speed digital computing, and hence finite element analysis has been widely applied to problems in bio-mechanics. The structure whose deformation is to be analyzed is subdivided into a suitable number of smaller elements called *finite elements*. In general, for a 3-D geometry, the finite elements will be eight-noded brick elements. The corners of each of the elements are known as *nodes* and the geometry of the whole structure is defined by the 3-D coordinates of each of the nodes with respect to a pre-defined coordinate system. For each of the finite elements, the displacements of any point within the element is assumed to have a functional relationship to the displacements of the nodal points. Based on the principles of mechanics, a governing equation for each of the finite elements is of the form:

$$\{F\} = [k]\{\delta\},$$

where $\{F\}$ is the vector of nodal forces (forces acting on the nodes), $\{\delta\}$ is the vector of nodal displacements, and $[k]$ is the stiffness matrix. The stiffness matrix contains information about the geometry of the structure (through the nodal coordinates) and the material properties of the structure. The governing equations for each of the individual finite elements are combined to obtain the global governing equations. Once the external loads acting on the structure are speci-fied, as well as the boundary conditions of restraints, the algebraic governing equations can be evaluated with the aid of a digital computer to solve for the nodal displacements. After the nodal displacements are obtained and making use of the relation between strain and displacements as well as stress and strain for a given material, the stress and strain distribution can be easily determined. The advantage of the finite element method lies in the fact that the 3-D geometry of a highly irregular structure can be represented by suitable division into finite elements. As the finite elements are made smaller, a better approximation of the actual geometry can be obtained. However, the total number of elements and hence the number of nodal points will increase accordingly resulting in round off and cumulative errors in the numerical solution procedure. Thus a judicious choice in the number and size of the finite elements must be exercised so that the solution errors are minimized and yet the actual geometry of the structure is approximated as closely as possible.

Since the material property is specified at the finite element level, regional variation in the material property can be easily incorporated into the solution procedures. Geometric and material non-linearity can be accounted for by using the appropriate constitutive relationship. Even though the method described above is for a static analysis, dynamic problems can also be solved by including mass and damping matrices and using the technique of mode superposition or direct integration.

A method of reconstruction of LV geometry from 2-D echocardiograms

Our method of reconstruction of the 3-D LV geometry from 2-D echocardiographic images and the generation of a finite element mesh will be briefly described. Further details may be found elsewhere (Nikravesh *et al.*, 1984). Several short-axis images from the base (mitral level) to the apex of the left ventricle are obtained with the transducer mounted in a 3-D articulated arm. A schematic of the articulated arm with six degrees of freedom, θ_1 through θ_6, is shown in Figure 2. The angle θ_7 (transducer mounting orientation) is fixed for a particular experiment. In the case of dog experiments, images of good quality are obtained if the transducer is aimed from below with the animal lying in the right lateral decubitus position on a specially-prepared table ($\theta_7 = 180°$) (Wyatt *et al.*, 1979). The position and orientation of the transducer are measured by the six potentiometers and the signals from the six channels are simultaneously digitized and recorded in a (LSI 11/23) microcomputer at the time of recording of each individual 2-D image. The LV intracavitary pressure, which is also simultaneously measured by a catheter-tip pressure transducer, is digitized and stored in the computer along with the ECG signal which serves as a time reference in the cardiac cycle. The 2-D echocardiographic images at early diastole (corresponding to the nadir of the LV pressure) and at end diastole (pre-'A' wave) are recorded onto videotape and subsequently are traced onto transparent sheets from stop-frame video images. The endocardial and epicardial outlines are then digitized using a (Summagraphics) digitizing tablet and entered into a minicomputer.

An interactive mesh generation program is used in the 3-D reconstruction procedure and is executed from a graphics terminal (Hewlett-Packard 2648A). Initially, the digitized values of the cardiac outlines are transformed from the coordinate axes of the digitizer to the coordinate axes of the base of the articulated arm, which is fixed to the examination table as schematically represented in Figure 2. The details of the transformation matrices involved in this step are given in Chandran *et al.* (1984). Subsequently, the digital values of the cardiac outlines are transformed to a coordinate system fixed to the LV chamber. The center of mass of the endocardial contour of the apical cross-section (most apical short-axis echocardiographic cross-section) is defined as the origin of the LV-fixed coordinate system. A line connecting the origin to the center of mass of the basal cross-section (at the mitral valve level) is taken as the Z-axis (long-axis) of the LV-fixed coordinate system. A line perpendicular to the Z-axis which passes through the posterior junction of the right ventricular free wall and ventricular septum at high-papillary muscle level (an anatomically well-defined point) is defined as the

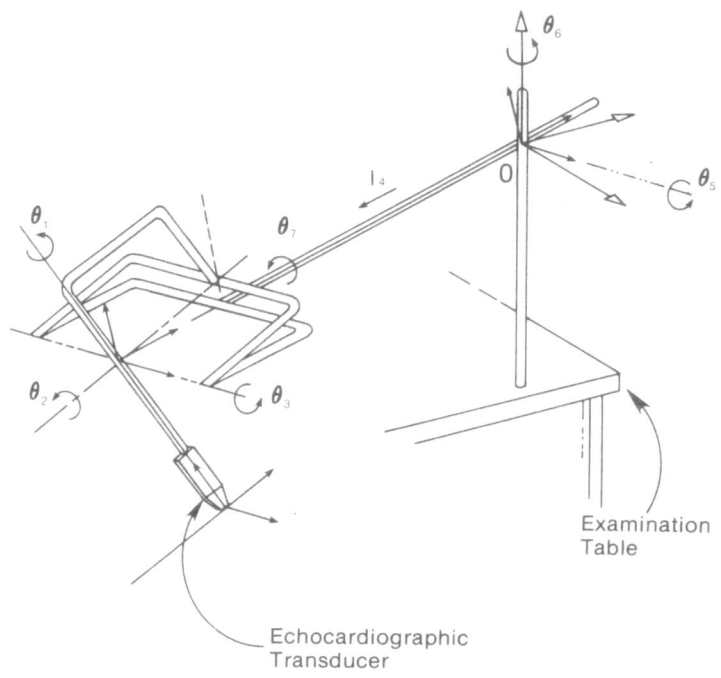

Figure 2. Diagram of the mechanical echocardiographic transducer position registration arm. The echocardiographic transducer is attached to a mechanical device with six degrees of freedom (θ_1–θ_6). This device, with its high resolution potentiometers, permits the position and orientation of the transducer relative to the post which connects the arm to the examination table to be recorded accurately for each 2-D echocardiographic image.

direction of the X-axis and then the Y-axis is selected to be mutually perpendicular to X- and Z-axes and to give a right-handed coordinate system. In the earlier reported version of our method (Chandran *et al.*, 1984), the origin of the LV-fixed coordinate system was fixed to the most apical point on the epicardial outline from a long-axis image. However, we subsequently found that our long-axis images did not always adequately visualize the apex and thus did not approximate the true LV long-axis.

A schematic of the coordinate system fixed to the LV chamber is shown in Figure 3. After the transformation of the cardiac outlines to the LV-fixed coordinate system, each of the short-axis contours is displayed on the screen of the graphics terminal with a predefined number of radial divisions emanating from the center of the cross-section as shown in Figure 4. The intersection points between the radial lines and the cardiac contours (endo- and epicardium) are selected as the nodal points. Once the X and Y coordinates of the nodal points are known, the corresponding Z coordinates are evaluated from the equation of the plane of the short-axis images. A least square or cubic spline curve is fitted

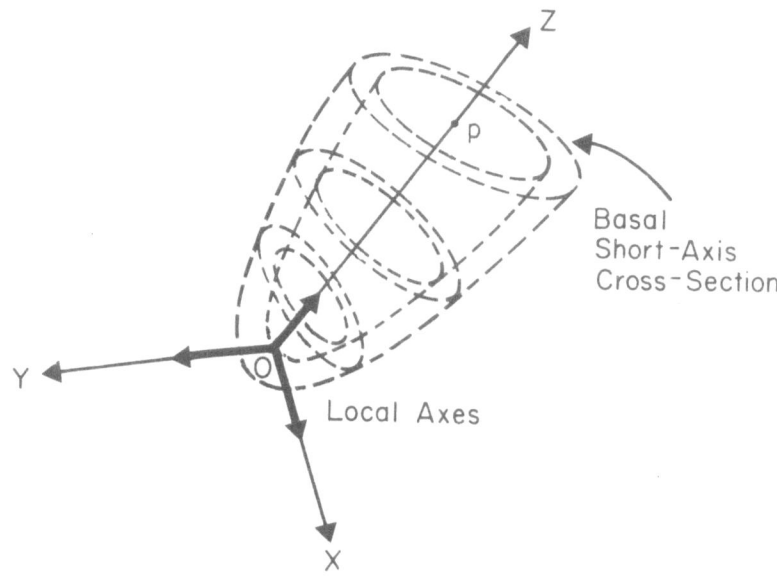

Figure 3. Definition of the three-dimensional coordinate axes as referenced to the left ventricular geometry. The long-axis (Z axis) of the heart passes through the centers of mass of basal and apical short-axis cross-sectional images. Details on the definition of the other two orthogonal axes are found in the text.

through a group of nodes along the long axis (Z) direction. This curve is employed to interpolate additional nodes so that the short-axis planes in the finite element mesh will be parallel to each other except for the basal cross-section which retains its inclination. The resulting information on the coordinates of the nodes as well as the assembly of nodes to form the finite elements is used to create input files for a general purpose finite element program and a 3-D graphics display and plot program (MOVIE–BYU, Brigham Young University). A typical 3-D plot of the reconstructed LV geometry is shown in Figure 5.

Finite element analysis and assessment of myocardial stiffness

Using the reconstruction technique described above, the 3-D geometry of the LV at early diastole and at late diastole are reconstructed. The finite element analysis is performed on the early diastolic geometry. The change in LV pressure during filling (the difference between the pressure at early and at late diastole) is the load at the endocardial surface of the LV chamber, with the load at the epicardial surface assumed to be zero in the open-chest preparation. The nodes at the basal layer are also fixed (boundary condition) for the finite element analysis. Eight-noded isoparametric 3-D brick elements are used in the finite element mesh

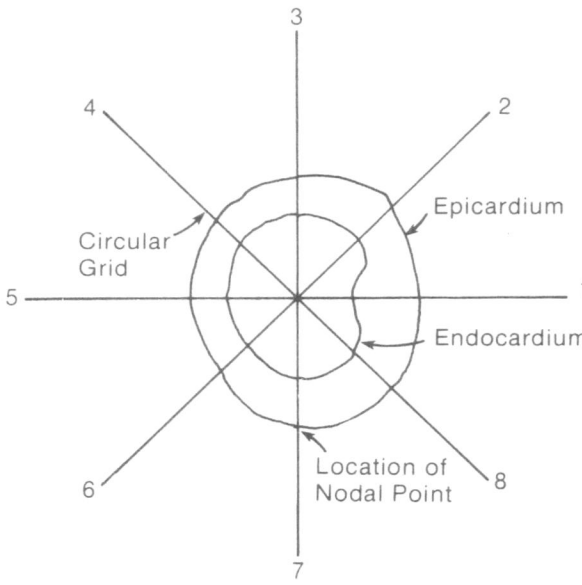

Figure 4. Projection of typical short-axis contours in the *x, y* plane. The endocardial and epicardial contours traced from a two-dimensional echocardiographic short-axis image are superimposed on a radial (circular) grid. The intersection points between the radii and cardiac contours identify the location of finite element nodal points.

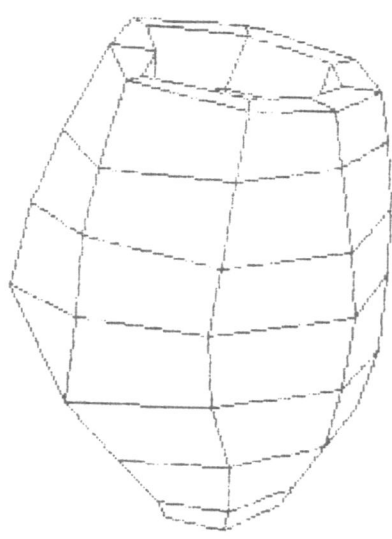

Figure 5. Three-dimensional finite element reconstruction of a dog left ventricle in early diastole. In this figure, hidden lines are removed.

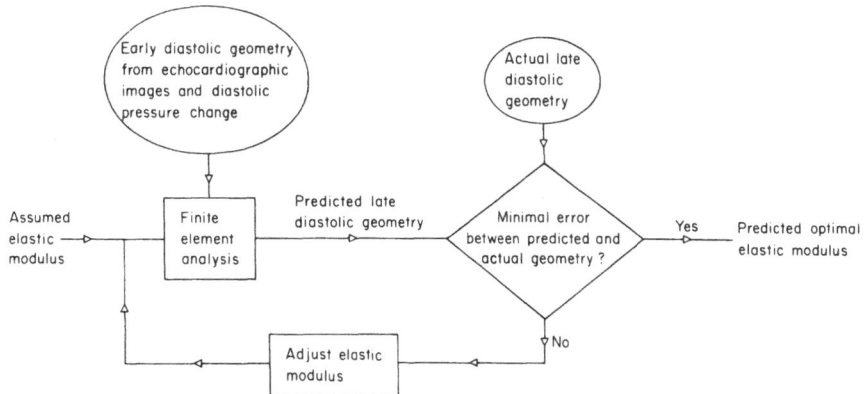

Figure 6. Method of estimation of the elastic modulus of the myocardium using echocardiographic and hemodynamic data. An assumed elastic modulus, the early diastolic geometry of the left ventricle obtained from the echocardiographic reconstruction, and the measured pressure change in the left ventricle during diastole are used to predict the late diastolic geometry of the ventricle. This predicted geometry is compared to the actual, reconstructed late diastolic geometry and this process is repeated until the difference between predicted and actual late diastolic geometries is minimized.

except near the apical region where six-noded elements are used. A total of 64 elements with 130 nodes are used in the analysis.

Assuming an initial value for the Young's modulus of the myocardium, the finite element analysis is performed to determine the predicted displacements of the nodal points. The late diastolic geometry of the LV chamber as predicted by the computer analysis is compared with the actual reconstructed late-diastolic geometry. The square root of the sum of the squares of differences in displacements between these two (in the three coordinate directions) is defined as an index of performance. In computing the index of performance, a different weighting function can be specified for each of the coordinate directions if desired. The assumed elastic modulus for the myocardium is modified, based on an optimization algorithm, and the value of the elastic modulus which yields the minimum value of the index of performance (i.e., the least difference between predicted and actual nodal displacements) is defined as the optimal value for the elastic modulus of the myocardium. A schematic of the steps involved in the estimation of the myocardial elastic modulus is shown in Figure 6. In this analysis, the myocardium is assumed to be an isotropic, homogeneous, linearly-elastic medium.

Preliminary results

We initially tested our method of estimating the regional LV elastic modulus by studying anesthetized dogs before and after acute occlusion of the circumflex

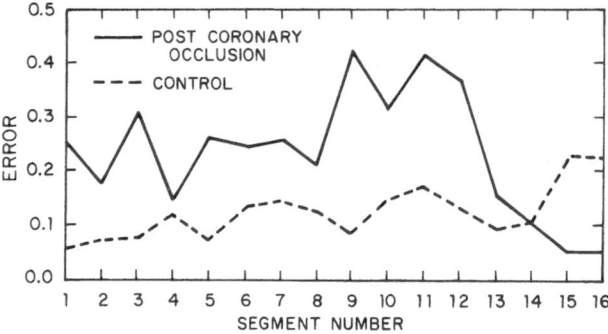

Figure 7. Regional variation in elastic modulus before and after acute coronary occlusion in the dog. The diagram indicates the error between computer-predicted and actual nodal displacements for each of 16 segments into which the reconstructed left ventricle was divided. The interrupted line indicates the variability in error (that is, variability in elastic modulus) found before coronary occlusion. The solid line indicates segmental errors after coronary occlusion. In segments 9–12, the error appears higher than that in other segments, suggesting a regional change in elastic modulus due to acute coronary occlusion.

coronary artery. The 3-D finite element mesh of the LV in this experiment consisted of 64 elements and was divided into 16 segments of 4 elements each for the presentation of results in a regional fashion. The index of performance (difference between predicted and actual late diastolic geometry) for each of the segments for the optimal value of the elastic modulus in one animal is plotted in Figure 7. The 'control' curve corresponds to experimental results obtained on the dog before coronary occlusion. After the control recordings were completed, the circumflex coronary artery was occluded to induce local ischemia in the posterior and posterolateral LV myocardium and the analysis was then repeated. The curves show a considerable increase in the error (index of performance) in selected segments (of the posterolateral LV) indicating a change in myocardial elastic modulus in the myocardial location corresponding to those segments.

Conclusions

The goal of 3-D echocardiography is to produce a computer-generated reassembly of multiple 2-D echocardiograph images into a 3-D representation of cardiac anatomy. Another use of echocardiographic reconstructions is the finite element analysis of cardiac diastolic biomechanical properties based on simultaneous hemodynamic and echocardiographic measurements. In this way physiological induces may be obtained which would not be possible without accurate 3-D reconstruction of the heart.

Acknowledgements

The authors wish to acknowledge Bob Kieso and Pam Hite for their technical assistance. The authors also expess their appreciation to Carolyn Frisbie, Rita Yeggy and Ann Aschoff for their expert preparation of this manuscript. This study was supported in part by the U.S. Veterans Administration, the National Heart, Lung and Blood Institute – Grant #1 R01 HL 27035 and the American Heart Association – Iowa Affiliate Grant #82–G–7. Dr. Skorton is a recipient of a U.S. Veterans Administration Research Associate Career Development Award.

References

Bonow RO, Bacharach SL, Grier MV *et al.* (1981) Impaired left ventricular diastolic filling in patients with coronary artery disease: assessment with radionuclide angiography. Circulation 64:315–323

Bunnell IL, Grant C, Greene DG (1965) Left ventricular function derived from the pressure-volume diagram. Am J Med 39:881–894

Chandran KB, Olshansky B, Attarwala YM, Skorton DJ (1984) Finite element analysis of three-dimensional echocardiographic data for the evaluation of diastolic left ventricular function. Automedica 5:151–169

Collins SM, Skorton DJ, Geiser EA *et al.* (1984) Computer-assisted edge detection in two-dimensional echocardiography: a comparison to anatomical data. Am J Cardiol 53:1380–1387

Cook RD (1981) Concepts and Applications of Finite Element Analysis, Second Edition, John Wiley and Sons, New York

Desai CS (1979) Elementary Finite Element Method. Englewood Cliffs, New Jersey: Prentice-Hall, Inc.

Garcia E, Gueret P, Bennett M *et al.* (1981) Real time computerization of two-dimensional echocardiography. Am Heart J 101:783

Geiser EA, Lupkiewicz SM, Christie LG *et al.* (1980) A framework for three-dimensional time-varying reconstruction of the human left ventricle: sources of error and estimation of their magnitude. Comput Biomed Res 13: 225–241

Grossman W, McLaurin LP (1976) Diastolic properties of the left ventricle. Ann Intern Med 84:316–326

Hirota Y (1980) A clinical study of left ventricular relaxation. Circulation 62: 756–763

Joskowicz G, Kliepera M, Pachinger O *et al.*, (1982) Computer-supported measurements of 2-D echocardiographic images. In: *Computers in Cardiology*. Los Angeles: IEEE Computer Society, p. 13

Maurer G, Ghosh A, Nanda NC (1981) Volume determination and three-dimensional reconstruction of echocardiographic images using rotation method (abstract). Circulation 64:IV–206

McLaurin LP, Grossman W, Stefadouros MA *et al.* (1973) A new technique for the study of left ventricular pressure volume relations in man. Circ Res 48:56–64

Moritz WE, Shreve PL (1974) A microprocessor-based spatial locating system for use with diagnostic ultrasound. Proceedings of IEEE 64:966

Moritz WE, Medema DK, Ainsworth M *et al.* (1980) Three-dimensional reconstruction and volume calculation from a series of nonparallel, real time ultrasonic images (abstract). Circulation 62:III–143

Nikravesh PE, Skorton DJ, Chandran KB, Attarwala YM, Pandian N, Kerber RE (1984) Computerized three-dimensional finite element reconstruction of the left ventricle from cross-sectional echocardiograms. Ultrasonic Imaging 6:48–59

Pao YC, Ritman EL (1980) Estimation of passive and active muscle properties of working heart. Proceedings of International Conference on Finite Elements in Biomechanics. Tucson, Arizona, USA, 2:657–672

Ray G, Chandran KB, Nikravesh PE, Ghista DN, Sandler H. (1976). Estimation of the local elastic modulus of the normal and infarcted left ventricle from angiographic data. In: Saha, S (ed) Proceedings of the 4th New England Bioengineering Conference, pp. 173–176

Ritman EL, Harris LD, Kinsey JH et al. (1980) Computed tomographic imaging of the heart: the dynamic spatial reconstructor. Radiol Clin North Am 18:547

Skorton DJ, McNary CA, Child JS et al. (1981) Digital image processing of two dimensional echocardiograms: identification of the endocardium. Am J Cardiol 48:479

Skorton DJ, Geiser EA (1983) Three-dimensional echocardiography: a geometric reconstruction. In: Talano JV, Gardin JM (eds) Textbook of Two-dimensional Echocardiography. New York: Grune & Stratton, pp 357–370

Ueda K, Kuwaki K, Inoue K (1980) Three-dimensional display and volume determination of the left ventricle by two-dimensional echocardiography (abstract) Am J Cardiol 45:471

Wyatt HL, Heng MK, Meerbaum S et al. (1979). Cross-sectional echocardiography. I. Analysis of mathematic models for quantifying mass of the left ventricle in dogs. Circulation 60:1104–1113

DISCUSSION

GESELOWITZ: I enjoyed your remark about the significant figures. This is something that really bothers me with students. Students have calculators and put out answers to all kind of significant figures. I think, as a professor of engineering, that if we don't make the student appreciate that the data are accurate to a certain number of significant figures, we're cranking out lousy engineers. In biological data we're often dealing with, at best, two significant figures. That is something we have to keep in mind. Have you attempted to do any sensitivity analysis were you change your geometry by, say 5%? What does this do to the calculation of the mechanical properties?

ANS: We would love to be able to do such a thing. The problem is that in sensitivity analysis you have to have a denominator, an independent variable. We don't have one. That is, we have no a priori knowledge of the precise in vivo geometry. We postulate that we can detect changes on the order of about 10%. I can't tell you what the sensitivity is for the detection of changes in the elastic modulus because I don't have a yardstick by which to compare the numbers that we get.

LANIR: I take it that you assume iostropy and small deformation in finite element. How does it compare to the actual deformation?

ANS: We assume linear elasticity and isotropic material properties. The only thing we didn't assume was that elasticity was homogenous throughout the myocardium. The fact that we assumed linear properties doesn't bother me because of the very limited portion of diastole which we examined.

LANIR: Can you compare to the actual measurement? How does it compare? What are the deformation gradients that you got from your echo?

ANS: The chamber volume actually changed by a few percent in this portion of the cycle.

LANIR: That is really beyond the scope of a small deformation. Your discrepancies may stem not from the stiffness changes, but from the fact that you assume isotrophy and small deformation.

ANS: It's possible. The only way to solve this would be to do it in a smaller animal model, from which we could take out pieces of normal and infarcted muscle, and superfuse them, and actually measure the elastic stiffness. We can't do this in a dog.

NEREM: You showed the 16 segment model. I thought that was to look at a particular ischemic case. I wondered if you had looked at the variability within the myocardium just for a normal functioning ventricle and what kind of differences do you see from segment to segment?

ANS: This is the only case we have so far completed. The differences that we found were what the solid line in Figure 17, the control line, shows. At least, in the control state, we do find this degree of variability. I believe that there probably are slight changes in normal elastic modulus from place to place because of differing fiber orientation, and the fact that collagen deposition in normal hearts is not perfectly uniform. I have to agree, however, that a lot of those changes may be due to errors in the reconstruction. So we'll have to do a few more of these studies to be able to give you a better answer on that.

ADAM: Could you comment about the error associated with the small angle between the transdusor rays and the myocardium? Between the ultrasonic ray and the border of the myocardium?

ANS: In areas in which the beam is not perpendicular? The error in visualizing the borders nearly parallel to the beam in single frames is important. We found, and so did DeMaria and others, that reproducibility for different observers tracing the echo from time to time, for example, may be relatively poor. Another way to answer is that we've done echos of excised fixed hearts, using the 3-D reconstruction system, then cut the hearts along the plane that we have imaged, then made calibrated photographs, traced the endocardial borders and compared them to our borders. We routinely have problems in tracing borders parallel to the beam, but there is liner correspondence between the measurements made from echo and the anatomy. There is usually an overestimation of wall thickness, and an underestimation of cavity size. Finally, it doesn't make too much difference in qualitative analysis if you are perpendicular or parallel to the beam because the whole differentiation in the echo textbooks about specular versus nonspecular reflectors is true for pieces of plastic, but nothing in the body is ever really completely specular; everyting is a little irregular and therefore scatters omnidirectionally to some degree. That's why you can see the borders to some degree at all points around a short-axis image.

Cardiac imaging and modelling

ROBERT M. HEETHAAR[1,2,3], JOHN HEETHAAR[4] and
JACQUES M. HUYGHE[3]
[1] *Department of Cardiology, University of Utrecht*
[2] *Department of Medical Physics, University of Utrecht*
[3] *Department of Biomedical Engineering, University of Technology, Twente*
[4] *Interuniversity Cardiology Institution, Utrecht, The Netherlands*

Abstract

In this paper a method is described to measure accurately the three-dimensional geometry of the isolated, working canine heart during the cardiac cycle. Times of flight of ultrasonic pulses are measured with high accuracy for many directions through the object under study. These transmissions times are then used to reconstruct the ultrasound velocity distribution in the plane of measurement.

Additional information about regional cardiac contraction, like the dynamic fibre shortening and fibre orientation are measured with help of radiopaque markers which are inserted in the cardiac walls at different places. The spatial positions of the markers throughout the cardiac cycle and thus also cardiac dimensions are determined with help of a biplane X-ray system.

The dimensional data of the heart, obtained with both methods will be basic input parameters of a finite element model of the heart that is being developed. With this model we aim to compute regional intramural wall stresses and strains in normal and pathological situations. An interesting feature of this model is that it will incorporate blood rheology into tissue mechanics. As a first step in this direction perfusion of blood in tissue with a rich vasculature is described by extending the law of Darcy (describing flow of a newtonian fluid through a porous medium) for the specific situation were venous and arterial bloodflow can exist simultaneously in a small volume element. Preliminary tests of this model look promising.

Introduction

To meet the demands of the body the heart propels the blood by cyclic contraction of its individual muscle fibres. During contraction these fibres develope forces, leading to stresses and strains in the cardiac walls, resulting into ventricular pressures and finally into ejection of blood into the systemic and pulmonary circulation. For a single cardiac fibre it is possible to express its contractile behaviour from its changes of length and from the forces generated during contraction in the so-called length-tension relationships. These basic quantitative measurements however cannot be made in the intact heart for many reasons, such as for instance the complex anatomic arrangement and electrical activation sequence of the cardiac fibres and the interaction of blood rheology and tissue mechanics.

Assessment of cardiac function of the intact heart often occurs on the bases of parameters, reflecting the integral contractile behaviour of all individual muscle fibres in their specific anatomic environment (such as ejection fraction, stroke volume etc.). However regional dysfunctioning of the heart cannot always be derived from these parameters as control mechanisms of the healthy muscle fibres can compensate for the impaired function of the affected zones (Kuijer, 1985). It is our belief that quantitatieve analysis of regional cardiac function can be performed on the bases of analysis of regional parameters such as wall thickness, myocardial deformations and intramural stresses and strains. As intramural stresses and strains cannot be measured directly in the intact heart models are often used to approximate these parameters. Cardiac geometry plays an important role (Heethaar *et al.*, 1977; Pao *et al.*, 1974). Besides it is a well known fact that many heart diseases alter ventricular geometry (Burton, 1957).

To study regional cardiac function we are developing a model that incorporates intramyocardial blood rheology into cardiac tissue mechanics. This model uses as input parameters the three dimensional geometry of the heart, intramural deformations and ventricular pressures (Huyghe, 1983).

Measurement of the 3-dimensional geometry is achieved by ultrasound velocity tomography (Mol, 1981; Mol *et al.*, 1981), whereas measurement of intramural, endo- and epicardial deformations is performed by measuring distances between implanted radiopaque or natural (bifurcations of coronory arteries) markers with help of a biplane X-ray system (Elshuraydeh, 1981; Elshuraydeh *et al.*, 1981).

Methods

Ultrasound tomography

Interaction between ultrasound and tissue can be characterized by a number of parameters like speed of propagation, attenuation, absorption coefficients etc. As ultrasound velocity is characteristic for a particular tissue the possibility is opened for ultrasound velocity tomography. The principles hereof and implications for medicine have been described by Greenleaf *et al.* (1975). In ultrasound velocity tomography transmitters and receivers are positioned around the object under study. Times of flight of ultrasonic pulses from transmitter to receiver are measured accurately. By rotating the transmitters and receivers in a plane around

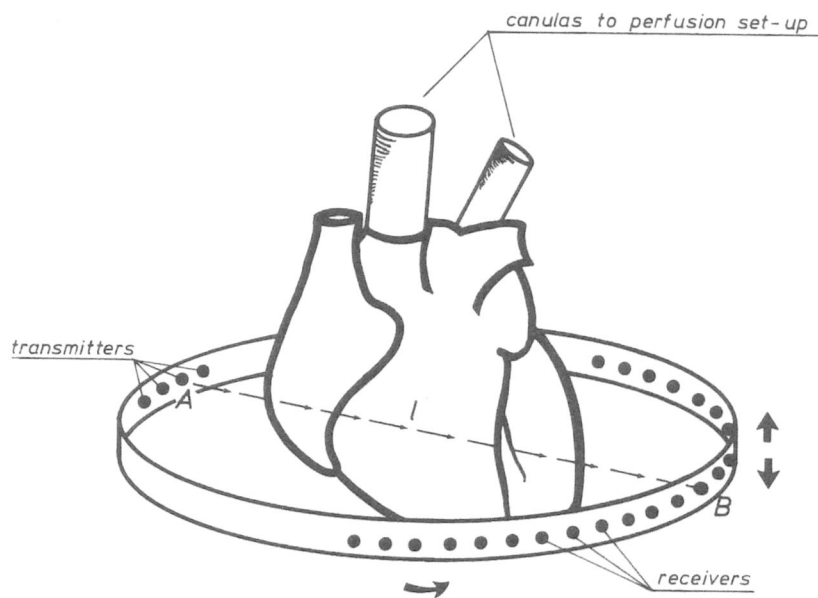

Figure 1. Schematic representation of the perfused, isolated working canine heart and the ring with ultrasound transmitters and receivers. l is the straight pathway between transmitter A and receiver B.

the object, measurements can be performed for a sufficiently large number of directions to allow a reconstruction of the ultrasound velocty distribution in the plane of measurement.

Ultrasound tomograph

An important part of the tomograph is a cylinder, which can be filled with a suitable fluid in which the isolated, working canine heart preparation is submerged. During the experiment the heart is perfused with blood and the left ventricle ejects blood against an adjustable impedance and compliance (Heethaar *et al.,* 1982). In the cylinder a ring is positioned around the heart containing 4 transmitters and 22 receivers (see Figure 1). The ring can be rotated around the heart to obtain the number of transmission times through the heart, required for reconstruction of the ultrasound velocity distribution in the transducer plane. Also vertical displacement of the ring is possible to obtain reconstructions of other cross sections between base and apex. Transmission times are measured within an accuracy of 4 ns. The selection of the transducers and the corresponding receivers, the rotation and translation of the ring and the collection of the data occur under control of a mini computer.

Principle of data collection

For a complete reconstruction of one cross section of the heart we use transmission time measurements from 200 different angles of view over 360°. In each direction 44 measurements of transmission times are performed resulting in 8800 measurements for one cross section. All measurements are performed sequentially. The heart is electrically stimulated to obtain a regular beating heart. The cardiac cycle is subdivided into periods of 20 ms. Within such a period it is assumed that the changes in cardiac geometry are limited. In this period 44 transmission times are measured. For such successive periods in one cardiac cycle the transmission times are digitized and stored on disk. Fourty milliseconds prior to a new heart beat the transducer ring is rotated over 1.8° and a new series of measurements is started. This procedure is carried out for 200 successive heart beats, after which all data over 360° are stored on disk. Next the data belonging to corresponding phases in the cardiac cycle are selected and used for reconstruction of the cross section studied. Other cross sections are obtained by repeating the above mentioned procedure after vertical displacement of the transducer ring to scan the appropriate cross section.

Reconstruction technique

With ultrasound velocity tomography the local speed of ultrasound in a cross section of the subject under study is computed from a large set of ultrasound transmission times. These calculations (reconstructions) are based upon a model that describes the propagation of ultrasound in a medium. In its simplest form the ultrasonic pulses are supposed to travel along straight pathways from transmitter to receiver. The measured transmission times depends on the velocity distribution $v(x, y)$ in the plane of reconstruction:

$$T_{AB} = \int_l \frac{1}{v(x, y)} ds, \tag{1}$$

where: T_{AB} represents the transmission time between transmitter A and receiver B;

l is the straight pathway between A and B (see Figure 1).

Equation (1) is approximated by a finite sum:

$$T_{AB} = \sum_{i=1}^{n} \frac{\Delta s}{v(x_i, y_i)}, \tag{2}$$

where: l is subdivided into n small segments Δs.

An important improvement of reconstructions can be obtained by selecting a more appropriate model and abandon the 'straight pathway approximation'. A more sophisticated model gives a description of the propagation of ultrasonic waves in a medium based upon the wave equation:

$$\nabla^2 \varphi \, (r, t) - \frac{1}{v^2 \, (r)} \cdot \frac{\partial^2 \varphi \, (r, t)}{\partial t^2} = 0, \tag{3}$$

where: $\varphi(r, t)$ = the local (tissue) pressure,
$v(r)$ = the local (complex) speed of ultrasound,
$\varphi(r, t_0) = f(r)$, with $f(r)$ a probing ultrasound pulse at time t_0.

Progress has been made in the field of applied mathematics to invert this relation for the application mentioned here by techniques that establish a transformation between the data and the characteristics of the operator that describes the development of the ultrasonic field. To give the reader some insight, a sketch of an appropriate procedure for relating the measured acoustic field to the data is presented. The medium is characterized by an acoustic profile:

$$O(r) = 1 - v_0^2 \, / \, v^2 \, (r), \tag{4}$$

where: v_0 = the speed of ultrasound in the fluid surrounding the heart and
$v(r)$ = the local speed of ultrasound in the heart.

For an insonifying wave it can be derived that:

$$\varphi(\varkappa, \omega) = f(k, \varkappa) \cdot \hat{O}(k(\mathbf{s} - \mathbf{s}_0)) \tag{5}$$

where: $\hat{\varphi} \, (\varkappa, \omega)$ = the one dimensional fourier transform of the field, measured along l,
$\hat{O}$ = the two-dimensional fourier transform of O,
f = a function of $k, \varkappa$ and the position of l,
$\mathbf{s}$ = a (unity) vector $(\varkappa/k, l/k \, \sqrt{k^2 - \varkappa^2})$
$\mathbf{s}_0$ = a (unity) vector pointing in the direction of the incident wave.

So the Fourier transform of the data equals the two-dimensional Fourier transform of the acoustical profile $O(r)$ on a halfcircle. By selecting different directions of s and l the Fourier transform of $O(r)$ can be found for a large number of points. The inverse transformation finally will lead to $O(r)$. For $k \to \infty$ (wavelength $\to 0$) the radii of the halfcircles tend to go to infinity and the well known result of reconstructive tomography is found: the one-dimensional fourier transform of the projected data is equal to a slice through the two-dimensional Fourier transform of the projected object.

Determination of ventricular dimensions, wall thickness and dynamic fibre orientation

For the measurement of ventricular dimensions, intramural deformations, fibre shortening and fibre orientation, radiopaque markers were implanted at various locations in the myocardium of a dog heart. Subepicardial markers were stitched onto the left ventricular wall after being inserted in the lumen of braided suture material. Subendocardial markers were implated with help of a hollow blunt needle (outer diameter 1.4 mm, inner diameter 1.0 mm) in which a platinum marker fitted tightly. The needle with a marker at its tip was inserted into the ventricular myocardium and pushed forward gently until the endocardial membrane was sensed. Then the marker was ejected by a stylet and the needle was withdrawn. By approaching the heart from different directions markers could be placed almost anywhere in the myocardium, even in the septum.

Usually 10–20 markers were implanted. Stimulation electrodes were stitched on the right atrium. After the thorax was closed the heart was paced and the motion of the markers was recorded on film with help of a biplane X-ray equipment at 84 frames per second. An electrogram, left ventricular and aortic pressures were recorded.

The X-ray films were analyzed with help of a digital videodensitometer interfaced to a computer. Markerprojections within a filmframe were pinpointed by lightpen, and their coordinates were computed as the centroids of density of a small area around the marker selected. Spatial markercoordinates were found by selecting the corresponding projections of a particular marker from its two orthogonally projected filmframes. Test fantoms containing platinum markers at precisely known distances showed an accuracy of the method of 0.2 mm.

From the spatial marker coordinates, ventricular dimensions, and dynamic fibre shortening and fibre orientation were calculated in a way described below.

Calculation of dynamic (epicardial) fibre shortening and fibre orientation
Dynamic fibre orientation and shortening were found by computing the largest deformation in a particular triangular element formed by three markers and the corresponding direction of the deformation. It is assumed that the fibre orientation corresponds to the direction of the maximal shortening. Within the triangle linear elastic deformations are considered. In that case the displacement of a point D ε ABC can be expressed as a linear function of its coordinates:

$$u = a_0 + a_1 x + a_2 y, \qquad (1)$$
$$v = b_0 + b_1 x + b_2 y, \qquad (7)$$

where: u is the displacement in x-direction, and
v is the displacement in y-direction.

These equations also hold for the markers in A, B and C. Substituting their measured displacements in x- and y-direction results in six equations from which a_0, a_1, a_2, b_0, b_1, and b_2 can be calculated (Zienkiewicz, 1977). From these coefficients the displacement of any point in the triangle can be computed. The strains in x- and y-direction (ε_x and ε_y) and the shear strain ε_{xy} are given by:

$$\varepsilon_x = \frac{\partial u}{\partial x}$$

$$\varepsilon_y = \frac{\partial v}{\partial y} \tag{8}$$

$$\varepsilon_{xy} = \frac{\partial u}{\partial y} + \frac{\partial u}{\partial x}$$

Through any point in the neigbourhood of (x,y) there passes one and only one quadric surface of the family (Love, 1927)

$$\varepsilon_x x^2 + \varepsilon_y y^2 + \varepsilon_{xy} xy = \text{const.} \tag{9}$$

Such a surface has the property that the reciprocal of the square of its central radius is proportional to the extension of a line in that direction. The lines in the unstrained state for which the extension is a maximum or a minimum or is stationary with being a true maximum or minimum are the principal axes of the strain and the extensions in the direction of these axes are the principal extensions. In our theoretical approach the direction of the largest shortening in the successive phases of the contraction is taken as the dynamic fibre orientation.

Model considerations

To compute regional intramural stresses and strains from the data measured a three-dimensional finite element model is being developed in which intramyocardial blood rheology is incorporated into cardiac tissue mechanics. It is a well known fact that intramyocardial stresses affect coronary blood flow (Hoffman, 1979). On the other hand some authors suggest that intramyocardial blood volume might play an important role in the viscous properties of the heart muscle (Hoffman, 1979). The large number of microvessels per unit ventricular volume does not allow to incorporate these vessels individually in a quantitative description of heart muscle. Therefore a statistical approach to the coronary circulation is chosen for, wherein pressure flow relationships are described in terms of average flow and pressure over a number of vessels. In our model this description is based on the law of Darcy for a newtonian fluid through a unit area of porous medium:

$$f_i = \sum_{j=1}^{3} - K_{ij} P_{,j} \quad \text{(for } i = 1, 2, 3\text{)}, \tag{10}$$

where: f_i = flow in x-, y- or z-direction for resp. $i = 1$, 2 or 3
P_j = pressure gradient in x-, y- or z-direction

K_{ij} = symmetric permeability tensor, dependent upon the geometry of the pores and the viscosity of the fluid.

The pressure P and the flow f_i at a point x_i are defined as averages over a number of pores surrounding x_i.

Application of this equation on the ventricular myocardium cannot be done without certain changes. As in the ventricle pressure differences in a small volume can exist in the venous and arterial system the above-mentioned equation is extended to:

$$f_i = \sum_{j=0}^{3} -K_{ij} P_{,j} \; (i = 0, 1, 2, 3) \tag{11}$$

It is assumed that a Poiseuille type pressure-flow relationship is valid for the individual vessels, whereby the apparent blood viscosity can be diameter dependent (Fahraeus-Lindqvist effect). The symmetric conductance tensor K_{ij} is dependent upon the density, the diameter and the orientation of blood vessel cross sections and the blood viscosity. The pressure derivative $P_{,0}$ represents the arteriovenous pressure gradient, whereas f_0 represents the total flow through all vessels with cross section x_0 within a myocardial unit volume. In particular, when choosing $x_0 = 0$ (capillairy level) f_0 represents regional blood perfusion. $P_{,i}$ and f_i ($i = 1,2,3$) represent pressure variation and flows between different myocardial regions. These parameters allow to model the transmural pressure gradient during the different phases of the cardiac cycle.

Results

Ultrasound Velocity Tomography

Experiments have been performed to record the three dimensional geometry of the working, isolated canine heart under various experimental conditions such as changes in heart rate, preload and afterload. An example of a set of reconstructions is shown in Figure 2 for two phases in the cardiac cycle (end-diastole (A) and systole (B)) for five different layers between base and apex. During the cardiac cycle distinct changes in geometry can be observed along with the motion of the papillary muscles. As in this experiment the filling of the right ventricle was not controlled, its free wall will occasionally coincide with the ventricular septum. Visual inspection of a sequence of these pictures (movie) reveals interesting facts about cardiac contraction. However quantitation of the observed phenomena is required to deepen the insight in cariac contraction in normal and pathological situations. An example of such a quantitation is presented in Figure 3, where the cross sectional area enclosed by the endocardial contour is plotted. Although this

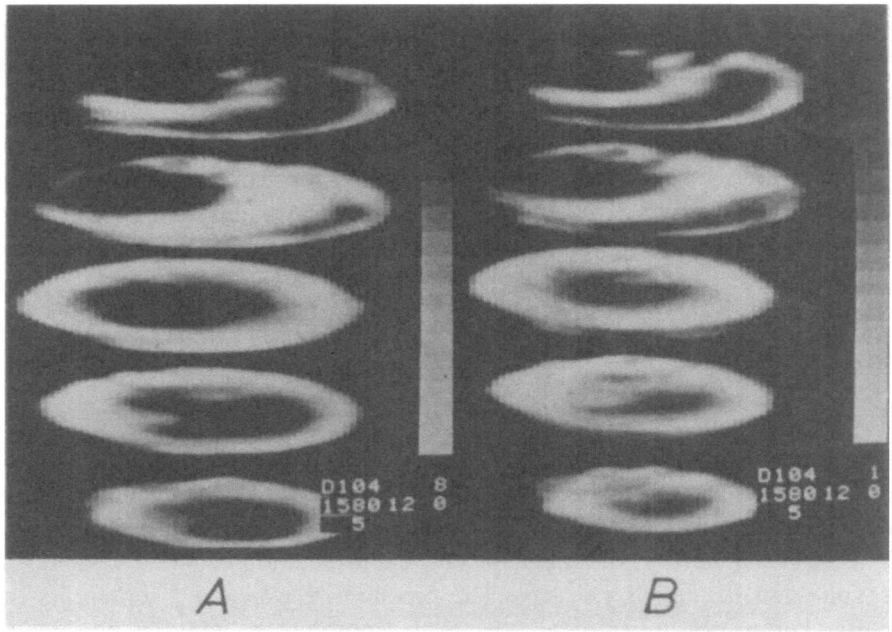

Figure 2. Reconstructed cross sections from base to apex of a beating heart for two phases in the cardiac cycle (panel A, end diastole; panel B, end systole).

parameter reflects mainly the integral effects of contraction and relaxation of muscle fibres at that particular level, regional differences can be seen. During the isovolumic contraction phase distinct changes in cardiac geometry occur. During ejection, contraction seems to start somewehere at midventricle and propagates with different speeds to base and apex. Also, during the isovolumic relaxation phase, pronounced changes in geometry occur, whereas in the filling period different relaxation velocities of myocardial tissue can be noticed.

Apart from visual inspection of (a movie of) cross sections of the heart additional information can be obtained by looking at the three-dimensional shape and shape changes of the heart during the cardiac cycle. Therefore we developed several mathematical interpolation procedures to obtain three dimensional images of the heart from the measured cross sections. In Figure 4 such an example is presented. Shown are the endocardial surfaces and some indications of the epicardial contours (dotted lines). In Figure 5 both epi- and endocardial surfaces are plotted in a diastolic phase of the heart. Additional mathematical procedures allow numerical vivisection of an arbitrairy segment of the heart. In this way visual inspection of the inside of the ventricles becomes possible. In Figure 6 a third way of representing the ventricles is shown. Now the ventricular myocardium is imaged with parts of the septum and the left and right ventricular walls being resected by mathematical scalpel.

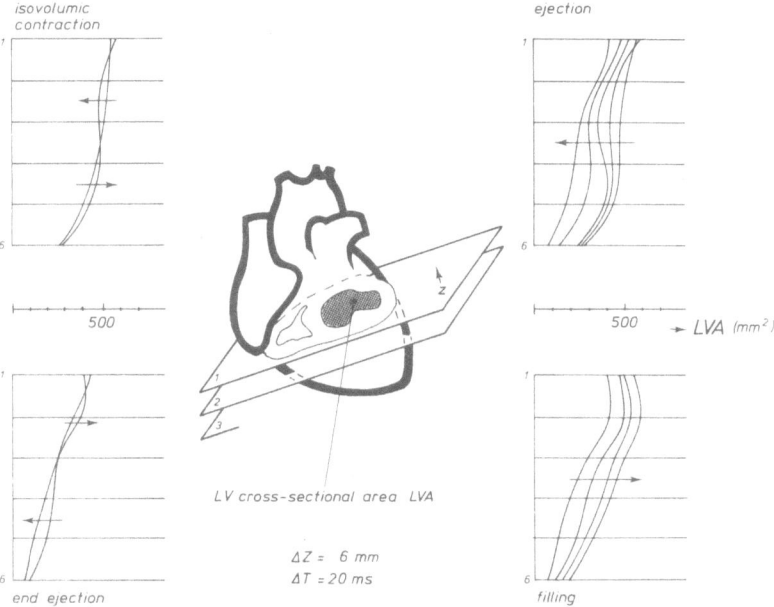

Figure 3. Left ventricular cross sectional area for different cross sections from base (1) to apex (6). The time interval between successive lines is 20 ms. Vertical distances between cross sections is 6 mm.

Radiopaque Ventricular Markers

By implanting various markers in the ventricular myocardium, dimensional data can be obtained such as inner and outer long axes, wall thickness, regional contraction and relaxation patterns, ventricular torsion and rotation and fibre orientation, and fibre shortening (Elshuraydeh, 1981). In Figure 7 a typical example of; fibre shortening (A), fibre orientation. (B), fibre strain perpendicular to the fibre (C), and layer thickening (D) is presented during a normal heart beat in the midwall of the left ventricular anterior free wall halfway between base and apex. In all experiments rate of shortening during contraction is markedly lower than rate of lengthening during relaxation. In Figure 8 an example is given of calculations of endocardial fibre strain (A), epicardial fibre strain (B) and epicardial fibre orientation (in radians) for four successive beats (two normal beats, an induced extrasystole and a controlled post extrasystole). Markers were placed in a region halfway between base and apex. Basic RR-interval was 500 ms, the induced extrasystolic interval 350 ms. As was compensated for changes in AV conduction time (due to changes in stimulation rate) the postextrasystolic RR-interval differed less than 2 ms from the basic RR-interval (controlled post-extra-systolic stimulation) (Kuijer *et al.*, 1978).

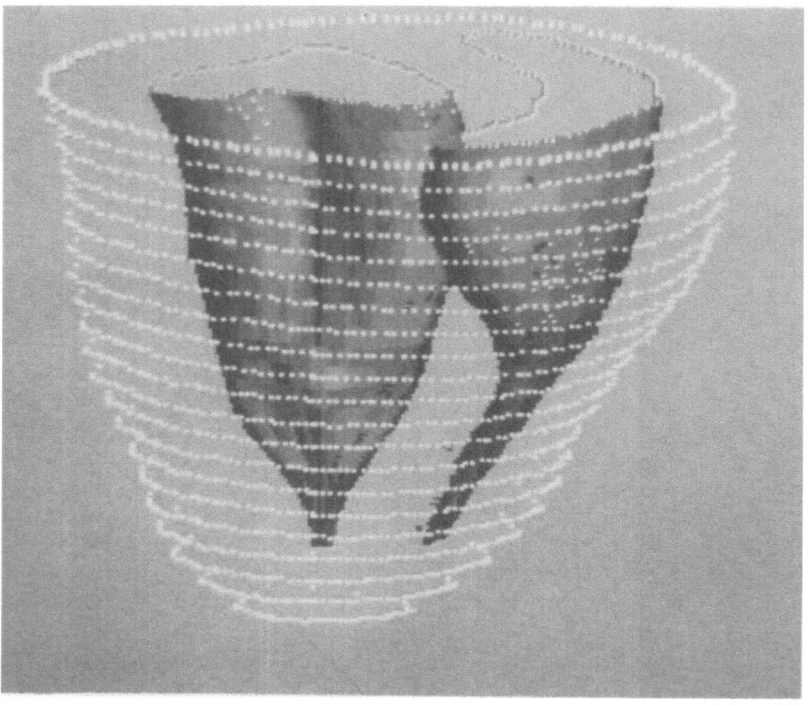

Figure 4. Interpolated reconstruction of the left and right ventricular endocardial surfaces and epicardial contours.

Model Considerations

As a first step to evaluate the extended Darcy equation it was applied to a 2-dimensional simulated arteriolar network, shown in Figure 9. At the branching point the parameter x_0 equals minus the average of the diameters of the two largest vessels leaving or reaching this branching point. Between two subsequent branching points x_0 varies linearly with distance. The K-tensor is taken constant over the x_0 ranges selected. (Table 1). The apparant blood viscosity is taken to be diameter dependant according to the data of Haynes (1960). For this branching network two pressure distributions P_1 and P_2 are chosen. The extended Darcy equation is applied for $(x_1, x_2) = (1, -0.3)$. The neigbourhood of this point is the volume $V = 3\,\text{mm}^3$ (Figure 9). Linear regression on the pressure distributions yields $P_{,0}$, $P_{,1}$ and $P_{,2}$ while the K-tensor is computed from the local blood viscosity and the vessel geometry. The flows f_0, f_1 and f_2 resulting from the extended Darcy equation are in fair agreement with the exact flows obtained by adding the flow contribution of each vessel taken seperately as is indicated in Table 1.

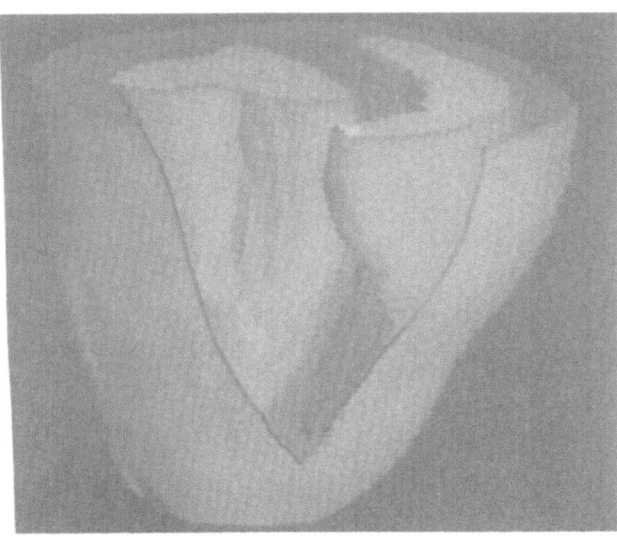

Figure 5. Interpolated reconstruction of left and right ventricular epi- and endocardial surfaces, with numerical resection of some regions of the cardiac walls.

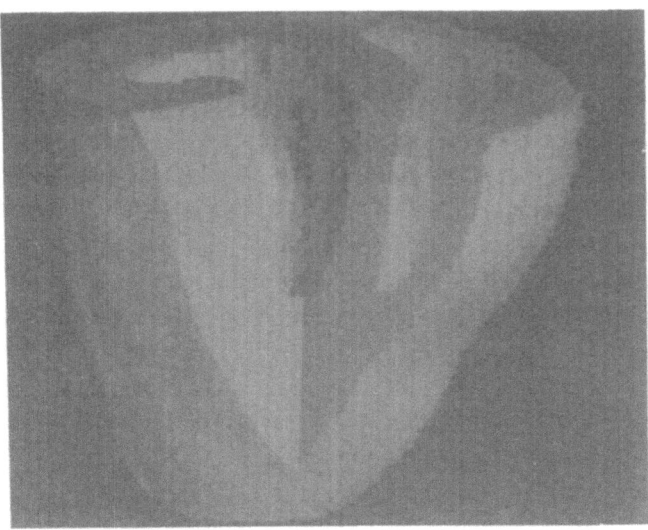

Figure 6. Interpolated reconstruction of left and right ventricular muscle walls, with numerical resection of parts of the septum and left and right ventricular walls.

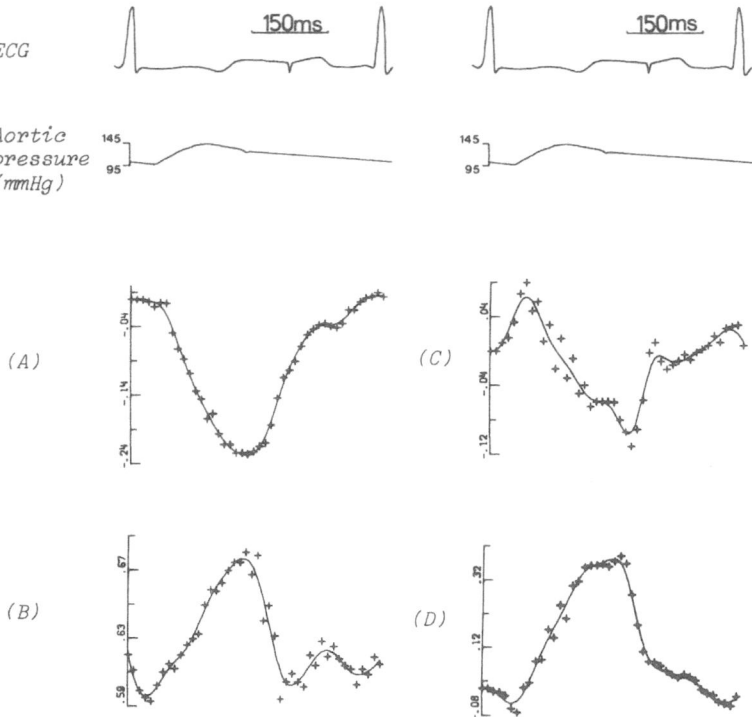

Figure 7. Results of calculations of fibre strain (A), fibre orientation (in radians) (B), strain perpendicular to the fibre (C), and layer thickening (D) during a normal heart beat in the midwall of the left ventricular anterior free wall at midventricle.

Discussion

Quantitative determination of cardiac function and cardiac reserve is still a major challenge in cardiology. In spite of the strong increase in diagnostic tools and technologies such as X-ray equipment, echocardiography, nuclear medicine and NMR there is a need to deepen the insight in the fundamentals of cardiac contraction in normal and pathological situations. This is of importance when surgical interventions are considered in order to correct abnormal hemodynamic loads imposed by ventricular lesions, aneurisms or abnormal shunts. Because of various compensatory mechanisms, loss of myocardial function may not become manifest in ventricular pump function until late in the course of the disease. Various indices derived from hemodynamic measurements have been used to assess quantitatively ventricular overall performance. However, these indices do not reflect regional contraction of the ventricular myocardium.

Stresses generated in the walls of the ventricle caused by contraction and relaxation of the individual muscle fibres may play an important role in the

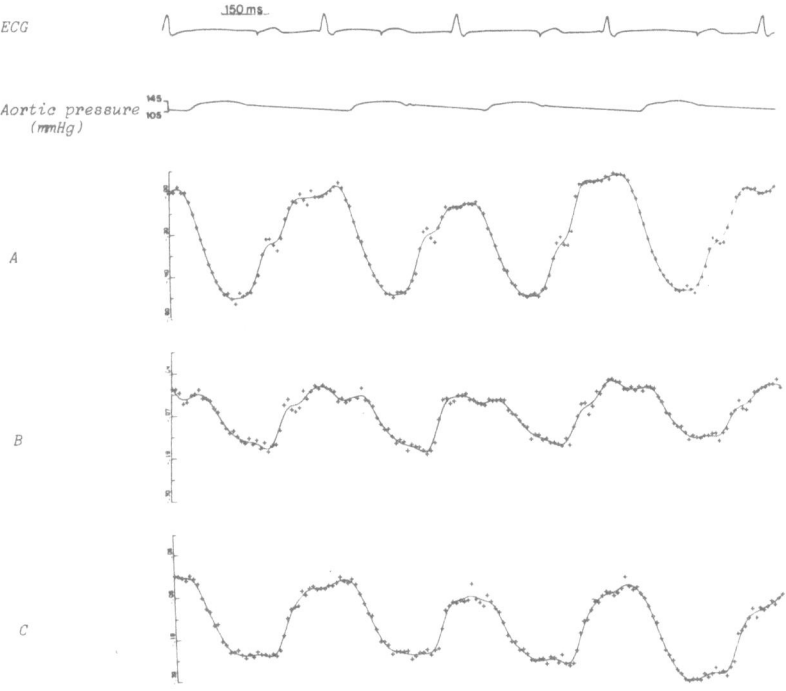

Figure 8. Calculated endocardial fibre strain (A), epicardial fibrestrain (B) and epicardial fibre orientation (C) during four cardiac cycles (two normal beats followed by an induced extrasystole and a controlled post extrasystole). Markers were inserted halfway between base and apex. Basic RR-interval is 500 ms, extrasystolic interval 350 ms.

assessment of regional cardiac function. For instance because of chronic volume and pressure overload on the ventricle, wall stress would increase; however, hypertrophy is a compensatory mechanism that increases wall thickness and therefore tends to maintain wall stresses within a particular window. In addition wall stress is one of the determinants of myocardial oxygen consumption and plays an important role in the behaviour of the coronary circulation. Because wall stress is a theoretical concept that cannot be measured directly, different investigators have tried to compute stresses with help of model studies of the heart and theories of elastic media. Frequently, approximate geometric forms such as spheroids or ellipsoids are taken for the ventricular shapes. Already in 1892, Woods applied the law of Laplace for the evaluation of wall stresses in the heart. In a later stage, Burch and associates (1952) and Burton (1957) demonstrated the importance of size and shape of the ventricle in relation to its performance. Since then many authors have calculated wall stresses under different assumptions of geometry, homogeneity, linear elasticity, and anisotropy of cardiac muscle (Heethaar *et al.*, 1977; Pao *et al.*, 1974; Sandler and Dodge, 1963; Mirsky, 1969;

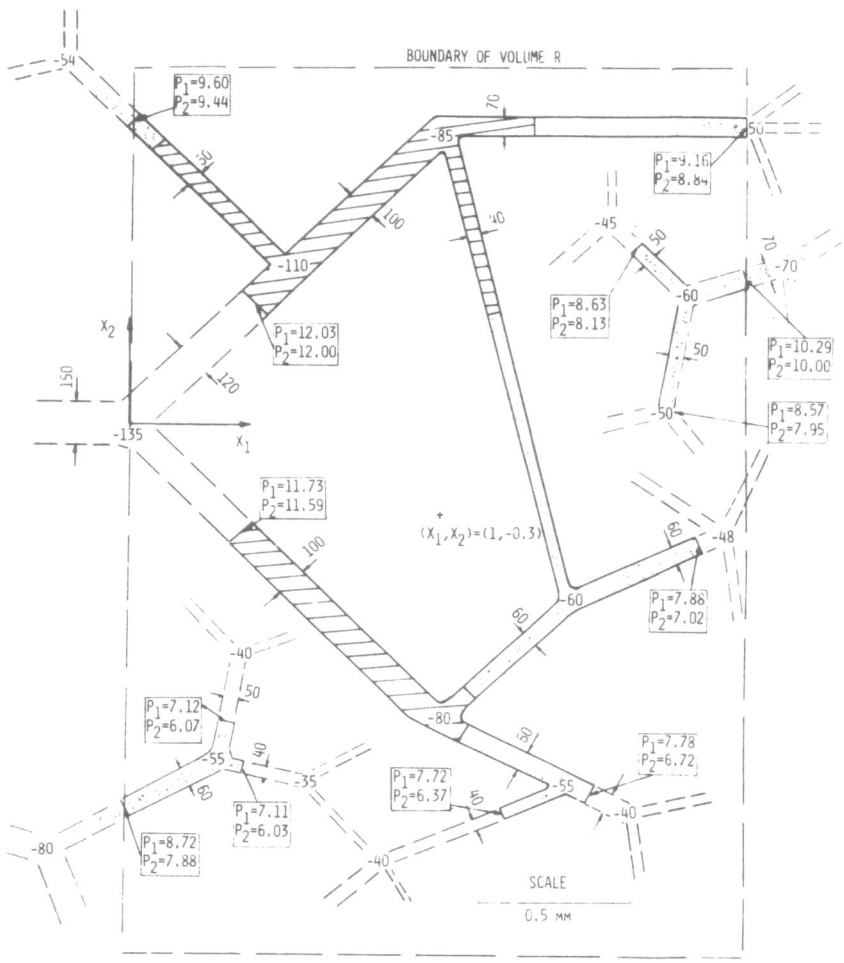

Figure 9. Schematic representation of the arteriolar network to test the extended Darcy equation. Two pressure distributions P_1 and P_2 are chosen. (pressures in kPa), diameters in um. Shaded area compartment with $-115 < x_0 < -75$, stippled area with $-75 < x_0 < -50$.

Gould *et al.*, 1972; Wong & Rautaharju, 1968). No completely satisfactory theory has yet been developed.

In our model we aim to incorporate the interrelationship between cardiac muscle mechanics and coronary blood perfusion. In this model geometry of the heart plays an essential role. The method of ultrasound velocity tomography can be useful, as is demonstrated to measure the three-dimensional geometry of the heart in the laboratory with sufficient accuracy. The accuracy (the spatial resolution) of the tomogram depends on the total number of measurements. As the set of equations (1b) can be solved only if the number of variables does not exceed the

Table 1. Application and verification of the extended Darcy equation for two narrow and two broader compartments of the branching network, shown in Figure 9. Two pressure distributions are chosen on this network, represented by 1 resp. 2

x_0	K-tensor (mm/kPA.s) K_{00} K_{01} K_{02} / K_{11} K_{12} K_{22}				Press. gradient (kPa/mm)			Extended Darcy flows (1/s)			Exact flows (l/s)		
(−115,	4.124	.399	.132	1	−.488	3.819	.215	.461	.044	.001	.461	.044	.001
−110)	.039	.014	.039	2	−.494	3.648	.369	.532	.051	−.002	.532	.051	−.002
(−75,	1.246	.079	.021	1	−.425	.666	.265	.471	.025	.008	.461	.032	.004
−70)	.013	−.001	.006	2	−.479	.644	.443	.537	.030	.008	.532	.038	.003
(−115,	2.902	.234	.017	1	−.243	1.039	.294	.457	.031	−.003	.461	.031	−.003
−75)	.026	.000	.024	2	−.266	1.024	.433	.526	.036	−.006	.532	.037	−.006
(−75,	1.290	.101	.009	1	−.483	.719	.351	.547	.036	.000	.535	.040	.002
−50)	.017	.002	.007	2	−.560	.822	.595	.634	.042	−.001	.623	.046	−.001

number of equations (measurements) it can be seen easily that the obtained resolution equals at best the area to be reconstructed devided by the number of measurements. So, if the size of the area to be reconstructed is 10*10 cm, at least 10.000 measurements are required for a resolution of 1 mm. Due to noise and model errors, the equations need not be exact and consistent so an even larger number of equations is needed to which only an approximate solution can be found.

A second reason to start the development of the ultrasound tomograph was the idea that contracted and relaxed muscle tissue should have a different speed of propagation for ultrasound on the basis of a supposed difference in elasticity. As the speed of ultrasonic waves is proportional to the square root of the ratio of elasticity coefficient and density (Wells, 1969) we assumed the possibility of finding a difference of ultrasound velocity in cardiac tissue as function of the state of contraction. According to this hypothesis reconstruction of the ultrasound velocity distributions should reveal the spread of mechanical contraction and relaxation throughout the ventricular myocardium and offers the possibility to relate it to the spread of electrical excitation. However extensive measurements did not reveal a systematic change in ultrasound velocity as function of the phase in the cardiac cycle. Although we do not yet clearly understand this phenemenon some factors may be responsible for the absence of a change in ultrasound velocity: like the changing density of the myocardium, which counteracts the effects of elasticity and the blood being squeezed out of the ventricular muscle.

A disadvantage of the method is the need for a stationary heart rhythm for at least 200 successive heart beats to image one cross section. Analysis of extra-systoles becomes hard as they require an even larger number of identical heartbeats.

Summary

The ultrasound velocity tomography allows measurement of cardiac geometries for various phases in the cardiac cycle. The present tomograph makes reconstructions at intervals of 20 ms. Because of a lack of clear (intramural) landmarks (except the roots of the papillairy muscle), it is difficult to pinpoint spatial trajectories of particular points in the heart. Therefore, a second method was developed of injecting radiopaque markers in the heart and following their motion patterns during the cardiac cycle with help of a biplane X-ray equipment. The data obtained with both methods can be implemented in our finite element model of the heart to compute intramural stresses and strains. The results obtained sofar with the extended Darcy equation to account for the interaction of blood rheology and tissue mechanics look promising. Further testing with more sophisticated subjects than mentioned in Figure 9 is required before it will be implemented in our finite element model of the heart.

We conclude that analysis of regional cardiac function, including regional myocardial blood flow, requires still a major research effort but the results obtained sofar justify, to our opinion, a continuation in this direction.

Acknowledgement

The authors acknowledge Dr. C. Borst and coworkers for doing the animal experiments and prof. Van Campen and dr. Grootenboer for their participation is some aspects of this work.

References

Burch GE, Ray CT, Cronvich JA (1952) Certain mechanical pecularities of the human cardiac pump in normal and diseased states. Circ 5:504–513

Burton AC (1957) The importance of the shape and size of the heart. Am Heart J 54:801–810

Elshuraydeh K (1981) Cardiac dimensions and intramural deformations. University Thesis, State University of Utrecht

Elshuraydeh K, Smits J, Heethaar RM, Denier van der Gon JJ (1981) Method for measuring cardiac dimensions and intramural deformations. J Biomed Eng 3:49–52

Greenleaf JF, Johnson SA, Samayoa WF, Duck FA, Wood EH (1975) Algebraic reconstruction of spatial distribution of acoustic velocities in tissue from their time of flight profiles. In: Booth N (ed) Acoustical Holography. New York, Plenum Press, pp 71–90

Gould P, Ghista D, Brombolich L, Mirsky I (1972) In vivo stresses in the human left ventricular wall: analysis accounting for the irregular 3-dimensional geometry and comparison with idealised geometry analyses. J Biomech 5:521–539

Haynes RH (1960) Physical basis of the dependence of blood viscosity on tube radius. Am J Physio 198:1193–1200

Heethaar RM, Pao YC, Ritman EL (1977) Computer aspects of three dimensional finite element analysis of stresses and strains in the intact heart. Comp Biomed Res 10:271–285

Heethaar RM, Mol CR, Elshuraydeh K, Heethaar J, Van Dort JMT, Batianen GW, Sneek JHJ, Borst C, Meijler FL (1982) Cardiac function fibre shortening and dynamic geometry. Mayo Clinic Proc suppl, 57:104–113

Hoffman JIE (1979) The effect of intramyocardial forces on the distribution of intramyocardial blood flow. J Biomed Eng 1:33–40

Huyghe JM, Grootenboer DH, Van Campen DH, Heethaar RM (1983) Intramyocardial blood rheology and heart muscle mechanics. In: Proc ASME Symp on Biomech 56:241–244

Kuijer PJP, Heethaar RM, Herbschleb JN, Zimmerman ANE, Meijler FL (1978) Post extrasystolic relaxation in the dog heart. Eur J Cardiology 7:133–145

Kuijer PJP (1985) Het effect van cen extrasystole op de postextrasystolische contractie en relaxatie van de linker ventrikel. University Thesis, State University of Utrecht

Love AEH (1927) A treatise on the mathematical theory of elasticity. New York, Dover Publ Inc

Mirsky I (1969) Left ventricular stresses in the intact human heart. Biophys J 9:189–208

Mol CR (1981) Ultrasound velocity tomography and dynamic cardiac geometry. University Thesis, State University of Utrecht

Pao YC, Ritman EL, Wood EH (1974) Finite element analysis of left ventricular myocardial stresses. J Biomech 7:469–477

Sandler H, Dodge HT (1963) Left ventricular tension and stress in man. Circ Res 13:91–104

Wells PNT (1969) Physical principles of ultrasonic diagnosis. London, Acad Press

Wong AYK, Rautaharju PM (1968) Stress distribution within the left ventricular wall aproximated as a thick ellipsoidal shell. Am Heart J 75:649–662

Woods RA (1892) A few applications of a physical theorem to membranes in the body in a state of tension. J Anat Physiol 26:362–370

Zienkiewicz OC (1977) The Finite Element Method, 3rd ed. McGraw Hill, London

A data acquisition and processing system for ultrasound- and video images and the reconstruction of 3-D images

WALTER AMELING

Technical University of Aachen, RWTH, Department of Electrical Engineering and Computer Science 5100 Aachen, F.R.G.

Abstract

The analysis of image sequences yields important functional parameters. But past applications indicates that scene analysis can be successful only if; (1) the class of scenes is a priori restricted to scenes and regions which are relevant for analyzing and (2) each image is available in a form suitable for processing. To ease clinical application we have developed the Modular Multi Mode-Microprocessor System (M5PS), an image acquisition and processing system which stores digitized input signals (ultrasonic or video signals).

In this paper the system, currently configured to store and process echo signals of phased array ultrasonic sector-scan systems in real time operation over a period of 20 s, is described and some results are presented. The paper also illustrates the computer aided reconstruction of two-dimensional data frames. As an example, the geometric modelling of a human heart from a set of different echocardiographical views is shown. To allow data evaluation with small computing facilities (microprocessor-systems), data processing is decomposed into data acquisition, segmentation, 3-D database formation, and selected two and three-dimensional object retrieval.

Introduction

Clinical applications require the analysis of image sequences from video or ultrasonic devices. In many cases processing should take place in real-time or within few minutes.

The evaluation of morphological data (Heintzen *et al.*, 1975) requires image enhancement and feature extraction. In order to achieve this, the analog signal is converted into discrete values, usually referred to as grey levels. Normally enhancement and feature extraction require multistep procedures. For example noise filtering, contrast modification and edge sharpening enhance a picture. Thresholding, edge detection, region growing are some approaches to obtain characteristic features of the image. To evaluate functional data (Brennecke *et al.*, 1980; Gramiak *et al.*, 1979; Heintzen *et al.*, 1975; Hoehne *et al.*, 1975; Kobayashi, 1978) these procedures must be applied to each frame of an image sequence and the results of every single frame must be mapped into one set of scene results. Image processing is therefore a problem of applying numerical algorithms which should be inexpensive in terms of memory space and computation time. For the application we have in mind, we decompose the overall task of processing image sequences into the following subtasks:

(a) real-time data acquisition for scenes,

(b) transient recording,

(c) image enhancement by real-time filtering, and

(d) fast off-line data processing.

During the recent seven years, the multiprocessor system M5PS was designed and developed (Ameling, 1982; Ameling *et al.*, 1977; Krings *et al.*, 1981, 1982; Milde *et al.*, 1982a; Li *et al.*, 1979). It was planned as a system of coupled subsystems (clusters), where each cluster by itself is a multiprocessor system. Several clusters with up to eight processor modules, connected to a common memory via a time-shared bus are realized. In order to evaluate the system performance, i.e. the processing speed, typical parallel problems have been programmed and measured by means of a measuring tool, which does not influence the system timing.

One reason for the development of parallel processor systems is to increase the performance and to overcome the limits of a sequential single processor system. (Brinch and Hansen, 1973; Dijkstra, 1968; Gargantini, 1982; Giloi, 1981; Hoener and Roehder, 1976, 1977)

In our image sequence processing system the data flow is adjusted to the transfer rate of disk drives by a 3-port multifunction frame memory supporting different input sources and output units. The three ports are used for video input/output, data transfer to disk drives, and image processing. By segmenting the memory of currently 256 K bytes into 16 K byte pages for a frame size of 512 × 512 pixels all three buses may simultaneously access different pages. In the data acquisition mode this feature together with FIFO queueing allows operation at the disk's maximum transfer rate. In the processing mode each page can be connected to a microcomputer or signal processor so that parallel processing for image analysis is possible. Look-up tables in the output channel of the video port allow pseudo color representation of the contents of the frame memory. Microprogramming principles assisted by a microcomputer at the console (man-machine-interface) are used to control the overall data flow.

Image sequence processing system

The overall system architecture of the Image Sequence Processing System is depicted in Figure 1.

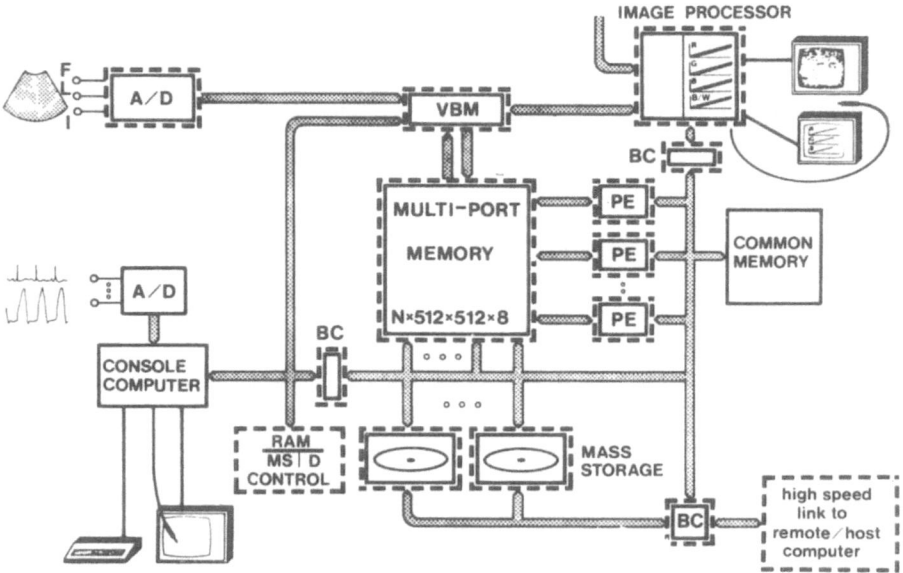

Figure 1. Image sequence processing system.

Opposed to conventional structures of data processing systems this architecture contains multi-port devices. By this we allow implementation of data flow concepts and parallel processing and we avoid the 'von Neumann bottleneck' due to a single link between memory and control/ operation units of classical computing systems. The most important component of the system is a 3–port paged memory which is used:

(a) to input digitized analog data or output data for video display,

(b) to transmit data to disk drives, and

(c) to allow the processing of image data by several processing elements (PE's) in parallel; possible operation modes are data flow. SIMD or MIMD.

If different pages are addressed, each port allows immediate access to the data. Arbitration logic is activated only in case of contention.

Dual-port fixed disks are used to permit reading and writing from a host computer. The host has also access to the multi-port memory. Each processing element contains a microprocessor with links to

(a) the multi-port memory,

(b) common memory,

(c) local private memory.

All operations in the Image Sequence Processing System are controlled by a

(a) direct control unit,

(b) microsequenced control unit.

In the second case a RAM functions as control store. Thus, control flow can be tailored to meet specific processing needs. With this architecture emphasis is put

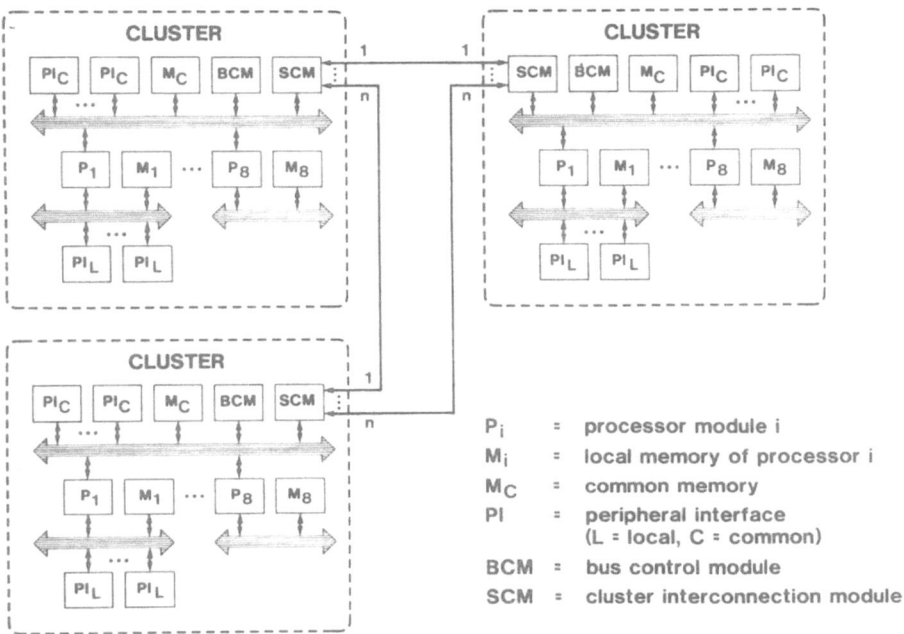

Figure 2. Structure of the Multiprocessor-System M5PS.

on real-time data acquisition at the highest possible transfer rate and on a continuous recording time of up to 20 s. More details are given when discussing the above mentioned subtasks.

The multiprocessor-system consists of identical processor modules with a ZILOG-Z80 CPU, 2 K private ROM, 2 K private RAM, private I/O in case of need, and a memory management device for paging and extended addressing up to 1 M Byte. The operating system runs in the common memory so that each functions can be performed by each of the processors of the symmetric system. The process management allows to start and to synchronize parallel tasks at the process-processor-assignment level (Hoehne *et al.*, 1979). Paralleslism at the instruction level is obtained by interlacing all memory- and I/O–operations on the common bus. Since all bus operations are of the same length (500 ns), the bus timing is divided into equidistant time slots. At the end of each slot the bus arbiter samples the bus request signals and gives an acknowledge to one of the contending processors, according to a bus allocation strategy.

The system can operate as an ensemble of identical processors having equal right (MIMD-mode) or as a SIMD-processor (SIMD-mode). Different subsets of processors also can operate simultaneously in MIMD- and SIMD-mode.

The operating system supports one user to run parallel processes. It is located in the common memory, and each operating system function is performed by the processor in need for it, i.e. there is no masterprocessor in the system. This concept allows great flexibility (e.g. automatical adaptation to the number of processors) and parallel execution of system functions. The user can start, stop and synchronize parallel processes, which are normally not dedicated to one special processor but can run on every available one. For special cases however it is also possible to define a fixed assignment of processes to processors.

A picture, which can be divided in n parts of equal length, has to be stored on a disk after some transformation is done by n processors. Each of them performes the same computation on a part of the picture. The transfer to the disk must be done by one processor. If the transformation is done in SIMD-mode, all processes finish their part of the transformation at the same time and the transfer to the disk can start without explicit synchronization. In MIMD-mode each transformation process has to indicate its end e.g. by an unlock-operation, and the disk process has to collect this messages e.g. by n *lock*-operations.

Real-time data acquisition

In the data acquisition mode the system has to sample and to store ultrasonic or video signals in real-time. Along with each pulse transmitted by the ultrasonic scanner a scan start signal (S) is generated, which initiates the sampling of the analog signal (I) and the storing of the digitized values into one of two FIFO buffers of the video bus module (VBM). The contents of a full buffer are transferred to the multi-port memory while the second buffer is filled with new data. The sampling process is shown in Figure 3.

By utilizing inactive sampling periods (i.e. retrace blanking) the memory input transfer rate may be adjusted between lines 1 and 2. For economical reasons it is desirable to use as low speed memory IC's as possible. 512 pixels per line can be displayed for video signals, if the video bus module and the multi-port memory

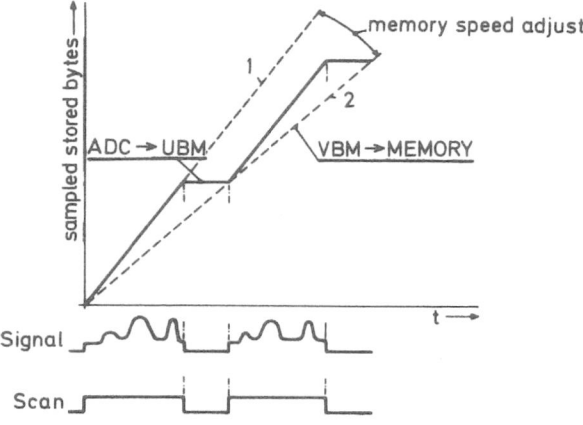

Figure 3. Asynchronous data transfer from ADC to memory.

operate at the maximum transfer rate. For phased array ultrasonic scanners the rate may be as low as 800 K kBytes/s, yielding 128 samples per reflected echo. The multi-port memory is subdivided into several pages. Together with the disks the memory serves as a large blocked FIFO-buffer. Data are transferred from memory to disks by handshake operation, considering timing characteristics of each disk drive. In the current configuration we use a microprocessor based arrhythmia detection system (Jensch *et al.*, 1979) as console computer. If the acquisition mode is activated the console computer is usually inactive, regarding control. Thus, the console computer can perform ECG and pressure analysis and mix the results thereof into the appropriate image data.

Transient recording

The system is prepared for transient recording at sample rates of up to 100 MHz. In such an operation mode the two separate modules 'image ADC' and VBM must be replaced by a video bus module with integrated ADC. All connections to the multi-port memory remain the same. Two high speed buffers in the video bus module serve as temporary storage and the multiport memory is the long time storage device in this mode of operation. Due to the extremely high sampling rate a burst mode recording is limited by the capacity of the buffer in the video bus module.

Image enhancement by real-time filtering

The image processor supports the representation of image frames held in the multiport memory (512 × 512 pixels). Simple contrast enhancement is achieved by appropriate contents of look-up tables. A mapping of pixel values into grey levels (for B/W-TV monitor) is performed by a B/W look-up table. Separate R–G–B look-up tables are used to obtain a pseudo color representation. The contents of these tables may be modified by the console computer. For operating convenience the contents of the look-up tables can be displayed as curves on a B/W-monitor and changes can be made by means of a light pen. The image processor also contains a line buffer which allows to display an intensity profile along frame lines, frame columns, or any curves defined by light pen. Besides these mapping capabilities the on-line image processor (OIP) is able to generate contrast enhanced images by applying several filtering methods. For 256 pixels per line the following real-time manipulations are implemented: low pass filtering, high pass filtering. In the 'global operating mode' of the system filtering parameters are constant; in the 'local mode' these parameters depend on characteristics of a region around each pixel. With this approach details will become visible within larger uniformly bright or dark areas and the enhancement can be adjusted to the resolution (x, y and intensity) of the display unit.

Fast off-line data processing

The image sequence processing system covers several possibilities of processing recorded image data. Data paths between the video bus module and the multi-port memory are bidirectional. Thus, images available in the multiport memory can be manipulated by the image processor and any changes in look-up tables are immediately visible. The image data in the multi-port memory are not affected by these changes. Operation speed is the same as in the case of real-time filtering. In addition to this feature image analysis can be performed concurrently by several processing elements (PE's). These PE's access separate pages of the multi-port memory and they can operate in the modes single instruction multiple data (SIMD) or multiple instructions multiple data (MIMD). As shown in (Jensch *et al.*, 1979) a high performance can be achieved by utilizing independent data paths and buses with arbitration logic. That is why the system structure around the processing elements is basically the same as in the console computer (arrhythmia detection system in our configuration). Each processor element has access to image data via two different paths. Thus, bidirectional processing loops are possible. This feature allows pipeline processing or data manipulation according to different data flow concepts (Jensch and Ameling, 1977). In order to assure that operations of the PE's do not interfere with concurrent operation of the image processor, bus connection units (BC) separate processing paths and loops. As a scene is recorded prior to processing and as each image can be directly addressed on the disks, loop movies of selectable image sequences are feasible.

Tailored configuration

For many applications the discussed system comprises too many features. If, for example, in the clinical routine only ECG and pressure data must be assigned to PD-ultrasonic images in order to evaluate the ejection fraction then a small system is sufficient. In this case there is no need for PE's and the multiport memory may be drastically reduced to only a few pages of 16 K Bytes each. For standard evaluations there is no need for a disk drive. Due to the flexible control, using microprogramming principles, it is easy, for example, to change sample rates or to switch from ultrasonic signal recording to video signal recording. All data paths are buses to which appropriate modules can be connected. Thus, there are many ways to assemble a system optimized for specific processing needs.

Application

Figures 4, 5 and 6 show some images obtained from a system configured for ultrasonic signal recording and processing. Figure 4 is an enhanced image. High

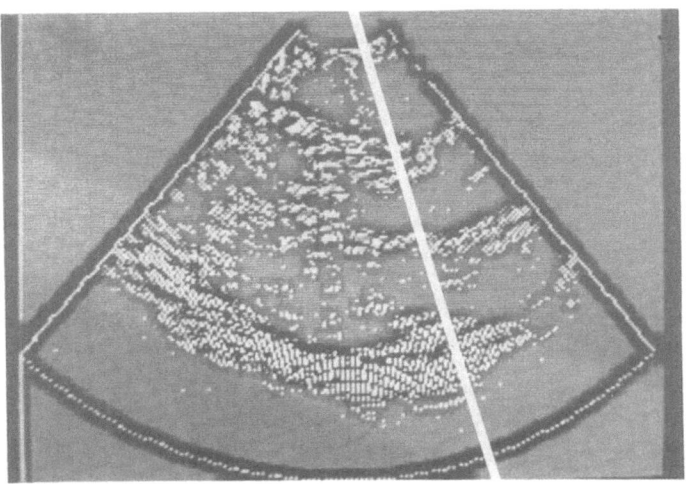

Figure 4. High pass filtered image.

pass filtering has been applied which imposes shades on the picture in order to give the impression of depth. Figure 5 depicts the intensity profile (pixel values) along the ray marked by the white line in Figure 4. This is identical to an A-scan. Further standard trajectories for intensity profiles are shown in Figure 6 if desired, an intensity profile can be obtained along any arbritary line defined by the light pen. Currently we use the representation of intensity profiles together with the pseudo color mapping in research for tissue characterization (Gramiak *et al.*, 1979; Joynt *et al.*, 1980).

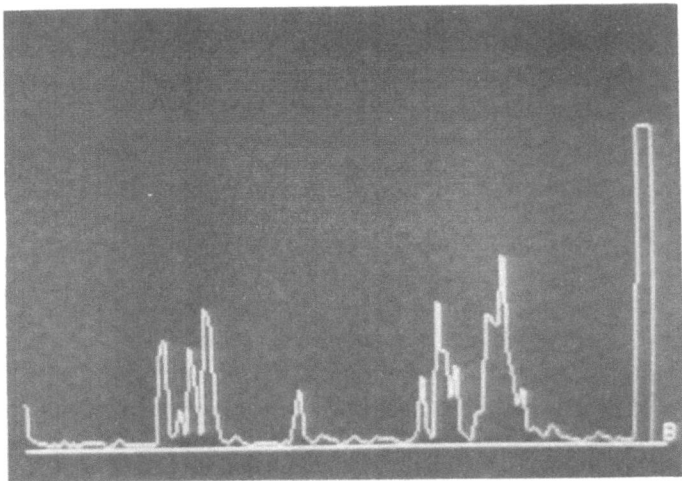

Figure 5. Intensity profile of a ray (white line of Figure 4).

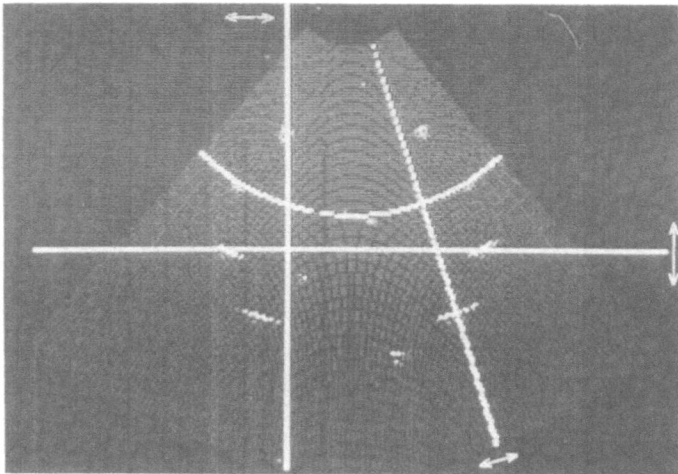

Figure 6. Standard trajectories for intensity profiles.

Reconstruction of 3D-images and selected cross-sections of the heart

Ultrasoundscanners can be used to produce sequences of echocardiograms. From such 2-D-scenes shape and structure of the heart as a 3-D-object can be visualized. Internal structures of a 3-D-object are obtained at arbitrary cross sections.

Two different approaches to the display of 3-D-information have been pursued. The first approach extracts information about boundary surfaces of an object from 2-D-images and reconstructs it as a wire model. In the second approach, the complete 3-D-information is displayed as a half-tone image giving the impression of space. At time of display the object can be rotated at any arbitrary angle and opened at any desired cross section plane to disclose inner structures. Our image sequence processing system (ISPS) allows recording of ultrasound signals directly supplied by an ultrasound scanner (Jensch *et al.*, 1980). Two approaches are provided:

(a) recording of two-dimensional cross section frames obtained from the usual ultrasound windows at different angles (*in vivo*)

(b) recording of parallel-cross section frames (e.g. anatomic specimen).

The analog output data of the scanner are digitized and stored in a mass storage device. In vivo digitization can be gated by a selectable point of the cardiac cycle to simulate a static object condition. Single objects, the cardiac chambers and large vessels, can be identified within the stored cross sections by segmentation. The boundaries are traced semi-automatically by first defining several reference points (anatomic landmarks) subsequently used to calculate a control polygon. This in return generates a B-spline curve interpolating the points to a smooth contour (Figure 7). To obtain a B-spline curve of desired shape, the reference points can be locally modified. Due to local behaviour of B-spline functions only a

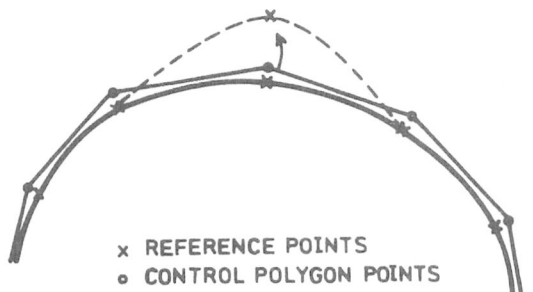

Figure 7. B-spline interpolation between a set of reference points.

few spans concerning the modified point will be changed, the other parts remain unaffected. Frames with proper contrast permit automatic segmentation. For contour smoothing digital filtering can be applied. To allow local corrections manual interaction is provided via a digitizer-tablet or a light-pen.

3-D-database

The segmentation procedure is repeated for each frame. Cross section frame data taken from an arbitrary but known position of the ultrasound transducer are transformed into their proper 3-D-coordinates and stored in a 3-D-database. This database is organized in a way to simplify retrieval processes. The combination of all stored cross section frames allows the three-dimensional reconstruction of the heart. Two approaches have been attempted:

Wire model with B-spline surface

A sculptured surface is obtained by interpolation with two-dimensional B-spline-functions. A B-spline surface is considered as a collection of surface patches and the whole surface is a mosaic of these patches linked together with proper continuity (Figure 9). Due to its computational efficiency a uniform bicubic B-spline surface has been implemented. The bicubic B-spline patch can be written in matrix form as

$$Q(u, v) = U\, B\, P\, B^t\, V^t,$$

where

218

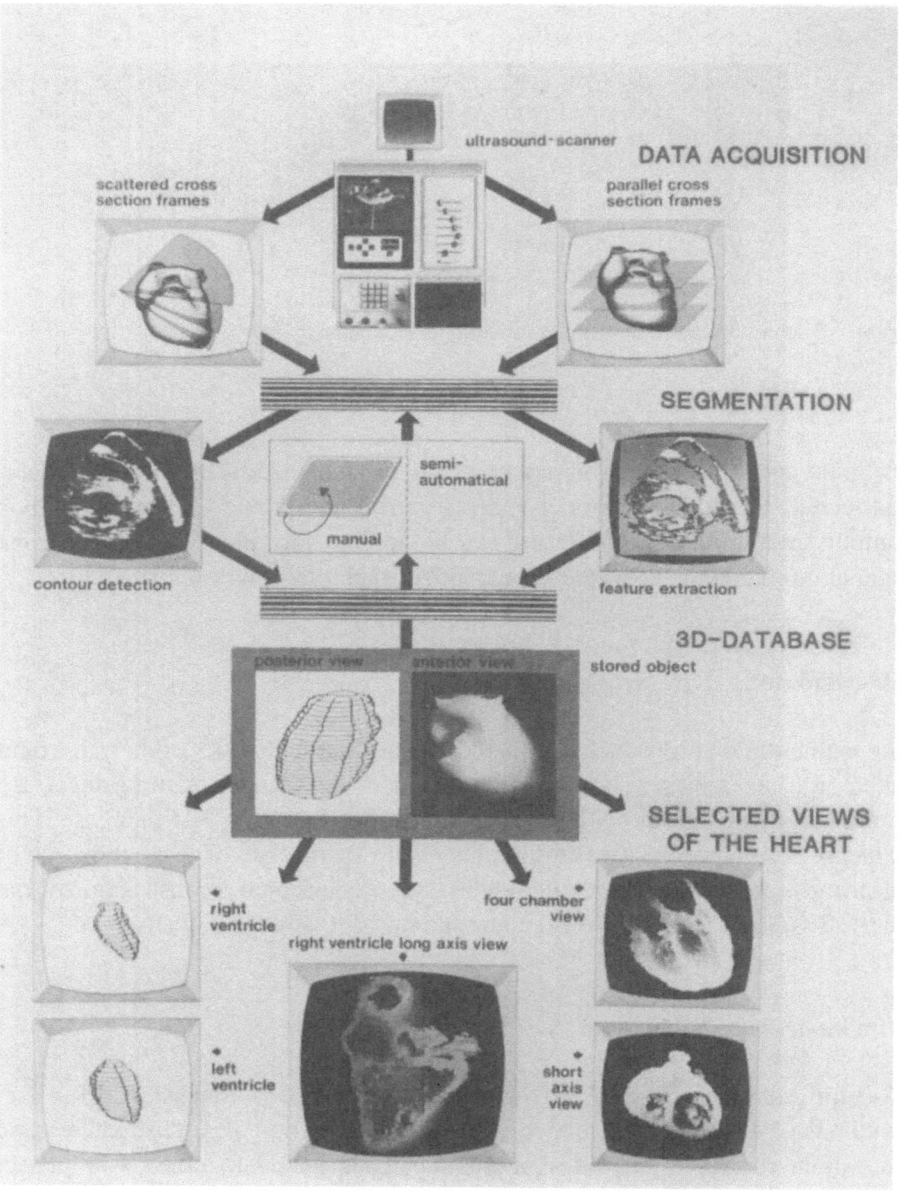

Figure 8. Data acquisition of echocardiograms, 3-D-reconstruction, and selected cross sections of the heart.

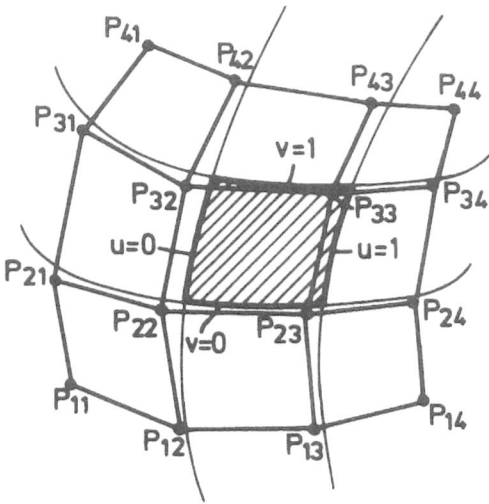

Figure 9. B-spline patch as a mosaic element of a surface.

$$B = 1/6 \begin{bmatrix} -1 & 3 & -3 & 1 \\ 3 & -6 & 3 & 0 \\ -3 & 0 & 3 & 0 \\ 1 & 4 & 1 & 0 \end{bmatrix}$$

is the B-spline basis matrix for cubics, and

$$P = \begin{bmatrix} P_{11} & P_{12} & P_{13} & P_{14} \\ P_{21} & P_{22} & P_{23} & P_{24} \\ P_{31} & P_{32} & P_{33} & P_{34} \\ P_{41} & P_{42} & P_{43} & P_{44} \end{bmatrix}$$

is the set of control points arranged on a topologically rectangularmesh, and

$$U = (u^3, u^2, u, 1) \quad \text{and} \quad V = (v^3, v^2, v, 1)$$

are the primitive basis vectors.

u, v are the normalized parametric coordinates and vary from 0 to 1 corresponding to the boundaries of the patch. These formulas are an extension of the above mentioned 2D-case. But for data processing, effective algorithms for data retrieval and evaluation are essential. The chosen algorithm is adjusted to the grid of a selected wire model and hidden line problems are also imbedded.

Full object representation

The stored object can be represented either as a wire model or as a half-tone (pseudo-coloured) image. The wire-model permits quantitative measurements whereas the half-tone image uncovers structures. Both representations may be superimposed and, furthermore, combined with functional values to represent a dynamic functional model. The representation as a half-tone image with all its details requires a lot more information than the wire model (Roger & Adams, 1976; Wu et al., 1977). Therefore the object is stored in a virtual cube shaped space (Meagher, 1982). This cube can be subdivided down to its atomic elements, the 'voxels' (volume elements as 'pixels', for picture elements), which finally hold binary object information.

The large amount of data required to store a complex object like a complete heart becomes evident when contemplating the desired resolution of the picture. In our approach this universe consists of $128 \times 128 \times 128 = 2M$ voxels. To be able to store the object at tenable expense and to handle data efficiently a modified hierarchical tree (octtree) datastructure has been implemented. To solve the hidden surface problem this list is sorted in order to output voxels most distant to the observer first. They may be overwritten by voxels closer to the observer which are output later. Once the database is created, any single chamber or any choosen cross section can be retrieved from the stored data, e.g. (Figure 8, bottom part):

    (a) inner parts of the whole object can be isolated separately (left and right ventricle), and

    (b) any kind of long axis views can be extracted if the originally recorded images were cross sections of short axis views.

A half-tone or pseudo-coloured image gives information about cavity, showing structures of inner parts of the heart. Selected cross sections of that kind reveal details not visible within the original echocardiograms.

Concluding remarks

The Image Sequence Processing System is a tool to analyze image scenes. Basically there are two modes of operation:

    (a) real-time recording and

    (b) fast processing.

A very high performance is obtained by an architecture allowing parallel data handling and processing due to multi-port devices (memory, disks, processing elements) and independent data paths.

References

Ameling W (1982) Parallelism in computer architecture. Proc 10th IMACS World Congress, Montreal, pp 275–180

Ameling W, Hoener S, Roehder W (1977) Interconnection structures for parallel processor system. In: Feilmeier M (ed) Parallel Computer – Parallel Mathem. Munich 189, ACM, pp 296–300

Brennecke R, Hahen HJ, Heintzen PH (1980) A multiprocessor-system for the acquisition and analysis of video image sequences. Informatik-Fachberichte 29:113–122

Brinch Hansen P (1973) Operating System Principles. Englewood Cliffs, New Jersey: Prentice Hall, Inc

Dijkstra W (1968) Cooperating sequential processes. In: Genuys F (ed) Programming Languages. New York: Academic Press

Gargantini I (1982) Linear octtrees for fast processing of three-dimensional objects. Comp Graphics and Image Processing 20: 365–374

Giloi WK (1981) Rechnerarchitektur. Berlin: Springer

Gramiak R, Waag RC, Schenk EA, Kee POK, Thomson K, Macintosh P (1979) Ultrasonic imaging of experimental myocardial infarcts. Echocardiology 99–106

Heintzen PH, Brennecke R, Bursch JH, Lange P, Malerczyk V, Moldenhauer K, Onnasch D (1975) Automated video-angiocardiographic image analysis. Computer (IEEE) 8:55–64

Hoehne KL, Boehm M, Nicalae (1979) The processing of X-ray image sequences. In: Stucki P (ed) Advances in Digital Image Processing. New York: Plenum Press, pp 147–163

Hoener S, Roehder W (1976) Modular multi-microprocessor architecture with virtual memory. Proc Euromicro, pp 99–108

Hoener S, Roehder W (1977) Efficiency of a multi-microprocessor system with time-shared buses. Proc Euromicro, pp 35–42

Horowitz SL, Budinger TF, Gebel MJ et al. (1979) Biomedical imaging and modeling. Biomed. pattern recogn. and image processing. Life sci. Res. Report, Verlag Chemie Weinheim 15:355–432

Jensch P, Ameling W (1977) A computer architecture for multiple data flow programs. In: Feilmeier M (ed) Parallel computers – parallel mathematics. Munich 189, ACM

Jensch P, Herzog H, Ameling W, Meyer J, Effert S (1979) Arrhythmia detection with a multi-microprocessor system for distributed and parallel processing. Comp in Card, Genf 1979, IEEE 79, CH 1462–1c, 63–66

Jensch P, Ameling W, Kubalski W, Heuck N, Meyer J, Effert S (1980) A data acquisition and processing system for sequences of ultrasound echoes and video images. Comp in Card, CH 1606:227–230

Joynt L, Martin R, Macovski K (1980) Techniques for in vivo tissue characterization. Acoust Imag 8:527–538

Kobayashi H (1978) Modeling and Analysis. Chapt 3–9. Addison-Wesley Publ Comp

Krings L, Milde J, Ameling W (1982) The influence of bus allocation algorithms on the system performance of multiprocessor systems with a time-shared bus. An Experience Report, 10th IMACS World Congress, Montreal

Krings L, Milde J, Ameling W (1981) An approach to performance measuring in multiprocessor systems with time-shared buses. Proc Euromicro. Paris, North-Holland Publ Co, pp 411–419

Li CC, Ameling W, Fu KS, DeMori R et al. (1979) Cardio-pulmonary system. Biomed. Pattern Recogn. and Image Processing, Life Sci. Res. Report, Verlag Chemie, Weinheim 15: 299–332

Meagher D (1982) Geometric modeling using octtree encoding. Comp Graphics and Image Processing 19:129–147

Milde J, Krings L, Ameling W (1982a) Architektur des Multiprozessorsystems M5PS und Auswertung einiger Anwendungen. Ulm, NTG-Gi Fachtagung

Milde J, Krings L, Ameling W (1982b) Realization of synchronization tools and their efficiency in the multiprocessorsystem M5PS. Proc 10th IMACS World Congress, Monteal

Rogers DF, Adams JA (1976) Mathematical Elements for Computer Graphics. McGraw-Hill

Wu SC, Abel JF, Greenberg DP (1977) An interactive computer graphics approach to surface representation. Communications of the ACM 20:10:703–712

The cardiac and vascular interactions in the regulation of cardiac output

Matthew N. Levy
Division of Investigative Medicine, The Mt. Sinai Medical Center, Case Western Reserve University, Cleveland, OH 44106, U.S.A.

Abstract

Cardiac output is determined by the following four factors: preload, afterload, heart rate, and myocardial contractility. The first two of these factors may be called coupling factors, because their magnitudes are determined by the characteristics of both the cardiac and vascular components of the cardiovascular system. The nature of the coupling between these two components can be analyzed by means of two characteristic curves. The first curve, the so-called cardiac function curve, reflects the Frank-Starling mechanism. It describes the cardiac output as a function of the cardiac filling pressure (or preload). The second curve, the so-called vascular function curve, reflects certain vascular characteristics, namely the peripheral resistance, arterial and venous compliances, and total blood volume. This curve describes the cardiac filling pressure as a function of the cardiac output. The equilibrium values of cardiac output and cardiac filling pressure are defined by the point of intersection of these two curves. The various humoral, neural, and pharmacological factors that affect the cardiovascular system will alter one or both of these curves. The effects of such factors on cardiac output and preload are defined by the point of intersection of the new cardiac and vascular function curves.

The four factors that determine the cardiac output are the preload, afterload, heart rate, and myocardial contractility. The heart rate and contractility are intrinsic characteristics of the cardiac tissues per se. The preload and afterload, on the other hand, reflect the characteristics of both the heart and the vascular system. The preload and afterload influence cardiac performance, but at the same time, the magnitudes of both these factors are determined by the cardiac function and vascular characteristics.

Only recently have we begun to appreciate fully that changes in the peripheral circulation are often just as important in determining the level of the cardiac output as are changes in cardiac function itself. Therefore, in order to understand the regulation of cardiac output, it is important to appreciate the nature of the

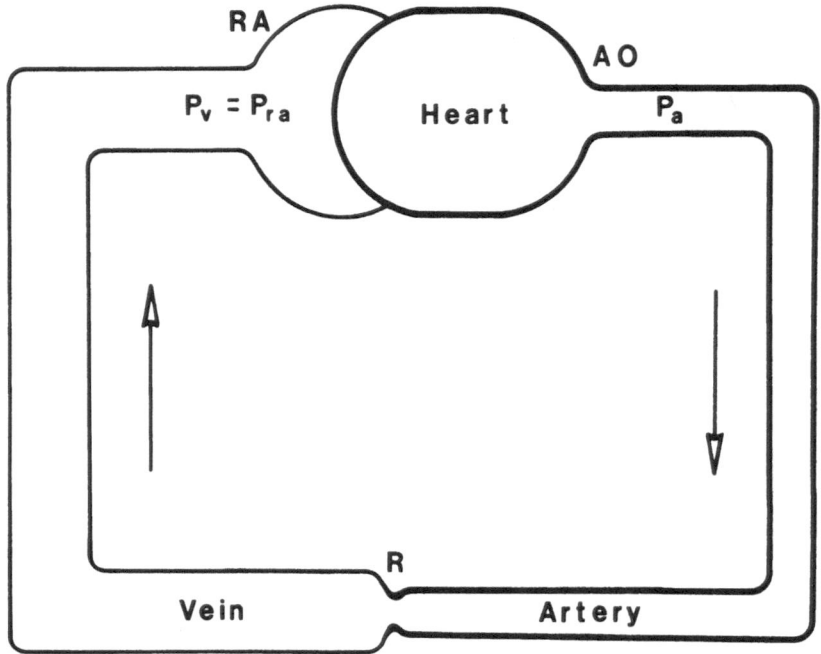

Figure 1. Simplified model of the cardiovascular system. Abbreviations: RA, right atrium; AO, aorta; R, systemic resistance; P_v, central venous pressure; P_{ra}, right atrial pressure; and P_a, arterial pressure. (From Levy, with permission of the American Heart Assoc., Inc.)

coupling between the heart and the vascular system. Much of the elucidation of the role of the vascular system in the control of cardiac output was accomplished by Guyton (1955) and Guyton *et al.* (1955a, 1955b, 1973).

Circulatory system model

In order to analyze the functional coupling between the heart and the blood vessels, we will use a model in which the cardiovascular system has been reduced to its simplest components (Levy, 1979; Berne and Levy, 1981). The model consists of a pump, an elastic arterial system, a peripheral resistance (R), and an elastic venous system (Figure 1). The relative ease of analysis of the interactions among the components of this simplified model permits the elucidation of certain basic principles. For many purposes the model is much too simple and potentially misleading. For such purposes, more complicated models must be used, such as those developed by Grodins and his coworkers (1959, 1960), Sagawa (1972), and Guyton *et al.* (1973).

The cardiovascular model shown in Figure 1 may be subdivided arbitrarily into cardiac and vascular components. Coupling between these components takes

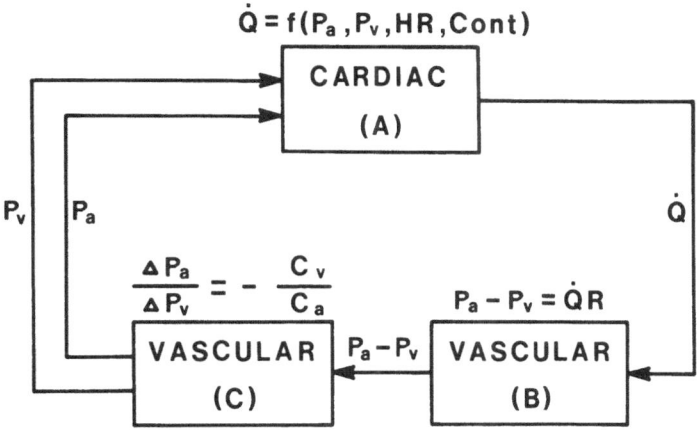

$$\dot{Q} = f(P_a, P_v, HR, Cont)$$

Figure 2. The feedback loop involved in the coupling of the cardiac and vascular portions of the circulatory system. Abbreviations: Q, systemic flow; P_a, arterial pressure; P_v, venous pressure; HR, heart rate; Cont, cardiac contractility; R, systemic resistance; C_a, arterial capacitance; and C_v, venous capacitance. (From Levy, with permission of the American Heart Assoc., Inc.)

place at the following two sites; (1) the right atrium connects the terminal veins to the input side of the pump and (2) the aortic origin connects the output side of the pump to the upstream end of the vascular system. The pressures in the aorta (P_a) and in the right atrium (P_{ra}) and central veins (P_v) comprise the mechanical feedback signals that coordinate the activities of the cardiac and vascular components of the circulatory system. In the model, the pressures in the right atrium and large central veins are considered to be equal; i.e., $P_{ra} = P_v$. The cardiac pumping action tends to establish the levels of P_a and P_v, which in turn influence the rate of blood flow through the vascular system. Concomitantly, the vascular characteristics also determine the levels of P_a and P_v, which in turn affect the volume of blood to be pumped by the heart each minute.

The block diagram depicted in Figure 2 outlines the manner in which the cardiac and vascular subunits of the circulatory system interact mechanically with each other. The elements in the diagram constitute a feedback loop. The block in the top half of the loop represents the cardiac behavior, whereas the two blocks in the bottom half of the loop represent the vascular function. A preliminary version of this block diagram has been presented previously by Fermoso *et al.* (1964), and a more detailed version has been developed by Grodins and his coworkers (1959, 1960).

Cardiac component

The heart is the energy source that is responsible for pumping the total blood flow (Q) around the body. As stated above, the preload, afterload, cardiac contractility, and heart rate are considered to be the factors that determine the output of the heart. P_{ra} is a cardinal determinant of right ventricular preload, and for convenience, P_{ra} is often equated with the preload. Similarly, P_a is an essential determinant of left ventricular afterload, and often is taken to be the afterload. Hence, in the 'cardiac function' block (A) in Figure 2, P_a and P_v are shown as two critical inputs that tend to determine Q. In general, Q varies directly with P_v and inversely with P_a. The effects of P_v and P_a on cardiac output have been analyzed in detail by Herndon and Sagawa (1969).

Vascular component

For the flow of a fluid through a system of tubes, the hydraulic equivalent of Ohm's law is:

$$Q = (P_1 - P_2)/R, \tag{1}$$

where Q is the flow, R is the total resistance, and $(P_1 - P_2)$ is the pressure gradient across that resistance.

For the vascular system model under consideration, the pressure gradient would be the arteriovenous pressure gradient, $P_a - P_v$. Substituting $(P_a - P_v)$ for $(P_1 - P_2)$ in Eq. (1) and rearranging, we obtain

$$P_a - P_v = QR. \tag{2}$$

From this equation, it is apparent that the magnitude of the arteriovenous pressure gradient at equilibrium is determined by the peripheral vascular resistance, R, and by the quantity of blood per minute being pumped by the heart, Q. A change in Q would evoke a proportionate change in the gradient. Assuming a constant R for the present purpose, and given that the energy source for the flow is derived from the pumping action of the heart, we may consider Q to be the independent variable in this relationship, and $(P_a - P_v)$ to be the dependent variable (block B, Figure 2).

The selection of the dependent and independent variables is often arbitrary. For example, the energy of cardiac contraction is involved in the development of pressure as well as flow. Therefore, for other purposes, the opposite assignment of dependent and independent variables might have been made.

The absolute levels of the two components (P_a and P_v) of the pressure gradient that would prevail with a given change in Q (Eq. 2) is determined by the elastic characteristics of the systemic circulation and by the blood volume. The arterial capacitance, C_a, is defined as dV_a/dP_a, where V_a and P_a are the blood volume and pressure, respectively, on the arterial side of the circuit. Similarly, the venous capacitance, C_v, is defined as dV_v/dP_v, where V_v and P_v are the venous volume and pressure, respectively. In our model (Figure 1), let C_a and C_v both be constant, i.e., independent of both pressure and volume. Under such conditions, it is also true that $C_a = \Delta V_a/\Delta P_a$, and $C_v = \Delta V_v/\Delta P_v$.

For the sake of simplicity, let the changes in blood volume take place only in the systemic arteries and veins. Given a constant total blood volume,

$$\Delta V_a = -\Delta V_v. \tag{3}$$

Hence, any increment in V_a is accompanied by an equal decrement in V_v, or vice versa. But $\Delta V_a = C_a \cdot \Delta P_a$, and $\Delta V_v = C_v \cdot \Delta P_v$. Substituting these values in Eq. (3) and rearranging, we obtain

$$\Delta P_a/\Delta P_v = -C_v/C_a. \tag{4}$$

For the static system (i.e., $Q = 0$)., pressures are equal throughout the circuit, and that pressure is a function only of the total volume of blood and the overall capacitance of the system. This static pressure has been termed the mean circulatory pressure (P_{mc}) by Guyton (1955). At normal blood volumes and with normal vessels, the magnitude of the mean circulatory pressure has been estimated to be about 7 mmHg (Guyton, 1955; Guyton et al., 1955a, 1955b, 1973).

When the flow around such a system is increased in a stepwise fashion, there is a progressive increase in P_a and a progressive reduction in P_v (Figure 3). If we let ΔP_a and ΔP_v in Eq. (4) equal $P_a - P_{mc}$ and $P_v - P_{mc}$, respectively, then the following equation defining P_v as a function of Q can be derived from (2) to (4):

$$P_v = -\frac{RC_a}{C_a + C_v} Q + P_{mc}. \tag{5}$$

A graph of P_v plotted as a function of Q (Figure 4) has been termed a 'vascular function curve' (Levy, 1979; Berne and Levy, 1981). From eq. 5, it is evident that the slope of the relationship between P_v and Q depends only on R, C_v and C_a. Changes in flow have an inverse effect on P_v; i.e., as Q is increased, there will be a proportionate decrease in P_v. There is a limit to the reduction of P_v that can be produced by an increase in Q, however. At some critical maximum value of Q, sufficient fluid will be translocated from the venous to the arterial side of the circuit such that P_v will drop below the ambient pressure. In a system of distensible tubes, the venous system will be collapsed by this negative transmural pressure (P_v minus ambient pressure). This will, of course, limit the maximum value of cardiac output regardless of the capabilities of the pump.

In the simplified schema depicted in Figure 1 the venous system was considered to be without resistance. In the body, however, there is a continuous pressure gradient from the venules to the right side of the heart. If an open-chest animal is placed on total heart bypass and if the pump output is progressively increased, the

228

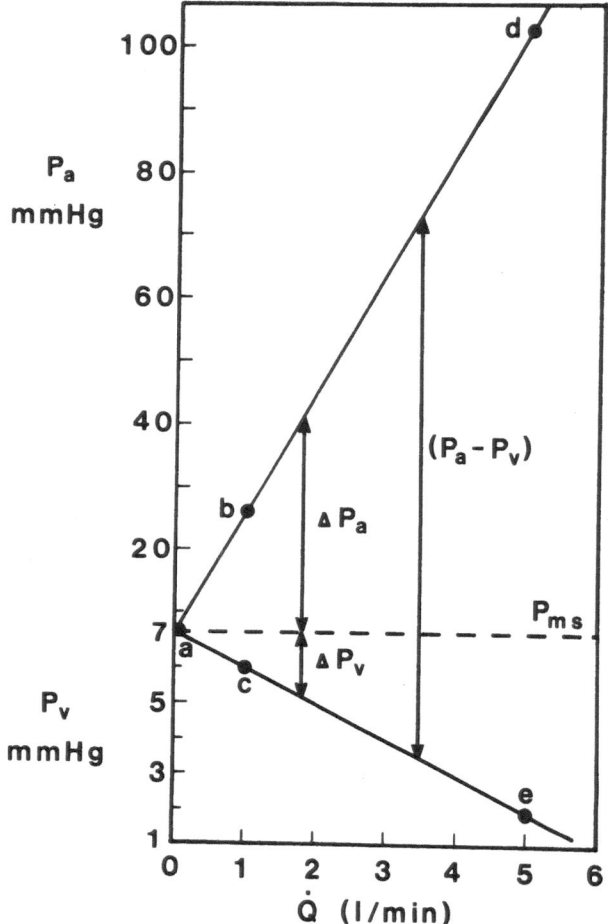

Figure 3. The arterial pressure (P_a) and central venous pressure (P_v) as functions of the systemic flow (Q) in the model depicted in Figure 1, where $R = 20$ and $C_v/C_a = 19$. Point a denotes the value of the mean systemic pressure (P_{ms}); i.e., the common value for P_a and p_v when $Q = 0$. Points b and c denote the values of P_a and P_v when $Q = 1$, and points d and e, the values of P_a and P_v when $Q = 5$. The deviations of P_a and P_v from P_{ms} are denoted by $\varDelta P_a$ and $\varDelta P_v$, respectively. Note that the scales for P_a and P_v are not the same. (From Levy, with permission of the American Heart Assoc., Inc.)

site of ultimate collapse will be at the junction of the venae cavae with the inflow port of the pump. In the normal, closed-chest animal, venous collapse occurs at the points of entry of the extrathoracic veins into the chest.

Equation (5) also shows that when $Q = 0$, P_v equals P_{mc}; i.e., P_{mc} is the pressure axis intercept of the vascular function curve. As stated above, one of the cardinal determinants of P_{mc} is the total blood volume. Hence, changes in total blood volume elicit changes in the pressure axis intercept (P_{mc}), but not in the slope, of the vascular function curve (Levy, 1959; Berne and Levy, 1981).

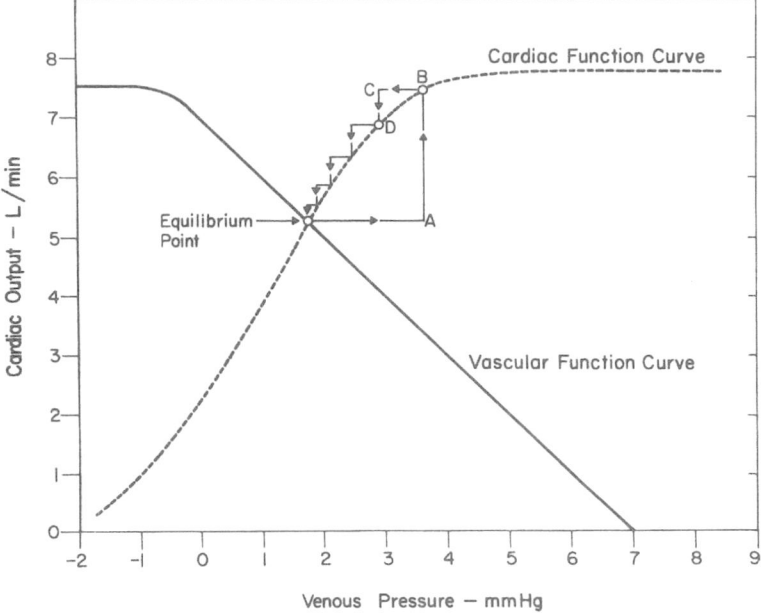

Figure 4. Hypothetical cardiac and vascular function curves. (From Berne and Levy.)

Coupling between the heart and the vasculature

In accordance with Starling's law of the heart, cardiac output is intimately dependent on P_{ra}. In our simplified model, we have let $P_v = P_{ra}$. In the discussion to follow, graphs of cardiac output as a function of P_v (Figure 4) will be called 'cardiac function curves'. Extrinsic regulatory influences may be expressed as shifts in such curves (Guyton *et al.*, 1973; Levy, 1979; Berne and Levy, 1981).

A typical cardiac function curve is plotted on the same coordinates as a normal vascular function curve in Figure 4. The cardiac function curve is plotted according to the usual convention; that is, the independent variable (P_v) is plotted along the abscissa, and the dependent variable Q is plotted along the ordinate. In accordance with the Frank-Starling mechanism, the cardiac function curve reveals that a rise in P_v is associated with an increase in Q. Conversely, the vascular function curve describes the inverse relationship between Q and P_v. Note that this is plotted contrary to the usual convention, in that the independent variable (Q) is plotted along the ordinate, whereas the dependent variable (P_v) is plotted along the abscissa. This breach of the convention is necessary in order to include both curves on the same graph. The equilibrium point of the system that is described by these two curves is defined by the point of intersection. The coordinates of this equilibrium point represent the values of Q and P_v at which such a system tends to operate. Only transient deviations from such values for Q and P_v are possible, as long as the given cardiac and vascular function curves accurately describe the system.

The tendency for the cardiovascular system to operate about such an equilibrium point may best be illustrated by examining its response to a sudden perturbation. Consider the changes elicited by a sudden rise in P_v from the equilibrium point to point A in Figure 4. Such a change might be induced experimentally by the transient opening of an arterio-venous shunt for just one cardiac cycle. Because of the Frank-Starling mechanism, the elevated P_v would elicit an increase in Q (point B) during the very next ventricular systole. The increased Q in turn, would accomplish a net transfer of blood from the venous to the arterial side of the circuit, with a consequent reduction in P_v (to point C). During the next cardiac contraction, Q would therefore be less (point D), although still above the equilibrium value. This process would continue in ever-diminishing steps until the equilibrium values for P_v and Q were re-established. This illustrates the negative feedback characteristics of the system depicted in Figure 2.

Interrelationships between cardiac output and venous return

Cardiac output and venous return are inextricably interdependent. Clearly, except for small, transient disparities, the heart will be unable to pump any more blood than is delivered to it through the venous system. Similarly, because the circulatory system is a closed circuit, the rate of venous return must equal the cardiac output under equilibrium conditions. The flow around the entire closed circuit depends upon the capability of the pump, the characteristics of the circuit, and the total volume of fluid in the system. Cardiac output and venous return are simply two terms for expressing the flow around the closed circuit. Cardiac output is the volume of blood being pumped by the heart per unit time. Venous return is the volume of blood returning to the heart per unit time. At equilibrium, these two flows are identical.

Acute changes in cardiac contractility, peripheral resistance, or blood volume may transiently exert differential effects on cardiac output and venous return. Except for such brief disparities, however, such factors simply alter flow around the entire circuit. It is irrelevant whether one thinks of that flow as 'cardiac output' or 'venous return.' All too frequently authors have ascribed the reduction in cardiac output during hemorrhage, for example, to a decrease in venous return. Such an explanation, of course, is a blatant example of circular reasoning, in its most literal sense. Hemorrhage reduces blood flow around the entire circuit, mainly because the diminished blood volume and generalized arteriolar constriction lead to a reduction in the cardiac preload. To attribute the reduction in cardiac output to a curtailment of venous return is equivalent to ascribing the decrease in systemic blood flow to a decrease in systemic blood flow!

Acknowledgement

This work was supported by United States Public Health Service Grant HL 10951.

References

Berne RM, Levy MN (1981) Cardiovascular Physiology, ed. 4. St. Louis: CV Mosby Co. pp 186–202
Fermoso JC, Richardson TQ, Guyton AC (1964) Mechanism of decrease in cardiac output caused by opening the chest. Am Physiol 207:1112–1116
Grodins FS (1959) Integrative cardiovascular physiology: A mathematical synthesis of cardiac and blood vessel hemodynamics. Quart Rev Biol 34:93–116
Grodins FS, Stuart WH, Veenstra RL (1960) Performance characteristics of the right heart bypass preparation. Am J Physiol 198:552–560
Guyton AC (1955) Determination of cardiac output by equating venous return curves with cardiac response curves. Physiol Rev 35:123–129
Guyton AC, Lindsey AW, Abernathy B, Richardson T (1955a) Venous return at various right atrial pressures and the normal venous return curve. Am J Physiol 189:609–615
Guyton AC, Jones CE, Coleman TG (1973) Circulatory Physiology: Cardiac Output and Its Regulation, ed. 2. Philadelphia: WB Saunders
Guyton AC, Lindsey AW, Kaufmann BN (1955b) Effect of mean circulatory filling pressure and other peripheral circulatory factors on cardiac output. Am J Physiol 180:463–468
Herndon CW, Sagawa K (1969) Combined effects of aortic and right atrial pressures on aortic flow. Am J Physiol 217:65–72
Levy MN (1979) The cardiac and vascular factors that determine systemic blood flow. Circ Res 44:739–746
Sagawa K (1972) The use of control theory and systems analysis in cardiovascular dynamics. *In*: DG Bergel (ed) Cardiovascular Fluid Dynamics, vol. 1. London: Academic Press, pp 116–171

Flow within the left ventricular cavity: relative significance of various hemodynamic effects

URI DINNAR

Dept. of Bio-Medical Engineering, Technion – Israel Institute of Technology, Haifa, Israel

Abstract

In the last decade a tremendous effort was directed into the use of clinical measurements and analytical analysis of left ventricular performance for the purpose of diagnosis, prognosis and physiological understanding. Numerical computations requires different schemes for the intraventricular flow-pressure solution and for the myocardial contraction-expansion solution. The matching boundary conditions for these two solutions is the ventricular pressure, which in most mathematical models is taken to be uniform. A simple analysis shows that pressure gradients of up to 20 mmHg might exist within the left ventricle. These gradients may not be evident in catheterization measurements, due to the method used. One must, therefore, be very carfull in analytical modeling of the left ventricle as to the exact matching boundary conditions for the elastic-flow problems. These deviations are characterised according to the various events occurring during the cardiac cycle.

Introduction

Next year will mark a century since Otto Frank (Frank, 1895) published his pressure-volume relationship for ventricular contraction and seventy years since Patterson *et al.*, 1914; Starling, 1918) introduced the relation between preload and stroke volume known as the Starling law of the heart. Most of the published work since then has demonstrated the variations of these relationship in health and disease. Only in the last two decased investigators have tried to obtain these relations by the use of more precise analytical models describing the pumping activity of the heart. Tremendous amount of work has been directed to obtain analytical expressions for the contracting properties of the myocardium yielding various constitutive relations for the cardiac muscle during each phase of the cardiac cycle. The force generated by the cardiac muscle was translated into ventricular pressure, assuming uniform pressure inside the ventricular cavity with negligible intraventricular pressure gradients. The flow inside the ventricle was considered in only a few publications, mainly in those interested in the nature of flow through the mitral or aortic valves. The goal of these investigations was to design better artificial valves and to obtain relations between the flow and intraventricular pressure. The intensive research of 3-D simulation of the cardiac cycle has triggered the idea of measuring noninvasivly the parameters used clinically to evaluate cardiac activity and pumping efficiency. Again, most of the attention has been directed to the description of myocardial contractility and muscle stiffness, and the flow parameters were mostly ignored. The pressure was assumed in these models to be the result of the elastic stress obtained from the model, or to be an input to the model taken from measurement of catheterization. The purpose of this presentation is to study the relative significance of ventricular flow in the determination of cardiac performance during each stage of the cardiac cycle. A better understanding of the atrioventricular dynamics and the relative contribution of myocardial stiffness and blood flow patterns may yield a new set of diagnostic mechanical indices that will be more sensitive to variations and more indicative of ventricular pumping efficiency than those used today.

Intraventricular parameters

The events of the cardiac cycle are determined by the positions of the valves and the contraction/relaxation of the muscles. These parameters are related to a variety of control mechanism both neural, chemical and mechanical. The mechanical control is achieved by the filling volume, the pressure of the ventricle prior to contraction and the build up of pressure which determine the opening and closure of the valves. To describe these parameters there are clinical significant volume and pressure values which serve as indications of cardiac performance. The volume parameters include the volume (amount of blood) of the ventricle just prior to systolic contraction defined as the end diastolic volume (EDV) and the volume of blood in the ventricle at the end of contraction, called end systolic volume (ESV). The difference between these volumes is the stroke volume, which multiplied by the heart rate will give the cardiac output. These parameters can be determined very easily from 3-D reconstruction of ventricular geometry. Thus if a spatial description of the left ventricle can be obtained by external noninvasive measurement (angiographic, ultrasonic or any other) these valves can be computed with same degree of accuracy as the measuring system. The pressure parameters used to describe the intraventricular activity are obtained from left ventricular pressure transducer. They include the pressure, p, and the peak rate of change in ventricular pressure during isometric contraction, $(\mathrm{d}p/\mathrm{d}t)_{\max}$. The last value gave an excellent indication of inotropic response of the ventricle (Linden, 1968). Pressure is measured by the insertion of tip manometer into the ventricle, and assuming that pressure is uniform throughout the ventricle. With this assumption it is not essential to exactly locate the manometer. It is also assumed that position of the probe relative to the fluid is not of importance, thus neglecting the dynamic pressure and the acceleration of blood. It is obvious that when the tip manometer is place 'heads on' to flow it will record the stagnation pressure, while in any other positions it will record the actual pressure and related parts of the dynamic and acceleration pressure components. Later in this presentation the relative significance of these terms will be discussed. The small changes in pressure recordings might not be crucial in clinical measurements due to the high variability between one human to another. However, if the 3-D geometrical shape is used to study the flow and determine the pressure by non-invasive techniques this intraventricular pressure is the matching boundary conditions between the muscle contraction with the resulting stress and the generation of flow yielding pressure gradients in the flow computation. The determination of intraventricular pressure will require the solution of the intraventricular fluid flow problem.

Intraventricular pressure or myocardial stress in diastole

In analytical models describing the cardiac cycle in both systole and diastole there is a tendency to consider either the elastic contraction of the myocardium or the intraventricular flow in isolation. The reason is the complexity of the dual system and the relative role of each phenomena during the different phases of the cycle. The interactions between both systems is physiologically understood but mathematically hard to use. Instead different investigators have used different laws for time varying properties of cardiac elastic parameters which depend on the phase and not on the mechanical events that take place in each specific period. The relations between pressure generating flow, change in cardiac muscle response and the effect of electrical activity of the active contracting or relaxing muscle must be carefully analysed during the entire cycle to yield a suitable mathematical model.

To study to pressure-flow event in the left ventricle, consider, for example, the ventricular diastole. The initial phase is the isometric relaxation phase, lasting some 0.08 s (in normal heart with 70 beats per minute). In this phase there is no change in ventricular volume and the only event is relaxation of the muscle and a decrease in intraventricular pressure. The governing equations for this phase must be the elastic myocardial equations leading to a decreased wall pressure. Since the pressure reduction is obtained at constant volume it can be assumed that there is a uniform pressure reduction throughout the ventricle with no flow. This phase ends when the atrial pressure exceeds that in the ventricle, thus opening the mitral valve. The opening of the valve causes blood to surge into the ventricle during a very short period of time, from 0.1 to 0.15 s. During this phase of rapid

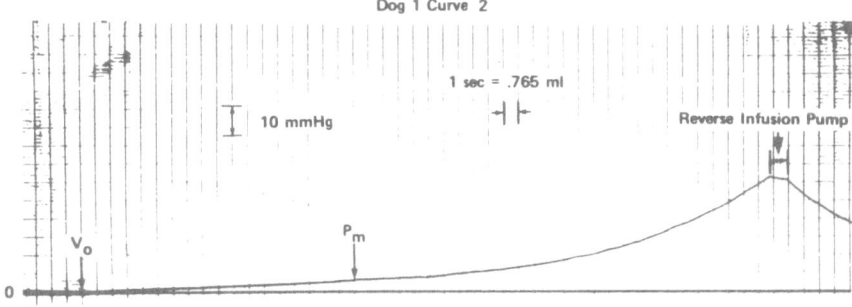

Figure 1. Pressure-volume curve measured in an excised dog heart by filling an excised ventricle with saline at a constant rate. At P_m the relations deviate from linear relationship. From Grantz (1980).

filling the fluid mechanics plays the major role. The muscle is still relaxing causing a further small decrease in pressure. It is, therefore, possible to neglect the elastic stiffness of the wall and to consider the flow alone. This phase is followed by a continuous filling of the ventricle at a slower rate, defined as the slow filling phase. During this phase the oncoming fluid is pushing the muscle, thus, increasing the stress slightly. If the pressure-volume curve for the rapid filling phase is linear, it tends to exhibit nonlinear relations at the slow filling phase. This relation for linear and nonlinear segments of pressure-volume relations is shown in Figure 1, taken from Glantz (Glantz, 1980). The force generating this ventricular expansion during late diastole is due to continued venous return and atrial contraction. The major problem at this stage is: what is the mechanism responsible for the closure of the mitral valve? (Caro *et al.*, 1978), is it the backflow through the mitralvalve?, is it the pressure generated by the expanding cardiac muscle?, is it the vortex formation behind the mitral valve cusps?, or is it the contraction of the pappillary muscles which pull the valve cusps? There are numerous theories that support these various mechanisms. This summary does not intend to solve this contraversy, but rather, to point out that by choosing one of the theories, one has to use a proper mathematical model to determine the termination of diastole. It is important not only from an analytical point of view, but also from a physiological point of view. Determination of the valve closure will determine the End Diastolic Volume (EDV) which determined the initial fiber length for ventricular systole and the initial intraventricular pressure.

Various mathematical models were suggested for the analysis of left ventricular diastole (Ghista *et al.*, 1969; Mirsky, 1973; Rabkin and HSU 1975, Ghista and Hamid 1977, Ghista and Ray 1980, a, b; Moskowitz, 1980). These models are directed toward either a part of diastole or toward analytical expressions for the cardiac elastic properties. Different parameters are used to describe the time varying behavior discussed earlier. They can be the general stiffness parameters, or parameters defined only for the need of the analysis, as for example the left ventricular medium's strain energy density (Mirsky, 1973) or others.

These parameters change in disease (Templeton *et al.*, 1975; Barry *et al.*, 1974; Mann *et al.*, 1979) and hence it is very hard to obtain a general expression which will cover the entire range of the diastole with a high degree of accuracy.

Left ventricular systole

At the beginning of diastole the mitral valves are closed and the pressures in both left atrium and left ventricle are equal. Due to electrical stimulation of the SA node, contraction begins. The pressure in the left ventricle is increased much more and at a faster rate than the atrial pressure. It is, therefore, clear that the contracting muscle and the amount of contracting muscle (determined by muscle thickness) are responsible for the activity of the ventricle and the intraventricular variations. As in the diastolic case, we distinguish here a phase of isometric contraction, where the chamber is closed and the net result of contraction is a build up of pressure. The end stage of this phase is determined by the opening of the aortic valves and the beginning of the ejection phase. In this phase the flow is extremely high, especially near the valve exit. It seems very clear that this phase is undoubtedly controlled by the elastic contractility of the heart and the pressure it generates within the ventricle. However, to determine the opening of the aortic valve and the termination of the isovolumetric contraction one must also consider the kinetic energy (dynamic pressure) and the acceleration term (associated with Newton's Second Law). These components will be determined by the flow conditions generated by the contracting muscles. Due to this interaction between contracting walls and valve opening a pattern of dynamics and accelerations will be formed, which will determine the stroke volume. However, as in the case of the mitral valve the rate of ejection depends, in the later stage of ejection, more on the dynamics of flow through the valve and the load of pressure existing in the aorta. Hence, it is evident that although the generating mechanism at the beginning of contraction is the contracting muscle, it must be determined what is the afterload and the valve mechanics to determine the conditions in the later stage of ventricular ejection. In healthy normal heart the contracting pattern will promote a favorable pressure gradient for the ventricular ejection. In pathological cases, this gradient may be altered, as shown in Figure 2, (from Ray *et al.*, 1979) for a patient with myocardial infarction. This will delay the opening of the aortic valve; thus, generating a larger isovolumic contraction period and smaller ejection phase leading to a smaller value of cardiac output. The figure also shows the pressure distribution in the same patient after coronary bypass surgery, with much smaller areas of reversed pressure gradients. This example which is based on numerical computation of the pressure field shows clearly the potential in using a real geometry simulation of ventricular performance. Such analysis might yield new indices and new direction in a diagnosis of cardiac performance. A variety of mathamatical models were suggested for the description of the systolic

PATIENT # 474701

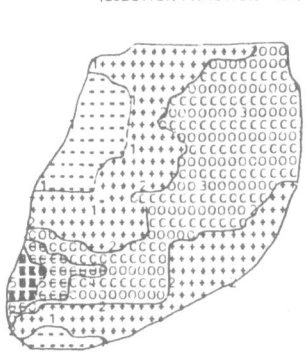

A. BEFORE CORONARY BYPASS
(EJECTION FRACTION = .65)

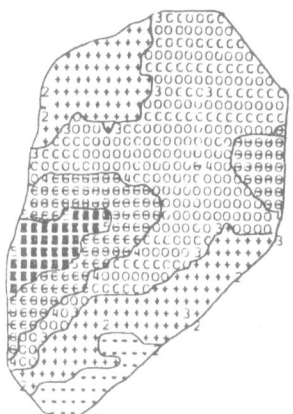

B. AFTER CORONARY BYPASS
(EJECTION FRACTION = .68)

NONDIMENSIONAL PRESSURE			% LV CHAMBER AREA AT PRESSURE LEVEL		COMMENTS (A NEO INTRINSIC MEAS- URE OF IMPROVED CONTRACTIVITY AFTER CORONARY BYPASS)
LEVEL	VALUE (P/P$_o$) (P$_o$ = 1, AT AV BOUNDARY OF LV CHAMBER)	SYMBOL	BEFORE BYPASS	AFTER BYPASS	
1	0.80 – 0.90	- - - - - - - - -	12.7 ⎫	5.8 ⎫	DECREASE OF ZONE OF LOW PRESSURE LEVEL (1 & 2) BY 23.9% AFTER BYPASS
2	0.90 – 0.98	+ + + + + + + + +	43.6 ⎭ = 56.3	26.6 ⎭ = 32.4	
3	0.98 – 1.02	0 0 0 0 0 0 0 0 0	38.0 = 38.0	45.1 = 45.1	INCREASE OF ZONE OF PRESSURE LEVEL (3) BY 7.1% AFTER BYPASS
4	1.02 – 1.08	𝘶 𝘶 𝘶 𝘶 𝘶 𝘶 𝘶 𝘶 𝘶	3.8 ⎫	17.4 ⎫	INCREASE OF ZONE OF HIGH PRESSURE LEVELS (4 & 5) BY 16.8% AFTER BYPASS
5	1.08 – 1.16	▪ ▪ ▪ ▪ ▪ ▪ ▪ ▪ ▪	1.9 ⎭ = 5.7	5.1 ⎭ = 22.5	

Figure 2. Pressure distribution in a patient with myocardial infarction before and after coronary bypass surgery. The measurement is taken just prior to ventricular ejection and shows a reversal of pressure gradients. From Ray *et al.* (1979).

phase. An excellent review paper was published recently (Sunagawa and Sagawa, 1982) describing the idea of time-varying elastance which describes the pump function of the left ventricle, and uses the end-diastolic volume to predict the stroke volume (or the end systolic volume). In this review, Sunagawa and Sagawa also compare their model with other models suggested for left ventricular systole. In addition they discuss the linkage between their model and the aortic interac-

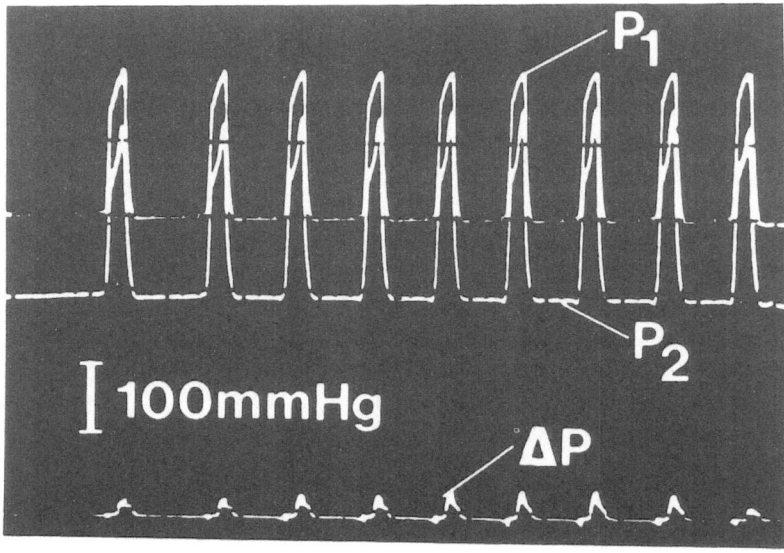

Figure 3. Recorded pressures in a dog's left ventricle. P_1 – pressure near the apex, and P_2 – pressure near the aortic value. The obtained pressure difference is 15–20 mmHg. From Ray *et al.* (1979).

tion by two mechanisms: the afterload determined by the aortic pressure and aortic valve performance; and the left-ventricular-aortic interaction through coronary circulation.

Matching boundary conditions

As was pointed out it is necessary to use simultaneously a model for the contracting muscle and a model for the intraventricular flow. Both models must be matched at each instant during the cardiac cycle. The matching boundary conditions must be determined on the endocardium, and the matching parameters is the pressure. As was pointed out before, most of the model considers the measured pressure measured at an inner point on the left ventricle, assuming uniform pressure inside the ventricular cavity. Two questions arise with respect to the measured pressure. The first one regards the type of measuring device used to measure the intraventricular pressure and the relative position of the pressure gauge with regard to ventricular flow. If the gauge is placed 'head on' to the flow it will measure static pressure. In most instances it will be at a certain angle to the flow thus giving a value somewhere between these values. The problem is to know the relative contribution of the dynamic pressure, the gravitational pressure and the effect of acceleration. The second problem is the distribution of these pressures. Due to the existence of the valve, the situation is not symmetrical and the pressure near the valves might be different from the pressure near the apex.

Ray et al. (1979) reported intraventricular pressure of as much as 15–20 mmHg between the apex and the aortic valve inside the left ventricle during ejection, Figure 3. They also showed that this pressure gradient is increased by administration of drugs (isoprotevenal), and decreased or even reversed after ligation of the left descending coronary artery of a dog after 18 and 35 min, respectively, Wang and Sonnenblick (1979) suggested numerical approximation for the peak pressure gradient using spherical geometry. They discovered the same phenomena. The model suggested by Wang and Sonnenblick can be used to give not only the differences that may occur in pressure measurements, but also the proper boundary conditions that must be applied to both elastic and fluid flow models. In the situations existing in the heart and the range of Reynolds number (or order 100) the viscous effects are confined to a thin layer near the endocardium, thus yielding a simple equation for the potential function inside the ventricle.

$$\nabla^2 \varphi = 0. \tag{1}$$

Assuming that the ventricle remains spherical with an unsteady radius $R(t)$, and a valve opening with orifice of solid angle α, thus having an area of $4\pi r^2 \alpha$ ($\alpha < 1$) and a flat velocity profile at the valve (aortic valve during ejection and mitral valve during filling) gives a solution described by spherical Legendre polynomial $Pn(\cos \theta)$ in the following form:

$$\varphi = R \frac{dR}{dt} \left\{ \sum_{n=1}^{\infty} \frac{2n + 1}{2n(n + 1)} \left(1 = \frac{1}{\alpha} \right) [(1 - 2\alpha)Pn(1 - 2\alpha) - \right.$$
$$\left. - Pn - 1(1 - 2\alpha)] \times \left(\frac{r}{R} \right)^n Pn(\cos \theta) - \frac{r\cos \theta}{R} \right\} \tag{2}$$

Bernoullis' law for unsteady flow of inviscid irrotational motion is given by (Goldstein, 1960)

$$\frac{P}{\rho} + \tfrac{1}{2} v^2 + gz + \frac{\partial \varphi}{\partial t} = F(t) \tag{3}$$

where, $\frac{1}{2}\rho v^2$ is the dynamic pressure, $\rho(\partial \varphi/\partial t)$ is the acceleration pressure and $\rho g z$ is the gravitational pressure. If the volume of the left ventricle is taken from a standard reference (Altman and Dittmer, 1971) as shown in Figure 4, and the corresponding spherical dimension is calculated for each step in time, Eq. (3) can be used to calculate the contribution of the additional pressure to the actual static pressure P. The value of P itself can not be calculated, but can be assumed from the known reference of peak systolic ventricular pressure. The results for $\alpha = 0.05$ are shown in figure 5 which describe the variations of dynamic and acceleration pressure at each point during the entire cycle. The gravitational pressure difference from base to apex is nearly 3 mmHg in the reversed direction. The

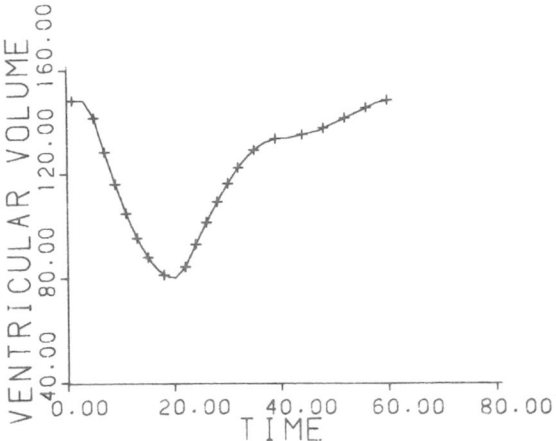

Figure 4. Variations of the left ventricular volume with time. Based on data from Altman and Dittmer (1971).

results show that nearly 20 mmHg difference in pressure can exist between apex and base during the ejection phase, and nearly 10 mmHg during the ventricular filling. These results point nearly 20% error by assuming uniform pressure during the ejection phase. In the ventricular filling phase this value can be much higher, reaching nearly 60% during peak pressure difference. These effects are inten-

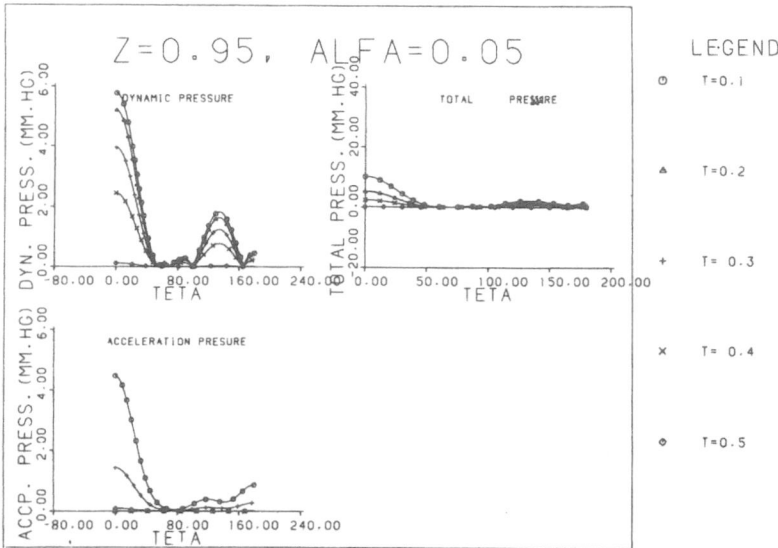

Figure 5. Distribution of dynamic, acceleration and total pressures with time during a cardiac cycle, at a distance of 0.95 from the radius of assumed sphere. TETA is the angle from the aortic valve and *T* is the normalized time.

sified in geometries other than spherical. The valves obtained in the computation process are very similar to those found in experiments, like the results of Ray *et al.* (1979). The error in measurements of $(dp/dt)_{max}$ is even more than the 20 mmHg value obtained for the pressure itself.

Discussion

In analytical analysis of left ventricular contraction, based on experimental measurement, and even more so in computations based on non-invasive measurement, one must be very careful as to what are the clinical parameters and how to use them in the numerical computation. The wall pressure distribution which is used as the matching parameters between the intraventricular solution and the myocardial contraction analysis must be specified to include the actual pressure and the dynamic and acceleration pressures. Solutions based on catheterization, which give total pressure, might therefore, show large deviation from reality.

In addition the events occurring in the cardiac cycle, like the opening and closure of the mitral and aortic valves must be determined from the computation. Many investigators use timing based on the heart rate and the knowledge of average duration of each phase. This may be true for normal heart, but will show a large deviation for diseased heart. A detailed solution can use pressure criterions for the opening and closing of the valve, and then correct the basic assumption by measurements.

References

Altman PL, Dittmer DS (ed) (1971) Federation of American Societies for Experimental Medicine. Respiration and Circulation. Bethesda, Maryland, p 304

Barry WM, Brooker JZ, Alderman EL, Harrison DC (1974) Changes in diastolic stiffness and bone of the left ventricle during angina pectoris. Circulation, 49:255–263

Caro CG, Pedley TJ, Schroter RC, Seed WA (1978) The mechanics of the circulation. New York and Toronto: Oxford University Press, pp 230–238

Frank O (1895) Zur Dynamik des Herzmuskels. Zeitschr. Biol 32:370–447. (Transl. by CB Chapman and E Wasserman in: Amer Heart J 58:282–317 and 467–478)

Ghista DN, Vago HW (1969) The time varying elastic properties of the left ventricular muscle. Bull Math Biophys 31:75–92

Ghista DN and Hamid S (1977) Finite elements analysis of the human left ventricle. Computer programs in Medicine 7:219

Ghista DN and Ray G (1980) Cardiac assessment mechanics: Left Ventricular mechanomyocardiography, a new approach to the detection of diseased myocardial elements and states. Med Biol Eng Comput 18:271–280

Ghista DN and Ray G (1980) Cardiac assessment mechanics: Left Ventricular mechanocardiography, a new approach to noninvasive intrinsic assessment of left ventricular pumping efficiency. Med Biol Eng Comput 18:344–352

242

Glantz SA (1980) Computing indices of diastolic stiffness has been counterproductive. Federation Proc. 39:162–168

Goldstein S (1960) Lectures on Fluid Mechanics. London; Intersciences Pub. Ltd, p 65

Linden AJ (1968) The heart-ventricular function. Anaesthesia, 23:566–584

Mann T, Goldberg S, Mudge GH Jr and Grossman W (1979) Factors contributing to altered left ventricular diastolic properties during angina pectoris. Circulation 59:14–20

Mirsky I (1973) Ventricular and arterial wall stress based on large deformation analysis. Biophysical J 13:1141–1159

Moskowitz SE (1980) On the mechanics of left ventricular diastole. J Biomechanics 13:301–311

Patterson SW, Piper H and Starling EH (1914) The regulation of the heart beat. J Physiol (London) 48:465–513

Rabkin SW and Hsu P.H. (1975): Mathematical and mechanical modeling of stress-strain relationship of pericardium. Amer J of Physiol 229:896–900

Ray G, Ghista DN and Sandler H. (1979): Left Ventricular Biomechanical Analysis for the Development of Indices Characterizing Normal-diseased Myocardium and Left Ventricular Pumping Efficiency. Adv Cardiovasc Phys Vol 4, Basel: Karger pp 161–178

Starling EH (1918) 'Law of the Heart' (Linacre Lecture 1915). London: Longmans Green

Sunagawa K and Sagawa K (1982) Models of Ventricular Contraction based on time-varying elastance. C.R.C Critical Reviews in Biomedical Engineering. Vol 10, pp 193–228.

Templeton GH, Wildenthal K, Willerson JT and Mitchell JH (1975) Influence of acute myocardial depression on left ventricular stiffness and its elastic and viscous components. J Clin Invest 56:278–285

Wang CY and Sonnenblick EH (1979) Dynamic pressure distribution inside a spherical ventricle. J Biomech 12:9–12

DISCUSSION

FEIGL: I'm a little mystified. The measurements that have been made across the mitral valve or the aortic valve show very small pressure gradients across normal vavalves, in the order of 1 mmHg. Is that correct?

ANS: Yes, for gradients across the valve. I was discussing intraventricular pressure gradients from the valves to the furthest point away from the valve.

FEIGL: I would think that the narrowest part of entering or exiting the LV were the valves. And if the peak gradient across the aortic valve, for example, is normally 1–2 mmHg, how can we have 20 mmHg inside the ventricle?

ANS: The pressure is about 6 or 7 mmHg; the pressure gradient is about 1 mmHg but it goes down. You may remember that Dr. Skorton pointed out that during the early part of rapid filling we still have a reduction in the pressure gradient within the ventricle. So there is a relation between pressure difference across the valve and the pressure between different parts within the ventricle.

FEIGL: I think that the ventricle is larger than the valve and therefore the gradients would tend to be smaller. And accelerations too.

SAGAWA: One factor with which Dr. Dinnar is probably so familiar that he forgot to draw our attention to it is the real nature of this pressure gradient. Dr. Feigl, for example, is probably primarily thinking of viscous resistance- induced pressure gradient, where large bore conductance interventricular lumen can create a gradient which is greater than that in the aortic orfice with a much more narrow diameter. The pressure gradient you presented is due to 2 factors: local acceleration pressure, or maybe interance pressure, and convective acceleration, or Bernoulli's pressure gradient, since blood flow must be accelerated by passing a narrow conduit. The energy for that acceleration has to be given by the ventricle wall and that is at least half of what Dr. Dinnar showed as a intraventricular pressure gradient. Norvil, for example, in England, did measure similar values, something like 6–10 mmHg of intraventricular pressure gradient.

ANS: Let me just add one thing. When I use the R vs t relations from the figure, from the regular chart, I insert here a kind of pumping activity due to the relaxation in the motion of the wall. It is very hard to define what is the mechanism of the pressure-volume relationship in diastole. Is it because the relaxation is expanding the volume or is it because the fluid is actually forcing the expansion of volume during the early parts of filling? We don't know the answer and this is part of the problem we have to solve for if we go to a detailed model.

RITMAN: About 7 years ago Falsetti and I measured considerable pressure gradients near the apex as well i.e. from one point to another near the apex.

A method for calculating time-dependent epicardial coronary blood flow

ROBERT M. NEREM, ELKANA ROOZ and THEODORE F. WIESNER

Physiological Fluid Mechanics Laboratory, Department of Mechanical Engineering, University of Houston, Houston, TX 77004, U.S.A.

Abstract

A computer model for calculating left epicardial coronary blood flow has been developed. This model employs a finite-branching geometry of the coronary vasculature together with the one-dimensional, unsteady equations for flow with friction. The epicardial coronary geometry includes the left main bifurcation and a selected number of smaller branches, each of which terminates in a resistance which is related to intramyocardial compression through a linear dependence on left ventricular pressure. The elastic properties of the epicardial arteries are taken to be non-linear and are prescribed by specifying the local small-disturbance wave speed. Calculations using this model predict pressure and flow waveform development and allow for the systematic investigation of the dependence of coronary flow on various parameters, e.g. peripheral resistance, wall properties, branching pattern, etc. Reasonable comparison between calculations and earlier experiments in horses has been obtained.

Introduction

The development of a real understanding of the fluid dynamic characteristics of epicardial coronary blood flow has been impeded by the general inaccessibility and small diameter of the coronary vessels and by limitations on instrumentation size. This is unfortunate for such an understanding and a detailed description of coronary fluid dynamics are necessary if we are to determine what the role of hemodynamics, i.e., fluid dynamics, is in coronary atherosclerosis.

In recent years, however, some progress has been made through model studies and through *in vivo* investigations in which point velocity measurements have been carried out in the coronary arteries of both dogs and horses using hot-film anemometer and pulsed ultrasonic Doppler systems. Unfortunately, and owing to the limited number of sites conveniently available for investigation experimentally, an overall picture of *in vivo* coronary flow and pressures waveform development based on aminal measurements is not possible. We have thus attempted to develop a mathematical treatment of epicardial coronary blood flow that qualitatively and, as far as possible, quantitatively reproduces the salient features of blood flow in the epicardial vessels as observed *in vivo*.

Several different types of mathematical models have been employed to study arterial blood flow. Among these have been the pure-resistance or steady-state perfusion models, the lumped-parameter or 'Windkessel' models, and linear models (McDonald, 1974). None of these approaches offers quantitatively the features desired here since they do not account for non-linear flow and wave propagation effects. Ling *et al.* (1972, 1973) have developed a two-dimensional nonlinear model of blood flow which is capable of predicting the flow as well as velocity profiles across a given artery section and which has been applied to both the dog aorta and the coronary arteries. However, *in vivo* measurements of the pressure gradient in the vessel section of interest are necessary as input data. This makes the model unsuitable for predicting flow in vessels where a prior knowledge of the pressure gradient is not available. Furthermore, it is difficult, if not impossible, to apply this method to an entire region of the vascular system such as is of interest here.

Another technique available for the prediction of arterial flow is to solve the non-linear, one-dimensional, unsteady equations of motion, using the method of characteristics. This method is an attractive one for this investigation since it intrinsically accounts for forward and backward running waves at each site in the physical plane. In using the one-dimensional equations, the pressure and flow are considered to be functions of only one spatial coordinate, i.e., distance along the vessel. Although such a one-dimensional model is in some ways more approximate than the two-dimensional models noted earlier, the effects of non-linear wave propagation and vessel branching, which are at least equally important, may be easily included.

Rockwell (1969) used the method of characteristics to solve the equations for a one-dimensional model of aortic blood flow. By specifying distal and proximal boundary conditions, Rockwell calculated the flow and pressure waveform development from the aortic valve to points as far distal as the abdominal aorta. Features such as the steepening of the aortic pressure waveform as one proceeds downstream of the valve were predicted and found to confirm *in vivo* results (McDonald, 1974). Womersley's (1957) original linear model failed to predict this, and Rockwell's results thus have established the importance of non-linear effects in modeling arterial flow. Van der Werff (1974) also used the method of characteristics to study aortic blood flow, but with a statement of only proximal boundary conditions (here both the pressure and flow waveforms are required as inputs) and employing the fact that the solution is periodic.

On the basis of the success of Rockwell and Van der Werff, the method-of-characteristics approach was chosen originally to solve the one-dimensional,

246

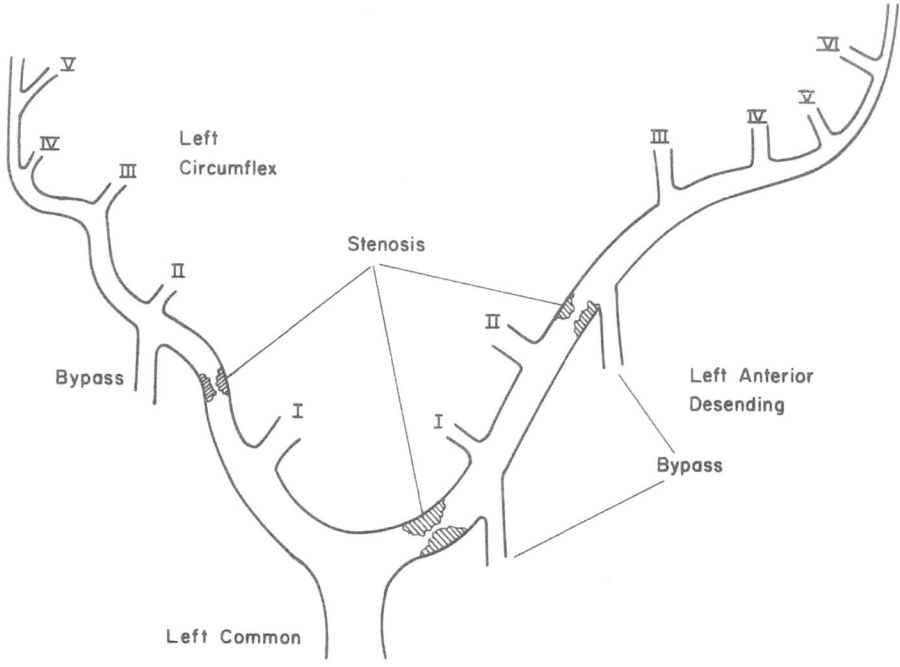

Figure 1. Finite-branching model of the left coronary system.

unsteady equations for flow in a leaky tube simulating an epicardial coronary vessel. This approach has recently been significantly modified, and it is this new model which is described here.

Model description

The calculations to be presented in the next section are based on a model which includes finite branching effects following the method employed by Stettler *et al.* (1981) for the aortic tree. The general geometry thus being used as a model for the left coronary system is shown in Figure 1. Here the branches in a given region, as denoted by number, are lumped together so that, with the exception of the bifurcation of the left common into the LAD and left circumflex coronary arteries, anywhere from 2–4 branches in a localized region have been collapsed into a single branch. In each such localized region a mass and momentum balance is written, and these two equations, together with appropriate boundary conditions, determine the flow conditions in the region of branching in a manner similar to that of Stettler *et al.* (1981).

Between major branch points, an epicardial artery is modelled as an elastic tube. The flow of blood in each such tube of the network is assumed to be that of an incompressible Newtonian fluid whose motion can be adequately described as unsteady and one-dimensional in nature. The vessel is assumed to be a straight, although possibly tapered, tube which allows for the continuous seepage of fluid through its walls to simulate losses due to small branches. The radial inertia of the tube and the fluid is neglected, and the effects of wall friction are accounted for only in an approximate manner. The elastic properties of the vessel are prescribed through specification of the propagation speed of small pressure waves through the system and the dependence of this wave speed on transmural pressure and spatial location.

The flow of blood is governed by the unsteady, one-dimensional continuity and momentum equations and by a relationship between the vessel cross-sectional area and pressure. These equations are as follows:

$$\frac{\partial S}{\partial t} + \frac{\partial (VS)}{\partial x} + \psi = 0, \tag{1}$$

$$\frac{\partial V}{\partial t} + V\frac{\partial V}{\partial x} + \frac{1}{\rho}\frac{\partial p}{\partial x} = f, \tag{2}$$

$$S = S(p,x). \tag{3}$$

$V(x,t)$ denotes the instantaneous flow velocity (averaged across the vessel), $p(x,t)$ the local pressure (reference to atmospheric), ψ the rate of volumetric outflow per unit length of the vessel (due to flow into small branch vessels), and f the force per unit mass representing the effect of wall friction. Both ψ and f are left unspecified at present.

Originally a method-of-characteristics mathematical approach was to be used (Rumberger and Nerem, 1977), and out of such a formulation there quite naturally arises a wavespeed, c, where

$$c^2 = \frac{S}{\rho\left(\frac{\partial S}{\partial p}\right)_x}. \tag{4}$$

Here c is the wave speed of a small disturbance in the fluid and is defined by a characteristic line whose slope dx/dt equals $V \pm c$ at any point on that characteristic. c thus is the local speed at which small disturbances travel relative to the fluid. In the case of a blood vessel, c is a function of transmural pressure and location, i.e., $c = c\,(p,x)$.

In the present formulation of the problem, the method of characteristics approach has not been used. Instead a type of finite-element-method approach has been employed (Rooz and Nerem, 1982). Inspite of this, Eq. (4) can still be used as a specification of the elastic characteristics of a blood vessel. Integration of Eq. (4) results in:

$$S = S\ (p_o, x)\ \exp\ [\frac{p - p_o}{\rho c\ (p, z)\ c\ (p_o, z)}]. \tag{5}$$

Here $S(p_0, x)$ is the cross-sectional area of the artery at a position denoted by x and a reference pressure p_0.

Intrinsic within this formulation is the assumption that certain geometric and mechanical relationships are known a priori for coronary arteries. In particular, the solution of the problem can be initiated only once the functional forms of the wave speed dependence, $c = c(p,x)$, and the cross-sectional area relationship, $S = S(p,x)$, are specified. Furthermore, the out-flow function, ψ, and the friction expression, f, must be expressed as explicit functions of $(p, V; z, t)$, together with appropriate initial and boundary conditions. These are all discussed in detail by Rumberger and Nerem (1977).

With regard to the friction factor, f, it is used to prescribe the frictional force per unit mass acting on the artery wall for a vessel circular in cross-section and of radius $(S/\pi)^{1/2}$. It is given by

$$f = \frac{2}{\rho} \left(\frac{\pi}{S}\right)^{\frac{1}{2}} \tau_w. \tag{6}$$

Here τ_w is the frictional shearing stress at the wall. The magnitude of this shear stress is a flow-dependent quantitity which has not been adequately described *in vivo* for any major blood vessel, let alone the coronary arteries. However, from *in vivo* velocity profile measurements using a hot-film anemometer probe in the major extramural vessels of the horse (Nerem *et al.*, 1976), it has been shown that the velocity profile rapidly approaches an almost fully developed, though skewed, character within a few vessel diameters distal to the left ostium. Furthermore, although time varying, at any instant of time and averaged over the vessel circumference, it is not totally unlike that of Poiseuille flow. Since it is only the average effect of wall friction on the velocity waveform development that is of interest here, it was felt that a laminar Poiseuille type of friction expression would be adequate at least initially to describe the viscous forces. However, the flow in the epicardial coronary system in fact corresponds more to an entrance region type flow (Nerem and Seed, 1983). This thus is one area where the model needs to be improved.

For each of the small branches shown in Figure 1, it is assumed that the branch terminates in a resistance which is related to the state of intramyocardial compression. This is done by expressing this resistance as being linearly and directly dependent on left ventricular pressure. Thus, during systole, when the heart is contracted, the resistance is high and during diastole, when the heart is relaxed, the resisitance is low. The mathematical form of this specification of the terminal resistance, R, is:

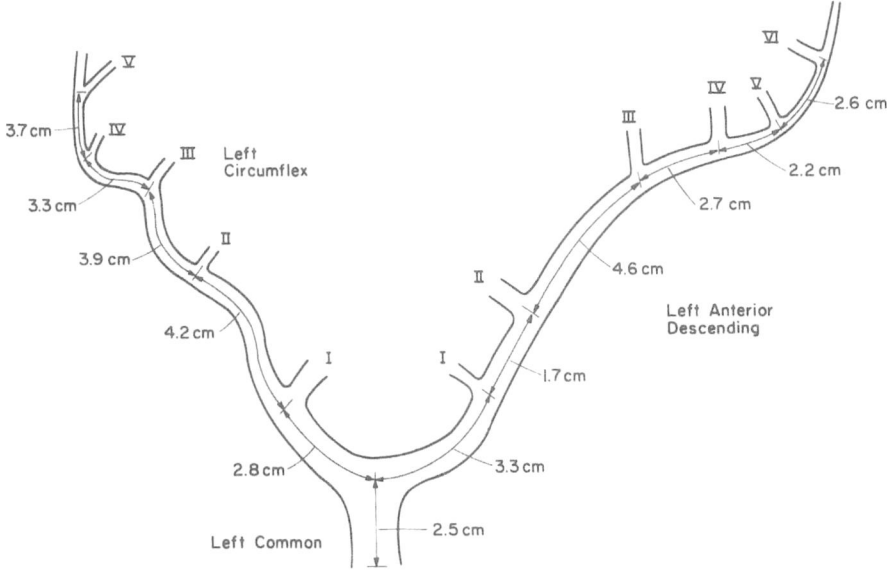

Figure 2. Model of Figure 1 applied to the left coronary system of the horse.

$$R = C_1 + C_2 \left[\frac{p_{LV} - p_{LVD}}{(p_{LV} - p_{LVD})_{max}} \right] \tag{7}$$

Here P_{LV} is the instantaneous left ventricular pressure, P_{LVD} is the minimum diastolic ventricular pressure, and $(P_{LV} - P_{LVD})_{max}$ is the maximum increase in left ventricular pressure. Equation (7) can be recast in the form

$$R = R_B(1 + U\bar{P}) \tag{8}$$

where R_B is the basal level of resistance, $U = C_2/C_1$, and $\bar{P}$ is the pressure function in brackets in Eq. (7) and ranges from zero to one. U represents the difference of the maximum intramyocardial resistance to the basal level of resistance.

Results

The calculations to be presented here have been carried out for the horse coronary geometry of Figure 2 for comparison with the experiments of Rumberger and Nerem (1979). The exact locations of the finite or discrete branches is shown in Figure 2, and in Figure 3 the cross-sectional areas at each branch point are indicated. Here S_1 is the proximal epicardial artery cross-sectional area, S_2 is

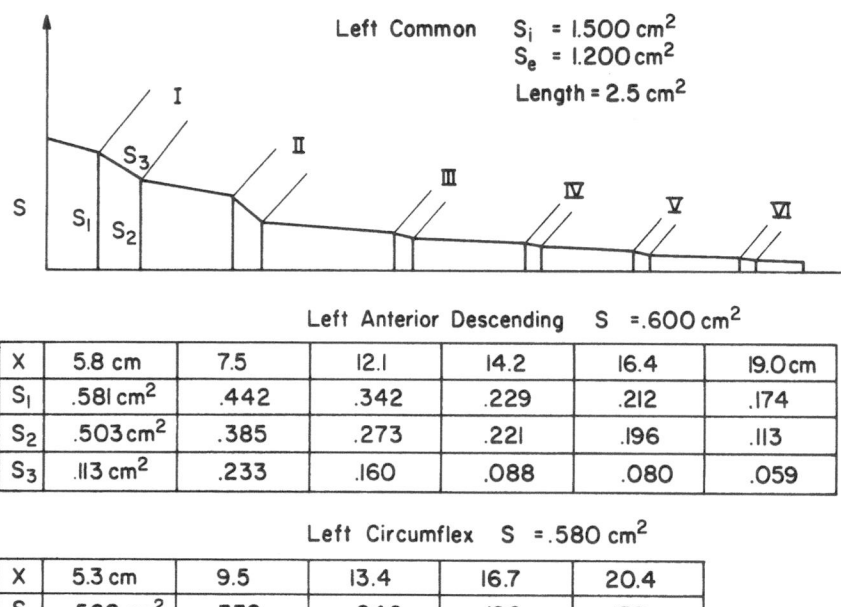

Left Common S_i = 1.500 cm^2
S_e = 1.200 cm^2

Length = 2.5 cm^2

Left Anterior Descending   S =.600 cm^2

X	5.8 cm	7.5	12.1	14.2	16.4	19.0 cm
S_1	.581 cm^2	.442	.342	.229	.212	.174
S_2	.503 cm^2	.385	.273	.221	.196	.113
S_3	.113 cm^2	.233	.160	.088	.080	.059

Left Circumflex   S =.580 cm^2

X	5.3 cm	9.5	13.4	16.7	20.4
S_1	.568 cm^2	.332	.246	.196	.159
S_2	.385 cm^2	.283	.212	.189	.062
S_3	.216 cm^2	.078	.066	.028	.110

Figure 3. Proximal and distal coronary artery and branch artery cross-sectional areas for the horse coronary geometry of Figure 2.

the distal epicardial artery cross-sectional area, and S_3 is the branch cross-sectional area. These areas are used in the mass and momentum balance carried out at each branch point. Each section of epicardial artery is assumed to taper linearly over its length.

The density of blood has been taken to be 1.055 gm/cm^3, ψ was set equal to zero, and f was evaluated from the following Poiseuille equation using a viscosity coefficient of 0.0365 Poise:

$$f = -\frac{8\mu V\pi}{\rho S}. \tag{9}$$

The wave speed, c, was taken from the work of Rumberger and Nerem (1979). In their experiments they found wave speeds in coronary arteries to range between 4 and 11 m·s^{-1}, and the data obtained indicate the wave speed to be highly dependent on both local intralumenal pressure and spatial location. A polynomial correlation was fit to the data using a least squares regression curve. The result is:

$$c = 1.57 + 3.63 \, p/p_0 + 0.125x - 0.0006xp/p_0. \tag{10}$$

Here p is the local coronary pressure and p_0 is a reference pressure ($p_0 = 13.3$ kPa $= 100$ mmHg), x is the distance in cm from the left ostium, and c is the wave speed in m·s^{-1}. The mean standard deviation of this correlation was 21 percent.

Rockwell (1969) based on the results of Anliker et al. (1968), used the same form for a correlation of wave speed results obtained in the dog aorta. The result was:

$$c = 0.97 + 2.03\, p/p_0 + 0.0194x + 0.04xp/p_0 \qquad (11)$$

Here p is local aortic pressure, p_0 is the previously noted reference pressure, and x is the distance from the aortic valve in cm. As may be seen, the pressure dependence derived here for the coronary arteries of the horse is on the order of twice that in Eq. (11) for the aorta of the dog. This is felt to reflect the less compliant character of the coronary vessels. It would have been desirable to obtain data such as presented in Rumberger et al. (1979) over a larger range in pressure. However, the pressure is determined by the carrier wave, i.e., the coronary pressure waveform, and although the range is limited, it is that of physiological interest.

There also appears to be on the average a stronger variation in wave speed with distance for the coronaries in comparison with the aorta. However, this result cannot be considered conclusive since this experimental investigation covered only the rather short region corresponding to the epicardial coronary vessels. It should be noted that the results obtained here are consistant with the measurements of the elastic properties of coronary vessels by Gow et al. (1974).

The boundary conditions used in the calculations are in the form of an upstream pressure and the downstream terminal resistances. The former is taken at the left coronary ostium to be equal to the aortic pressure, and the latter is as previously described. Left ventricular pressure must also be specified since it governs the time history of the terminal resistances. Figure 4 shows typical left ventricular and aortic pressure waveforms based on *in vivo* measurements. Also shown is the calculated left main coronary blood flow.

Figure 5 and 6 show calculated pressure and flow waveforms for the same case as Figure 4 and for four different locations. These are the coronary ostium, in the left anterior descending (LAD) coronary artery just distal to the left main bifurcation into the LAD and left circumflex (CFX) coronary arteries, mid-way along the LAD, and at the terminal end of the LAD. Of these two figures, the most striking are those results presented in Figure 5 where one sees a marked deterioration of the pressure waveform as it propagates along the LAD. This deterioration is in the form of the development of low frequency oscillations with a frequency on the order of 5 Hz. As will be discussed in the next section, this is in agreement with experiment.

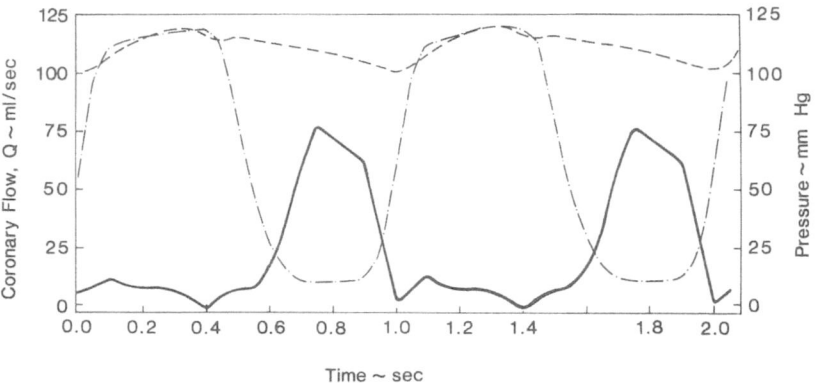

Figure 4. Aortic pressure, left ventricular pressure, and predicted left common coronary blood flow for the horse geometry of Figures 2 and 3.

Discussion

The development of the epicardial coronary flow model described herein is part of an overall approach to the prediction of coronary fluid dynamics including the rather detailed local flow characteristics. This approach separates the problem into the following two parts:

(1) the prediction of one-dimensional, unsteady flow in a network of elastic tubes representing the vascular system; and

(2) the prediction of three-dimensional, unsteady flow in a rigid geometry representing a local vascular region of branching or sharp curvature.

The purpose of the former is to predict the development of pressure and flow waveforms in the vascular system or some general region of the system, while the purpose of the latter is to predict some of the more subtle fluid dynamic features

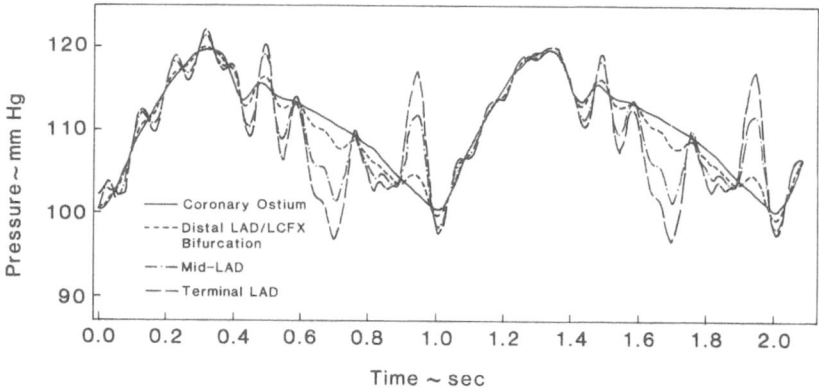

Figure 5. Calculated pressure wave forms for the horse coronary geometry of Figures 2 and 3 at four locations: coronary ostium, just distal to the left main bifurcation, mid-LAD, and terminal LAD.

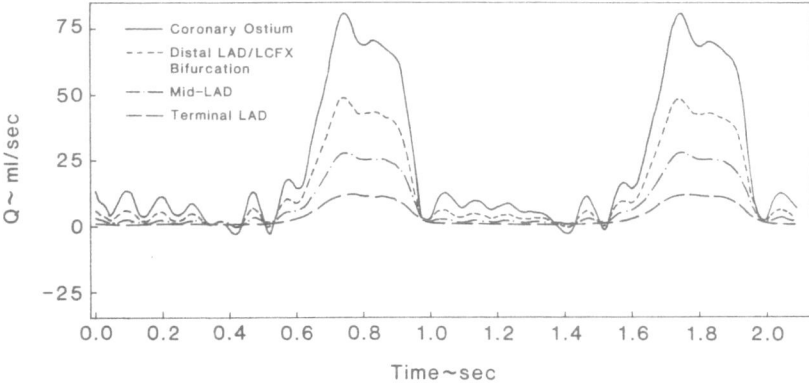

Figure 6. Calculated flow waveforms for the horse coronary geometry of Figures 2 and 3 at four locations: coronary ostium, just distal to the left main bifurcation, mid-LAD, and terminal LAD.

in a localized region where there may be asymmetric velocity profiles, secondary motions, and local flow separation. For the former, an important characteristic is the elastic properties of the blood vessels making up the system, i.e., wall elasticity is of primary importance in the establishment of the basic coronary arterial pressure pulse. However, from a computational point of view, once pressure, and thus the pressure gradient, is known as a function of position along the artery and with time, then the effects of wall elasticity would be of secondary importance in terms of the calculation of local flow details. The use of a rigid tube model for the local, three-dimensional, unsteady flow calculations then would appear to be justified, and one could calculate the local flow details neglecting the distensibility of the arteries, i.e., for a rigid geometry. However, the latter problem of three-dimensional, unsteady flow is difficult enough even for such a rigid geometry.

The present effort addresses only the first part of what we have presented as a two-step approach. In this, the prediction of waveforms through the calculation of one-dimensional, unsteady flow in a network of non-linear elastic tubes has been carried out using a model of the epicardial coronary vessels. The geometric model that has been employed is one which can be tailored to a specific coronary geometry. This is important because the results of Nerem and Seed (1983) indicate that human coronary vascular geometry is highly individualistic. Thus, in order to develop an understanding of epicardial coronary flow, it most likely will be necessary to deal with individual cases as opposed to some statistically representative model of coronary geometry.

Using this model, calculations which predict waveform development in the coronary system can be carried out for both animals and man. One such case is shown here, and as was seen, the pressure waveform is predicted to develop low-frequency oscillations as it propagates down the left main and the LAD coronary arteries. This is exactly as observed experimentally by Rumberger *et al.* (1979).

This was also predicted by our earlier method-of-characteristics coronary blood flow model (Rumberger and Nerem, 1977), and there is a suggestion in the results that the oscillations will have a frequency of approximately five times the heart rate. Thus, with increasing animal species size, the heart rate and the frequency of these oscillations both appear to decrease.

This suggests one use for a model such as presented here. This is to systematically investigate the sensitivity of coronary blood flow to various parameters, e.g. peripheral resistance, wall properties, geometric branching pattern, etc. Such a parametric ananalysis can be extended as the model is expanded. One possible modification to the model is to include somewhat more detail on the venous side of the coronary system. Also, as is indicated by Figure 1, it is possible to insert into the calculation multiple stenoses as well as to allow for the presence of multiple aorto-coronary bypass grafts. In the latter case, it is necessary to separately specify the wave-speed characteristics of any such grafts.

With this type of capability and with the model being able to treat an individual coronary geometry, one can foresee the day when one could input geometric data from a patient's coronary angiogram, carry out calculations of coronary blood flow for a coronary system with multiple stenoses of either the critical or non-critical type, make predictions for such a diseased system incorporating various bypass graft arrangements, and thus possibly even provide one additional piece of information – or at least a different perspective – which might be helpful in making clinical decisions relative to cardiac disease.

Acknowledgment

This research was supported by National Science Foundation Grant MEA-8200344.

References

Anliker M, Histand MB, Ogden E (1969) Dispersion and attenuation of small artificial pressure waves in the canine aorta. Circ Res 23:539–551

Gow BS, Schonfield D, Patal DJ (1974) The dynamic elastic properties of the canine left cirumflex coronary artery. J Biomech 7:389–395

Ling SC, Atabek HB (1972) Non-linear analysis of pulsatile flow in arteries. J Fluid Mech 55:493

Ling SC, Atabek HB, Letzing WG, Patel DJ (1973) Nonlinear analysis of aortic flow in living dogs. Circ Res 33:198

McDonald DA (1979) Blood Flow in Arteries. 2nd ed. London: Edward Arnold

Nerem RM, Rumber JA, Gross DR, Muir WW, Geiger GL (1976) Hot-film coronary artery velocity meaurements in horses. Cardiovasc Res 3:310–313

Nerem RM, Seed WQ (1983) Coronary artery geometry and its fluid mechanical implications. In: Schettler G et al. (eds) Fluid Dynamics as a Localizing Factor for Atherosclerosis. Springer-Verlag: Heidelberg, FRG

Rockwell RL (1969) Nonlinear analysis of pressure shock waves in blood vessels. Ph.D. Dissertation, Stanford University

Rooz E, Nerem RM (1982) A computerized model of coronary flow. Proc 34th Ann Conf Eng Med Biol, Sept 21–23, 1981, Houston, Texas, 372

Rumberger JA, Nerem RM (1977) A method of characteristics evaluation of coronary blood flow. J Fluid Mech 28:429–448

Rumberger JA, Nerem RM, Muir WW (1979) Coronary artery pressure development and wave transmission characteristics in the horse. Cardiovasc Res 13:413–419

Stettler JC, Niederer P, Anliker M (1981) Theoretical analysis of arterial hemodynamics including the influence of bifurcations. Ann Biomed Eng 9, 2:145–165

Van der Werff T (1974) Significant parameters in arterial pressure and velocity development. J Biomech 7:347

Womersley JE (1957) Elastic tube theory of pulse transmission and oscillatory flow in mammalian arteries. Tech Rept WADC-TR. Dayton, Ohio, Wright Air Development Center, pp 56–614

DISCUSSION

JARON: I'm interested in the relationship in your model between those terminal resistors and the pressure in the LV.

ANS: It is basically the simplest thing one could think of. The resistance is written as a sum of two constants multiplied by a linear pressure function. The pressure function is equal to one at peak LV pressure. At minimum LV pressure, the pressure function is zero.

JARON: I am not sure I understood you. You mean that the vessel closes during systole, i.e., the resistance is infinite?

ANS: No. It is not infinite as we can adjust the ratio of the 2 constants in Eq. (7).

JARON: How do you adjust them?

ANS: That's an input. It is based on insight and comparison with experimental data. We need to examine and find out exactly how sensitive the system is to changing inputs like that. This will give us an idea as to what kind of experiments we need to do in order to have a more realistic model.

SIDEMAN: We have seen here two models related to the coronary distribution, one by yourself and one by Professor Heethaar. Your model does not go deeply into the muscle. So my question is more related to Dr. Heethaar. It is logical that whatever the distribution of the ventricles, they should be almost evenly, homogenously, distributed. Why do you have to check the directions? Ultimately, the blood goes everywhere and comes back. So what is the point in measuring the direction. What would you gain that you don't know by assuming an even distribution?

HEETHAAR: We do not find an even distribution in all directions. There are directions which are preferable to other directions, especially when you go from the larger arteries. Also, we distinguished between arterial and venous blood flow. In one little myocardial element, you have the arteries, the arterioles and the venules, and blood is going successively through them and there are different pressures in the arterioles and capillaries. That is the reason we take them into consideration.

SIDEMAN: The network goes in a certain way, with a defined form and a finite direction. But eventually one stops being able to do the network. You start there. As long as you see directions. Dr. Nerem should be able to calculate it.

HEETHAAR: I think that this is the main difference. We can deal with many, many little vessels.

NEREM: Realistically speaking, in terms of computer time, there is a limit to how many vessels you can have. Thus, one can only follow the network so far. At some point, you have to go to something that is either modelled in terms of an electric analogue as a resistance or to a porous media approach.

HEETHAAR: The porous media approach was the starting point. There is a deviation from the porous medium in that you have distinct vessels in which the blood flows so it is not possible for a blood particle to go in all directions with equal probability.

SIDEMAN: Your matrix is actually multidirectional, including the fine vessels.

HEETHAAR: That's right. Actually we have introduced one particular parameer, (Kij, Eq. (10), these Proceedings). With a negative filling in the arteries, it has a value of 0, (in the capillaries) and then it gradually takes a positive value when blood goes into the veins. At the zero point you can approximately compare it to the diameter of the vessels. By introducing this particular parameter, we can express effects of orientation.

SIDEMAN: Does the zero state correspond to the porous media, and the rest is multidirectional?

HEETHAAR: Even the zero state has a component of direction in it. I would like to add to the work of Dr. Nerem. We have just finished a study of about 20 patients in which we didn't measure the pressures, but we measured the diameter of the different coronary arteries during the cardiac cycle. The surprise is that we found small oscillations. There were about 4 times the frequency of the cardiac cycle.

ANS: Our experience is with animal experiments. We have not done human measurement, but only horses and smaller animals. In general, as you go to a smaller species, the amplitude of the oscillation goes down and the frequency goes up. And because the amplitude goes down, depending on the exact condition, anaesthesia, etc., you may be able to see these oscillations in smaller species, and you may not.

HEETHAAR: Our data was obtained from patients during catherizations so they were awake.

NEREM: That's an interesting observation which is encouraging in terms of our model.

GOTTESMAN: We just studied about 300 patients, looking at their coronary anatomy and the sites of obstruction. The major problem seems to be the shearing stress on the intima. The real question is whether atheroma is caused by the destruction of the intimal cells, or whether, in fact, it is the additional layers which are added on in the buffer zones where there is very low flow. We showed that it favored proxmality; the more proxmal you are, not the more distal you are. What you've shown is multiple vibrations in the distal vessels rather than in the proxmal arteries, unless you are talking about segment length. And secondly, we showed, as everybody else has shown, that atheroma occurs at bifurcations. The interesting question is whether it's the increased pressure which is causing the destruction of the intima, or whether it's the zones of low pressure, as you showed in your bifurcation study, where you get your accretion of material, with layers being laid on each other? Curvature simply changes the stress at a particular area although the pressure is constant. It changes the actual shearing stress on the intima.

ANS: I would have to say that I'm a believer in the low shear hypothesis. However, I do not believe that it is due to an accretion of materials with layers being added, at least not during atherogenesis. I do believe that the influence of shearing stresses on endothelial cells is important. We're doing some corollary work to this in which we are looking at the effect of mechanical forces on endothelial cells and speculation at this point would be that in low shear stress regions, you have higher endothelial cell turnover. You also have more rounded endothelial cells. One of the things we found is that they are much more elongated in high shear regions than in low shear regions and there's a suggestion in the literature that these endothelial cells have a higher cell turnover rate, and in effect, a shorter lifetime. We don't know how that is related to the disease process. Perhaps during the turnover process, there would be an enhanced lipid influx; however, whatever the mechanism, I would argue in favour of the low shear type hypothesis.

EINAV: We did quite a few experiments on both high shear and low shear studies and found both of them to be important in the process. In other words, it's not the shape of the endothelial cell but the injury to the intima which is important at high shear. So let me represent the high shear group although I fully agree with Dr. Nerem that low shear has its importance as well.

ANS: All the human data I am aware of supports the low shear hypothesis.

JARON: You made an assumption, that the flow has a parabolic profile. Since this is such a highly branching system, and since there is really not enough room for the profile to develop, how good is this assumption and would there be a difference if you made a different assumption?

ANS: We intend to try a different assumption. You're are quite right that because of the branching nature of the system, you are more typically in an entrance region than you are in a fully developed region. One can in some ad hoc way include an entrance effect in this model and this is one of the things we are going do.

BASSINGTHWAIGHTE: I suspect that you are in a higher shear stress region than you are thinking, or rather a higher Reynolds number at the surface. Namely, you should take into account the shear dependent viscosity and the fact that one actually has at the endothelial surface, at least partially, a red cell free region with a lower viscosity than in the center. This is really related to Dr. Jaron's question. If you then use a profile that is more blunt than parabolic, as seems to be indicated, you would have higher shear rates at the wall. Secondly, you have presumed taper along those vessels, between branches. There is some other data in the literature that suggests that there is no serious amount of taper between branches but that the shrinkage in diameter occurs at branch points. That again would change your view of the flow profile, quite apart from the entrance effect, which is obviously fairly dominant.

ANS: We have the capability of including taper but have done calculations both ways. Our geometry is based on actual vascular casts. With regard to your other comment, it is very important in terms of local details. I'm still not convinced in my own mind that, in terms of the system characteristics, an accounting of the change in velocity profile and a plasma-free layer would be particularly important. The friction is important enough, so we need to have it in the calculation, but it's not a dominant factor in the calculation.

BASSINGTHWAIGHTE: You are probably right. There is a check, though, on whether your profiles are reasonable or not. And that is the dispersion that occurs for tracer labelled systems. If you look at the dispersion of an indicator of red cell or plasma labels between points in the system, you get ever so much less dispersion than would be anticipated from a parabolic profile. That could be used locally if experimentally accessible to give an assessment of how close you are to a parabolic profile in an arterial branching system.

ANS: Of course, we have been measuring profiles directly with our pulsed ultrasonic Doppler system and we see a number of non-parabolic type features. But in this calculation, the assumption of Newtonian flow is needed only to calculate an average value for the friction factor. That's the only question pertinent to the model at this point.

WELKOWITZ: When looking at the aorta, one of the interesting things with regard to your friction term is that the hydraulic loss, which is what essentially results from the friction, is very much greater, say 10 or 20 times, the Poiseuille type number. What would happen in your particular calculation if you had the same kind of ratio?

ANS: That would be a major effect. But you are not going to have that kind of ratio in a coronary artery because of the Reynolds number there as compared to the aorta. It's well known that in the aorta there is anything but a parabolic situation. Our own measurements in coronary arteries in a number of animals suggest it's reasonably close, i.e. a parabolic velocity profile is a reasonable approximation.

Multidimensional activation of the heart: The effect of anisotropy in conductivity of cardiac tissue

ROBERT PLONSEY and ROGER C. BARR

Department of Biomedical Engineering, Duke University, Durham, NC 27706, U.S.A.

Abstract

This paper examines the current flow patterns and excitation isochrones of a two-dimensional cardiac tissue with anisotropic intracellular and interstitial conductivity parameters. Only when the anisotrophy ratios in intracellular and interstitial space are equal does the behavior of current flow extrapolate from one dimensional cable theory. For realistic (measured) conductivities a component of action current flow is characterized by wide loops and multiple membrane crossings. Furthermore the transmembrane current at any site depend on transmembrane potential in the entire surrounding region. Isochrone simulation based on Hodgkin-Huxley rising phase shows that the assumption of local plane wave behavior is not generally acceptable. This is not surprising in view of the current flow patterns which do not correspond to simple one-dimensional flow, locally. The consequences of this study is that simulation of activation in real cardiac tissue must recognize the effects of anisotropy. The implications could be important not only for normal activation patterns but for studies of arrhythmias as well.

Introduction

An extensive body of knowledge has developed on the electrophysiology of the single fiber (axon). Its behavior is well described by the linear core-conductor model in which each membrane patch is represented by a Hodgkin-Huxley style formulation.

Cardiac tissue, however, is not one-dimensional but three-dimensional. But since all intracellular space is electrically interconnected and all interstitial space also interconnected it is as if the heart were a single cell whose behavior could consequently be derived as a simple extension of one-dimensional studies. The characterization of the myocardium as a syncytium is a recognition of its behavior being comparable to that of a single cell. And, in fact, most models of cardiac activation are based on ideas derived from continuous (one-dimensional) cable theory.

There are two limitations in this approach which have come to light in recent years. Once concerns the assumption that cardiac tissue is continuous hence overlooking the effect of discontinuities in conductivity (such as at the gap junctions between cells). The second is the assumption of isotropicity, an assumption which is inescapable in one-dimensional models but which is unsupported in three dimensional preparations where anisotropy in conductivity both in intracellular as well as interstitial space is well documented experimentally (Spach and Kootsey, 1983). It is this latter factor, the influence of cardiac anisotropy on its electrophysiological behavior, that this paper is concerned with.

Measurements of cardiac tissue tensor conductivities are reported on in only three papers, and these values are not in complete agreement (Clerc, 1976; Roberts et al., 1979; 1980). All agree, however, that conductivity along the fiber axis exceeds that across the fiber axis by a substantial factor. Furthermore, this factor (the anisotropy ratio) is substantially different in intracellular vs. interstitial space.

We have investigated and report here, the effect of different anisotropy conductivities on current flow patterns and on activation isochrones. We shall see that these results are not consonant with simple extensions of one-dimensional behavior.

For simplicity our model has ignored structural discontinuities such as the gap junctions. The conductivity of such elements are considered here only by their inclusion into the averaged (macroscopic) conductivity values. The latter correspond to those obtained in typical macroscopic conductivity measurements. The effect of discontinuities are not unimportant and studies of their influence are presented elsewhere (Spach et al., 1979; 1982).

Since our model recognizes the separate intracellular and interstitial domains that characterize cardiac tissue, it adopts the formal structure known as the *biodomain* model (Tung, 1978; Miller and Gezelowitz, 1978). In this model both intracellular and interstitial spaces are assumed to be continuous and congruent ('interpenetrating') (Schmitt, 1969) but separated everywhere by the cell membrane. These ideas are made more concrete in the following mathematical description.

The model

The lowest dimension for which anisotropy can be studied is two. Although our objective is an investigation of three-dimensional cardiac tissue the difficulties in simulation are great enough that we chose, as an initial step, to examine a uniform anisotrophic two-dimensional preparation. (We considered a square block of tissue 8 mm on a side). The bidomain model leads to, and is described by, the following equations

$$\bar{J}_i = - [g_{ix} \, \partial\varphi_i/\partial x \, \bar{a}_x + g_{iy} \, \partial\varphi_i/\partial y \, \bar{a}_y], \tag{1}$$

$$\bar{J}_o = - [g_{ox} \, \partial\varphi_o/\partial x \, \bar{a}_x + g_{oy} \, \partial\varphi_o/\partial y \, \bar{a}_y], \tag{2}$$

where $\bar{J}$ is the longitudinal current in the intracellular (subscript i) or interstitial (subscript o) space, g_{ix} is the intracellular conductivity in the x direction etc., and $\bar{a}_x$ is unit vector in the x direction etc., while φ is the electrical potential. Note that all physical quantities are defined on the same space and that the tissue conductivity, in general, requires specifications of four parameters. (While potentials and currents are functions of position they reflect only a spatial average about that position. These values are the ones which are, presumably, retrieved in typical (macroscopic) measurements.)

Continuity of current requires that current leaving intracellular space enter interstitial space, and vice versa. This is expressed by

$$- \nabla \cdot \bar{J}_i = \nabla \cdot \bar{J}_o = I_M, \tag{3}$$

where I_M is the transmembrane current (per unit volume). Using the definition of transmembrane potential $V_m = \varphi_i - \varphi_o$ and Eq. (1)–(3) enables one to derive

$$(g_{ix} + g_{ox}) \, \partial^2\varphi_i/\partial x^2 + (g_{iy} + g_{oy}) \, \partial^2\varphi_i/\partial y^2 = \\ g_{ox} \, \partial^2 V_m/\partial x^2 + g_{oy} \, \partial^2 V_m/\partial y^2 \tag{4}$$

which is a partial differential equation for φ_i based on V_m in the role of a source function. One can transform variables to put (4) into a standard Poisson's equation and solve for φ_i as a function of V_m. Then using (1) and (3) one can obtain the following expression for transmembrane current

$$I_M = \frac{(\lambda_x - \lambda_y)}{2\pi G(1 + \lambda_x)(1 + \lambda_y)} \int [g_{ox} \, \partial^2 V_m/\partial x'^2 + g_{oy} \, \partial^2 V_m/\partial y^2].$$

$$\frac{\dfrac{(x - x')^2}{G_x} - \dfrac{(y - y')^2}{G_y}}{\left[\dfrac{(x - x')^2}{G_x} - \dfrac{(y - y')^2}{G_y} \right]^2} \; dx'dy', \tag{5}$$

where $G_x = g_{ix} + g_{ox}$, $G_y = g_{iy} + g_{oy}$, $G = \sqrt{G_x G_y}$, $\lambda_x = g_{ox}/g_{ix}$ and $\lambda_y = g_{oy}/g_{iy}$. The integral is taken over the entire tissue but, in fact, need only be taken over the active region since elsewhere the partial derivities of V_m are zero or negligible.

Anisotropic properties

When the intracellular and extracellular anisotropy ratios are equal then $\lambda_x = \lambda_y = \lambda$ (this includes the isotropic condition when $\lambda_x = \lambda_y = 1$). In this case Eq. (5) reduces to zero except for the contribution from integration over the neighborhood of $x' = x$, $y' = y$. Once can show that the quantity in brackets is, in fact, a delta-function so that the result is

$$I_M = \left(\frac{1}{1 + \lambda}\right)(g_{ox}\, \partial^2 V_m/\partial x^2 + g_{oy}\, \partial^2 V_m/\partial y^2). \tag{6}$$

But this result is an extrapolation of the familiar Hodgkin and Rushton (1946) one-dimensional cable equation to two dimensions. Furthermore one can also determine that

$$\Phi_o = -\left(\frac{1}{1 + \lambda}\right) V_m, \tag{7}$$

$$\Phi_i = \left(\frac{\lambda}{1 + \lambda}\right) V_m \tag{8}$$

and

$$\bar{J}_i = -J_o \tag{9}$$

which are further generalizations of (one-dimensional) continuous cable theory to two dimensions.

Since the extension of continuous (one-dimensional) cable theory to two (or more) dimensions requires isotropicity or equal anisotropy ratios and since equal anisotropy ratios are not seen experimentally one expects that the evaluation of transmembrane current at a particular site for real tissue does not depend solely on derivatives of V_m at that site (as in Eq (6)) but rather requires a spatial integral of derivatives of V_m about that site. Eq. (5) describes this spatial integration. In examining (5) one recognizes that the second derivatives of V_m with respect to x and to y contribute through the weighting function in the brackets. For equal anisotropy ratios this behaves like a delta function but otherwise it simply accentuates the closer-in points more than distant points.

Simulation

We have investigated the electrophysiological behavior of three basic types of tissue namely, isotropic, nominally normal, and reciprocal. Table 1 gives the assumed conductivity parameters as well as those measured by Clerc (1976).

*Table 1.*Conductivity values (Siemens/mm)

S/mm	Clerc (1976)	Nominal	Isotropic	Reciprocal
g_{ix}	1.74×10^{-4}	2×10^{-4}	1×10^{-4}	2×10^{-4}
g_{iy}	1.93×10^{-5}	2×10^{-5}	1×10^{-4}	2×10^{-5}
g_{ox}	6.25×10^{-4}	8×10^{-4}	1×10^{-4}	2×10^{-5}
g_{oy}	2.36×10^{-4}	2×10^{-4}	1×10^{-4}	2×10^{-6}

The nominally normal values approximates those that were measured, while the reciprocal was chosen to exaggerate certain behavior which is contained in the nominally normal case.

We have carried out simulations under two different conditions. In the first a circular isochrone with an assumed spatial rising phase for V_m is assumed and the resulting transmembrane and longitudinal currents determined for each conductivity case. The objective was to hold all conditions constant except the conductivities to see the effect of the latter on patterns of current flow. (In this we tactily assume that the initial transmembrane potential distribution, while based on observed waveforms, could be specified arbitrarily).

In the second simultation a transthreshold stimulus was applied at the coordinate origin and the membrane action potential determined. For this it was assumed that the membrane obeyed the Hodgkin-Huxley equations during the rising phase (with an idealized plateau following activation). In this way the activation pattern (isochrones) could be derived and followed as a function of time. The procedure is basically similar to that followed in one-dimensional simulation. The transmembrane current at a particular membrane patch is first determined from its Hodgkin-Huxley ionic contributions plus the capacitive component that depends on time variations in V_m. This, in turn, is equated to the current as evaluated numerically from Eq. (5), which depends on the values of V_m at neighboring nodes as well as (to a lesser extent) more distant nodes (which enter the spatial integration specified in Eq. (5)). An iterative procedure is followed which permits moving from one time step to the next for all nodes under active consideration.

Numerical techniques

Space does not permit an extensive discussion of the computational procedures and the reader is referred to Plonsey and Barr (1984) and Barr and Plonsey (1984) for additional details. We mention here the use of two innovative ideas to help keep computation within bounds.

In the first, the integration of Eq. (5) must be carried out by discretization of the area surrounding the point at which I_M is to be evaluated. The greatest

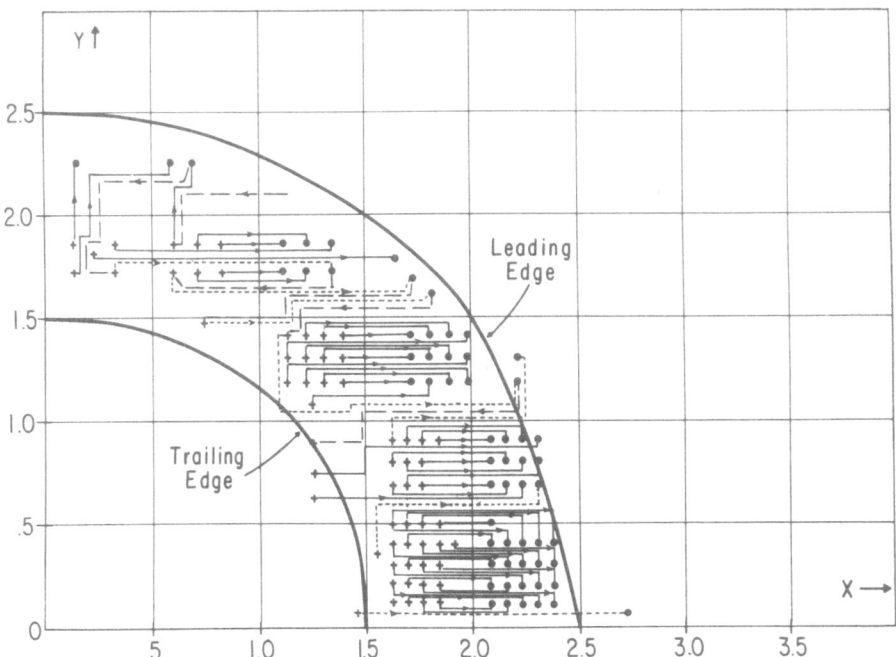

Figure 1. Nominal ($g_{ix} = 2 \times 10^{-4}$ Siemens/mm, $g_{iy} = 2 \times 10^{-5}$, $g_{ox} = 8 \times 10^{-4}$, $g_{oy} = 2 \times 10^{-4}$). ●
outward transmembrane current + inward transmembrane current —— intracellular current for
which equal and opposite interstitial current is not shown. - - - - longitudinal interstitial current ······
longitudinal intracellular current. Each line represents 10,000 (relative) units of current. Source field
is a circular isochrone centered at $r = 2.0$ mm with the transmembrane potential variation along any
radius given by equation (10). [Reproduced from the Biophysical Journal 45:557–571 (1984) by
copyright permission of the Biophysical Society].

contribution is the self-term and this was evaluated analytically. Surrounding this
was a near-zone in which the mesh size was adaptively reduced in size until the
variation of the integrand throughout a mesh was sufficiently small. In the far
region the contributions was relatively small and a fixed algorithm could be used.
A measure of the computational efficiency of this adaptive methodology is that
between 10,000 and 30,000 squares were required, whereas for a uniform division
at the smallest squares used a total of 4,000,000 squares would be required.

A second innovation, utilized in connection with the simulation of activation,
was to retain under consideration only those membrane patches in which some
activity or contribution to an adjacent patch activity was present. Thus as soon as
a patch was slightly depolarized it was added to the active list. And upon
maintaining the plateau for a period of time it is removed from the active list. In
this way it is not necessary to be burdened with patches that do not significantly
contribute in any way (since they are either completely at rest or completely in a
plateau state).

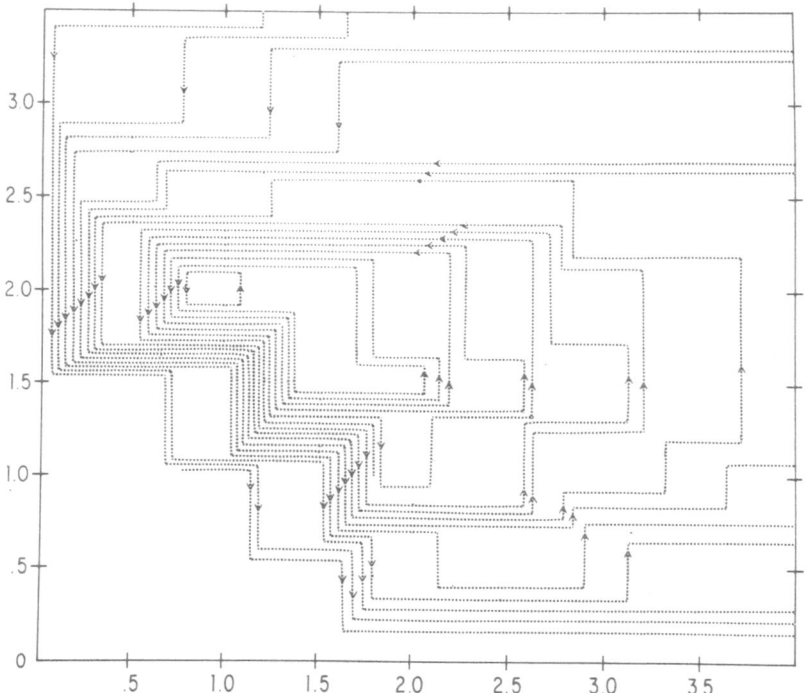

Figure 2. Difference current for nominal conductivities (see caption for Figure 1), as defined in Eqs. (11) and (12). No assignment of result to intracellular or interstitial path is made on the figure. Each line represents 1000 (relative)units of current (compare with Figure 1). Source field is described in caption for Figure 1. [Reproduced from the Biophysical Journal 45:557–571 (1984) by copyright permission of the Biophysical Society].

Results

Figure 1 is the current flow map for a two-dimensional cardiac tissue with nominal conductivity that arises from an assumed circular isochrone, where the rising phase of the transmembrane action potential in the radial direction was assumed to follow a 'typical behavior' as given by the equation

$$V_m = 52 \tanh [5.4(2 - r)] - 38\, mv, \tag{10}$$

where r is in mm. The center of the isochrone defined by (10) is along a radius $r = 2.0$ mm; as noted earlier a tissue of 8 mm × 8 mm was examined and the upper right quadrant is shown in Figure 1. To keep the figure as simple as possible we determined the total current crossing the sides of each .5 mm × .5 mm square, or found the transmembrane current associated with this area. This simplification also introduces a quantization effect which must be taken into account when interpreting the figure.

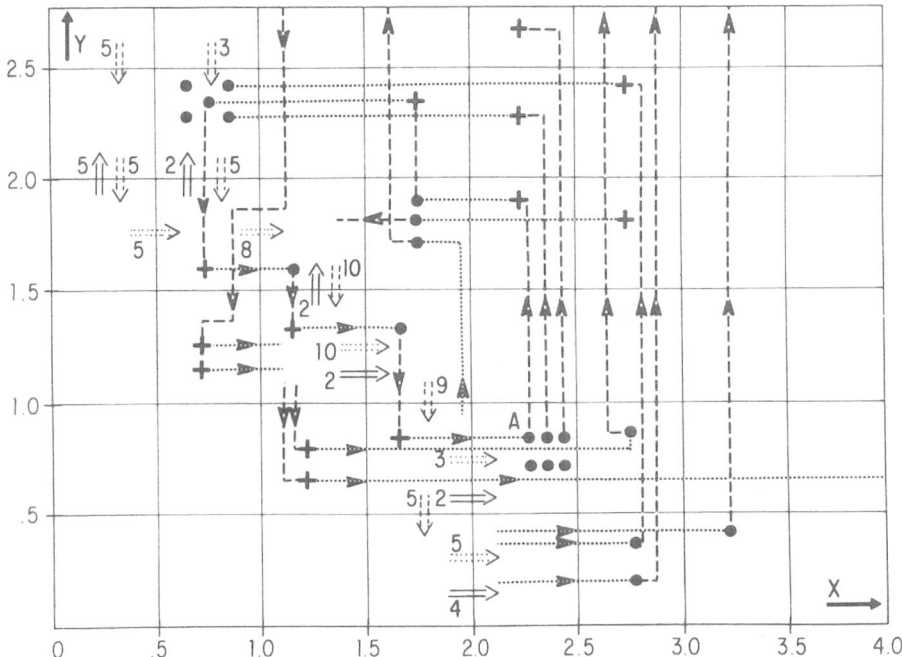

Figure 3. Current flow map for reciprocal anisotropy ($g_{ix} = 2 \times 10^{-4}$ Siemens/mm, $g_{iy} = 2 \times 10^{-5}$, $g_{ox} = 2 \times 10^{-5}$, $g_{oy} = 2 \times 10^{-4}$). Intracellular, interstitial and transmembrane currents are shown. ● outward transmembrane current + inward transmembrane current —— intracellular current for which equal and opposite interstitial current is not shown ---- longitudinal interstitial currents ······ longitudinal intracellular current. Large numbered arrows represent the (numbered) additional current (lines) crossing the respective square (.5 mm × .5 mm) boundary. Transmembrane current in the active region shown only in part. Each line represents 5000 (relative) units of current. [Reproduced from the Biophysical Journal 45:557–571 (1984) by copyright permission of the Biophysical Society].

In examining the current flow patterns in this figure we note greater current densities near the x axis in contrast to those along the y axis and this reflects the higher x conductivity (this is the fiber direction) compared to that for y (the cross-fiber direction). While this difference reflects the anisotropy in conductivity the measure of the deviation from a simple extension of one to two-dimensional behavior is the amount by which intracellular longitudinal current fails to be equal and opposite to extracellular longitudinal currents. To highlight this quantity we define 'difference currents' I_d as:

$$I_{dx} = I_{ox} + I_{ix}, \tag{11}$$

$$I_{dy} = I_{oy} + I_{iy}, \tag{12}$$

and, clearly $I_{dx} = I_{dy} = 0$ for isotropic and equal anisotropy conditions. When I_d

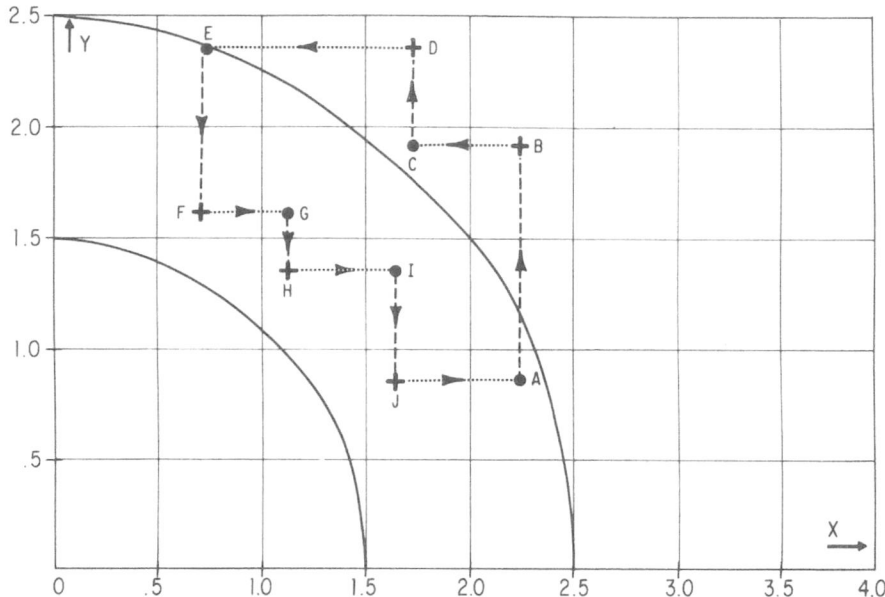

Figure 4. *A closed current pathway for reciprocal* anisotropy (see caption for Figure 3). Membrane is crossed at A, B, C, D, E, F, G, H, I, J. ● outward transmembrane current + inward transmembrane current ---- longitudinal interstitial current ⋯⋯ longitudinal intracellular current. [Reproduced from the Biophysical Journal 45:557–571 (1984) by copyright permission of the Biophysical Society].

$\neq 0$ its behavior reflects the nature and degree of current flow pattern that go beyond simple cable theory extrapolated to higher dimensions. One can show that the current $\bar{I}_d$ is solenoidal and in Figure 2 we plot $\bar{I}_d$ for the conditions of nominal conductivity as described in Figure 1. The scale of current density in Figure 2 is 10% that in Figure 1 so the effect shown in Figure 2 is not the dominant one. Yet there is a significant component of current which is solenoidal – not because intra- and extracellular currents are equal and opposite – but rather because there are loops of current which can be fairly extensive.

This phenomena is seen more sharply in the case of reciprocal conductivity, where in the intracellular space the x conductivity is ten times greater than y while in the interstitial space the y conductivity is ten times greater than x. While admittedly non-physiological it demonstrates in exaggerated form phenomena that exists to lesser degree under realistic conditions. The current flow pattern is shown in Figure 3, and of particular interest, are the extensive current loop paths that involve multiple membrane crossings. (One specific path is identified and exhibited in Figure 4.) In such paths the current lies in the intracellular space when flow is in the x direction and in interstitial space when its direction is along y – hence taking advantage of the relatively high conductivities encountered in this way. We note that to the extent that current tends to flow in such open loops, the local currents at a segment of isochrone are not those which arise were the

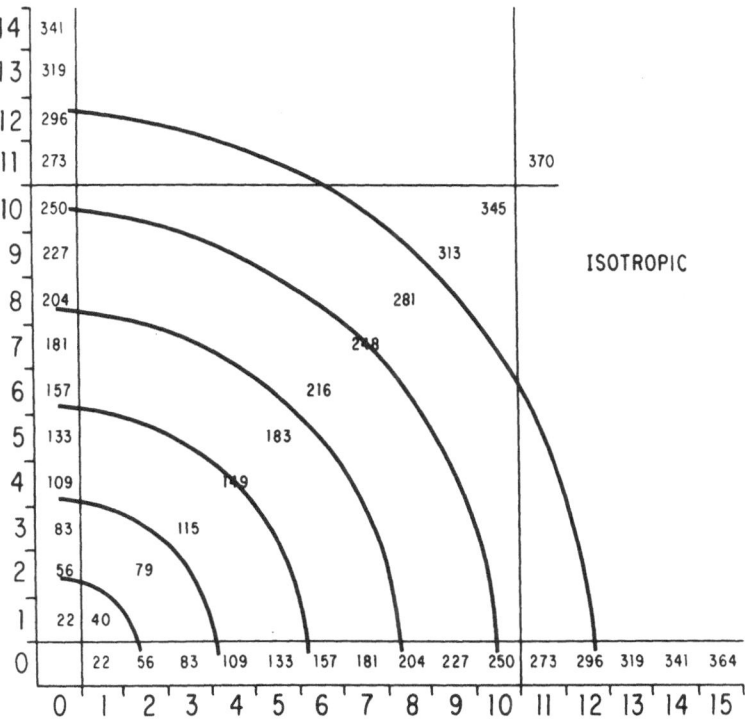

Figure 5. Isotropic conductivities. All intracellular and extracellular conductivities were equal. From the computed values, the number of time steps from the time origin to the activation time of each node was transcribed onto the grid layout of the figure. The large numbers on the bottom and left indicate the *i, j* grid indices. They may be converted to the *x, y* coordinate position by multiplying by d*x* and d*y*. For clarity in the figure, the time steps are shown only along the *x* axis, *y* axis and diagonal, although on the original a time step was present for every node. Further, although the results are shown for one quadrant only, the simulation itself used all four quadrants. (All four were needed to perform the spatial integration for I_M.) Isochrones were added manually at multiples of 50 time steps (heavy black lines). As expected the isochrones are circles. Other straight lines on the grid (lighter black) were added to the figure to make it easier, visually, to judge the relative isochrone positions along *x, y,* and the diagonal; these lines had nothing to do with the calculation. The time origin was chosen arbitrarily to be 0.2 ms after the onset of the stimulus. The time interval from the onset of the stimulus to the activation time of any node can be computed as the number of time steps given on the figure times the interval between steps (Δt), plus 0.2 ms. Here $g_{ix}, g_{ox}, g_{iy}, g_{oy}$ all equal 0.2 mSiemens/mm; $\Delta t = 0.01$ ms; d*x*, d*y* = 0.10 mm. [Reproduced from the Biophysical Journal 45:831–850 (1984) by copyright permission of the Biophysical Society].

isochrone part of a plane wave; the local currents for the latter lie in tight loops of equal and opposite intracellular and interstitial currents. Accordingly, theories of isochrone shape based on the assumption of local plane wave behavior (Muler and Markin, 1978) could not be expected to be fully correct, particularly in the case of extreme anisotropy conditions.

To examine, specifically, the isochrone shape arising from central stimulation of two-dimensional tissue with isotropic, nominal, and reciprocal conductivities a

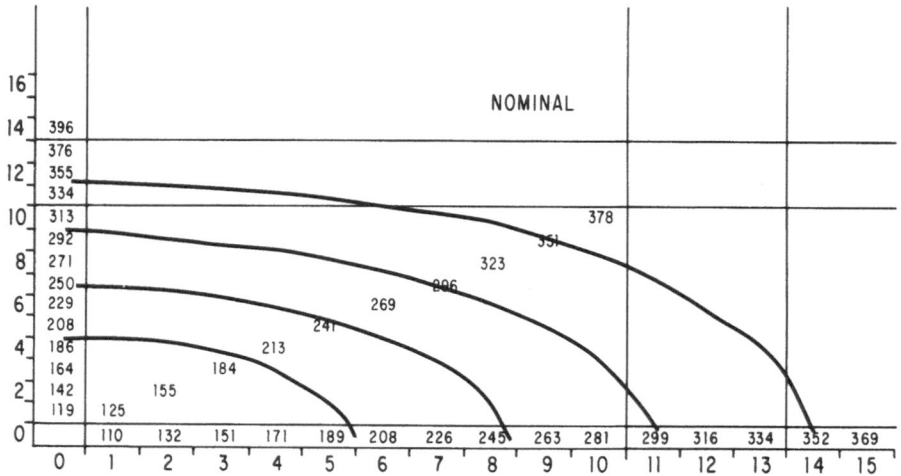

Figure 6. Nominal conductivities. Computed times and isochrones for nominal conductivities. The same format as Figure 5 is used. These elliptical patterns were close but not quite equal to those expected from the Muler-Markin, 1978 predictions. Here g_{ix}, $g_{oy} = 0.2$, $g_{ox} = 0.8$, $g_{iy} = 0.02$; $\Delta t = 0.01$ ms; $dx = 0.10$ mm, $dy = 0.04$ mm. [Reproduced from the Biophysical Journal 45:831–850 (1984) by copyright permission of the Biophysical Society].

simulation was performed with the membrane assigned Hodgkin-Huxley properties – as noted earlier. It has been shown that although developed for the squid axon the Hodgkin-Huxley activation phase involves sodium dynamics that corresponds correctly to that arising in cardiac muscle. Since Hodgkin-Huxley equations do not reflect cardiac muscle recovery our simulation algorithm simply holds the transmembrane potential at a constant, fully depolarized, value – hence reflecting an expected (idealized) plateau. Consequently, in this way, activation isochrones and rising phase phenomena could be correctly simulated while using equations which are well known and documented.

In Figure 5 the expected circular isochrone arising from isotropic tissue is shown. A propagation velocity of 29.4 cm/s is measured at the outset increasing to a steady value of 43.5 cm/s. These are, generally, good 'ballpark' values.

In Figure 6 we show successive isochrones for the nominal conductivities. The results are elliptical-like shapes not unlike that seen experimentally (Spach *et al.*, 1979). An x velocity of 57 cm/s and a y velocity of 19 cm/s is in the order of values determined in these experiments.

The reciprocal conductivity tissue yielded isochrones which are shown in Figure 7. Since this is non-physiological there is no experimental evidence for comparison. However, Muler and Markin (1978) determined isochrone shapes for this condition based on the assumption that each isochrone element behaves as if it were part of an infinite plane wavefront. Their result is also a square-like shape but rotated 90°. As noted above there is reason to believe that the plane

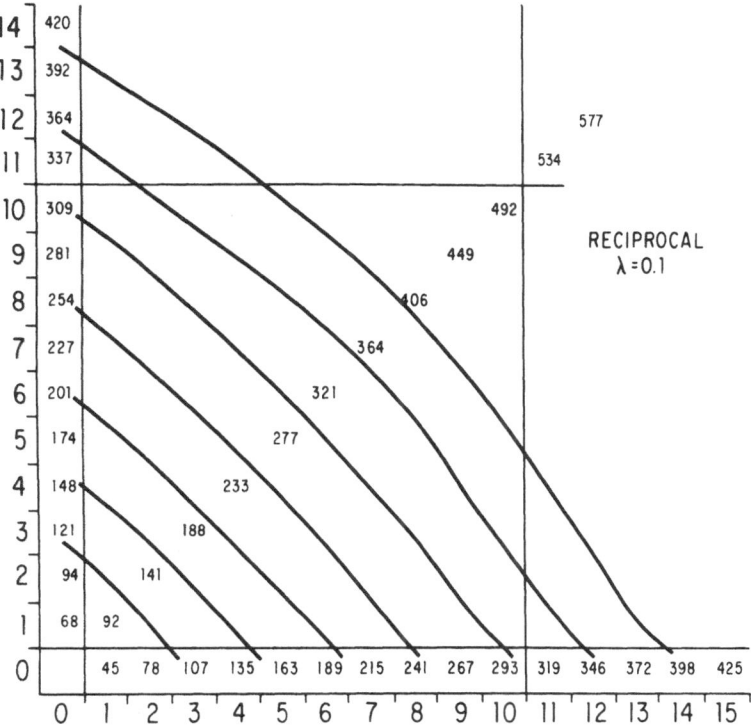

Figure 7. Reciprocal conductivities, $\lambda = 0.10$. The computed times and isochrones (heavy lines) were markedly different from the shape of isochrones predicted theoretically by Muler and Markin, 1978 which more closely approximated the box formed by the lighter straight lines at $i, j = 10$; presumably the discrepancy occurred because they assumed plane-wave current flow patterns. Same format as Figure 5. Note that excitation times are not precisely symmetric between the x, y axes, a discrepancy that must arise from numerical error. Here $g_{ix}, g_{oy} = 0.20, g_{ox}, g_{iy} = 0.02$ mSiemens/mm; $\Delta t = 0.01$ ms; $dx, dy = 0.10$ mm. [Reproduced from the Biophysical Journal 45:831–850 (1984) by copyright permission of the Biophysical Society].

front approximation will not be satisfactory because of the extensive local current loops that arise in this type of anisotropy.

Discussion and conclusions

This paper examines the current flow and propagation properties of two-dimensional anisotropic cardiac tissue through a simulation based on a bidomain model with the Hodgkin-Huxley equations describing the membrane-rising phase properties. The results make clear in a number of ways that one-dimensional cable theory can be extrapolated to higher dimensions only in the case of equal anisotropy ratios. When the condition does not exists then components of action currents will form open loops characterized by membrane crossings in excess of two. The result may cause the isochrone shape to deviate significantly from that expected under simple considerations. This different behavior is not surprising when one examines the mathematical formulation of Eq. (5) and notes that the transmembrane volume conductor current at a specific site is linked to the transmembrane potential behavior over the entire surrounding region (rather than to its behavior at the point alone). It is also clear in the computed action current distribution itself that action currents range over larger distances than expected in linear cable theory. The full consequences of this phenomena avaits further study – it is clearly important for both normal activation as well as for studies of arrhythmia.

Acknowledgement

This work was supported in full by grants HL31286, HL11307, and HL6128 from the National Institutes of Health.

References

Barr RC, Plonsey R (1984) Propagation of excitation in idealized anisotropic two-dimensional tissue. Biophys J 45:831–850

Clerc L (1976) Directional differences of impulse spread in trabecular muscle from mammalian heart. J Physiol 255:335–346

Hodgkin AL, Rushton WA (1946) The electrical constants of a crustacean nerve fiber. Proc Royal Soc 133:444–479

Miller WT, Geselowitz DB (1978) Simulation studies of the electrocardiogram. Circ Res 43:301–315

Muler AL, Markin VS (1978) Electrical properties of anistropic nerve-muscle syncytia. III. Steady form of the excitation front. Biophys 22:699–704

Plonsey R, Barr RC (1984) Current flow patterns in two-dimensional anisotropic bisyncytia with normal and extreme conductivities. Biophys 45:557–571

Roberts DL, Scher AM (1982) Effect of tissue anisotrophy on extra-cellular potential fields in canine myocardium in situ. Circ Res 50:342–351

Roberts DL, Hersh LT, Scher AM (1979) Influence of cardiac fiber orientation on wavefront voltage, conduction velocity and tissue resistivity in the dog. Circ Res 44:701–712

Schmitt O (1969) Biological information processing using the concept of interpenetrating domains. In: Leibovic KN (ed) Information Processing in the Nervous System, Springer-Verlag New York NY 325–331

Spach MS (1982) The electrical representation of cardiac muscle based on discontinuities of axial resistivity at a microscopic and macroscopic level. In: de Carvalho A Paes, Hoffman BE, Lieberman M (eds) Normal and Abnormal Conduction in the Heart, Mt. Kisco NY: Futura Publishing Co.

Spach MS, Kootsey JM (1983) The nature of electrical propagation in cardiac muscle. Amer J Physiol 244:H3–H22

Spach MS, Miller III WT, Miller-Jones E, Warren RB, Barr RC (1979) Extracellular potentials related to intracellular action potentials during impulse conduction in anisotropic cardiac muscle. Circ Res 45:188–204

Tung L (1978) A bidomain model for describing ischemic myocardial DC potentials. Ph.D. dissertation Mass Inst Tech Cambridge MA

A bidomain model of the ECG: Time integrals and the inverse problem

DAVID B. GESELOWITZ

Bioengineering Program, Pennsylvania State University, Electrical Engineering West Building, University Park, PA 16802, U.S.A

Abstract

With use of a bisyncitial model of the heart, it is shown that time integrals of QRS and QSR-T are related to the amplitude (A), area (μ), and activation time (τ) of the cellular action potential (AP) on the closed surface surrounding the ventricles. For the normal heart, solution of the inverse problem would give μ and τ on the heart surface, and by interpolation in the myocardium, allowing reconstruction of the AP. In the case of ischemia and infarction, μ and A_r would be available, which, while not defining the AP, might provide valuable information. Necrosis introduces an unknown perturbation.

Introduction

Miller and Geselowitz (1978a) have presented a model of the electrocardiogram (ECG) based on a bisyncitial (bidomain) model of the heart. The heart is considered to consist of two interpenetrating syncytia: an intracellular domain and an extracellular domain. Current passes from one domain to the other through the cell membrane. The model predicts that the bioelectric sources in the heart are proportional to the spatial gradient of the transmembrane action potential (AP) (Geselowitz and Miller, 1982; Geselowitz et al., 1982). It has been quite successful in accounting for the human electrocardiogram and magnetocardiogram for the normal and ischemic heart (Miller and Geselowitz, 1978a; 1978b) as well as for potentials in a tissue bath preparation (Geselowitz et al., 1982).

The ventricular gradient is defined as the area under the QRS-T waveform (Wilson et al., 1934). Other time integrals, such as the area under QRS, can also be considered. With use of the heart model, these time integrals can be shown to be related to three parameters of the action potential: amplitude, activation time, and area. The present paper derives these results and explores some of their consequences with regard to the inverse problem.

Model

Let σ_i and σ_e be the effective conductivity of intracellular and extracellular (interstitial) space respectively, where the intracellular and interstitial compartments are each taken to occupy the entire tissue space. The current density, J, is then

$$J = -\sigma_i \nabla \varphi_i - \sigma_e \nabla \varphi_e, \tag{1}$$

where J is a macroscopic current density, and φ_i and φ_e are macroscopic potentials in intracellular and interstitial space respectively. Macroscopic quantities may be considered to be averages over small volumes of tissue including several cells.

The transmembrane potential, φ_m, is

$$\varphi_m = \varphi_i - \varphi_e. \tag{2}$$

Hence

$$J = -\sigma_i \nabla \varphi_m - (\sigma_i + \sigma_e) \nabla \sigma_e = -\sigma_i \nabla \Phi_m - \sigma \nabla \varphi_{em} \tag{3}$$

where σ, the sum of σ_i and σ_e, is the bulk conductivity of the myocardium. In the present analysis the conductivities will be taken to be isotropic.

The potential φ_e can be considered to arise from cardiac electromotive forces which can be represented by impressed currents (Geselowitz, 1967). If j^i is the impressed current density at a point, then the total current J is given by

$$J = J^i - \sigma \nabla \varphi_e \tag{4}$$

A comparison of Eqs. (3) and (4) leads to the result

$$J^i = -\sigma_i \nabla \varphi_m \tag{5}$$

J^i is unaffected if a constant is added to φ_m. It is convenient to select this constant so that the transmembrane potential is measured with respect to the resting potential of a normal cell.

Let us restrict our attention to the ventricles. The ventricular myocardial volume may be considered to be enclosed by a surface which encompasses the endocardial and epicardial surfaces of the ventricles. The endocardial surface is normally in contact with the intraventricular blood mass, while the epicardial surface is in contact with the lungs and other tissues of the thoracic volume conductor.

If the entire surface of the heart, S_H, is surrounded by an insulator, then the normal component of J must vanish everywhere on this surface. Since the volume conductor problem of electrocardiography is a quasi-static one the divergence of J must vanish. Consider the following expression for φ_e:

$$\varphi_e = - (\sigma_i/\sigma)\varphi_m = - (\sigma_i/\sigma_e)\varphi_i. \tag{6}$$

Note that the divergence of J is then zero. Indeed J itself is zero, with current in intracellular space equal and opposite to current in extracellular space. Hence the normal component of J vanishes on the heart surface. Therefore Eq. (6) gives the expression for φ_e when the heart is insulated. It is also the solution for all instants when φ_m is zero on the heart surface. The model therefore predicts that φ_e is zero ahead of the activation wavefront until either epicardial or endocardial break-through has occurred. For excitation originating in the Purkinje system, however, breakthrough would occur almost immediately.

If heart muscle is anisotropic, the conductivity ratio depends on direction, and Eq. (6) is no longer valid.

As long as σ_i and σ_e do not depend on J, the volume conductor is linear and superposition holds. The potential, φ, in the volume conductor, and its value, V, on the surface, can be expressed as a weighted sum or integral of the sources throughout the myocardium.

$$V = \int J^i \cdot Z dv = - \int \sigma_i Z \cdot \nabla \varphi_m dv, \tag{7}$$

where Z is the transfer impendence relating the potential at the observation point to the source at the element of volume, dv, in the heart.

From considerations of reciprocity, Z is equal of the lead field, that is the electric field in the heart arising from unit current injected into the lead, V (McFee and Johnston, 1953). Therefore,

$$\nabla \cdot Z = 0 \tag{8}$$

except at surfaces separating regions of differing conductivity. Equation (8) is assumed to hold in the heart.

$$\int \nabla \cdot (Z\varphi_m) dv = \int Z\varphi_m \cdot dS_H = \int (\varphi_m \nabla \cdot Z + Z \cdot \nabla \varphi_m) dv \tag{9}$$

where S_H is the surface which bounds the heart. From Eqs. (7), (8), (9)

$$V = - \sigma_i \int \varphi_m Z \cdot dS_H. \tag{10}$$

During periods of no ventricular activity all cells are at their resting potential, φ_r. The corresponding surface potential, V_0, will be designated the baseline.

$$V_0 = - \sigma_i \int (\varphi_m - \varphi_r) Z \cdot dS_H. \tag{11}$$

Since the ECG is generally recorded with a–c coupled amplifiers, the absolute value of C_0 is not known. Henceforth we will take V to be the departure from the baseline, and, consistent with Eq. (11), φ_m for each cell will be measured with respect to its individual resting potential.

Consider now the area under the ECG waveform.

$$\int_0^T V \mathrm{d}t = - \sigma_i \int [\int_0^T \varphi_m \mathrm{d}t] \, Z \cdot \mathrm{d}S_H, \tag{12}$$

If T is chosen to include QRS, then to a good approximation, except perhaps for the very first cells to repolarize,

$$\varphi_m = A \, u(t - \tau), \tag{13}$$

where A is the amplitude of the upstoke of the action potential, u is the unit step function, and τ is the excitation time of the point on the heart surface. Then

$$\int_0^{T_1} V \mathrm{d}t = - \sigma_i \int A(T_1 - \tau) \, Z \cdot \mathrm{d}S_H. \tag{14}$$

Note that

$$\int Z \cdot \mathrm{d}S_H = \int \nabla \cdot Z \, \mathrm{d}v = 0 \tag{15}$$

Therefore

$$\int_0^{T_1} V \mathrm{d}t = \sigma_i A \int \tau \, Z \cdot \mathrm{d}S_H \tag{16}$$

If T is chosen to include QRS-T, them φ_m is the entire action potential. Let μ be the area under the action potential. Then

$$\int_0^{T_2} V \mathrm{d}t = - \sigma_i \int \mu \, Z \cdot \mathrm{d}S_H. \tag{17}$$

Note that A and μ are to be taken with respect to the resting potential of the individual cell.

Hence the surface ECG is related to the distribution of φ_m on S_H, the area under QRS is related to the distribution of excitation time on S_H, while the area under QRS-T (ventricular gradient) is related to the distribution of μ on S_H. The forms of all three equations are the same. For the normal heart, φ_m varies only in duration. Hence μ is a monotonic function of duration.

If Eqs. (16) and (17) can be inverted, then one would have τ and μ everywhere on the heart surface. Since τ and μ vary smoothly throughout the heart, it should then be possible to estimate their values everywhere by interpolation, and thus to reconstruct φ_m everywhere. The inverse problem would then be solved.

Discussion

Eq. (10) indicates that the sources in the heart can be replaced by an equivalent double layer on the surface of the heart. From a theorem of Helmholtz, this double layer should be σ times the voltage which would appear on the surface of the heart when it is insulated (Helmholtz, 1853) (Thevenin's theorem in circuit theory is a special case of Helmholtz' theorem.) From Eq. (6) it is evident that Eq. (10) is consistent with Helmholtz' theorem.

It should be noted that S_H includes the endocardial surfaces. The result that φ_e on the insulated epicardium is proportional to φ_m is only valid if the inner surface is also insulated. If the surface of the heart is exposed *in vivo,* the endocardial surface will be in contact with blood, and therefore epicardial potentials will not obey Eq. (6).

The result that φ_m on the heart surface completely determines potentials outside the heart serves to clarify the nature of the inverse problem. Geselowitz and Miller (1984) have previously shown that this double layer is unique (Cuppen, 1984). The arguments above indicate that the two parameters which characterize φ_m for the normal heart, namely activation time and duration, can be obtained on the heart surface by considering two time integrals of the ECG waveform. But φ_m in the walls of the heart is completely undetermined. In the normal heart, however, activation time and duration are known to vary smoothly from endocardium to epicardium. Hence if they can be determined on the heart surface it would appear likely that their values in the myocardium could be extimated rather accurately by use of an appropriate interpolation scheme. Furthermore Cuppen (1984) and van Oosterom & Cuppen (1982) have recently shown very encouraging results with a solution to the inverse problem of Eq. (16). They also derived the result of Eq. (16) using an argument that during activation the cardiac source is a uniform double layer on the excitation isochrone.

The effects of the assumption of isotropy remain to be explored.

What about the abnormal heart? We will identify here several possibly serious difficulties with the inverse problem which arise in the case of pathology.

First of all, μ, the area under the AP, is no longer simply related to the AP duration. Ischemic cells, for example, show a range of changes including an elevation of resting potential, a decrease in amplitude, a shortening or prolongation of the action potential, and a slower upstroke. Each of these changes affects μ, while a change in resting potential or in amplitude affects A. Variation in A means that the inversion of Eq. (16) is no longer simply related to τ, but involves the product $A\tau$. Variation in AP waveshape means that μ obtained from inverting Eq. (17) is no longer uniquely associated with a particular AP waveform. Nonetheless, determination of μ and $A\tau$ might still provide valuable information.

Both τ and μ may be expected to vary much less smoothly in the abnormal case. Indeed an injury may be expected to be confined to one or more limited regions of the heart. Since τ and μ are determined only on S_H it may be more difficult to extrapolate to the interior, although knowledge of their values on S_H might well provide sufficient information concerning the injury. Note that if an injury is entirely intramyocardial, it will not be evident outside the heart since the extra-cardiac potentials depend only on φ_m on S_H. Such a 'silent' injury appears unlikely.

In the case of necrosis, internal surfaces appear. A double layer equal to $\sigma_i \varphi_m$ on each such surface then acts a source in addition to the double layer on the heart surface. A solution to the inverse problem will then yield values of τ and μ which are a superposition of their values for the surface cells and an effective value reflecting the internal surfaces. These values on S_H are still unique. If, however, the internal surfaces are unknown (their existance is probably not known) then interpretation of the values of τ and μ obtained from the inverse solution becomes more difficult. If an internal necrotic volume is small, it will act approx-imately as a dipole whose moment is the integral of the double layer over the internal surface.

From Eq. (10) the inverse problem could be solved in principle at each instant of time to give φ_m during the cardiac cycle. The advantage of using integrals of the waveform is that the inverse problem need be solved only twice to provide a complete solution, at least for the normal heart. Furthermore, it may be that the inverse solution for the time integrals is better behaved (less 'ill-posed') than for φ_m.

There are practical difficulties to be considered in evaluating the integrals. For example, accurate determination of the area under QRS requires a knowledge of where QRS begins and ends. Identification of the end of QRS may be difficult in the presence of ST segment shifts. Both integrals depend on the accurate deter-mination of the baseline.

Summary

Consequences of a bisyncitial model of the heart are explored. The model posits that cardiac sources are proportional to the gradient of the cellular action poten-tial throughout the myocardium. In the absence of necrosis, an equivalent source for the surface electrocardiogram is a double layer on the heart surface whose moment is proportional to the cellular action potential on the surface. The time integral of QRS depends on the product of activation time and amplitude of the AP on S_H, while the time integral of QRS-T depends on the area under the AP on S_H. For the normal heart, where A is constant, the integral of QRS is then directly related to τ, while the integral of QRS-T is directly related to AP duration. Solution of the inverse problem would then completely determine φ_m.

In the case of ischemia, the ventricular gradient gives information about μ which, in turn, depends on the degree of ischemia. The time integral of QRS depends on $A\tau$ where A may vary. If the inverse problem can be solved, these parameters will be known on the inner and outer surfaces of the ventricles, thus providing considerable information, albeit ambiguous, about cellular action potentials throughout the ventricular myocardium. The presence of regions of necrosis adds a perturbation to the double layer on S_H, and hence to $A\tau$ and μ.

Acknowledgment

This work was supported in part by the National Science Foundation under grant ECS-8018168.

References

Cuppen JJM (1984) Calculating the isochrones of ventricular depolarization. SIAM J Sci Stat Comput, 5:105–120

Geselowitz DB (1967) On bioelectric potentials in an inhomogenous volume conductor. Biophys J 7:1–11

Geselowitz DB, Barr RC, Spach MS, Miller III WT (1982) The impact of adjacent isotropic fluids on electrograms from anisotropic cardiac muscle. Circ Res 51:602–613

Geselowitz DB, Miller III WT (1982) Active electric properties of cardiac muscle. Bioelectromagnetics 3:127–132

Geselowitz DB, Miller III WT (1984) A bi-domain model for anisotropic cardiac muscle. Ann Biomed Engrg. In press

Helmholtz H (1853) Uber einege gesetze der vertheilung elektrischer strome in korperlischen leitern mit anwendung auf die thierisch elektrischen versuche. Pogg Ann Bd 89:S211–213, S353–357

McFee R, Johnston FD (1953) Electrocardiographic leads: I. Introduction. Circ 8:554–568

Miller III WT, Geselowitz DB (1978a) Simulation studies of the electrocardiogram: I. The normal heart. Circ Res 43:301–315

Miller III WT, Geselowitz DB (1978b) Simulation studies of the electrocardiogram: II. Ischemia and infarction. Circ Res 43: 315–323

van Oosterom A, Cuppen JJM (1982) Computing the depolarization sequence at the ventricular surface from body surface potentials. In Antaloczy Z, Preda I (eds) Budapest: Academia Kiado; Amsterdam: Excerpta Medica, pp 101–106

Wilson FN, MacLeod AG, Barker PS, Johnston FD (1934) The determination and the significance of the areas of the ventricular deflections of the electrocardiogram. Amer Heart J 10:46–61

Critical aspects of the forward and inverse problems in electrocardiography

YORAM RUDY

Dept. of Biomedical Engineering, Case Western Reserve University, Cleveland, OH 44106, U.S.A.

Abstract

Selected model studies of various aspects of the electrocardiographic process are described.
  (1) A one-dimensional model of propagation in cardiac muscle which incorporates discontinuities on the cellular level (intercalated discs) was developed. The discrete structure causes propagation to be discontinuous, with small sources traveling inside the cell at 10 times the average velocity over many cells, and very large, persistent sources present at the discs. The discontinuous nature of propagation is reflected in the extracellular potential field close to the fiber, but these effects are smoothed-out at distances greater than 10 times the fiber radius.
  (2) The effects of the torso volume conductor on the electrocardiographic potential distribution were examined utilizing an eccentric spheres model. The effects of the blood cavity, lung region, and the surface muscle layer are described. The importance of interactions between the various torso compartments in determining the potential distribution is demonstrated.
  (3) Properties of the inverse reconstruction of epicardial potentials from body surface data are discussed. It is shown that epicardial potentials accurately reflect details of the underlying myocardial sources, and are only minimally affected by body shape and by torso inhomogeneities. Initial results demonstrate the ability of the inverse procedure to accurately reconstruct multiple local cardiac events from the low resolution, smooth surface potential data.

Introduction

As a result of the electrical activity of the heart, electrical potentials appear at all points of the body surface. These potentials reflect both the electrical sources within the heart, and the electrical properties of the torso volume conductor. The

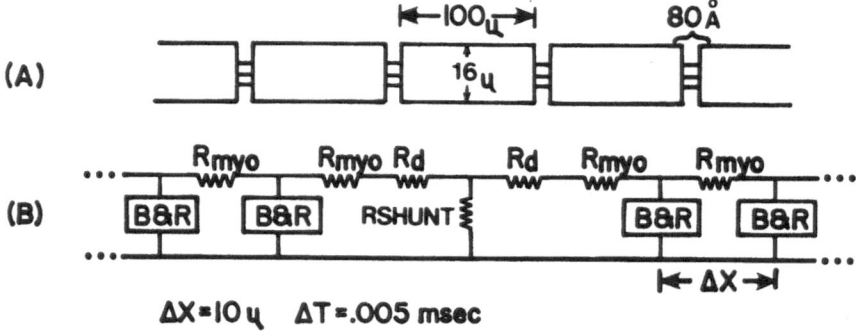

Figure 1. (A) Discrete cable model of cylindrical cardiac cells, each 100μ in length and 16μ in diameter, interconnected by an intercalated disc structure of 80Å. (B) Core conductor network utilized for the intercalated disc interaction between two adjacent cells.

goal of electrocardiography is to relate the body surface potential data to the underlying electrical activity within the heart. The understanding of the relationships between body surface potentials and the cardiac electrical events (cardiac sources) can be greatly enhanced through the use of theoretical models. This paper is a brief review of selected model simulation results, which address various aspects of the electrocardiographic process. These include; (A) Effects of myocardial structure on the cardiac sources; (B) The forward problem – volume conductor effects and (C) The inverse problem – reconstruction of epicardial potentials from body surface potential distributions.

Effects of myocardial structure on the cardiac sources

The anatomical structure of the myocardium as an assembly of discrete cells separated by a periodic intercalated disc structure was established in 1954. However, until recently the propagation of electrical excitation in cardiac muscle has been characterized as though it occurred in a syncytium, and the structural discontinuities introduced by the discs were not icluded in activation models. We have examined the structural effects using a model which incorporates microscopic discontinuities (intercelated discs) at the cellular level. The model (Figure 1) consists of a one dimensional fiber made up of 50 cells (cell length = 100μ, cell diameter = 16μ). Neighboring cells are connected by an intercalated disc structure modelled as a T-resistance network (two axial resistances representing the intercytoplasmic channels, and a radial leakage resistance to the extracellular space). Each cell is discretized into ten membrane patches represented by the ventricular action potential of Beeler and Reuter (1977). This number of patches provides the high resolution necessary for the study of spatial variations within a single cell.

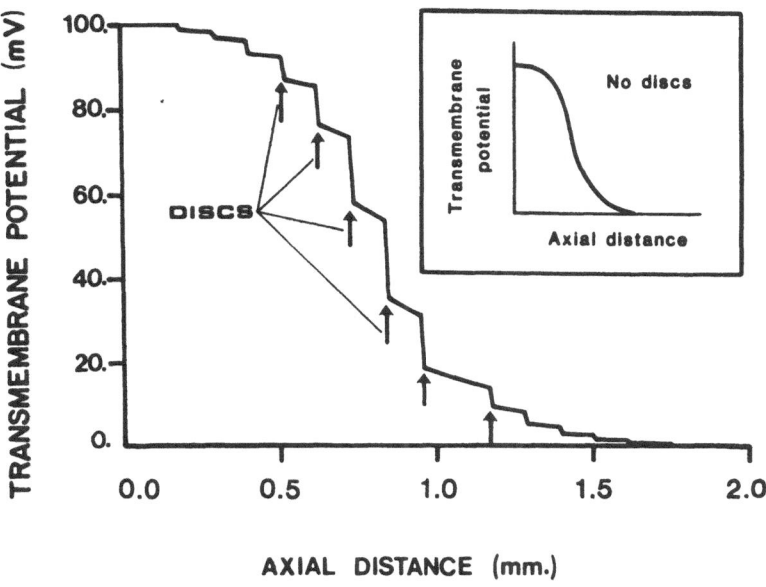

Figure 2. Spatial action potential wavefront obtained from the discontinuous model. Note major discontinuities in leading edge (arrows). A smooth action potential is shown for comparison (insert).

The presence of the structural discontinuities (discs) has a major effect on the nature of electrical propagation and source distribution in cardiac muscle. The rising phase of a spatial propagating action potential obtained from the model is shown in Figure 2. Note the sharp discontinuities introduced at each intercalated disc location (arrows). In contrast, the action potential computed from a continuous model (no discs included) is smooth, and does not show sharp changes in slope (insert to Figure 2). The equivalent dipole source distribution arising from the 'discontinuous' spatial waveform (proportional to the slope dv_m/dz) includes very strong concentrated sources at each disc location due to these discontinuities in the spatial wavefront. A schematic description of the equivalent dipole source distribution in the fiber (labelled A), related spatially to the propagating action potential (labelled B) is shown in Figure 3. The dipole densities within the cell are much smaller than at the intercalated discs. In addition, due to a 0.45 ms delay in propagation across the disc (for 1Ω cm^2 disc resistance), propagation inside the cell (i.e. between discs) is 10 times faster than the average propagation velocity in the fiber (over many cells). The propagation is therefore discontinuous, saltatory in nature, with very large sources 'jumping' from disc to disc.

The discontinuous nature of propagation is reflected as 'notches' in the spatial extracellular potential field close to the fiber (Figure 4). At radial distances of 10 times the fiber radius or greater, the computed spatial field is a smooth bi-phasic waveshape (Figure 5), and does not reflect the discontinuous distribution of the sources at all. These results imply that while at the tissue level the structural discontinuities affect the extracellular potential field, for global forward prob-

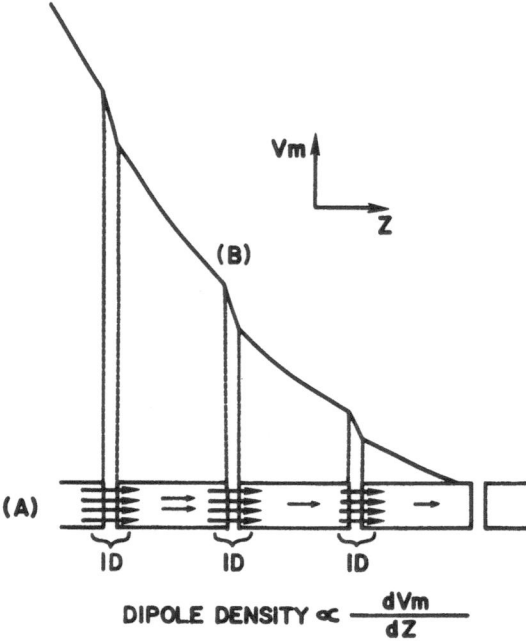

Figure 3. Schematic representation of equivalent dipole sources arising from discontinuities in the leading edge of the action potential.

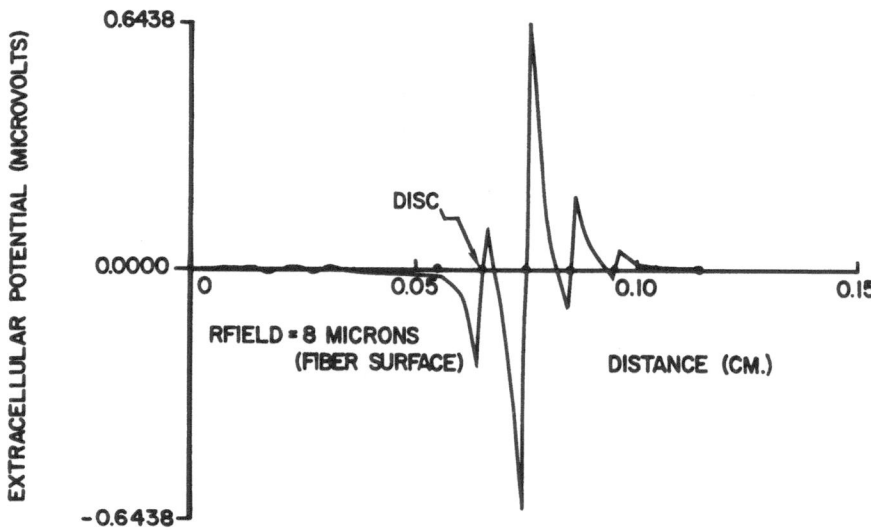

Figure 4. Spatial extracellular potential computed on the surface of the fiber. Dots on abcissa indicate disc locations within the leading edge.

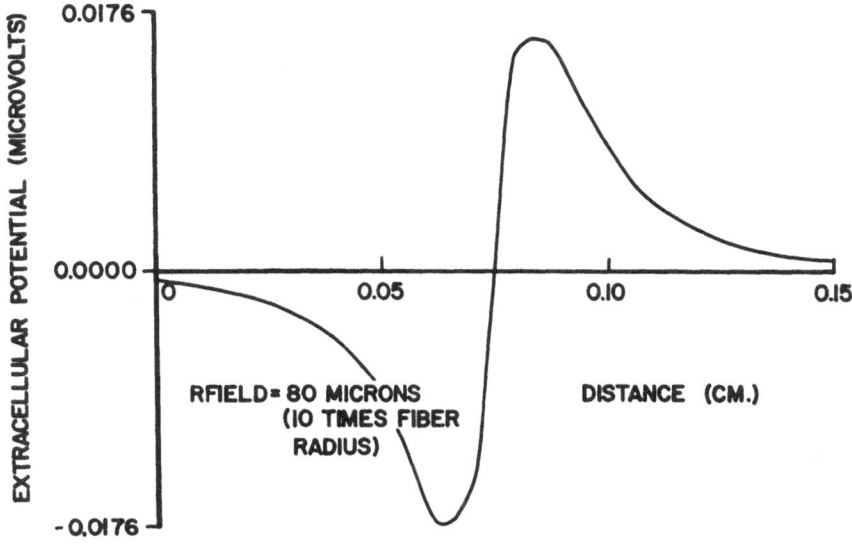

Figure 5. Spatial extracellular field at a distance of 10 radii $(80\,\mu)$.

lems (such as the computation of potentials in the volume conductor surrounding the heart) these effects can be averaged, and a smoothly-propagating activation front can serve as a good approximation to the cardiac sources (Dürer *et al.*, 1970).

It should be mentioned, that the incorporation of the intercalated discs in the model completely changes classical relationships obtained from continuous ('Hodgkin-Huxley') cable theory. For example, the inverse square root relationship between velocity and axial resistance does not hold, and an increase in $\dot{V}_{max}$ accompanies slow conduction caused by high disc resistance. These deviations from classical continuous cable theory are further discussed elsewhere (Diaz *et al.*, 1983; Rudy *et al.*, 1983).

The forward problem – volume conductor effects

The body surface potential distribution is determined by both the cardiac sources and the torso volume conductor. To study the volume conductor effects on the potential distribution, an eccentric spheres model of the heart – torso system was developed (Rudy and Plonsey, 1979; Rudy *et al.*, 1979). This idealized forward model includes all important torso inhomogeneities, and yet is simple enough to permit analytic solutions for both body surface and epicardial potentials. In the model (Figure 6), the heart is represented as a sphere consisting of a central blood volume bounded by a spherical heart-muscle shell and pericardium; the heart, in turn, is located eccentrically within a spherical torso, where the latter consists of a lung region bounded by muscle and fat layers. The eccentric location of the heart is an important property of the model, reflecting the asymmetry with which the lungs envelope the heart. The source is a double layer spherical cap which lies within the myocardium and represents an idealized activation wave. The model permits altering the conductivities of the intracavitary blood, heart-muscle, lungs, surface muscle layer, subcutaneous fat, and pericardium. The thickness of each of the layers present can be varied as well. The model also allows adjustment of the location of the heart and its relative size in the torso. In addition, the location of the double layer myocardial source and its extent can be varied. The idealized spherical geometry is necessary to obtain an analytic solution that includes the aforementioned complexities, and permits the easy manipulation of the various parameters. The expressions for epicardial (φ_E) and body surface potentials (φ_S) as series expansions in Legendre polynomials (P_l) are shown below.

$$
\Phi_E (r_2, \theta) = 2\pi a^2 \left\{ \sum_{l=1}^{\infty} F_l \left(\frac{1}{l+1} \right) \left(\frac{r_0^{l-1}}{r_2^{l+1}} \right) P_l' (\cos \theta_0) \right.
$$

$$
\left. + G_l \frac{1}{l} \left(\frac{r_2^l}{r_0^{l+2}} \right) P_l' (\cos \theta_0) \right\} P_l (\cos \theta), \text{ and}
$$

(1)

$$
\Phi_s (r_5, \theta) =
$$
$$
2\pi a^2 \left\{ \sum_{s=1}^{\infty} \left[\left(\frac{d}{r_5} \right)^{s+1} \sum_{l=1}^{s} M_l \frac{r_0^{l-1} P_l' (\cos \theta_0)}{l+1} \right. \right.
$$
$$
\cdot \frac{1}{d^{l+1}} \cdot \frac{s!}{l! \, (s-l)!} + \left(\frac{r_5}{d} \right)^s \sum_{l=s}^{\infty} N_l \frac{P_l' (\cos \theta_0)}{l r_0^{l+2}}
$$
$$
\left. \cdot d^l \cdot \frac{(-1)^{l-s} \, l!}{s!(l-s)!} \right] P_s (\cos \theta)
$$
$$
\left. + \sum_{l=1}^{\infty} N_l \frac{P_l' (\cos \theta_0)}{l r_0^{l+2}} \cdot d^l \cdot (-1)^l \right\},
$$

(2)

A summary of some of the results follows.

(1) Combined effect of the inhomogeneities

The inhomogeneities augment the surface potentials. For an endocardial location of the double layer, with all inhomogeneities included in the model, the peak surface potential value is almost twice the value obtained for the homogeneous case (conductivity everywhere the same and equal to the conductivity of the myocardium). The augmentation is caused by the blood cavity and (for anterior points on the torso) by the lungs. The pericardium and surface muscle layer

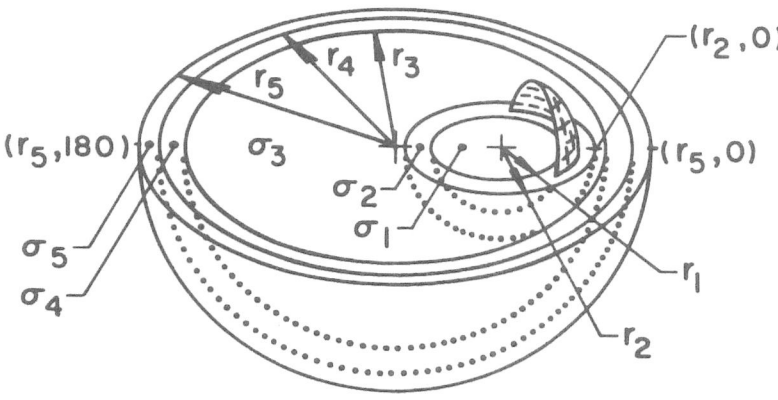

Figure 6. Eccentric spherical model of the inhomogeneous torso. Double-layer source is marked by + and − signs on its positive and negative surfaces, respectively. Typical values of the geometrical parameters are $r_1 = 4$ cm, $r_2 = 5$ cm, $r_3 = 11$ cm, $r_4 = 12$ cm, and $r_5 = 12.5$ cm. Eccentricity (distance between heart center and torso center) is typically 5 cm. σ_i is the conductivity of region (i). 1-blood cavity, 2-myocardium, 3-lung region, 4-muscle, 5-fat. The pericardium is represented by a resistive membrane at r_2.

attenuate the surface potential. Similar augmentation effect is observed at the epicardium with the augmentation factor for the peak epicardial potential being 2.22.

(2) Blood cavity

For a double layer source located endocardially, the surface potential increases by 46.4% when the intracavitary blood is included in the inhomogeneous model. An interesting observation is that when the blood is added to an otherwise homogeneous model (conductivity everywhere equal to the myocardial conductivity), the enhancement of surface potentials is 71.9%. This result shows that the remaining torso compartments (lung, skeletal muscle, fat, pericardium) act to diminish the augmentation effect of the blood. The result also demonstrates the importance of interactions between the various torso compartments in determining the surface potential distribution. This observation implies that combined models, rather than models which isolate single compartments of the torso volume conductor should be used. Regarding variations in blood conductivity (caused clinically by changes in hematocrit), the model predicts an increase in potential with increasing conductivity (decreasing hematocrit). This behavior was observed both experimentally (Nelson, 1972), and clinically (Rosenthal, 1971) in patients with anemia and polycythemia.

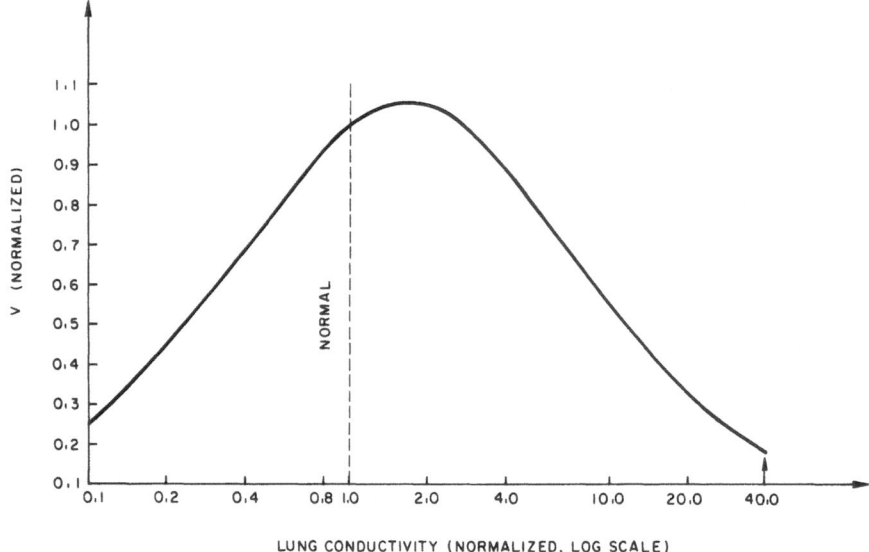

Figure 7. The effect of variations in lung conductivity on the magnitude of anterior surface potential (*V*). *V* is normalized to a value of unity at the typical lung conductivity (Normal). The conductivity of physiologic saline is indicated by an arrow.

(3) Lung region

The effect of variations in lung conductivity on the surface potential magnitude is shown in Figure 7. The behavior is bell-shaped with low potentials obtained for high as well as low conductivity values. This non-monotonic behavior is determined by the lung interaction with the surrounding muscle layer. In the absence of the muscle layer, the surface potential increases monotonically with decreasing lung conductivity. This observation demonstrates again the importance of interactions between the various torso compartments in determining the potential distribution. It should be mentioned that experimental results (Toyama, 1974) as well as clinical findings of low ECG potentials in patients with obstructive lung disease (low lung conductivity) are in keeping with the model prediction. On the other end of the spectrum, the model results of low surface potentials for abnormally *high* lung conductivity (such as occur clinically in cases of pulmonary edema) were confirmed experimentally by our recent study in patients undergoing bronchopulmonary lavage with saline solution (a high conductivity fluid) (Rudy *et al.*, 1982). The non-monotonic behavior predicted by the model is therefore in agreement with both experimental results and clinical observations. It should be mentioned that intuitive predictions favored a monotonic behavior, arguing that high lung conductivity permits more current flow to the surface, resulting in high voltages. The failure of the intuitive prediction is not surprising since it does not consider the complex effect of the lung-surface muscle interac-

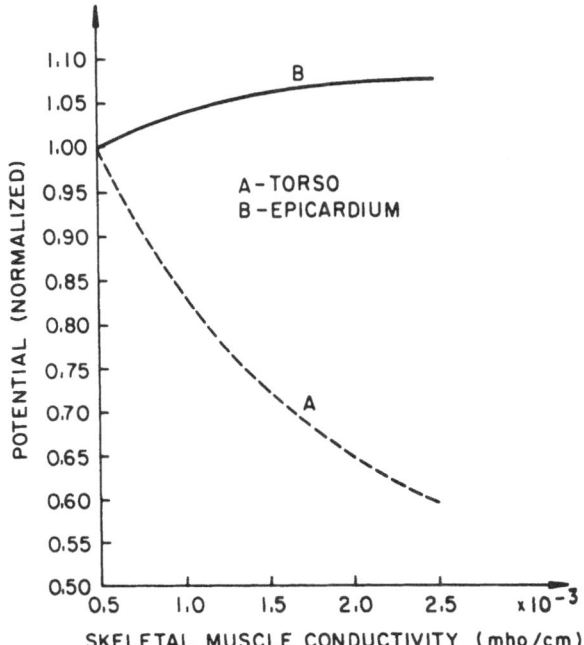

Figure 8. The effect of variations in the conductivity of the skeletal muscle layer on body surface (A) and epicardial (B) potentials. The potentials are adjusted so that a value of unity is obtained for a conductivity equal to that of the underlying lung region (0.005 mho/cm). The typical conductivity of skeletal muscle is 0.00125 mho/cm.

tion. As explained above, this interaction determines the non-monotonic behavior.

(4) Surface muscle layer

Body surface and epicardial potentials are shown in Figure 6 as a function of skeletal-muscle conductivity. The muscle layer attenuates surface potentials (by 25%), and is a major contributor to the 'smoothing effect' of the torso volume conductor (see below). The surface potential decreases with increasing muscle conductivity, and a 5-fold increase in conductivity (from 0.0005 to 0.0025 mho/cm) causes the potential to decrease by 40.5%. In contrast, epicardial potentials are not strongly affected by the presence of the muscle layer. A 5-fold increase in muscle conductivity causes a slight increase of only 8% in epicardial potential (see Figure 8).

The results described above, and the fact that the muscle layer controls the functional dependence of the surface potential on the conductivity of the lungs, demonstrate the importance of the muscle in determining the torso surface potential distribution.

The effect of the muscle layer on epicardial potentials requires further discussion. Intuitively, it could be argued that the surface muscle layer should have no effect on the epicardial distribution. The argument is that the epicardium, being part of the heart, reflects the primary cardiac sources independently of any torso effects. It should be emphasized that the potential field generated by the primary sources gives rise to secondary sources at the lung-muscle interface (the secondary source strength is proportional to the discontinuity in conductivity at the interface). These secondary sources, in turn, affect the potential field everywhere, and in particular on the epicardial surface. As shown in Figure 8, the effect is small.

(5) Size of the heart

The effect of dilation of the heart is to augment surface potentials. The potential is augmented by 82.3% when the radius of the heart is increased from 5 to 8 cm (the area occupied by the activation wavefront is proportionately increased as well). This theoretical prediction is opposite to the results of a clinical study (Ishikawa, 1971) of patients with congestive heart failure, which showed a decrease in potentials with increasing cardiothoracic ratio. The model simulations which permit the separation of interactive processes provide a possible explanation to this apparent discrepency. The congestive heart failure is accompanied by pulmonary edema, bringing about an increase in lung conductivity. As discussed above,

$\longrightarrow$

Figure 9. Examples of regional cardiac events that are reflected in the body surface potential distribution. The surface potential distributions shown in the figure were obtained with our 180-electrode mapping system. Potential levels are displayed as different colors (the color scale is given in microvolts). Each map is divided into four segments, from left to right: right chest, left chest, left back, and right back. The time from the beginning of the QRS (in ms), and the maximum and minimum potential values (in microvolts) are displayed below each map.

1: The appearance of a 'notch' in the anterior positive potential region (26 ms), and its development into a very localized anterior minimum (28–32 ms) reflect right ventricular breakthrough.

2: The three discrete potential maxima (50 ms) reflect activation fronts in three regions of the heart. From left to right: right ventricular outflow tract; anterior wall of left ventricle; posterior wall of left ventricle.

3 and 4: RBBB – The two distinct (posterior and anterior) potential maxima reflect depolarization of the right ventricle and of the left ventricle respectively. While the posterior maximum diminishes in amplitude (reflecting completion of depolarization of left ventricle), the anterior maximum increases in amplitude, reflecting the late onset of right ventricular depolarization and the sequential nature of cardiac events (right ventricle after left ventricle) in RBBB.

5 and 6: WPW Syndrome – The potential distribution in 5 reflects an activation front traveling from right to left. The right-anterior location of the potential minimum corresponds to an accessory pathway located at the lateral-inferior portion of the right A-V groove. In 6, the posterior location of the minimum reflects a pre-excitation site on the postero-basal wall. The predicted locations of the accessory pathways were confirmed during surgery.

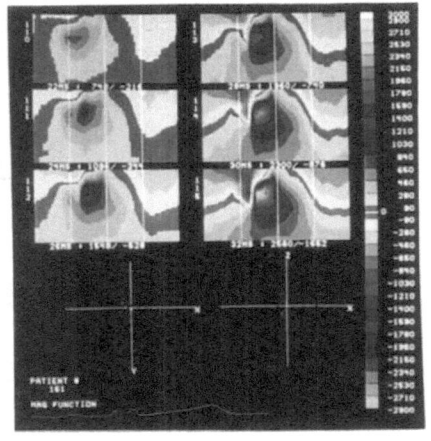

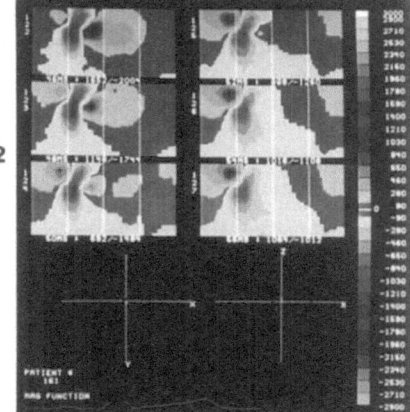

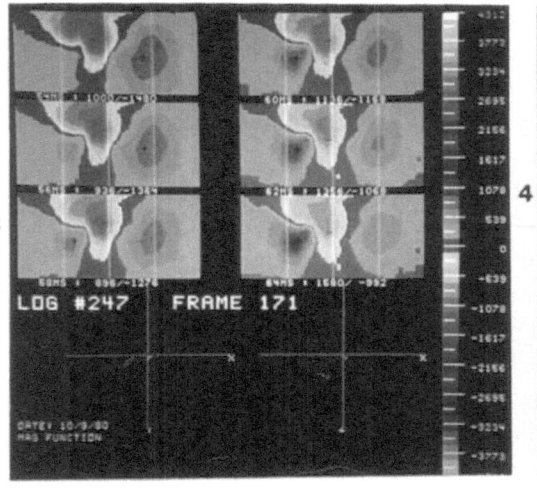

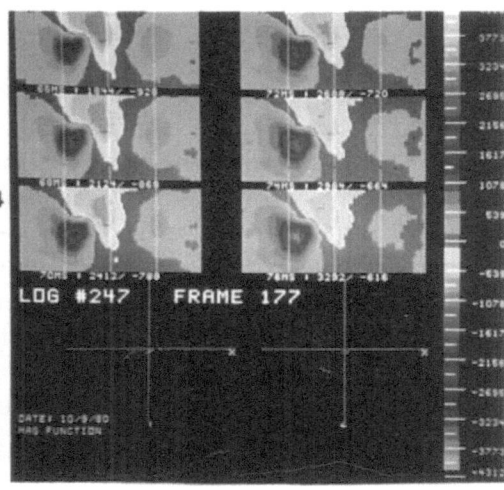

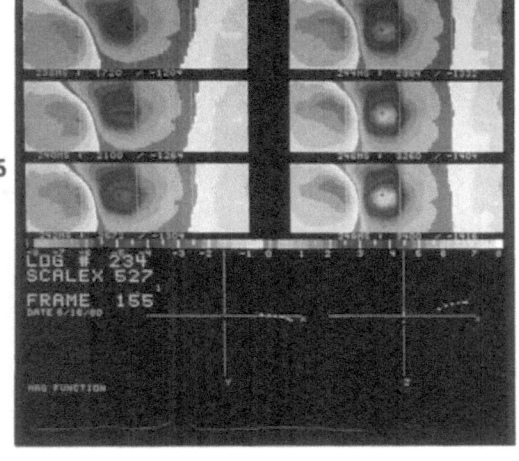

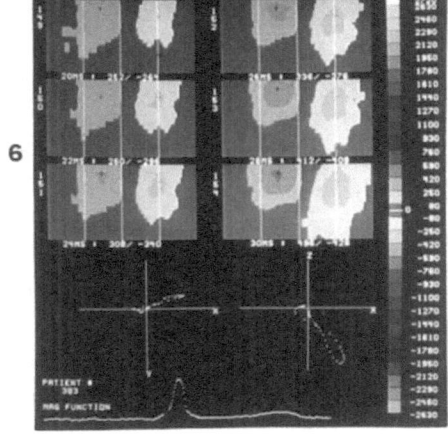

the effect of high lung conductivity is to attenuate surface potentials, an opposite effect to that produced by dilatation. It is likely that this attenuation effect of the lungs predominates over the augmentation due to dilatation so that low potentials result *in spite* of the enlarged heart.

The inverse problem – reconstruction of epicardial potentials from body surface potential distributions

At each instant of time throughout the cardiac cycle, the potential distribution over the entrie torso constitutes the complete set of data in non-invasive electrocardiography. As mentioned above, these potentials reflect both the cardiac sources and the torso volume conductor. The potential distribution over the entire torso permits the detection and identification of regional electrical events in the heart in a fashion that is not possible from standard ECG and VCG. In fact, VCG is based on the assumption that the cardiac sources can be lumped into a single equivalent dipole, located at the center of the heart. This dipole results from the total cardiac electrical activity, can not reflect simultaneous multiple wave fronts in different regions of the heart, and cannot be related to local electrophysiological events. Examples of local events that are reflected at the body surface are shown in Figure 9. These include right ventricular breakthrough, multiple activation fronts during late QRS, separation of simultaneous activation fronts in the right and left ventricles in right bundle branch block, and determination of the general location of pre-excitation in Wolff-Parkinson-White (WPW) syndrome.

The ability to non-invasively relate surface potential patterns to regional cardiac events is of great physiological and clinical importance. An example of a clinical application already in use is the approximate localization of the accessory atrio-ventricular pathway in WPW syndrome prior to surgery. However, as will be shown below, the body surface potential distribution is an integrated, smoothed-out, low resolution reflection of the underlying cardiac events (Spach *et al.*, 1977; 1978; Ramsey *et al.*, 1977; King *et al.*, 1972; Rudy and Plonsey, 1980). Moreover, it is modified by the inhomogeneous thoracic volume conductor. As a result, the ability to accurately describe cardiac events from surface potentials based on observation alone is limited.

In contrast, epicardial potentials accurately mirror details of the electrical events within the myocardium with high resolution. This property is demonstrated below by our eccentric spheres model simulations. In these simulations, when two activation waves in the anterior part of a spherical myocardium are separated by less than 100°, two discrete maxima arise on the epicardium, whereas a single broad maximum appears on the body surface. For a separation greater than 100°, two discrete maxima are apparent on the body surface as well (see Figure 10). Note, however, that the fact that the single surface potential max-

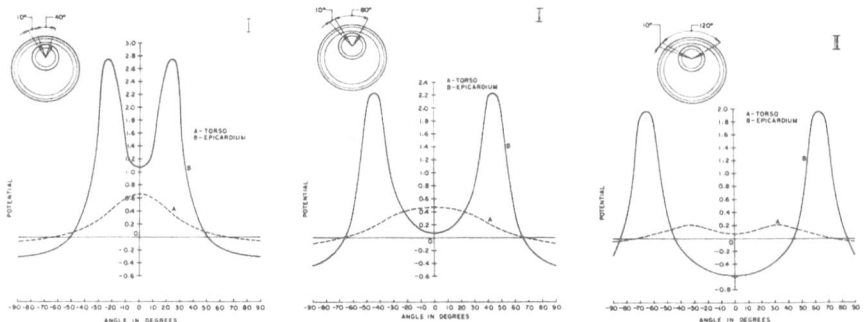

Figure 10. Comparison of body surface (A) and epicardial (B) potentials originating from two discrete activation wave fronts located in the myocardium. The central angles of the two activation waves are 10°. The separation between the wave fronts is I-40°, II-80°, III-120°. The geometry is illustrated by the cross section of the model in the left upper corner of each graph.

imum shown in Figure 10, I originated from a specific multiple source configuration is reflected in its specific amplitude and shape (spatial extent of the maximum and low level 'tails'), in contrast with the single maximum in 10, II, which arises from a different multiple source configuration. Even when two maxima appear on the surface (Figure 10, III), their location does not correspond to the location of the wavefronts. In contrast, the location of the epicardial maxima accurately reflects the location of the underlying activation waves so that in this example, the epicardial potential map is an accurate reflection of the myocardial sources.

Another property of epicardial potentials is demonstrated in Figure 11. Our simulations show that these potentials (Figure 11B) are almost completely independent of the location of the heart within the torso, while surface potentials (Figure 11A) are greatly affected by heart position. When the eccentricity is increased from 1 to 5 cm, the torso potential is almost doubled (97% increase). In

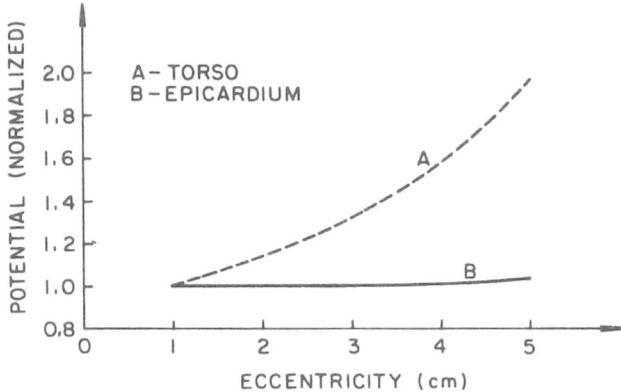

Figure 11. The effects of variations in the eccentricity of the heart on body surface (A) and epicardial (B) potentials. The potentials are nomalized to unity at an eccentricity of 1.0 cm.

contrast, the same change in eccentricity produces a potential increase of only 3.8% at the epicardium. This implies that epicardial maps are not sensitive to variations in the location of the heart caused by different postures of the subject, and are almost completely free from effects of body shape and size. In this sense, a transformation from surface to epicardial maps serves both as a normalization procedure as well as enhancing resolution of intracardiac events, and therefore is of great biophysical and clinical importance. It should be added (Rudy and Plonsey, 1980), that in contrast to surface potentials, epicardial potentials are only minimally affected by the torso inhomogeneities, a property which makes them a better, more faithful reflection of the cardiac sources.

As previously discussed (Martin and Pilkington, 1972; Martin et al., 1975; Barr et al., 1977; Barr and Spach, 1976) the formulation of the inverse problem in terms of epicardial potentials has several advantages over the equivalent generator approach. The solution is unique, and can be more directly related to underlying physiological processes. The formulation in terms of potentials does not require restrictive assumptions regarding the nature of the sources to be made. The intracavitary blood inhomogeneity is taken into account implicitly in the potential formulation. In addition, inverse solutions in terms of potentials can be evaluated by a direct comparison with epicardial measurements, such as those obtained simultaneously with surface potentials in an experimental anima (Barr and Spach, 1978).

A very important consequence of potential theory is that in principle, epicardial potentials can be recovered from body surface data. Based on this capability, there is hope that epicardial data may be available noninvasively through computations based on body surface potentials (obtained by mapping techniques) and body geometry. The availability of the potential distribution over the entire torso (nearly a closed surface) permits such inverse transformation to be investigated.

Initial inverse calculations of epicardial potentials were performed utilizing the eccentric spheres model of the inhomogeneous torso. The inverse-computed epicardial potentials are given by the following expression where c_n and b_n are expansion coefficients, determined by surface integration of the torso potential data (Geselowitz, 1960), and boundary conditions at interfaces between torso inhomogeneities.

$$V_{epi} = \frac{1}{4\pi\sigma_3} \left\{ \sum_{s=1}^{\infty} \left[(\frac{d}{r_2})^{s1} \sum_{n=1}^{s} C_n \cdot \frac{1}{d^{n+1}} \cdot \frac{s!}{n!\,(s-n)!} + (\frac{r_2^s}{d}) \sum_{n=s}^{\infty} b_n \cdot d^n \cdot \frac{(-1)^{n-s} n!}{s!\,(n-s)!} \right] P_s(\cos\theta) + \sum_{n=1}^{\infty} b_n \cdot d^n \cdot (-1)^n \right\}$$

The surface integration was performed using a Gaussian quadrature technique of order 48. The data were the forward – computed surface potentials with all inhomogeneities present. Good convergence was obtained with 35 terms in the orthogonal series expansion representing the epicardial potentials (20 terms

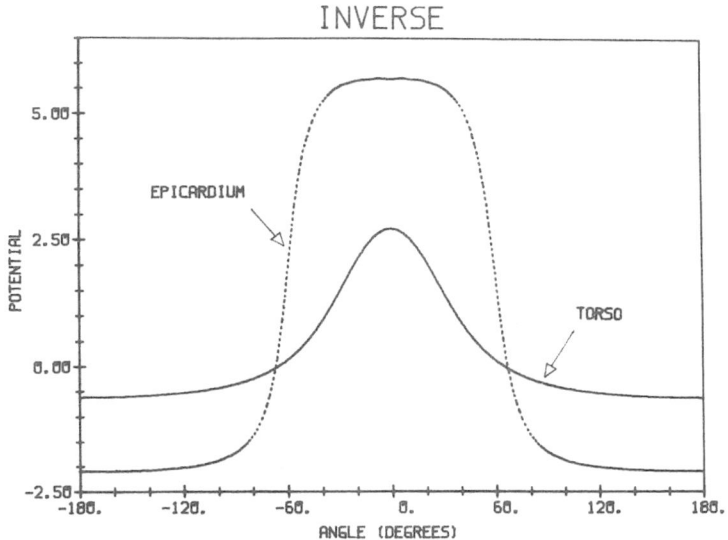

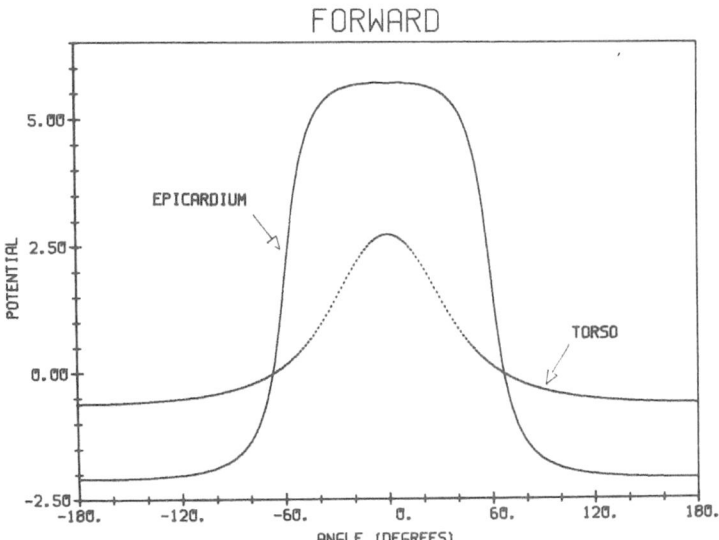

Figure 12. Figure 12 (top): Inverse reconstructed epicardial potentials (Epicardium) together with the surface data (Surface) from which they were computed. The actual forward-computed potentials are shown in Figure 12 (bottom) for comparison.

produced 3% error). The inverse – computed results were compared to the forward – computed epicardial potentials for a variety of source configurations within the (spherical) heart wall. Some of the results obtained are shown below (Figures 12 and 13).

The inverse – computed epicardial potentials together with the surface potentials from which they are computed are shown in Figure 12 (top). The calculations are for a double layer source 60° in extent (see Figure 6 for definition of geometrical parameters). The actual epicardial potentials, computed from the underlying source, are shown in Figure 12 (bottom). The agreement between the inverse – computed epicardial distribution and the actual forward – computed one is excellent. Note that the inverse – computed epicardial potentials provide a very 'sharp' reflection of the underlying source, depicting its exact location and extent. In contrast, the surface distribution is much smoother, and the extent of the surface potential maximum does not correspond to the extent of the underlying double layer.

Figure 13 shows similar results but for a different source configuration. There are two activation fronts, one extending from 20° to 30°, and the other from −20° to −30°. Figure 13 (top) shows the surface data and the inverse-reconstructed epicardial potentials. Figure 13 (bottom) shows the actual forward-computed epicardial and body surface potentials for comparison. The surface distribution exhibits only a single potential maximum and does not reflect the two discrete activation fronts. The inverse-reconstructed epicardial potentials, on the other hand, contain two separate maxima which clearly reflect the true nature of the source. The location of the activation fronts and their extent are accurately reflected in the location and extent of the reconstructed maxima. This result demonstrates the capability of the inverse procedure to accurately reconstruct multiple local cardiac events from the low resolution, smooth surface potential data. As already mentioned, this property of the inverse procedure permits detailed examination of regional electrical events within the heart in a fashion that is not possible directly from the body surface potential distribution.

It should be mentioned that the inverse solutions shown above were computed from accurate, noise-free surface data that was generated by the eccentric spheres model. This type of 'synthetic' data is useful for the study of many aspects of the inverse procedure (sensitivity to geometrical parameters and torso inhomogeneities, sensitivity to the number of surface data points, performance of various interpolation methods, etc.). In the presence of noise, regularization schemes must be utilized due to the ill-posed nature of the inverse problem (Tikhonov and Arsenin, 1977). Our derivation of stability estimates to the problem (Rudy, 1981) demonstrate the strong dependence of the solution on an *a priori* bound for the magnitude of the epicardial potential. This result suggests that by incorporating *a priori* knowledge of epicardial potentials into the regularization scheme to be used, one can greatly improve the accuracy of inverse computations.

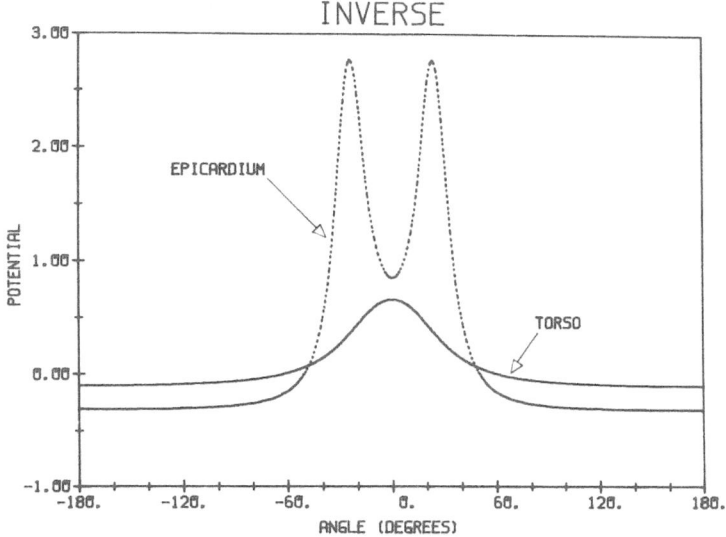

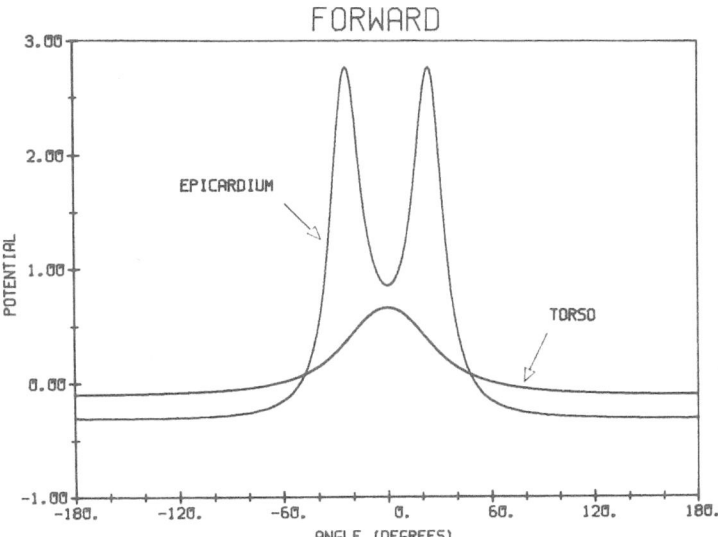

Figure 13. Figure 13 (top): Inverse reconstructed epicardial potentials (Epicardium) together with the surface data (Surface) from which they were computed. The actual forward-computed potentials are shown in Figure 13 (bottom) for comparison. Note the ability of the inverse transformation to reconstruct two distinct epicardial peaks from a single peak at the surface.

Acknowledgement

This study was supported by the National Institute of Health Grants HL 23645 and HL 17931, and by Grant HANEO-4426 from the American Heart Association, North East Ohio Affiliate, Inc.

References

Barr RC, Spach MS (1978) Inverse calculations of QRS-T epicardial potentials from body surface potential distributions for normal and ectopic beats in the intact dog. Circ Res 42:661

Barr RC, Spach MS (1976) Inverse solutions directly in terms of potentials. In: Nelson CV, Geselowitz DB (eds) The Theoretical Basis of Electrocardiology. Oxford Clarendon Press: pp 294–304

Barr RC, Ramsey M, Spach MS (1977) Relating epicardial to body surface potential distributions by means of transfer coefficients based on geometry measurements. IEEE Trans Biomed Eng 24:1–11

Beeler GW, Reuter H (1977) Reconstruction of the action potential of ventricular myocardial fibers. J Physiol London 286:177

Diaz P, Rudy Y, Plonsey R (1983) The intercalated discs as a cause for discontinuous propagation in cardiac muscle: A theoretical simulation. Ann Biomed Eng 11:177–190

Durrer D, Van Dam R Th, Freud GE, Janse MJ, Meijler FL, Arzbaecher RC (1970) Total escitation of the isolated human heart. Circ 41:899

Geselowitz DB (1960) Multiple representation for an equivalent cardiac generator. Proc of IRE 48:75–79

Ishikawa K, Berson AS, Pipberger HV (1971) Electrocardiographic changes due to cardiac enlargment. Am Heart J 81:638

King TD, Barr RC, Herman-Giddens GS, Boaz DE, Spach MS (1972) Isopotential body surface maps and their relationship to atrial potentials in the dog. Circ Res 20:393–405

Martin RO, Pilkington TC (1972) Unconstrained inverse electrocardiography: Epicardial potentials. IEEE Trans Biomed Eng 19:276–285

Martin RO, Pilkington TC, Morrow MN (1975) Statistically constrained inverse electrocardiography. IEEE Trans Biomed Eng 22:487

Nelson CV, Rand PW, Angelakos ET, Hugenholtz PG (1972) Effect of intracardiac blood on the spatial vectorcardiogram. 1. Results in the dog. Circ Res 31:95

Ramsey III M, Barr RC, Spach MS (1977) Comparison of measured torso potentials with those simulated from epicardial potentials for ventricular depolarization and repolarization in the intact dog. Circ Res 41:660

Rosenthal A, Restieaux NJ, Feig SA (1971) Influence of acute variations in hematocrit on the QRS complex of the Frank electrocardiogram. Circ 44:456

Rudy Y (1981) Inverse computation of cardiac potentials: an ill-posed problem. Proc 34th ACEMB, pp 123

Rudy Y, Diaz P, Plonsey R (1983) Discontinuous propagation of excitation in cardiac muscle: A theoretical study. Proc 10th Int Cong Electrocardiology, Bratislava, Czechoslovakia, in press

Rudy Y, Plonsey R (1980) A comparison of volume conductor and source geometry effects on body surface and epicardial potentials. Circ Res 46:283–291

Rudy Y, Plonsey R (1979) The eccentric spheres model as the basis for a study of the role of geometry and inhomogeneities in electrocardiography. IEEE Trans Biomed Eng 26:392

Rudy Y, Plonsey R, Liebman J (1979) The effects of variations in conductivity and geometrical parameters on the electrocardiogram, using an eccentric spheres model. Circ Res 44:104–111

Rudy Y, Wood R, Plonsey R, Liebman J (1982) The effect of high lung conductivity on electrocardiographic potentials: Results from human subjects undergoing bronchopulmonary lavage. Circ 65:440

Spach MS, Barr RC, Lanning CF (1978) Experimental basis for QRS and T wave potential distributions in the intact chimpanzee. Circ Res 42:103–118

Spach MS, Barr RC, Lanning CF, Tucek PC (1977) Origin of body surface QRS and T wave potentials from epicardial potential distributions in the intact chimpanzee. Circ 55:268

Tikhonov AN, Arsenin VY (1977) Solutions of ill-posed problems. Winston, Wiley

Toyama J, Okada A, Nagata Y, Okajima M, Yamada K (1974) Electrocardiographic changes in pulmonary emphysema: Effects of experimentally induced overinflation of the lungs on QRS complexes. Amer Heart J 87:606

DISCUSSION

ADAM: On one of the slides you showed the epicardial potentials and how they are related to the conductivity of the muscle tissue; and on the other hand, you showed another slide in which there is nearly no effect of the placement of your inner sphere. Can you explain the differences?

ANS: Two independent effects contribute to the epicardial potentials. The first is the effect of high conductivity skeletal muscle encircling the very low conductivity lung region, for a given location of the heart. Thus, variation in skeletal muscle conductivity for this geometry causes tremendous changes in surface potentials, but has much less effect on the potentials on the epicardium. The second effect we examined was the effect of varying the eccentricity of the heart within the torso for a given skeletal muscle conductivity. As the heart is moved closer to the lung-skeletal muscle junction, the secondary sources at that interface contribute to a 3% change in the potential on the epicardium.

GESELOWITZ: There's a corallary to that question, and that is, that in terms of the inverse problem, you have to know an awful lot about where the heart is.

ANS: We are presently investigating that issue. From the forward problem, we know that for a given source distribution within the heart, moving the heart between the two extremes causes large changes in torso potentials, but only a 3% change in the epicardial potential. For the inverse problem, we are interested in the sensitivity of the epicardial potentials to uncertainties in heart position for a given potential distribution on the torso.

BEYAR: I'm very pleased, as a physician, to see that you can resolve potentials on the heart from the surface, but I'm trying to see what the uncertaininies are. One unknown factor is the lung conductivity, for example, in a specific patient. What is the sensitivity of the inverse problem to these parameters?

ANS: The sensitivity of the inverse problem to uncertainties in heart position and in conductivities of the volume conductor can be studied using the model presented here. Althoug results presented here were only for the ideal, noisefree situation, we are continuing our studies of the effects of uncertainties on the epicarial potentials.

DINNAR: I want to ask you about the inverse problem right here. Is the absolute level of any significance, or just the relative changes? And if it is, how constant is it for a patient and what is the variation from one patient to another?

ANS: You are asking how sensitive is the inverse problem to a priori knowledge of the amplitude and distribution of potentials on the epicardium. From stability estimates of the inverse problem, derived with the help of Bob Grossman from Princeton, using an integral operator approach to the inverse problem, I can answer that the inverse problem is very sensitive to a priori information. Although the epicardial potentials are sensitive to noise on the torso, the solution of the inverse problem is even more sensitive to the a priori bounds that you impose on the epicardial potentials.

That is, the more you know, the better you can stabilize the problem and the more accurately you can estimate the solution.

DINNAR: Is it dependent on the shape, or does it depend on the absolute value? The difference between your figures is that there is a change in the center where there is also a shift upwards; and this will, probably, depend on lung properties and other properties.

ANS: Yes, that is correct. The potentials on both the epicardium and the surface are determined by the sources and by the effects of the inhomogeneities throughout the entire volume conductor.

RITMAN: I noticed in your inverse solutions that you get little upswings at the edges.

ANS: These are artifacts resulting from the truncation of an infinite series expansion to a finite number of terms. If we add 5–8 terms, the artifact disappears. Note that the deviations in the epicardial solutions are present only in the more difficult situation of two activation fronts on the posterior of the heart. The posterior of the heart is farther from the torso surface than is the anterior of the heart, and the surface potentials are correspondingly lower. The inverse solution is more difficult in the case where the information on the torso consists of low potentials with very smooth gradients. Nevertheless, accurate solutions are obtained with a higher number of multipoles.

FEIGL: Looking at this presentation and others on scanners; why cannot a technique like the convolution technique from a scanning system be used by you, since basically the scanning technique holds for sources in terms of positron emission and you have a surface; it is true the surface is irregular but Dr. Geselowitz, for example, assumed that the conductivity in the intervening region is uniform. Why can you not use a technique like that?

ANS: In principle, you may. Our mathematical treatment in terms of integral operators is similar to what is done in CAT scanning. In CAT scanning, and other scanning techniques, Radon transforms are used. The source is known, and it is projected along a ray whose path is known and can be controlled. In our situation, we use a Bergman operator that obeys Laplace's equation. The sources arise independently within the heart. As you heard from Dr. Plonsey, a very complicated pattern of propagation arises in the heart, and the resulting fields must obey Laplace's equation in an inhomogeneous torso. The simple, predictable directionality of the rays used in scanning techniques permits very accurate inverse-type solutions. Our case is much more complicated, however, because of the origin of the sources and because of the complexity of the field distribution within the torso.

Simulation of the cardiac electrical activity sequence using 3-D stochastically distributed parameters

DAN ADAM

The Julius Silver Institute, Department of Biomedical Engineering, Technion, Israel Institute of Technology, Haifa 32000, Israel

Abstract

This report outlines our efforts, present and future, of studying a model of the cardiac electrical propagation processes. The objectives of the study are: (1) to develop a model of the cardiac conduction system and the myocardial cellular electrical activity, in which the cell parameters obey a predetermined random distribution, (2) simulate the propagation of the electrical activity in the 3-D true geometry model of the left ventricle (LV), (3) test the sensitivity of the model parameters in the range of values reported for normal hearts, (4) generate pathological activities, like premature beats, tachycardia, alternans and fibrillation, by introducing cellular parameters found in a diseased hearts, (5) determine the time of activation of each point in the myocardial space, (6) calculate the body surface potential maps according to reported transfer characteristics, (7) evaluate the model's performance by comparing its sequence of body surface potential maps to experimentally and clinically generated maps. Results of down-scaled elemental models demonstrate that such models with randomly distributed parameters may initiate unpredictably premature beats, tachycardias and other pathologies. Thus, the 3-D polygonal model is expected to generate, with great spatial detail, the normal as well as pathological unstable electrical activities, and under these conditions represent the different patterns of dynamic, time varying body surface potential maps.

Introduction

The major clinical use of ECG analysis, in all its forms, has been restricted to diagnosis alone. The efforts of many researchers, as well as that of industry, has been devoted quite successfully to the interpretation of the morphology of a single beat from a single (or multiple) lead ECG, or of a single 'frame' of a body surface potential map. An impressive effort has also been invested in the analysis of ECG strips for arrhythmia analysis. The analytical techniques are based on a huge body of experimental work which was designed to study how the electrical fields are being generated and how the related potentials are determined inside the myocardium, the epicardium and on the body surface. The history of the electrocardiographic studies dates back to 1856 when the two German physiologists Kolliker and Muller were able to discern between the depolarization activity and repolatization activity by attaching the cut end of the frog's sciatic nerve to the epicardium and watch the gastrocnemius muscle twitch twice. Since then, concurrent with the advancement of the experimental work, simulation studies have shown us different models which try to explain how 'the system works'. These studies produced quantitative relationships between different potentials (measured or estimated) and the electrical generators which produced them.

The challenge which confronts us these days, after the diagnostic value of the ECG has been well proven, is to prove the prognostic value of the ECG in all its forms. The importance of such a non-invasive, inexpensive, tool cannot be overemphasized. The best way known to use electrocardiography as a prognostic tool is as an alarm of the vulnerability of the heart to dysrhythmia and fibrillation.

When trying to establish the feasibility of the ECG as a prognostic utility, it is desirable to examine the different mechanisms which lead to increased susceptibility to dysrhythmia and thus to a higher risk of mortality. In the 60's many studies (Han and Moe, 1964; Han et al., 1964; Han, 1969; Moe et al., 1964) reported that the variety of cardiac states, in which the vulnerability is high – are characterized by increased disparity of recovery times, thus coining the phrase 'Dispersion of Refractoriness' hypothesis. As it became clearer that the synchronization of the repolarization process is one of the determinants of the ST–T waveform (through measurements and models), it seemed plausible that states of increased susceptibility may be recognized from ECG waveforms. Some clinical investigations support this possibility (Zalter and Sadik, 1961; Wilson et al., 1973; Nielsen, 1973; Mandel et al., 1968).

A body of evidence was also established through animal experiments (Adam et al., 1981; 1982) in which fluctuations in T–wave morphology indicated and correlated with increased vulnerability to dysrhythmia. Although most studies today were based on single lead or orthogonal three lead systems, it seems likely that a broad, useful index of susceptibility should be based on a multiple cardiographic lead system. Body surface potential maps are the best tool for processing regional cardiac examination and thus detecting locally disparate ventricular recovery, in specified cardiac area. Wilson et al. (1934) suggested the measurement of the QRST area (ventricular gradient) as an index of recovery properties, and this index was later modified (Abildskov et al., 1980) to generate QRST iso-area maps and thus serve as local recovery index.

When trying to establish the ECG as a prognostic utility, the huge amount of existing physiological data must be supported by quantitative formulation of the relationship between the measurable surface potentials and the intracardiac events. Solving the forward problem, or alternatively simulating the generation of Body Surface Potential Maps (BSPM) accurately throughout the cardiac cycle of a normal and a sick heart, will produce quantitative indices and quantitative predictable ECG for different cardiac pathologies. The main purpose of this report is to introduce a model of the electrical conduction and activation sequence from the AV node, the HIS and Bundle branches and the Purkinje fibers to the myocardium itself. The simulation of this activity generates the electropotential wavefronts from which the myocardial dipoles and then the BSPM are calculated according to previously reported methods.

Methods

Model description

The myocardial volume of the LV (and, later, the whole heart) is sectioned into about 1 mm^3 polygons (14 faced truncated octahedron) which are stacked up to fill the whole space. The polygons are small enough to fill the space evenly and create smooth layers at the boundaries. Each polygon is a center of concentric spheres – the smallest one being the 14 polygons which touch the 14 faces of the center polygon; there is a periodicity of the radiuses which describes the larger, containing spheres. Thus, a spheric spread of excitation is simulated.

Each polygon, or cell, is characterized by a set of properties: action potential shape, orientation, different conduction velocities for each direction. The action potential is described by a few parameters in a way similar to that of Miller and Geselowitz (1978): the conduction delay a, is followed by a sharp risetime b, a phase 2 of time length $c + d$, and a phase 3 repolarization of time length e. Each of these variables is attributed a value according to a Gaussian distribution with predetermined value for the mean and Standard Error. The mean value of the effective refractory period $(c + d)$, for instance, depends on the distance of the particular cell from the center of the left ventricle, as this value was reported to change (decrease) its value from the endocardium to the epicardium. Once all values are determined, simulation produces normal activation sequences. Pathological conditions, like increased sympathetic tone, hypothermia, Digitalis toxicity, etc., produce a change in the given distributions. Under such conditions the simulation produces normal activity until an incident occurs, like premature beat, ventricular tachycardia or fibrillation. In the modeled system this might mean 'sudden death'.

Each simulation study starts with certain cells being depolarized, or paced. Under normal conditions the pacing starts along the conduction system, i.e., through the left and right bundle branches and the Purkinje fibers. These fibers are modeled by series of polygons, touching each other and set along predetermined lines (or tracks) similar to those of the conduction system of the ventricle.

These particular sets of polygons have different properties similar to those of the conduction system. The spread of activity, from one polygon to all its polarized neighbors, generates the activation wavefronts, or intra-myocardial potential maps (PM).

Generation of surface potentials

The simulation of the mathematical model generates outputs which are the intramyocardial PM as a function of time (within one beat and from beat-to-beat). These maps are of great interest and use by their own merit, i.e. for generating the time of activation of the mechanical model. On the other hand, model evaluation and use may be applied only if the model does simulate results which are comparable to data which is acquired non-invasively during experiments and clinical trials. BSPM seems to be the best technique for this purpose. The generation of BSPM from intramyocardial PM was reported by many groups (Miller and Geselowitz, 1978; Barr *et al.*, 1977; Cuffin and Geselowitz, 1977). Different methods have been suggested, and their sensitivities to many variables were tested. Many of these methods are based on developing a set of dipoles which are assumed to characterize the myocardial electrical activity; transfer coefficients are then calculated or measured, and from these the BSPM are calculated.

In our simulation studies, the models of BSPM generation, as reported by Geselowitz's group, are implemented. The models are modified to our particular needs, but retain the ideas and concepts of the original reports. These models generate the surface potentials at any given point on the 'torso' surface, and may produce also the potentials simultaneously in an array of 30 electrodes.

Interpolation is used to connect all points of similar potential at any given instant. Usually the maps are calculated and represented at 10 msec steps with voltage resolution of 10 Vm. Isochrones may also be constructed if so desired.

Results

Several models, primitive and down scaled from the one described in this report, have been tried. The most relevant model to the one presented here is that of Smith (1982) which was done in collaboration with the author of this report. In this model, which is comprised of a cylindrical, single layer of macrocells, the idea of implementing randomly distributed parameters was successfully used. The model generates normal single lead surface ECG when its parameters are within normal range. On the other hand, when one of the parameters, e.g. mean refractory period, was increased to simulate pathological conditions – normal ECG was generated for some time until unpredictably sustained VT or fibrillation occurred. Our 3-D multilayer model was constructed only recently and while no ECG was produced, the tendency of the myocardial activity to produce instabilities was observed. The ability of our model to produce circular movement of activity in more than one surface, increases its sensitivity to produce pathological behavior.

Discussion

Traditionally, the 'forward problem' (usually restricted to the ventricular depolarization and the QRS complex), has been separated to different topics:

(1) The cellular electrical activity, as associated with membrane depolarization and repolarization (Plonsey, 1974; Muler and Markin, 1978)

(2) The sequence of activation propagating from cell to cell (Young, 1957; 1956; Spach and Barr, 1975).

(3) The representation of this sequence as a single dipole (probably first described by Einthoven, 1913, as explained by Burger *et al.*, 1946, Brody *et al.*, 1964, and representing the sequence as multiple dipoles: Horan *et al.*, 1978, Selvester *et al.*, 1968; 1965, Holt *et al.*, 1969, Miller and Geselowitz, 1978, and many others.)

(4) The generation of potentials at different locations on the epicardium and the myocardium itself (Spach and Barr, 1975a; 1975b).

(5) The generation of surface ECG or body surface potential maps *directly* or through transfer coefficients from the epicardium to the body surface (Hersh *et al.*, 1978; Barr *et al.* 1977; Spach *et al.*, 1975a; 1975b; 1977).

Most investigators agree upon the several last topics, in one way or another. It is acceptable to represent the electrical activity by multiple (8, 20, 23 etc.) dipoles; the geometry of the torso as well as its inhomogeneity have a smaller effect on the generated ECG.

This report focuses on probably the most important and unclear issue of the 'forward problem' – that of the cellular electrical activity and the sequence of activity through the conduction system and the myocardial cells. Many reports focus the attention on a single cell, and the spread of activity from one cell to another. Usually the results depend heavily on the cellular geometry and many assumptions concerning the extracellular media. When trying to directly relate cardiac depolarization to torso electrocardiographic potentials most reports use a different approach to avoid computational complexity. The common approach is, therefore, that of a uniform macroscopic dipole-sheet approximation. The complexity of the interconnections among the cells, their axial orientation etc., is reduced to a single homomorphic sheet. The 'uniform' (or 'Byplane') hypothesis approximation is based on assuming a sharply defined, smooth, continuous boundary between the resting and depolarized myocardial tissue – behaving as a uniform double-layer current source as reported by Frank (1952). A segment of this surface behaves as a current dipole, pointing perpendicular to that surface – in the direction of propagation.

The 'uniform' hypothesis has been useful – and very popular – in providing a rough visualization of the origin of the electrical fields and generating the surface potentials. The validity of this hypothesis is challenged when one tries to establish the ECG (or maps) as a prognostic utility. As stated before, the accuracy needed to define prognostic indices, cannot be based on assuming identical cells in terms of action potentials, morphology direction etc. The 'dispersion' hypothesis is, therefore, used. Once this hypothesis is used to provide the activation sequence, a model similar to that of Miller and Geselowitz (1978) is used to generate the different dipoles and their associated epicardial potentials. The Barr and Spach transfer coefficients are used to generate the body surface potential maps, which are compared to measured experimental data.

The 'dispersion' hypothesis assumes that the myocardial cells are not identical in their contribution to the excitation wavefront, and in other electrical properties like the refractory period. The non-identical properties are enhanced when different perturbations are considered. There is a wide body of evidence in support of that contention, as for example, Yanovitz *et al.*, 1966, demonstrated the functional distribution of sympathetic innervation to the ventricles, and also the effect of that distribution on the ECG. Schwartz and Malliani, 1975 reported of clinical and experimental evidence of this distributed effect.

Our model is therefore based on true 3-D geometry (as defined by the mechanical model and verified by the echo scanner, 3-D reconstruction procedure). Each cell is characterized by a set of properties; each property of a cell is assigned a random value from a Gaussian distribution, the mean of which changes according to the physical location of the particular cell and also with time. Conduction velocity will be assigned different mean values according to the direction of propagation (to account for the 2:1 or even 3:1 anisotropy), and whether the cell is part of the conduction system or the myocardium itself.

We believe that such a model will produce normal as well as pathological surface potentials, when the distributions are modeled in a similar way to what occurs in disease. The model inherently contains the possibility for generating dysrhythmia and fibrillation when conditions change. It may therefore be useful in establishing the surface potentials as a prognostic utility.

References

Abildskov JA, Evans AK, Burgess MJ (1980) Ventricular recovery properties and QRST deflection in cardiac electrograms. A J Physiol 239:H227–231

Adam DR, Akselrod S, Cohen RJ (1981) Estimation of ventricular vulnerability to fibrillation through T-wave time series analysis. Comp in Card 307–310

Adam DR, Powell AO, Gordon H, Cohen RJ (1982) Ventricular fibrillation and fluctuations in the magnitude of the repolarization vector. Comp in Card 241–244

Barr RC, Ramsey M, Spach MS (1977) Relating epicardial to body surface potential distributions by means of transfer coefficients based on geometry measurements. IEEE Trans. Bio-Med Eng BME-24:1–11

Brody D, Arzbaecher R (1964) A comparative analysis of severall correlated vectorcardiographic leads. Circulation 39:533–542

Burger HC, van Milaan JB (1946) Heart vector and leads. British Heart J 8:157

Cuffin BN, Geselowitz DB (1977) Studies of the electrocardiogram using realistic cardiac and torso models. IEEE Trans Bio-Med Eng. BME-24:242–252

Durrer D, van Dam RT, Freud GE, Janse MJ, Meijler FL, Arzbaecher RC (1970) Total excitation of the isolated human heart. Circulation 41:899–912

Einthoven W, Farh G, deWaart A (1913) Pflugers Arch ges Physiol., 150:275–315

Frank E (1952) Electric potential produced by two point sources in a homogeneous conducting sphere. J Appl Phys 23:1225–1228

Han J (1969) Ventricular vulnerability during acute coronary occlusion. Am J Card 24:857–864

Han J, Moe GK (1964) Nonuniform recovery of excitability in ventricular muscle. Circ Res 14:44–60

Han J, de-Jalon PG, Moe GK (1964) Adrenergic effects on ventricular vulnerability. Circ Res 14:516–520

Han J, Millet D, Chizzonitti B, Moe GK (1966) Temporal dispersion of recovery of excitability in atrium and ventricle as function of heart rate. Am Hear J 71:481–487

Hersh LT, Barr RC, Spach MS (1978) An analysis of transfer coefficients calculated directly from epicardial and body surface potential measurements in the intact dog. IEEE Trans Bio-Med Eng BME-25:446–461

Holt JH, Barnard ACL, Lynn MS (1969) A study of the human heart as a multiple dipole electrical source. Circulation 40:697–710

Horan LG, Hand C, Johnson JC, Sridharan MR, Rankin TB, Flowers NC (1978) A theoretical examination of ventricular repolarization and the secondary T wave. Circ Res 42:750–757

Mandel WJ, Burgess MJ, Neville J, Abildskov JA (1968) Analysis of T waveform abnormalities associated with myocardial infarction using a theoretical model. Circulation 38:178–188

Moe GK, Abildskov JA, Han J (1964) Factors responsible for initiation and maintenance of ventricular fibrillation. In 'Sudden Cardiac Death', NY Grune & Stratton 56–63

Nielsen BL (1973) ST-segment elevation in acute myocardial infarction: Prognostic importance. Circulation 48:338–345

Miller WT, Geselowitz DB (1978) Simulation studies of the electrocardiogram. Circ Res 43:301–315

Muler AL, Markin VS (1978) Electrical properties of anisotropic nerve-muscle syncytia. Biophysic 22:536–541

Plonsey R (1974) The formulation of bioelectric source-field relationships in terms of surface discontinuities. J Franklin Inst 297:317–324

Ramsey III, Barr RC, Spach MS (1977) Comparison of measured torso potentials with those simulated from epicardial potentials for ventricular depolarization and repolarization in the intact dog. Circ Res 41:660–672

Scher AM, Young AC (1956) The pathway of ventricular depolarization in the dog. Circ Res 4:461–469

Scher AM, Young AC (1956–7) Ventricular depolarization and the genesis of QRS. Ann NY Acad Sci 65:768

Schwarz PJ, Malliani A (1975) Electrical alternation of the T wave. Am Heart J 89:45–50

Selvester RH, Solomon JC, Gillespie TL (1968) Digital Computer model of a total body electrocardiographic surface map. Circ 38:684–690

Selvester RH, Kalaba E, Collier CR, Bellman R, Kajiwada H (1965) Simulated myocardial infarction with a mathematical model of the heart containing distance and boundary effects. Proc LI Symp on Vector-cardiography, Queens, NY

Smith JM (1982) Finite element model of ventricular dysrhythmias. MSc thesis, MIT Cambridge, Mass

Spach MS, Barr RC (1975a) Ventricular intramural and epicardial potential distributions during ventricular activation and repolarization in the intact dog. Circ Res 37:243–257

Spach MS, Barr RC (1975b) Analysis of ventricular activation and repolarization from intramural and epicardial potential distributions for ectopic beats in the intact dog. Circ Res 37:830–843

Spach MS, Barr RC, Lanning CF (1977) Experimental basis for QRS and T wave potentials in the WPW syndrome. Circ Res 42:103–118

Wilson FN, Macleod AG, Barker PS, Johnson FD (1934) The determination and significance of the areas of the ventricular deflections of the electrocardiogram. Am Heart J 10:46–61

Wilson C, Pantridge JF (1973) ST-segment displacement and early hospital discharge in acute myocardial infarction. Lancet 2:1284–1288

Yanowitz F, Preston JB, Abildskov JA (1966) Function distribution of right and left stellate innervation to the ventricles. Circ. Res. 18:416–428

Zalter R, Sadik E (1961) Prognostic significance of the magnitude of ST segment shift in myocardial infarction. Circulation 24:1075–1076

DISCUSSION

RUDY: I have a question about the finite element electrical model of the heart. Do you plan on incorporating the actual conduction system as part of it? Or how would you establish isochrones and the sequence of activation?

ANS: The sequence of activation is generally received by the formulation that Dr. Geselowitz used in his paper. The main difference is in the production of those potentials, i.e., the laws of the propagation of the electrical activity through the conduction system and myocardial cells.

RUDY: In an ischemic state, the ischemic myocardium would affect the action potential of that region but may also affect the order of propogation and may interact with the order of propogation as determined by the conduction system. So even in ischemia there is another effect which is not just the effect of changing action potentials but also one affecting the order of propogation. Therefore it is not the complete picture. You have to incorporate the conduction system in order to incorporate changes in the order of the activation sequence.

ANS: We will incorporate it, but as a second stage in the construction of our model due to the complexity and uncertainty involved. Your comment means that there is a general change in conduction properties in diseased condition. This can be incorporated by the delayed time parameter, A, that can be increased or changed according to different needs. This means that now each cell does not excite the next one at each time interval of simulation, but at some point after a time delay.

RUDY: You want to incorporate different activation sequences by incorporating different delays.

ANS: Yes, this is one parameter among others that we plan to modify to generate different activation sequences. The conduction system in a diseased heart is a very complicated issue because of all the computations needed to do that. It's just a matter of patience and time in order to give the particular cells their different physiological and spatial properties. One can do that and we plan to do that.

AKSELROD: It should be quite easy to do. You can decide upon a certain strain of fibers, give them a certain refractory period, and give all the rest the Gaussian distribution. It would be as easy as giving the Gaussian distribution to all the other cells of the myocardium

ANS: I'm sure that's the way to do it but its's not that easy, because you need to follow predetermined spatial, 3-D conduction pathways.

RUDY: The problem is really to accurately know the geometry of the conduction system. There is also a second problem: there are certain electrophysiological properties to the conduction system, other than the velocity of propogation (which is, say, five times as high). There is this controversy about how the conduction system acts once you enter it not in the proper way. If you come from the AV node, the signal spreads through the conduction sytem and seems to leave the conduction system at terminations, which is, of course, complicated by the geometry. That's the reason why you create activation fronts that are parallel to the cavity, going perpendicularly from endocardium to epicardium. For the adnormal situation, when you excite the heart somewhere else, it's not very well understood what effect the conduction system has under those conditions, whether you penetrate it at all, or not. This is a difficult case, physiologically, to simulate at this point, mainly because we don't know how it operates under those conditions. In a normal situation we know more. It is an important part of the model because that's the main factor in determining the sequence of activation. If you then want to simulate an abnormal activation sequence, you have to have that because that gives you the initial conditions for what happens in the myocardium after that.

GESELOWITZ: How many cells do you have in your model at this point?

ANS: Same as in your model; to simulate the propagation in the myocardium alone.

GESELOWITZ: In our model, incidently, we put in by hand the activation time based on Durrer's model. If you want to simulate activation, the evidence of people who tried it is that you need of the order of 2 million points. These models have always intrigued me. They can give us a lot of insight. There is a kind of background caution one has to have in terms of understanding what is really going on in terms of the model. The first study of this kind that I am aware of was by Van der Paul who basically used a variation of the Van der Paulian equation. It's a non linear equation and non linear systems have all kinds of behaviour. The Van der Paul equation which has no relation to cardiac electrophysiology gives you all kinds of strange oscillations that are observed in the heart. So, you can build in all these refractory periods and so forth which presumably have an electrophysiological basis, and of course, they are going to give results that you can see in the heart. Is it really corresponding to what's going on? I think we are getting closer to that but my point is that with a non linear system, almost any non linear equation can give all this bizarre behaviour, and the heart exhibits all kind of bizarre behaviour.

Plonsey: Since your goal is to determine the activation sequence, I don't think you achieved your goal if you require in a sense too much information. If you require for your model to know the activation sequence, if you have to put that into the model to get the activation sequence, then the model hasn't generated anything you didn't already know. I don't see how you can generate an activation sequence unless you put in somewhere the membrane properties. Otherwise all you put into your model is some kind of algorithm which is just assumed and answered in a way.

ANS: Your comment is very true, as a model does not generate anything new if it requires the same amount of information as the amount it produces. But I do not think this is the case here. Our model does not require knowing the activation sequence. All it needs are some rules by which to play – the geometry (of the ventricular myocardium, of the basic cell and of the conduction system), how one cell affects its neighbours and the shape of the distribution of the different parameters. As the parameters may vary with time and the initial conditions are different for each beat – a wide range of activation sequence patterns is generated. The same model, obeying the same rules, produces normal activation fronts parallel to the cavity while some time later it may produce chaotic patterns. Although it is, no doubt, an ad hoc model, we may gain from it a lot of insight about how myocardial instability is produced, about the sensitivity of the normal myoelectrical activity to the different cellular parameters and their spatial distribution and about the accuracy and usefulness of the laws by which the activity propagates.

RUDY: I agree completely with Dr. Plonsey and Dr. Geselowitz but I don't think that it means we shouldn't try to incorporate these kinds of algorithms into our models. It is true that we have to try and understand everything that is going on in the membrane, but as you reported today, when you go to two dimensions and it is very complex, then you have to give up and average the properties by assigning to one point in space the properties of the intracellular, extracellular and so on. You average everything out. On the other hand, you have to go back to one dimension in order to include the structure of discontinuities. I think it will take many years before we actually incorporate the membrane properties. On top of that there are microscopic structural discontinuities like the ones that Madison Spach has been talking about in terms of connective tissues septa in the muscle and so on. We can continue to learn a lot of the underlying basic mechanism from these kinds of models. At the same time we can incorporate all the knowledge that is obtained from those models into what Bob Plonsey justifiably calls ad hoc models. Ad hoc models can produce some interesting important results and that is the level at which we are now, at which we can incorporate the conduction system to create different activation sequences. There is a certain work by Okagima. They divided the heart into, say twelve finite elements, and assigned ad hoc different conduction velocities to parts which model the conduction system and they managed to get very nice results. They managed to duplicate the Durrer's isochrones with a very good accuracy. It's again an ad hoc model but is has its benefits.

PALTI: Let me just add to those who are interested in the membrane mechanisms, with which I am more familiar. We now have here in Haifa specific antibodies to ionic channels in the heart. In other words, we can block specific channels, like sodium channels, in the heart by specific antibodies in mammals. So whoever feels he may make use of these kinds of things, we will try to help him.

Metabolic control of coronary blood flow

ROBERT M. BERNE
*Department of Physiology, University of Virginia School of Medicine,
Charlottesville, VA 22908, U.S.A.*

Abstract

Coronary blood flow is closely linked to the metabolic activity of the heart under a variety of physiological conditions. Several agents have been suggested as messengers between the parenchymal tissue and the vascular smooth muscle of the coronary resistance vessels. Among these are oxygen tension, carbon dioxide, lactic acid, adenosine, osmolarity and prostaglandin. A decrease in pH produces only a small decrease in coronary resistance, an increase in osmolarity has a negligible effect on coronary blood flow, oxygen tension, probably acts indirectly via release of a vasodilator substance and the prostaglandins have not been shown to play a physiological role in the regulation of coronary blood flow. Adenosine fulfills many of the criteria for a mediator of metabolically linked coronary vasodilation. Adenosine is produced by and released from the myocardial cells when the oxygen supply becomes inadequate for the oxygen needs of the myocardium under physiological and pathophysiological conditions. Hence, adenosine is a major factor but not the only factor involved in the metabolic regulation of coronary blood flow.

Introduction

For over one hundred years it has been recognized that a parallelism exists between tissue metabolic activity and blood flow. In the case of the heart, this relationship was clearly demonstrated by Eckenhoff *et al.* (1947) who observed a good correlation between myocardial oxygen consumption ($M\dot{V}O_2$) and coronary blood flow (CBF) under basal conditions and with several different experimental interventions that increased cardiac oxygen utilization. This correlation is of course not unexpected since the oxygen content of coronary venous blood is quite small and enhanced oxygen requirements must be met chiefly by an increase in CBF.

Another well established observation that supports a cause and effect relationship (within certain limits) between $M\dot{V}O_2$ and CBF is the parallelism between the duration of brief (ca. 5–180 s) coronary artery occlusions and the duration of the reactive hyperemia that occurs upon release of the occlusion. The prevailing concept is that with an inadequate oxygen supply for the needs of the heart, whether this be a reduced oxygen delivery resulting from hypoxemia or ischemia, or an increase oxygen demand caused by enhanced myocardial activity, a vasodilator substance is released by the parenchymal tissue. This substance enters the interstitial fluid and reaches the vascular smooth muscle of the resistance vessels where it elicits relaxation. This concept is predicated on the existence of nonneurogenic vascular smooth muscle tone, for which there is abundant evidence. The nature of the vasodilator agent that serves as messenger from the parenchymal tissue to the resistance vessels has been the objective of numerous studies. Several substances have been proposed as the mediator of metabolic vasodilation and the most important of these will be evaluated.

Mediators of metabolic vasodilation

Oxygen tension

An increase in oxygen tension of arterial blood (PaO_2) as produced by inhalation of 100% oxygen, results in an increase in coronary vascular resistance (Sobol *et al.*, 1962), whereas a decrease in PaO_2 elicits coronary vasodilation (Hilton and Eichholtz, 1925). Similar effects in response to changes in PO_2 have been observed with helical strips of coronary arteries (Gellai *et al.*, 1973). In a dog heart-lung preparation Hilton and Eichholtz (1925) observed a marked increase in CBF with hypoxemia which they attributed to a direct effect of oxygen lack on the vascular smooth muscle of the coronary vessels. However, hypoxemia in the open-chest dog, in which myocardial oxygen supply was maintained by hyperperfusion (high coronary perfusion pressure) did not elicit coronary vasodilation (Berne *et al.*, 1957). In brief, PO_2 per se did not influence coronary vascular resistance, whereas a reduction in cardiac oxygen supply decreased it. In these experiments (Berne *et al.*, 1957), a progressive decrease in coronary arterial blood oxygen content did not affect coronary resistance until coronary sinus oxygen levels fell below about 5.5 vol. % (Figure 1).

Another observation that militates against a direct effect of PO_2 on vascular smooth muscle is that within 1–2 s, after the onset of reactive hyperemia, the coronary venous blood becomes bright red (high PO_2). If PO_2 directly affected coronary resistance one would expect a prompt return of CBF to control levels after release of a brief (10–60 s) coronary occlusion. Hence, it is evident that the decrease in coronary vascular resistance observed with hypoxemia is probably secondary to the release of a vasodilator substance triggered by an inadequate oxygen supply to the myocardium.

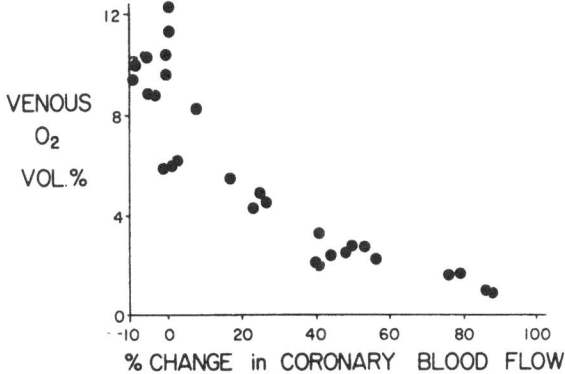

Figure 1. Relationship of oxygen content of coronary sinus blood to coronary blood flow during progressive hypoxemia. (Reproduced by permission from the Journal of Clinical Investigation 36:1101, 1957.)

Carbon dioxide and lactic acid – pH effects

There is general agreement that a decrease in pH produces coronary vasodilation and an increase elicits the opposite effect. However, the changes in CBF with changes in pH are small relative to what one observes under conditions of altered myocardial metabolic activity. In studies with a heart-lung preparation an increase in level of CO_2 produced only a small increment in CBF (Hilton and Eichholtz, 1925). More recently greater changes in CBF were observed with an increase in PCO_2 (Case *et al.*, 1978), but the levels of CO_2 were quite high and there is no good evidence that PCO_2 reaches such high levels under physiological conditions. There is also no evidence that lactic acid is released by the heart unless there is an impairment of oxygen supply. In short, a decrease in pH can produce coronary vasodilation but the effect is small and not of paramount importance.

Potassium

In 1938 Katz and Lindner showed that a small increase in arterial K^+ levels produced coronary vasodilation, whereas a large increase produced coronary vasoconstriction. In 1941, Dawes suggested that K^+ might serve as a physiological mediator of metabolically-induced vasodilation. Under steady state conditions Driscol and Berne (1957) observed only a small increase in CBF with intracoronary infusion of KCl sufficient to elevate K^+ levels 2–4 fold. Furthermore, procedures that produced increases in CBF (such as aortic constriction, asphyxia, catecholamine or dinitrophenol administration) failed to cause a measurable release of K^+ from the myocardium. Transient increments in CBF have been elicited by intracoronary injection of KCl (Murray and Sparks, 1978) and in helical strips of coronary arteries, K^+ only elicited an unsustained relaxation of the vessel (Gellai and Detar, 1974). Hence, K^+ could only account for the initial increase in CBF that occurs with enhanced myocardial metabolism. In addition, coronary sinus blood collected during myocardial hypoxia or increased cardiac work did not elicit vasodilation when it was reoxygenated and infused into a test coronary artery (Jelliffe *et al.*, 1957). If K^+ were a physiological coronary vasodilator one would not expect the action to be destroyed or inactivated by reoxygenation of the cardiac venous blood.

Adenosine

The nucleoside adenosine meets many of the requirements of a mediator of metabolic regulation of CBF (Berne, 1980). Early analysis of cardiac effluent collected under conditions of reduced oxygen supply revealed only the presence of nonvasoactive degradative products of adenosine. Subsequently, with the availability of better methods, adenosine was recovered in the venous effluents of isolated and in situ hypoxic hearts (Katori and Berne, 1966; Rubio *et al.*, 1969). The effect of ischemia on the adenosine content of rat hearts is depicted in Figure 2. This hearts were frozen in situ in the open-chest rat following different periods of cross-clamping at the atrioventricular groove. Significant increases in myocardial adenosine levels occurred within 5 s, peaked at about 22 s and then leveled off at about 3 times control levels (Berne and Rubio, 1979). When hypoxemia was produced in open-chest rats by changing ventilating gas from room air to 10% O_2, the myocardial content of adenosine almost tripled (Berne *et al.*, 1970), and in the isolated perfused guinea pig heart adenosine release, cardiac adenosine content and coronary flow increased in a parallel fashion with progressive reduction of the oxygen content of the perfusion fluid (Rubio *et al.*, 1974). Even during a single cardiac cycle, significant changes in the cardiac levels of adenosine occurred; peak levels of myocardial adenosine coincided with midsystole and lowest levels were found in mid diastole (Thompson *et al.*, 1980). From the adenosine studies discussed above it is apparent that an inadequate myocardial oxygen supply results in adenosine production. However, if oxygen is supplied in excess of myocardial needs, such as by administration of nitroglycerin, the increase in coronary flow is associated with a decrease in cardiac adenosine levels (Berne *et al.*, 1983B). This is illustrated in Figure 3.

Since oxygen supply is usually unimpaired under physiological conditions, whereas oxygen demand can be quite variable, it is of critical importance to study the relationship of coronary flow and adenosine formation with altered levels of myocardial metabolic activity. Experiments were conducted in the open-chest rat in which cardiac work was increased by constriction of the thoracic aorta just above the diaphragm (Foley *et al.*, 1978). The increased pressure work of the left ventricle was associated with an increase in the adenosine content of the myocardium (Figure 4). If the sum of adenosine and its degradative products, inosine and

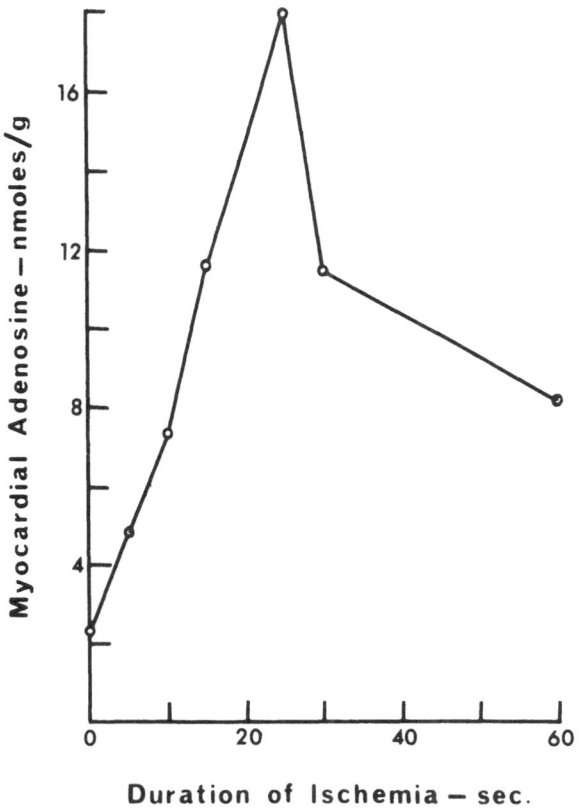

Figure 2. Effect of ischemia on myocardial adenosine levels in the rat heart. (Reproduced by permission of the American Heart Association from Circulation Research 34:109 (Suppl III) 1974.)

hypoxanthine are plotted against cardiac work an even greater significant change is observed (Figure 5). In these aortic constriction experiments, the coronary vessels were also exposed to the high perfusion pressure resulting from aortic constriction, and hence it is very unlikely that the oxygen supply is compromised.

In another series of experiments the effects of various interventions (stellate ganglion stimulation, aortic constriction, pacing, norepinephrine or calcium administration) were performed in the anesthetized open-chest dog while CBF, arterial and coronary sinus blood oxygen contents and cardiac adenosine release were monitored (Miller *et al.*, 1979; Knabb *et al.*, 1983a). Adenosine release from the epicardial surface of the heart was determined by injecting warm Krebs-Henseleit solution into the pericardial space immediately before the onset of each control and experimental period and then removing it after 4.5 min and measuring its content of adenosine. This method provides only a crude estimate of adenosine release but the correlations among the 3 variables ($M\dot{V}O_2$, CBF, and adenosine release) were significant with all interventions.

314

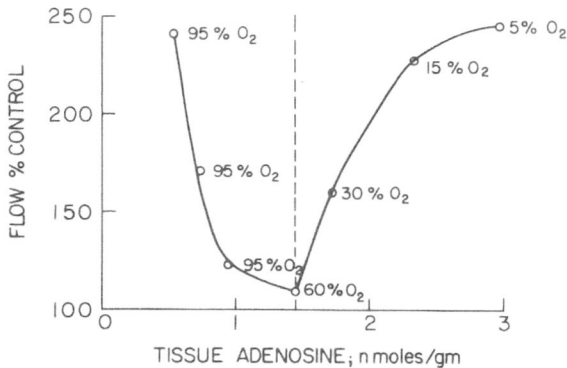

Figure 3. An increase in coronary flow is associated with either an increase or decrease in adenosine tissue levels in isolated guinea pig hearts perfused with Krebs-Henseleit solution. The points to the right of the vertical broken line were obtained by perfusing the hearts with solutions equilibrated with gas mixtures containing various amounts of O_2 (numbers beside each point). The points to the left of the vertical broken line show an increase in blood flow by infusion of various concentrations of nitroglycerin in solutions equilibrated with 95% O_2. (Reproduced by permission from Progress in Cardiovascular Disease 24:243, 1981.)

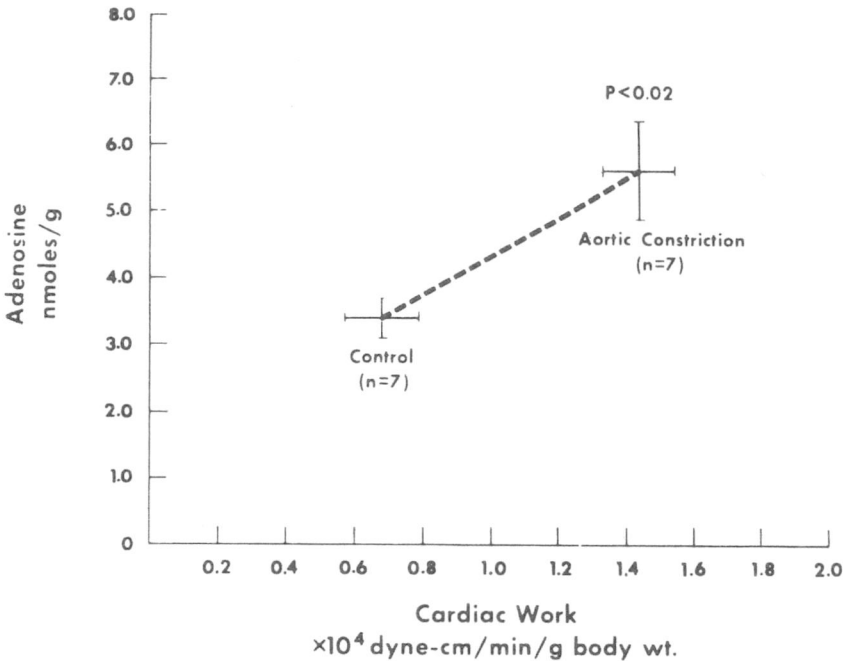

Figure 4. Effect of increased external cardiac work produced by thoracic aortic constriction on the myocardial adenosine content of the rat heart.

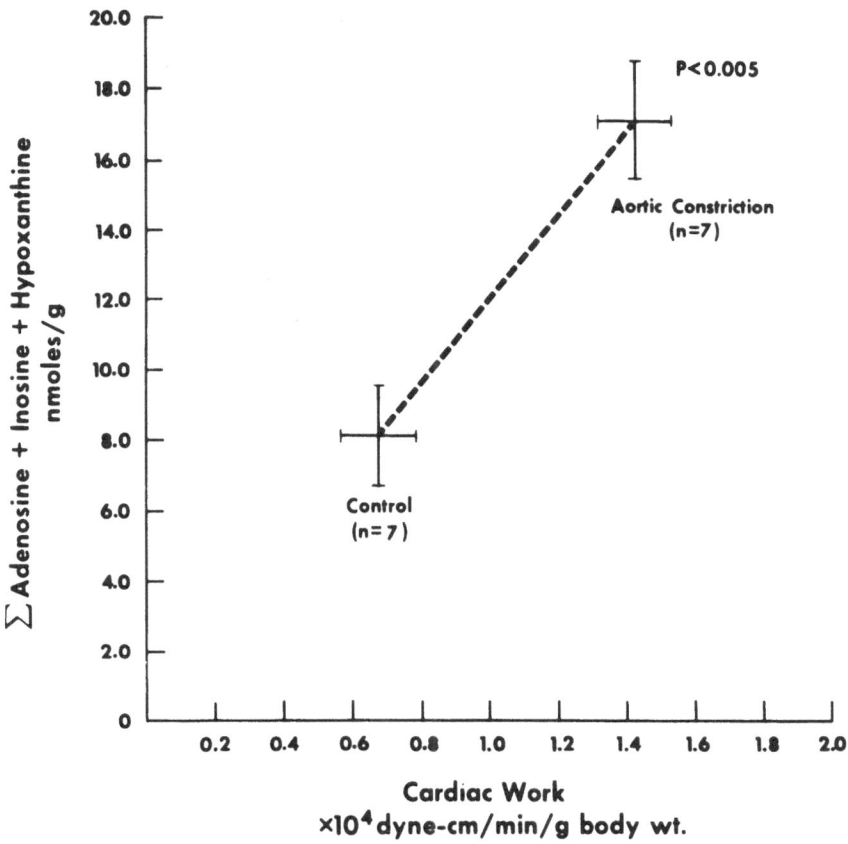

Figure 5. Effect of increased external cardiac work produced by thoracic aortic constriction on the sum of the myocardial adenosine, inosine and hypoxanthine contents of the rat heart.

The studies on anesthetized dogs were followed by experiments on un-anesthetized dogs. Under pentobarbital anesthesia, flow probes, catheters and tubes were appropriately placed and their connectors were exteriorized at the back of the animal. The dogs wore vests to protect the wires and tubes, and after about 2 weeks, when the animals were completely recovered from the surgery and trained to run on a treadmill, the studies were begun. Three physiological stimuli were employed, running on a treadmill at 2 and 4 m.p.h. at a grade of 10%, excitement produced by a loud noise, and feeding after a 24 h fast (Bacchus *et al.*, 1982). The results of these experiments are shown in Figure 6 and are essentially the same as those obtained with other interventions in the anesthetized dog.

In 1970 Kübler *et al.* demonstrated that treatment of the isolated perfused dog heart with dipyridamole resulted in an increase in the myocardial concentration of adenosine and a decrease in the release of the nucleoside in the venous effluent. Similar findings were obtained in the isolated perfused guinea pig heart by Degenring *et al.* (1976). One interpretation of these observations is that dipyridamole, which is known to block uptake of adenosine, also blocks release

316

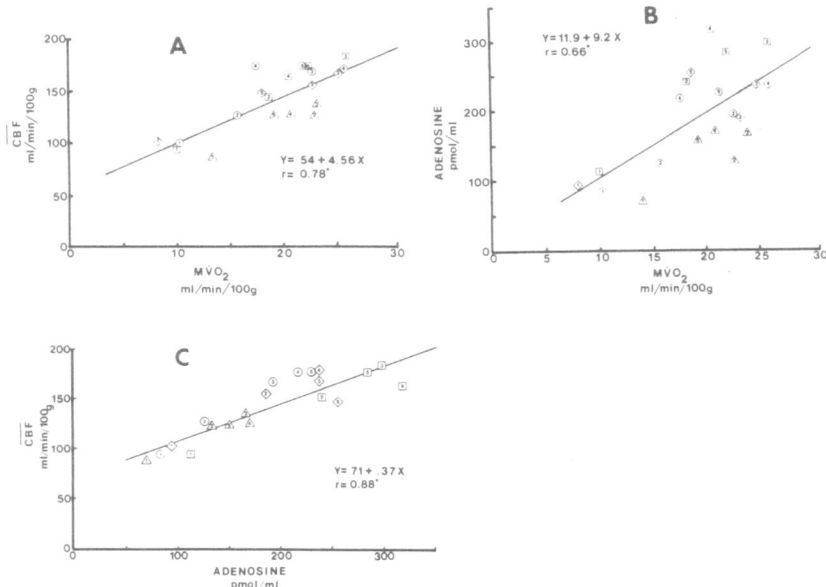

Figure 6. Relationship between A, myocardial oxygen consumption ($M\dot{V}O_2$) and mean coronary blood flow ($\overline{CBF}$), B – $M\dot{V}O_2$ and adenosine concentration in pericardial infusate, C – adenosine concentration in pericardial perfusate and $\overline{CBF}$. The different symbols represent different dogs. Numbers within symbols represent experimental maneuvers where 1 is control, 2 is 2 mph, 3 is 4 mph, 4 is excitement, and 5 is feeding. * Denotes that correlation coefficient (r) is statistically significant, n = 20. (Reproduced by permission from the American Journal of Physiology 243:H628, 1982.)

of the nucleoside, and that the high tissue levels of adenosine and the decreased release into the cardiac effluents produced by dipyridamole are due to trapping and accumulation of adenosine in the cardiac myocytes (Kübler *et al.*, 1970). If this is true then adenosine could not be a mediator of the coronary vasodilation caused by dipyridamole. Another interpretation is that dipyridamole blocks uptake but not release of adenosine from myocardial cells, a conclusion that is supported by the findings of Mustafa *et al.* (1975) that in cultured chick embryo heart cells adenosine uptake is blocked by dipyridamole but release is unaffected by the drug. Hence, it is possible that the enhanced adenosine formation produced by hypoxia is released into the interstitial space and accumulates there because the dipyridamole inhibits uptake into the myocardium as well as transport into the vascular compartment. This interpretation is quite speculative but is consonant with the experimental observations.

Recently, the effect of dipyridamole on the relationships among CBF, $M\dot{V}O_2$ and adenosine release were studied in the open-chest dog under basal conditions (Table 1) and during several different interventions that increase the rate of cardiac metabolism (Berne *et al.*, 1983a; Knabb *et al.*, 1983b). Adenosine release was measured in a pericardial infusate by the method described above. As shown in Table 1 and Figure 7, the relationship between $M\dot{V}O_2$ and CBF as well as that

Table 1. Effects of dipyridamole on cardiac adenosine release and coronary blood flow during basal conditions in the open-chest dog

Parameter[a]	Control	Dipyridamole
CBF, ml/(min · 100 g)	39.7 ± 1.6[b]	50.9 ± 1.7[c]
MVO$_2$, ml/(min · 100 g)	6.6 ± 0.4	6.5 ± 0.4
PCI ADO, pmol/ml	45.4 ± 5.2	80.6 ± 7.0[c]
CVR, peripheral resistance units/100 g	2.68 ± 0.14	1.94 ± 0.13[c]
O$_2$ EXT, ml/dl	16.8 ± 1.0	12.9 ± 0.8[d]
CSO$_2$, ml/dl	3.8 ± 0.1	8.0 ± 0.7[c]

[a] CBF, coronary blood flow, MVO$_2$, myocardial oxygen consumption; PCI ADO, pericardial infusate adenosien concentration (see text for details); CVR, coronary resistance; O$_2$ EXT, oxygen extraction by the heart; CSO$_2$, coronary sinus blood oxygen levels. [b] Values are means ± SEM. [c] Difference between control and dipyridamole treatment $P<0.01$. [d] $P<0.5$. (Reproduced by permission from Fed Proc 42:3136, 1983).

between MVO$_2$ and pericardial adenosine levels were significantly altered by dipyridamole. In brief, for any given level of MVO$_2$, the CBF and adenosine release were greater after the administration of dipyridamole. However, the relationship between pericardial adenosine levels and CBF was unchanged by dipyridamole. This suggests a cause and effect relation between adenosine release and CBF, regardless of the level of MVO$_2$.

Another observation that is in agreement with the adenosine hypothesis for the metabolic regulation of CBF is that administration of adenosine deaminase (the enzyme that deaminates adenosine to inactive inosine) reduces the coronary flow increment as well as the cardiac adenosine levels produced by hypoxia (Berne *et al.*, 1983b).

How adenosine induces relaxation of vascular smooth muscle is conjectural, although there is some evidence that the nucleoside blocks calcium uptake and/or prevents calcium from reaching the contractile machinery of the target tissue (Fenton *et al.*, 1982). It is also conceivable that adenosine may act by increasing cyclic AMP levels in the vascular smooth muscle and thereby inhibiting constriction. However, evidence in support of this concept is lacking (Herlihy *et al.*, 1976). It appears that the activity of 5'-nucleotidase (the enzyme that dephosphorylates AMP to form adenosine) is inhibited *in vivo* since it is 100 times more active *in vitro* than *in vivo*. The factor or factors that regulate 5'-nucleotidase activity are not known, although it is known that ATP, ADP and creatine phosphate inhibit the enzyme, whereas free magnesium potentiates its activity.

318

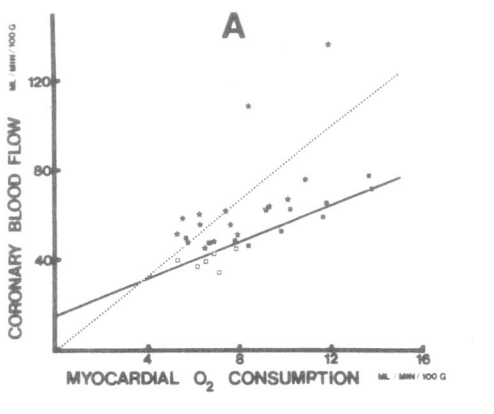

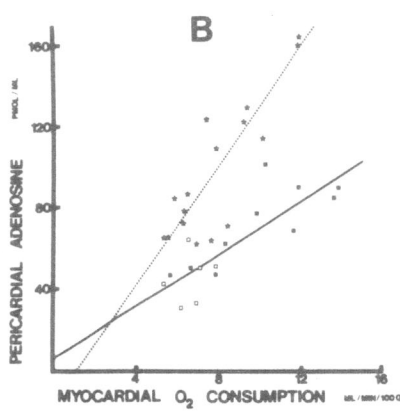

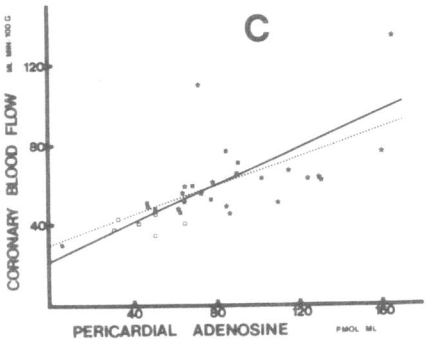

Figure 7. Effect of dipyridamole on the interrelationships between myocardial oxygen consumption and coronary blood flow (A), myocardial oxygen consumption and pericardial infusate concentration of adenosine (B), and pericardial infusate concentration of adenosine and coronary blood flow (C) in the anesthetized open-chest untreated dog (solid lines) during basal conditions (open squares) and interventions (open stars), such as aortic constriction, calcium infusion, norepinephrine infusion, and atrial pacing. The closed squares and stars represent the control and experimental procedures, respectively, when carried out in the presence of dipyridamole (dotted lines). Note that in A and B, dipyridamole shifts the curves to the left (greater flow for the same oxygen consumption). In C, the close parallelism between adenosine release and coronary blood flow is unaffected by dipyridamole. (Reproduced by permission of Martinus Nijhoff publishing, Boston, *The Regulatory Function of Adenosine,* In Berne RM, Rall TW, Rubio R (eds), p. 293, 1983).

Other factors

An increase in osmolarity that can occur during increased muscle activity has been suggested as a mechanism for the local metabolic regulation of blood flow (Mellander and Lundvall, 1971). However, in the case of the heart, the data do not support osmotic control of CBF (Scott and Radawski, 1971). Another potential agent for the role of regulator of coronary resistance is prostaglandin. The prostaglandins fail to fulfill several of the criteria for such a mediator but more data are needed to definitely rule them in or out.

Conclusions

In all likelihood no single factor is responsible for the link between myocardial metabolic activity and CBF. Adenosine probably plays a major role but other known or unknown factors undoubtedly participate in the physiological regulation of CBF.

Acknowledgement

Much of the research reported in this paper was supported by grant HL10384.

References

Bacchus AN, Ely SW, Knabb RM, Rubio R, Berne RM (1982) Adenosine and coronary blood flow in conscious dogs during normal physiological stimuli. Am J Physiol 243:H628–H633

Berne RM (1980) The role of adenosine in the regulation of coronary blood flow. Circ Res 47:807–813

Berne RM, Blackmon JR, Gardner TH (1957) Hypoxemia and coronary blood flow. J Clin Invest 36:1101–1106

Berne RM, Rubio R, Duling BR, Wiedmeier VT (1970) Effects of acute and chronic hypoxia on coronary blood flow. Adv Cardiol 5:56–66

Berne RM, Knabb RM, Ely SW, Rubio R (1983a) Adenosine in the local regulation of blood flow: A brief overview. Federation Proc 42:3136:3142

Berne RM, Rubio R (1974) Adenine nucleotide metabolism in the heart. Circ Res 34 and 35 (Suppl. III):109–120

Berne RM, Winn HR, Knabb RM, Ely SW, Rubio R (1983b) Blood flow regulation by adenosine in heart, brain, and skeletal muscle. In: Berne RM, Rall TW, Rubio R (eds) Regulatory Function of Adenosine. Boston: Martinus Nijhoff Publishing

Case RB, Felix A, Wachter M, Kyriakidis G, Castellana F (1978) Relative effect of CO_2 on canine coronary vascular resistance. Circ Res 42:410–418

Dawes GS (1941) The vaso-dilator action of potassium. J Physiol London 99:224–238

Degenring FH, Curnish RR, Rubio R, Berne RM (1976 Effect of dipyridamole on myocardial adenosine metabolism and coronary flow in hypoxia and reactive hyperemia in the isolated perfused guinea pig heart. J Molec Cell Cardiol 8:877–888

Driscol TE, Berne RM (1957) Role of potassium in regulation of coronary blood flow. Proc Soc Exptl Biol Med 96:505–508

Eckenhoff JE, Hafkenschiel JH, Harmel MH, Goodale WT, Lubin M, Bing RJ, Kety SS (1948) Measurement of coronary blood flow by the nitrous oxide method. Am J Physiol 152:356–364

Fenton RA, Bruttig SP, Rubio R, Berne RM (1982) Effect of adenosine on calcium uptake by intact and cultured vascular smooth muscle. Am J Physiol 242:H797–H804

Foley DH, Herlihy JT, Thompson CI, Rubio R, Berne RM (1978) Increased adenosine formation by rat myocardium with acute aortic constriction. J Mol Cellular Cardiol 10: 293–300

Gellai M, Detar R (1974) Evidence in support of hypoxia but against high potassium and hyperosmolarity as possible mediators of sustained vasodilation in rabbit cardiac and skeletal muscle. Circ Res 35:681–691

Gellai M, Norton JM, Detar R (1973) Evidence for direct control of coronary vascular tone by oxygen. Circ Res 32:279–289

Herlihy JT, Bockman EL, Berne RM, Rubio R (1976) Adenosine relaxation of isolated vascular smooth muscle. Am J Physiol 230:1239–1243

Hilton R, Eichholtz F (1925) The influence of chemical factors on the coronary circulation. J Physiol London 59:413–425

Jelliffe RW, Wolf CR, Berne RM, Eckstein RW (1957) Absence of vasoactive and cardiotropic substances in coronary sinus blood of dogs. Circ Res 5:382–387

Katori M, Berne RM (1966) Release of adenosine from anoxic hearts: Relationship to coronary flow. Circ Res 19:420–425

Katz LN, Lindner E (1938) The action of excess *Na, Ca* and *K* on the coronary vessels. Am J Physiol 124:155–160

Knabb RM, Ely SW, Bacchus AN, Rubio R, Berne RM (1983a) Consistent parallel relationships among myocardial oxygen consumption, coronary blood flow, and pericardial infusate adenosine concentration with various interventions and β-blockade in the dog. Circ Res 53:33–41

Knabb RM, Gidday JM, Ely SW, Rubio R, Berne RM (1983b) Effects of dipyridamole on pericardial infusate and coronary plasma adenosine. Federation Proc 42:462 (abstract)

Kübler WP, Spieckermann PG, Bretschneider HJ (1970) Influence of dipyridamole (Persantin) on myocardial adenosine metabolism. J Mol Cellular Cardiol 1:23–38

Mellander S, Lundvall J (1971) Role of tissue hyperosmolality in exercise hyperemia. Circ Res 28 and 29 (Suppl. I):39–45

Miller WL, Belardinelli L, Bacchus A, Foley DH, Rubio R, Berne RM (1979) Canine myocardial adenosine and lactate production, oxygen consumption, and coronary blood flow during stellate ganglia stimulation. Circ Res 45:708–718

Murray PA, Sparks HV (1978) The mechanism of K^+-induced vasodilation of the coronary vascular bed of the dog. Circ Res 42:35–42

Mustafa SJ, Berne RM, Rubio R (1975) Adenosine metabolism in cultured chick-embryo heart cells. Am J Physiol 228:1474–1478

Rubio R, Berne RM, Katori M (1969) Release of adenosine in reactive hyperemia of the dog heart. Am J Physiol 216:56–62

Rubio R, Wiedmeier VT, Berne RM (1974) Relationships between coronary flow and adenosine production and release. J Mol Cellular Cardiol 6:561–566

Scott JB, Radawski D (1971) Role of hyperosmolarity in the genesis of active and reactive hyperemia. Circ Res 28 and 29 (Suppl. I):26–32

Sobol BJ, Wanlass SA, Joseph EB, Azarshahy I (1962) Alteration of coronary blood flow in the dog by inhalation of 100 per cent oxygen. Circ Res 11:797–802

Thompson CI, Rubio R, Berne RM (1980) Changes in adenosine and glycogen phosphorylase activity during the cardiac cycle. Am J Physiol 238:H389–H398

DISCUSSION

DINNAR: What is the time scale of changes? If you induce a metabolic demand, how fast will you see the first reaction, and how long will it take you to reach a steady state in all these experiments?

ANS: The changes occur in seconds, or even less than a second. Do you remember that one experiment with only a single cardiac contraction? There was a significant increase in the amount of adenosine present in the myocardium during that single contraction.

DINNAR: You mentioned in some of the experiments that you waited about 10 min. After 10 min, are there other reactions coming into play? You mentioned that the reaction occurs within one second, and you also waited about 10 min in some of the experiments.

ANS: In those experiments in which we waited for a longer period of time we wanted to get a steady state situation. For example, the unanaesthetized dogs which we let run on the treadmill at 2 and 4 miles per hour, were essentially in a steady state condition and we obtained reasonable estimates of the amount of adenosine formed in, and released from, the heart. Whereas with the excitement and feeding, we do not know when to take the sample. We can take it over a period of time but I would not want to put any bets on the accuracy of quantitation. We could only get directional changes with the nonsteady state interventions.

BEYAR: Regarding the locus of control. Is there any idea where exactly the control of the coronary resistance takes place? Is this the direct effect on the smooth muscle or maybe a secondary effect from other sources of metabolic substances?

ANS: We think that the direct effect is primarily on the vascular smooth muscle of the arterioles (the resistance vessels). Dr. Duling has isolated resistance vessels, from several tissues (but not the heart), and can show a dilator or constrictor effect on these microscopic vessels with the application of appropriate vasoactive agents.

EDUD: Would you comment on the role of the prostaglandins on the regulation of the coronary blood flow?

ANS: We have not studied these agents except to see whether prostaglandin synthesis affected coronary blood flow. The administration of indomethacin did not alter the pressure-flow relationship of the coronary cirulation.

WILLIAMSON: Can I come to the issue of what you consider the oxygen sensor? As you perhaps know from my work, the increase of coronary flow comes before there is any evidence of tissue hypoxia. The issue is what really triggers the source in the myocardium. Our very recent work shows that there is, what I call, microheterogeneity. I was recently impressed by a demonstration by Sparks *et al.* that the mitochondria have nucleotides. So it makes sense to me that the very first indication in the cell of the limitation of oxygen would be in the mitochondria where the GTP level is most sensitive. This would increase AMP in the mitochondria and that would be the organelle responsible for the initial phase of adenosine production.

ANS: If you would have asked me that question about 2 or 3 years ago, I would not have agreed with you because I would have said that 5'-nucleotidase is a membrane enzyme (an ectoenzyme). I once thought that adenosine was formed at the cell membrane and was released into the interstitial fluid where it acts on the vasculature. This is a nice model. However, I now feel quite differently because of data from several sources, particularly on leukocytes, that the 5'-nucleotidase that is responsible for the formation of the adenosine in response to enhanced metabolism is intracellular possibly in the mitochondria. This is compatible with your concept.

BASSINGTHWAIGHTE: You proposed that the adenosine concentration in interstitial fluid rose with dipyridamole because cell reuptake was blocked, and I observed in your slide that increased released from the epicardial layer was at least observable, and in fact, large. What seemed contradictatory was your statement that the release into the vascular system was diminished. You didn't show data on that point, but that would seem not at all obvious. For example, if dipyridamole has no apparent effect on the permeation of the capillary membrane for intravascular molecules, it would be very strange if adenosine were being blocked in going from the interstitium to the blood stream.

ANS: I did not show the data. There is definitely a decrease in the release of adenosine into the effluent. The idea is purely hypothetical, in an attempt to account for the increase in the pericardial adenosine concentration in the presence of a decrease in release into the venous efferent. I have no data to answer the question you raised about how dipyridamole affects the transport of adenosine across the capillary membrane. These are experiments that we can do (and will do) with isolated arterioles, but I am at a loss to explain the findings by another mechanism.

BASSINGTHWAIGHTE: The only possibility I can see mechanistically is that you may block the uptake by muscle cells or cardiac or smooth muscle but increase uptake in endothelial cells.

ANS: We know from studies of several investigators that endothelial cells will avidly take up adenosine and store large amounts of it. The question is does dipyridamole enhance the uptake. This is not yet known but I doubt it.

BASSINGTHWAIGHTE: It is clear from our experiments that it does not differ from the lumenal side. It would have to be a strenuous difference between the lumenal and anti-lumenal surface of the endothelial cell.

QUESTION: Do you think the answer might be that dipyridamole blocks the adenosine receptor?

ANS: I do not know. There are different types of adenosine receptors. We have no evidence that the receptors are involved, in the sense that the pharmacologists believe on the basis of studies with a variety of adenosine analogues. Many investigators use the level of adenylate cyclase activity as an index of adenosine activity. The effects that I have shown you are the physiological effects that do not involve changes in cycle AMP. Hence, it must be via a different mechanism.

Neural control of coronary blood flow

ERIC O. FEIGL
Department of Physiology and Biophysics, University of Washington, Seattle, WA 98195, U.S.A.

Abstract

Coronary physiology has recently been reviewed where a more extensive list of references may be found (Feigl, 1983).

The coronary vessels are innervated by both the parasympathetic and sympathetic divisions of the autonomic nervous system, as demonstrated by light microscope (Woollard, 1926) and electron microscope (Lever *et al.*, 1965; Malor *et al.*, 1973). Cholinergic innervation has been demonstrated with the acetylcholinesterase-staining technique (Denn and Stone, 1976; Gerova *et al.*, 1979) and adrenergic innervation has been shown with flourescent histochemical methods (Denn and Stone 1976; Dolezel *et al.*, 1978, Nielsen and Owman, 1968).

Parasympathetic coronary control

Electrical stimulation of the cardiac end of the cut vagus nerve produces bradycardia, diminished atrial and ventricular contractility and a fall in aortic blood pressure, accompanied by a decrease in coronary blood flow. Under these conditions it is difficult to interpret the direct action of the vagus on coronary resistance since the net decrease in coronary flow is secondary to the fall in myocardial metabolism and aortic blood pressure. Katz and Jochim (1939) were the first to study coronary blood flow during vagal stimulation without bradycardia, by employing a fibrillating heart preparation. Electrical stimulation of the vagus nerves resulted in coronary vasodilation in the fibrillating heart. Subsequently parasympathetic coronary vasodilation has been demonstrated in beating heart preparations where the ventricular rate was held constant with electrical pacing (Berne *et al.*, 1965; Daggett *et al.*, 1967; Feigl, 1969; Bhagat *et al.*, 1976; Tiedt and Religa, 1979).

Reflex parasympathetic coronary vasodilation was first demonstrated by Hashimoto and co-workers (1964) in a fibrillating heart preparation where intracarotid injections of nicotine were used to stimulate carotid body chemoreceptors. Carotid body chemoreceptor reflex coronary vasodilation excited with nicotine injections, has been observed in paced open chest (Hackett *et al.*, 1972) and unanesthetized preparations (Vatner and McRitchie, 1975). However, Ehrhart *et al.* (1975) failed to find reflex coronary vasodilation when the carotid bodies were stimulated with hypoxic and hypercarbic blood, indicating that chemoreceptor reflexes do not control coronary blood flow with physiological stimuli. Unfortunately the reflex responsiveness of the anesthetized preparation was not tested with nicotine.

Recently our laboratory (Ito and Feigl, 1984b) has reinvestigated the question of carotid body chemoreceptor reflex parasympathetic coronary vasodilation in an anesthetized, beta receptor blocked, closed-chest preparation with the isolated carotid arteries perfused with hypoxic and hypercapnic blood. Vagal bradycardia was prevented by atrio-ventricular heart block and ventricular pacing. Graded levels of hypoxia and hypercapnia produced a transient coronary vasodilation that was blocked by atropine. The active vasodilation was in excess of any change in myocardial metabolism, as indicated by an augmented coronary sinus venous oxygen tension.

The conclusion at this time is that, hypoxic and hypercapnic perfusion of the carotid body chemoreceptors produces transient reflex parasympathetic coronary vasodilation. The importance of this reflex parasympathetic control of coronary blood flow in overall coronary regulation remains to be determined.

Electrical stimulation of the afferent carotid sinus nerve mimicing baroreceptor activation, results in vagal bradycardia and peripheral vasodilation by inhibition of sympathetic discharge. When carotid sinus nerve stimulation is employed in a preparation with the ventricles paced at a constant rate reflex parasympathetic coronary vasodilation is observed in anesthetized (Hackett *et al.*, 1972; Religa *et al.*, 1972) and unanesthetized preparations (Vatner *et al.*, 1970). However, it is difficult to equate a given nerve stimulation frequency with the carotid sinus pressure that physiologically activates baroreceptors.

Our laboratory has recently investigated the reflex effects of carotid sinus hypertension on the coronary circulation (Ito and Feigl, 1984a). The carotid sinuses were vascularly isolated and perfused with a servo controlled pressure pump. The aortic depressor nerves were cut bilaterally to prevent aortic arch baroreceptor reflexes from buffering carotid sinus reflexes. The left main coronary artery was perfused at constant pressure, and the ventricles were paced at a constant rate following the production of heart block in a closed-chest preparation. Aortic pressure was stabilized with a pressure reservoir and propranolol was administered to block reflex sympathetic effects to the myocardium. Step increases in carotid sinus pressure resulted in graded reflex coronary vasodilation accompanied by increases in coronary sinus oxygen tension. Atropine administration demonstrated that the major portion of the reflex vasodilation was due to parasympathetic activation. These results indicate that parasympathetic coronary vasodilation is part of the carotid sinus baroreceptor reflex.

Excitation of left ventricular receptors with intracoronary injections of veratridine results in the Bezold-Jarisch reflex producing vagal bradycardia and peripheral vasodilation. An examination of Bezold-Jarisch reflex with the heart paced at a constant rate revealed that parasympathetic coronary vasodilation is also part of this reflex (Feigl, 1975b). Intracoronary veratridine injections produce a nonspecific excitation of cardiac receptors and it remains to be determined if this reflex can be elicited by physiological rather than pharmacological stimuli.

Sympathetic coronary control

Stimulation of the sympathetic innervation to the heart results in tachycardia, augmented myocardial contractility, and increased aortic blood pressure, accompanied by an increase in coronary blood flow. The increase in coronary blood flow is secondary to the augmented myocardial oxygen consumption mediated by a local metabolic mechanism. However the direct effect of activation of sympathetic fibers to the cornary vessels is predominantly coronary vasoconstriction mediated by adrenergic alpha receptors.

The direct coronary vasoconstrictor effect of sympathetic activation can be unmasked by beta receptor blockade with propranolol that blunts the increase in myocardial metabolism due to sympathetic activation (Feigl, 1975a). After pretreatment with propranolol electrical stimulation of the sympathetic fibers to the heart results in an increase in coronary resistance and a fall in coronary sinus venous oxygen tension. Both the coronary vasoconstriction and the fall in coronary sinus oxygen tension during sympathetic stimulation were prevented by subsequent alpha receptor blockade.

The competition between local metabolic vasodilation and alpha receptor coronary vasoconstriction due to sympathetic activation was examined in a preparation without beta receptor blockade (Mohrman and Feigl, 1978). The coronary circulation was perfused at constant pressure during graded sympathetic activations produced by intracoronary norepinephrine infusions or activation of the carotid sinus baroreflex by lowering carotid sinus pressure. The relationship between coronary flow and myocardial oxygen consumption was examined before and after adrenergic alpha receptor blockade. For any given increment in myocardial oxygen consumption the increase in coronary blood flow was about 30% greater after alpha receptor blockade than before. This indicates that under normal circumstances without alpha or beta receptor blockade sympathetic activation of the heart produces a sympathetic vasoconstrictor influence that competes with the local metabolic vasodilator effects. Net coronary blood flow increases, but not in proportion to the increase in metabolism so that oxygen extraction across the coronary circulation increases.

It is interesting to note that the competition between alpha receptor vasoconstriction and metabolic vasodilation also occurs during the sympathetic activation that accompanies exercise (Murray and Vatner, 1979; Gwirtz and Stone, 1981; Heyndricks *et al.*, 1982).

The above results indicate that there is a competion between coronary alpha receptor vasoconstriction and local metabolic vasodilation during physiological conditions. Our laboratory has recently been investigating whether sympathetic coronary vasoconstriction is also present during hypoperfusion as occurs in the presence of coronary artery stenosis (Buffington and Feigl, 1981). An artificial 70% area stenosis was placed in the coronary circulation and graded intracoronary doses of norepinephrine were administered to activate coronary and myocardial adrenergic receptors. Myocardial oxygen and lactate extraction, coronary sinus blood oxygen tension, and coronary resistance were compared at equal levels of myocardial oxygen consumption before and after coronary alpha receptor blockade. In the presence of coronary stenosis, intracoronary norepinephrine infusion decreased coronary sinus oxygen content and increased myocardial oxygen extraction. At comparable myocardial oxygen consumptions coronary vascular resistance was greater with alpha receptors intact than after alpha receptor blockade. The increase in myocardial oxygen extraction was prevented by alpha receptor blockade. These data indicate that a sympathetic alpha receptor-mediated coronary vasoconstrictor influence operates, even in the presence of coronary stenosis, to limit oxygen delivery to the heart and increase myocardial oxygen extraction to the point of cardiac failure, but that this vasoconstrictor effect does not result in net myocardial lactate production.

There is also evidence that sympathetic coronary vasoconstriction occurs in patients with coronary artery stenosis (Mudge *et al.*, 1976; Mudge *et al.*, 1979). A recent animal study indicates that the effects of sympathetic coronary vasoconstriction may be amplified in the presence of severe coronary stenosis (Heusch and Deussen, 1983).

The combined effects of underperfusion and sympathetic coronary vasoconstriction on transmural coronary blood flow were examined in a closed chest preparation (Buffington and Feigl, 1983). One region of the left ventricle was selectively treated with an alpha receptor blocking agent while the untreated region served as a control. Both regions were progressively underperfused by lowering coronary artery pressure and sympathetic activation was produced with intracoronary norepinephrine infusion. Transmural blood flow was measured with radioactive microspheres. Uniform transmural alpha receptor coronary vasoconstriction was observed at normal coronary artery pressures but sympathetic vasoconstriction was lost during severe hypoperfusion when coronary artery pressure was 38 mmHg. At an intermediate coronary pressure of 50 mmHg significant alpha receptor coronary vasoconstriction was observed in the outer subepicardial layer of the left ventricle but the vasoconstriction was marginal in the inner subendocardial layer. These data suggest that sympathetic coronary vasoconstriction may help preserve uniform transmural blood flow in the left ventricular wall during hypoperfusion. These results are in agreement with other studies where uniform transmural coronary vasoconstriction has been observed at the normal pressures (Johannsen *et al.*, 1982).

Currently our laboratory is investigating the hypothesis that sympathetic coronary vasoconstriction acts to prevent a transmural steal from subendocardium to subepicardium during hypoperfusion by a sustained constriction in the outer layer of ventricle. An experimental preparation was employed where alpha receptor blocked and unblocked regions of the left ventricle are compared during graded reductions in flow to both regions. Preliminary results indicate that the transmural inner/outer blood flow ratio is better preserved in the area with alpha receptors intact than in the alpha receptor blocked region during comparable reductions in coronary flow. These preliminary results indicate that the teleological function of sympathetic coronary vasoconstriction may be to preserve subendocardial blood flow during stressful conditions.

Summary

The coronary vessels are innervated by both parasympathetic vasodilator, and sympathetic vasoconstrictor fibers. When the heart is paced at a constant rate, vagal stimulation produces coronary vasodilation. Parasympathetic coronary vasodilation has been observed in the baroreceptor reflex elicited by carotid sinus hypertension, the chemoreceptor reflex elicited by hypoxia or hypercarbia, and the Bezold-Jarisch reflex elicited by intracoronary injections of veratridine. Stimulation of the sympathetic fibers to the heart activates myocardial beta receptors producing tachycardia and an increase in contractility that augments myocardial metabolism. At the same time coronary vascular alpha receptors are activated producing a vasoconstrictor influence that competes with the metabolic vasodilation. This competition has been observed in the baroreflex elicited by carotid sinus hypotension and during exercise. Sympathetic coronary vasoconstriction is active during myocardial hypoperfusion and may help to preserve subendocardial blood flow.

Acknowledgement

This work was supported by NIH Grant HL 16910.

References

Berne RM, DeGeest H, Levy MN (1965) Influence of the cardiac nerves on coronary resistance. Am J Physiol 208:763–769

Bhagat CI, Maharaj RR, Reid JVO (1976) Differential effect of right and left vagal stimulation on right and left circumflex coronary arteries. S Afr Med J 50:1591–1594

Buffington CW, Feigl EO (1981) Adrenergic coronary vasoconstriction in the presence of coronary stenosis in the dog. Circ Res 48:416–423

Buffington CW, Feigl EO (1983) Effect of coronary artery pressure on transmural distribution of adrenergic coronary vasoconstriction in the dog. Circ Res 53:613–621

Dagget WM, Nugent GC, Carr PW, Powers PC, Harada Y (1967) Influence of vagal stimulation on ventricular contractility, O_2 consumption, and coronary flow. Am J Physiol 212:8–18

Denn MJ, Stone HL (1976) Autonomic innervation of dog coronary arteries. J Appl Physiol 41:30–35

Dolezel S, Gerova M, Gero J, Sladek T, Vasku J (1978) Adrenergic innervation of the coronary arteries and the myocardium. Acta Anat 100:306–316

Ehrhart IC, Parker PE, Weidner WJ, Dabney JM, Scott JB, Haddy FJ (1975) Coronary vascular and myocardial responses to carotid body stimulation in the dog. Am J Physiol 299:754–760

Feigl EO (1969) Parasympathetic control of coronary blood flow in dogs. Circ Res 25:509–519

Feigl EO (1975a) Control of myocardial oxygen tension by sympathetic coronary vasoconstriction in the dog. Circ Res 37:88–95

Feigl EO (1975b) Reflex parasympathetic coronary vasodilation elicited from cardiac receptors in the dog. Circ Res 37:175–182

Feigl EO (1983) Coronary physiology. Physiol Rev 63:1–205

Gerova M, Dolezel S, Gero J, Barta E (1979) Role of the vagus in control of the major conduit coronary artery in the dog. Physiol Bohemoslov 28:299–307

Gwirtz PA, Stone HL (1981) Coronary blood flow and myocardial oxygen consumption after α-adrenergic blockade during submaximal exercise. J Pharmacol Exp Ther 217:92–98

Hackett JG, Abboud FM, Mark AL, Schmid PG, Heistad DD (1972) Coronary vascular responses to stimulation of chemoreceptors and baroreceptors. Evidence for reflex activation of vagal cholinergic innervation. Circ Res 31:8–17

Hashimoto K, Igarashi S, Uei I, Kumakura S (1964) Carotid chemoreceptor reflex effects on coronary flow and heart rate. Am J Physiol 206:536–540

Heusch G, Deussen A (1983) The effects of cardiac sympathetic nerve stimulation on perfusion of stenotic coronary arteries in the dog. Circ Res 53:8–15

Heyndrickx GR, Muylaert P, Pannier JL (1982) α-Adrenergic control of oxygen delivery to myocardium during exercise in conscious dogs. Am J Physiol 242:H805–H809

Ito BR, Feigl EO (1984a) Carotid sinus baroreceptor reflex coronary vasodilation. In preparation

Ito BR, Feigl EO (1984b) Carotid body chemoreceptor reflex parasympathetic coronary vasodilation. In preparation

Johannsen UJ, Mark AL, Marcus ML (1982) Responsiveness to cardiac sympathetic nerve stimulation during maximal coronary dilation produced by adenosine. Circ Res 50:510–517

Katz LN, Jochim K (1939) Observations on the innervation of the coronary vessels of the dog. Am J Physiol 126:395–401

Lever JD, Ahmed M, Irvine G (1965) Neuro-muscular and intercellular relationships in the coronary arterioles. A morphological and quantitative study by light and electron microscopy. J Anat 99:829–840

Malor R, Griffin CJ, Taylor S (1973) Innervation of the blood vessels in guinea-pig atria. Cardiovasc Res 7:95–104

Mohrman DE, Feigl EO (1978) Competition between sympathetic vasoconstriction and metabolic vasodilation in the canine coronary circulation. Circ Res 42:79–86

Mudge GH Jr, Grossman W, Mills RM Jr, Lesch M, Braunwald E (1976) Reflex increase in coronary vascular resistance in patients with ischemic heart disease. N E J Med 295:1333–1337

Mudge GH Jr, Goldberg S, Gunther S, Mann T, Grossman W (1979) Comparison of metabolic and vasoconstrictor stimuli on coronary vascular resistance in man. Circulation 59:544–550

Murray PA, Vatner SF (1979) α-Adrenoceptor attenuation of the coronary vascular response to severe exercise in the conscious dog. Circ Res 45:654–660

Nielsen KC, Owman C (1968) Difference in cardiac adrenergic innervation between hibernators and non-hibernating mammals. Acta Physiol Scan Suppl 316:1–30

Religa Z, Trzebski A, Religa A, Glowienki A (1972) Effect of the stimulation of afferent fibers in Hering's nerve on the blood flow and resistance in the coronary vessels of dogs. Pol Med J 11:632–641

Teidt N, Religa A (1979) Vagal control of coronary blood flow in dogs. Basic Res Cardiol 74:267–276

Vatner SF, Franklin D, Van Citters RL, Braunwald E (1970) Effects of carotid sinus nerve stimulation on the coronary circulation of the conscious dog. Circ Res 27:11–21

Vatner SF, McRitchie RJ (1975) Interaction of the chemoreflex and the pulmonary inflation reflex in the regulation of coronary circulation in conscious dogs. Circ Res 37:664–673

Woollard HH (1926) The innervation of the heart. J Anat Physiol 60:345–373

DISCUSSION

SAGAWA: With reference to sympathetic innervation, is there any morphological evidence for your interesting idea that of alpha receptor control might be stronger, or primarily only on the epicardial vessels?

ANS: There is no evidence and part of the data that I showed would indicate that there is no functional evidence either. In the situation with constant pressure, where there is no chance for steal, these data indicate that there is a uniform transmural alpha vasoconstrictor effect. If there is a potential for steal in the experimental preparation, then alpha constriction is favoured in the sub-epicardium because of the more intense metabolic vasodilation in the subendocardium. That is a long hypothesis, and not all the points have been checked. It is our working hypothesis and I think it is logically sound but it needs several steps.

BASSINGTHWAIGHTE: Is there any evidence that impairment of the flow to the subendocarial layers will eventually result in the impairment of the subepicardial layers flow and if so, how would this fit in with your findings?

ANS: Are you asking about ischemia? Ischemia manifests first in the subendocardium. As it gets worse, it moves outward and reaches the epicardium and then, if it gets even worse and you get increasing ischemic areas move laterally.

JARON: I have a question about the steal syndrome in the coronary flow. Do you find it only in stenotic coronaries or can you play with the model in nonstenotic cases?

ANS: First of all, we have no model, in the sense that it is being used in this conference. Steal, in the usual vascular sense, only occurs in the presence of a stenosis. There are steal phenomenon which also include a collateral vessel. The principle is the same. That is, there are two resistors distal to a third stenosis upstream and those two resistors interact because there is a pressure drop across the upstream stenosis. It can cause subclavian steal, for example, where there are cerebral effects or it can cause transmural steal in the heart. That is, if there is a coronary stenosis, the epicardium steals from the endocardium and therefore the inner/outer ratio is below unity. This is thought of as a steal phenomenon.

JARON: Is there a kind of critical stenosis which initiates the steal phenomenon?

ANS: Yes, there is. At resting metabolic levels it is a diameter reduction of about 80 or 90%. The initial value is variable because the metabolism of the heart changes. So stenosis that is not critical at rest becomes critical and restricts flow during augemented metabolism. If the metabolism doubles, then flow may be restricted. This is the problem the angina patient has; he's all right at rest but he can't walk up a flight of stairs.

JANICKI: Why do you think your chemo-receptor effect was transient, and do you think you would have had a longer lasting effect if you had stimulated the aortic arch chemo-receptors?

ANS: We haven't investigated the aortic arch receptors. The technical problem of separating the coronary circulation from the aortic arch receptors is rather difficult.

LEVY: I wonder if you had tried those same experiments while controlling ventilation because other studies by Michael Daly and others, have shown that the most dramatic effect of chemoreceptor stimulation is to increase pulmonary ventilation. In experiments where the increase in pulmonary ventilation is prevented, there is a much greater and a more prolonged vagal discharge. It would have been interesting to see if that would have happened if you controlled ventilation. I would suspect that you would get a much greater and a much more prolonged reflex parasympathetic effect on coronary circulation, in conditions where you did control ventilation.

ANS: Just right. I tried to review a large topic and did not give all the experimental details. These animals were paralyzed and ventilated. The bradycardia was more sustained than the coronary vasodilation.

SIDEMAN: There is a difference between the slide you showed relating the endo to the epicardial ratio of blood flow and the calculated values that Dr. Beyar just showed. Your data indicated that this ratio of endo/epi approaches one as the heart rate goes up. His calculation does not indicate it. Could you comment on it?

ANS: Our data do not pertain exactly to heart rate. Other people's data do. In exercise, tachycardia, with flow measured with microspheres, the endo/epi, or the inner/outer, ratio tends to fall. Typically, at low heart rates, the endo/epi blood flow rates is about 1.15 and decreases to about 1.0 during exercise, as observed in Greenfield's laboratory. I think that the flow measurements are reliable and they don't agree with the model at the moment so there is some adjustment wanted in the model.

ADAM: I have a question about the data you presented concerning the stimulation of the sympathetic system. It's well known from electrical measurements that there is a different effect when you stimulate the left or the right stellate ganglia. I was wondering what procedure you have, and if you found any such results?

ANS: We've never compared the effects of stimulating the left and right stellate ganglia. In one experiment that I described, the left stellate ganglian was stimulated. In the other experiments either catecholamine infusion or reflex activation was employed. What I like best, as a physiologist, is the reflex activation.

ADAM: Did you ever measure the activity in the sympathetic trunk?

ANS: No.

The interrelationship between the left ventricular contraction, transmural blood perfusion and spatial energy balance: A new model of the cardiac system

R. BEYAR and S. SIDEMAN
The Julius Silver Institute, Departments of Chemical and Biomedical Engineering, Technion-Israel Institute of Technology Haifa 32000, Israel

Abstract

A model of the left ventricle (LV), which combines the distributed transmural mechanical parameters with the distributed energy demand and coronary perfusion parameters has been developed. The model is used for quantitative evaluation of various loading conditions and different pathologic states such as anemia, hypoxia and aortic stenosis.

Introduction

The contraction of the left ventricle (LV) is a complex phenomenon which depends on the interrelationships between the mechanics of the myocardium, the energy demand of the metabolic processes within the myocardium and the energy supply to the myocardium via the coronary arteries. Hormonal and neurogenic autoregulatory mechanisms play a major role in controlling these interrelationships.

Various models have been proposed to describe the LV mechanics (Diamond *et al.*, 1971; Feit *et al.*, 1979; Ghista and Hamid, 1977; Janz and Grimm, 1973; Janz *et al.*, 1974; Mirsky, 1970, 1974; Moskowitz, 1979; Pao *et al.*, 1974, 1980; Pao and Ritman, 1977; Pierce, 1981; Streeter *et al.*, 1970; Van der Broek and Van der Broek, 1979). The simpler models assume an equal stress distribution within the LV wall while the more detailed ones include a transmural stress distribution which relates to the stipulated anatomical construction of the LV. The correlation between the mechanical aspects of the contraction phenomenon and the overall energy demand of the cardiac muscle was intensively studied (Baller *et al.*, 1979; Binak *et al.*, 1967; Bing *et al.*, 1949; Braunwald, 1971; Bretschneider, 1979; Burns and Covell, 1972; Gamble *et al.*, 1974; Gibbs *et al.*, 1979; Graham *et al.*, 1968; Skelton *et al.*, 1970, 1974); Strauser, 1979; Monroe, 1972; Parmley, 1976; McKeever, 1958; Messer, 1962; Weber, 1979; Weber and Janicki, 1979; Weiss *et*

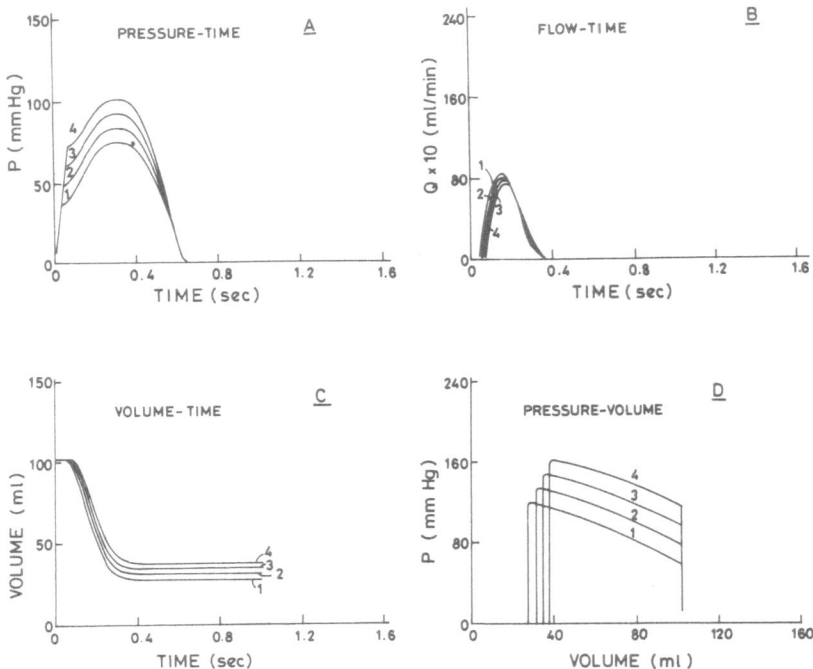

Figure 1. Calculated pressure-time, volume-time, flow-time and pressure volume relationship for different after loading conditions.

al., 1978). Furthermore, a huge number of experimental studies explaining different aspects of the coronary circulation have been published and are summarized by Berne and Rubio (1979) and Feigl (1983).

In general, none of these studies relates the spatial energy demand throughout the myocardium to the spatial and time dependent features of the cardiac mechanics. Obviously, knowledge of the myocardial blood flow distribution is required in order to link the energy demand to the energy supply.

A spheroidal model of the LV which incorporates the fibers' spatial architecture and the physiological fiber mechanics together with a simulated radial electrical propagation pattern was recently used to describe the LV cycle (Beyar and Sideman 1984b). Utilizing the sliding filament kinetics theory, the local mechanical phenomena was related (Beyar and Sideman 1984d) to the local energy demand. An extension of the mechanical model, which accounts for the effect of the pressure distribution within the wall and the autoregulatory response, was then used to describe the coronary blood flow distribution within the LV wall (Beyar and Sideman, 1984c).

It is the purpose of the present study to develop a general model of the LV which relates the mechanical determinants of cardiac contraction to the spatial myocardial energetics and the local coronary perfusion during the cardiac cycle. It is hoped that the model will help in the understanding and the quantification of the various processes involved in the cardiac cycle in normal and pathological states.

The mathematical model

The general model developed here is best demonstrated by detailing each of its building blocks separately, with particular emphasis on the assumptions used to formulate the model.

The mechanical model

The mechanical model is based on the following assumptions:
- (a) The LV is made of spheroidal nested shells, constructed of fibers with a linear fiber angle distribution, from $-60°$ to $+60°$, as described by Streeter et al. (1969).
- (b) A linear stress-(sarcomere) length (Pollack and Kruger 1978), and a linear stress-strain rate relationships (Ross et al., 1966) for the muscle fibers, are applicable.
- (c) The electrical activation front propagates radially from the endocardium to the epicardium.
- (d) The time dependent activation function is in the form of (half) a sinusoidal wave.
- (e) The diastole is viscoelastic and the viscosity coefficient of the cardiac muscle is adjusted so that the heart cavity fills during diastole to the previous end-diastolic-volume, at a constant LV filling pressure of 7 mmHg.
- (f) A force interval relationship (Johnson, 1975) relates the isovolumic stress to the heart rate. The duration of the isometric twitch is also heart-rate dependent.

The model can be used to determine the systolic mechanical parameters of the LV which include the stress and pressure distributions within the myocardial wall as a function of time, as well as the associated strain, strain rate, volumes and blood flows. The mathematical equations characterizing these phenomena are given in Appendix A. Some calculated results for a typical set of initial conditions are shown in Figure 1.

The energy demand model

The distribution of the energy demand within the LV wall is calculated by utilizing the mechanical parameters given by the mechanical model and the theory of cross-bridges kinetics across the actin and myosin fibers of the sar-

334

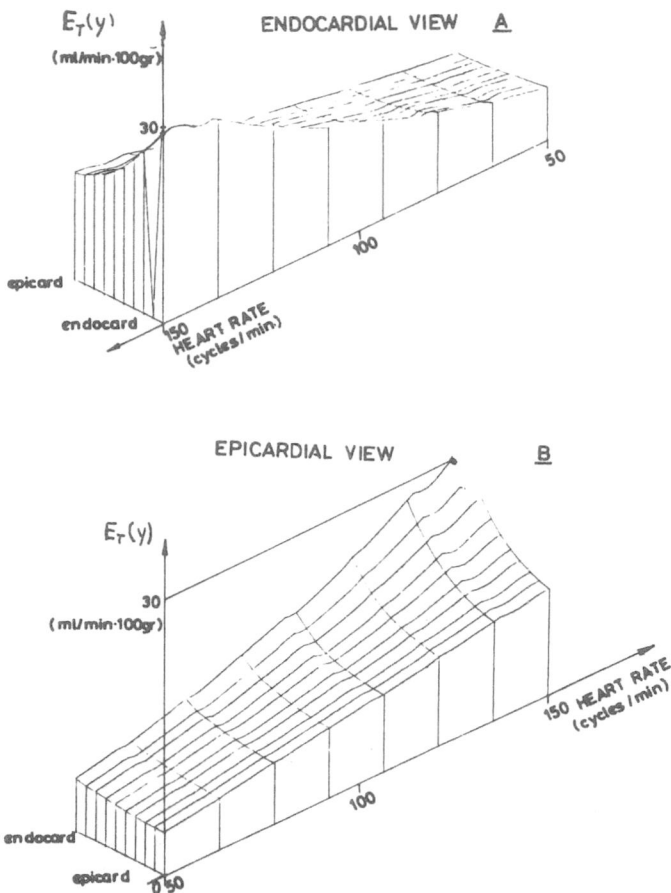

Figure 2. The energy demand $E_T(y)$ (in terms of oxygen demand) calculated by the LV model

comeres. The difference in the energy demand of the different layers stems from the fact that the sarcomere length, the stress, strain and strain rate are different at each layer. The energy demand of each layer $E_T(y)$ is related to the stress integral, stress development, strain rate and the basal metabolism by a set of constants.

The following assumptions are used in deriving the energy demand:

(a) The basal metabolism corresponds to 30% of the total consumption under normal conditions.

(b) The active stress development component corresponds to 15% of the total myocardial oxygen demand.

(c) The stress maintenance, or stress integral, under normal conditions corresponds to 40% of the myocardial oxygen demand.

(d) The external work done by the fibers corresponds to 15% of the total oxygen demand at basal conditions.

(e) The stress relaxation energy expenditure is negligible.

The mathematical equations are given in Appendix B. A typical presentation of the calculated energy demand for a set of initial conditions is given in Figure 2.

The myocardial blood flow

The pressure distribution within the wall, $P_w(y, t)$ is used as the input parameter in the calculation of the time dependent coronary blood flow distribution within the LV wall. The following assumptions are used

(a) A minimal pressure driving force, denoted as the critical closing pressure, is needed to affect the capillary flow.

(b) No flow occurs when the transmural pressure in the blood vessel is negative due to vascular collapse.

(c) The resistance of the coronary bed is inversely proportional to the transmural wall pressure, subject to the geometrical changes accompanying transmural pressure changes.

(d) The tonus of the coronary bed is represented by an arbitrary function $0 \leq T_{wf}(y) \leq 1$. The tonus of the small vessels modifies the coronary resistance according to local control mechanisms, so that the oxygen supply meets the metabolic demands. $T_{wf}(y) = 0$ means maximum vasodilatation and is associated with a minimum resistance value, $R_{min}(y)$, while $T_{wf}(y) = 1$ denotes maximum vasodilatation and associated with a maximum resistance value $R_{max}(y)$.

A detailed mathematical description of the model is given in Appendix C. A representation of the calculated blood flow distribution in the myocardium is given below.

The integrated general model

The above models yield quantitative descriptions of the local stress, strain and strain rate within the muscle as well as the instantaneous sarcomere length distribution. The local intramural pressure $P_w(y, t)$, together with the tonus of the small vessels $T_{wf}(y)$, determine the resistance of the coronary bed and thus determine the nature and magnitude of the coronary flow in the wall. The local energy demand is calculated from the local stress, strain rate and sarcomere length and, assuming aerobic metabolism, is expressed here in terms of the oxygen demand.

It is well-known that various local factors strongly affect the coronary perfusion. For instance, the oxygen tension, PO_2, is recognized as the major determinant of the coronary blood flow. Similarly, PCO_2 and pH have a direct effect on the coronary blood flow. It is assumed here that the oxygen tension at the

336

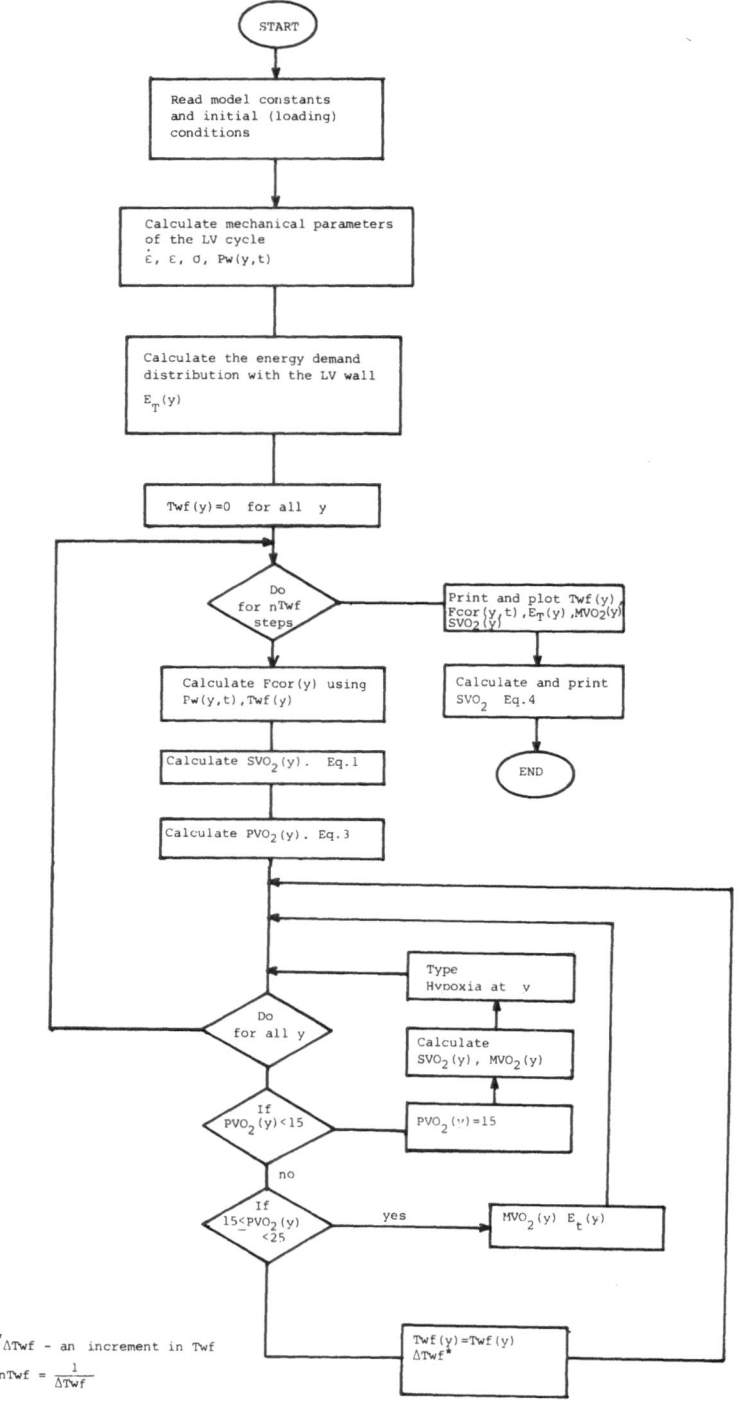

Figure 3. A schematic flow chart of the computer program.

Table 1. The relation between the heart rate and ejection parameters of the LV

HR [min⁻¹]	Oxygen consumption (ml/min 100 gm)	EF [%]	$[dp/dt]_{max}$ [mmHg/s]	Cardiac output [ml/min]
60	8.08	66	1672	4096
90	11.5	72	2511	6654
120	15.6	76	3159	9349
150	21.1	79	3253	12160

The end diastolic aortic pressure = 85 mmHg
The end diastolic LV volume = 101 ml.

capillary wall affects the tonus of the smooth muscle at the microvessels wall. A local control loop is thus formed at each layer which tends to keep the venous PO_2 at a level corresponding to an oxygen extraction ratio of 60–70% under normal conditions (Hoffman, 1978). As also noted by Hoffman, at extreme condition the heart muscle can extract up to 80% of the arterial blood oxygen content, corresponding to PO_2 of 15 mmHg.

Assuming aerobic metabolism, the relationship between the local energy demand $E_T(y)$ (which is equal to the oxygen consumption $MVO_2(y)$ when oxygen supply suffices), the time averaged coronary flow $\bar{F}_{cor}(y)$ and the arterial and venous oxygen saturation SAO_2, $SVO_2(y)$ is given by:

$$SVO_2(y) = SAO_2 - \frac{E_T(y)}{F_{cor}(y) \cdot Hb \cdot BC} \tag{1}$$

where Hb is the hemoglobin concentration (in gr/ml), and BC is the oxygen binding capacity of the hemoglobin molecules (= 1.3 ml O_2/gmHb at normal atmospheric conditions). The dissolved oxygen content under normal conditions

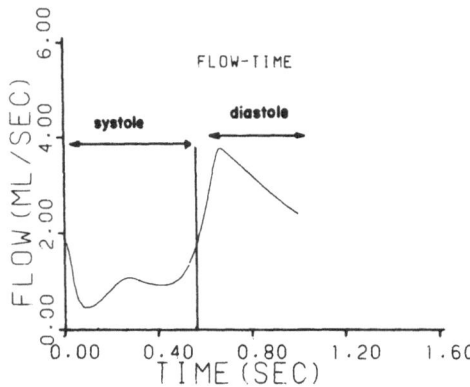

Figure 4. The coronary flow-time plot. HR = 60 cpm. LV muscle volume = 172 g.

338

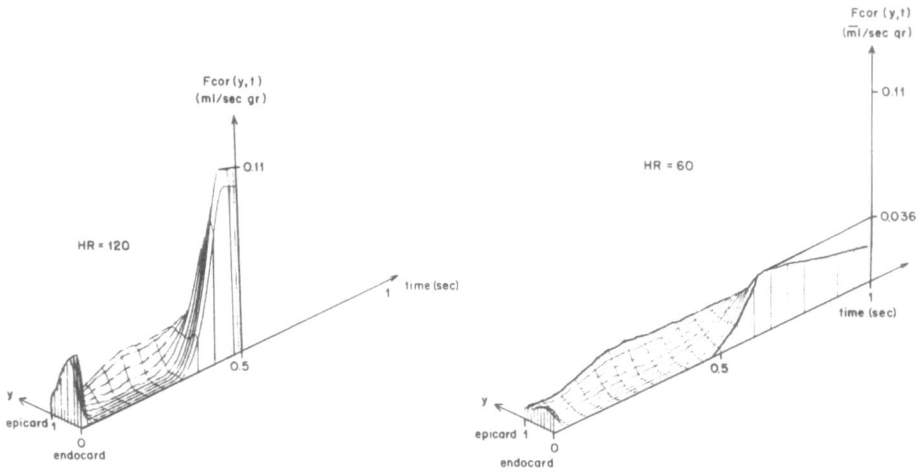

Figure 5. Time dependent coronary blood flow distributioning in the LV wall at heart rates, HR = 60, HR = 120 cycles per min.

is about 0.3 ml/100 cc solution (Ruch and Patton, 1974) and is thus assumed negligible by comparison to the amount of the oxygen bound to the hemoglobin.

The relationship between the hemoglobin saturation SO_2 (denoting either SAO_2 or SVO_2) and the blood oxygen tension is given by Hill's equation (West *et al.*, 1966):

$$SO_2 = \frac{(PO_2/P_{50})^n}{1 + (PO_2/P_{50})^n} \tag{2}$$

where n = 2.7 is the cooperation coefficient of hemoglobin and P_{50} is the oxygen tension at which half of the hemoglobin is saturated (=26 mmHg).

The PO_2 of the venous blood at each layer, $PVO_2 (y)$, is calculated from Eqs. (1) and (2):

$$PVO_2 (y) = P_{50} \sqrt[n]{\frac{SAO_2 \cdot F_{cor} (y) \cdot Hb \cdot BC - E_T (y)}{(1 - SAO_2) F_{cor} (y) Hb \cdot BC + E_T (y)}} \tag{3}$$

The calculation procedure is based on seeking, for each layer, a value of $T_{wf} (y)$ which corresponds to $PVO_2 (y) = 20$ mmHg. This represents a control mechanism which affects the coronary resistance by changing the microvascular tonus according to the local PO_2 value. No hypoxia is assumed to occur (i.e. $E_T (y) = MVO_2 (y)$) when $PVO_2 (y)$ is between 20 mmHg and 15 mmHg, even at maximum vasodilatation, when $T_{wf} (y) = 0$. However, values of $PVO_2 (y)$ lower than 15 mmHg are not permitted and, at $PVO_2 (y) = 15$ mmHg, an upper limit is set to the oxygen consumption $MVO_2 (y)$. Tissue hypoxia develops when the oxygen

Table 2. The effect of heart rate on the coronary flow and related parameters

HR [min⁻¹]	Coronary flow [ml/min 100 gm]	Venous PO_2 ($\bar{P}VO_2$) ×mHg]	Oxygen extraction [%]	Hypoxic part of myocardium
60	65	21	62	–
120	109	18	72	–
150	144	18	72	–

Hemoglobin cotent = 0.15 gm/ml
Arterial PO_2 = 100 mmHg
End diastolic aortic pressure = 85 mmHg
End diastolic LV volume = 101 ml

demand $E_T(y)$ is higher than this upper value of $MVO_2(y)$. Lactic acid which is then formed by the anaerobic metabolism pathways, is an indication for myocardial hypoxia.

The venous blood from the different layers, which contain different oxygen levels, is mixed in the major coronary veins. The average oxygen saturation of the blood $\bar{S}VO_2$, is given by:

$$\bar{SVO_2} = \frac{\int_0^h SVO_2(y) \cdot \bar{F}_{cor}(y) \cdot S(y)\,dy}{\int_0^h \bar{F}_{cor}(y) \cdot S(y)\,dy} \tag{4}$$

where $S(y)$ is the surface area of a spheroid at a distance y from the endocardium.

The computer program

The computer program was written in Fortran and run on an IBM 370 computer. The calculations were done in single precision and in time steps of 0.01 s. The myocardium was divided into ten layers of equal thickness at the unstressed state. A schematic flow chart of the computer program is shown in Figure 3. The mechanical parameters of the LV cycle were calculated first. Based on the calculated local strain ε, strain rate $\dot{\varepsilon}$ stress σ, and the basal metabolism, the oxygen demand of the myocardium was calculated for each layer. Utilizing the calculated wall pressure distribution $P_w(y, t)$ the coronary flow distribution was calculated, assuming maximum vasodilatation ($T_{wf}(y) = 0$). The value of $T_{wf}(y)$ was then gradually increased (vasoconstriction) and the PO_2 of the venous blood in each layer calculated, assuming an oxygen supply which equals the oxygen demand. $T_{wf}(y)$ was fixed for each layer when the local value $PVO_2(y)$ decreased below 20 mmHg or when maximum vasoconstriction occurred at a certain layer.

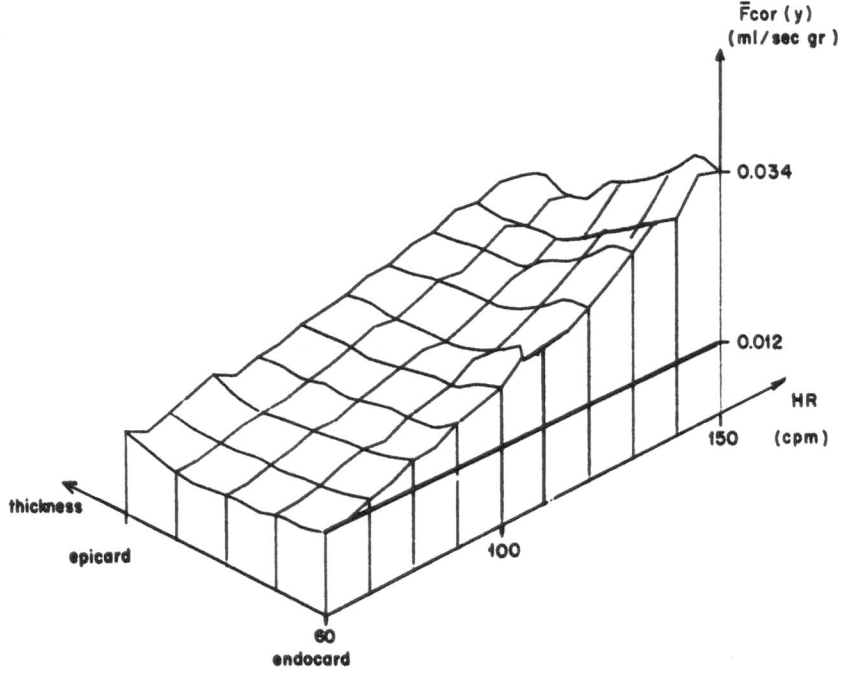

Figure 6. Coronary flow distribution as a function of the heart rate.

If PVO_2 (y) was less than 20 mmHg, in spite of maximum vasodilatation, the model allowed for increased oxygen extraction up to a minimum PVO_2 (y) of 15 mmHg.

After the distribution of the transmural vascular tonus, T_{wf} (y) , was determined, the spatial distribution of the time dependent and time-averaged coronary blood flow were calculated and plotted. The calculated relations between the average coronary flow, the coronary venous oxygen tension and the oxygen content are summarized below.

Results

General

The calculated dependence of the LV ejection parameters, and the oxygen consumption on the heart rate are presented in Table 1. As seen, the increase in heart rate is associated with an increase in the cardiac output, $(dp/dt)_{max}$ and the ejection fraction EF. For a constant preload, the relationship between the heart rate and the oxygen consumption is linear.

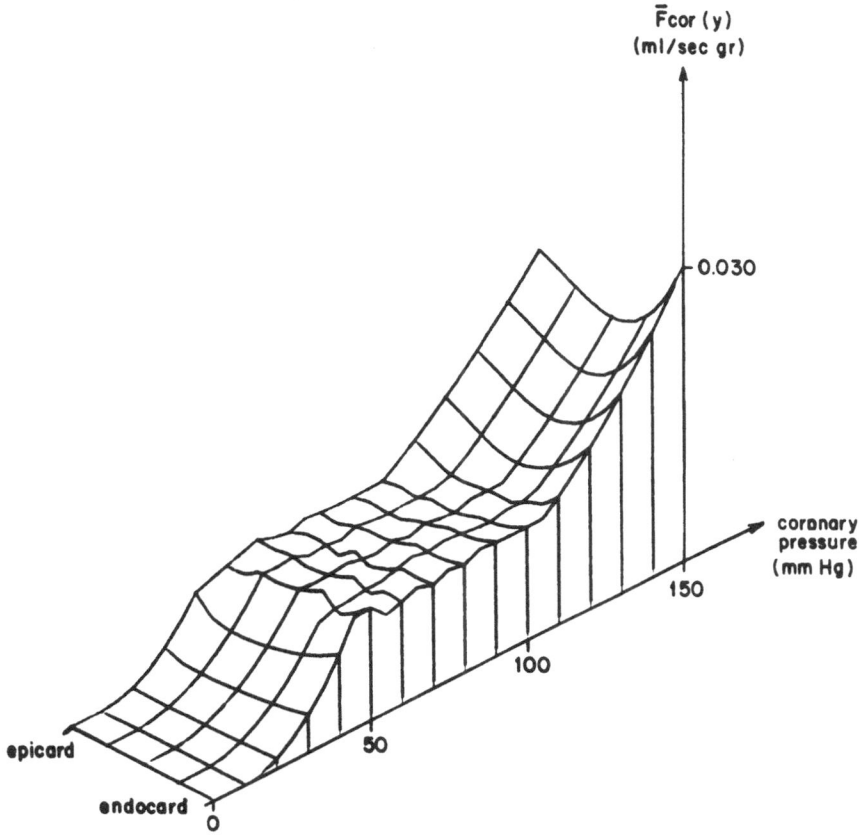

Figure 7. Coronary flow distribution versus coronary pressure.

The total LV myocardial flow, as a function of time, is shown in Figure 4. This is consistent with the well-known fact that most of the coronary flow occurs during diastole while the systolic flow is below 20% of the diastolic flow (Hoffman, 1978). A three dimensional plot of the coronary flow distribution during the complete cardiac cycle is shown in Figure 5. It is noted that the flow to the endocardial layers ceases during systole while the epicardial flow continues throughout the cycle. The effect of the heart rate on the total coronary flow at normal condition is seen in Table 2. The calculated oxygen extraction fraction of 62% at a basal heart rate of 60 cycles per minute is in good agreement with the literature (Klocke, 1976). Increasing the heart rate decreases the coronary venous oxygen tension (and oxygen content) and increases both the oxygen extraction fraction and the coronary flow. Thus, it is seen that almost all of the autoregulation of oxygen supply to the myocardium is done by increasing the flow, through some of the increased oxygen transfer is attributed to an increase of the oxygen

Table 3. The effect of anemia on the coronary flow. Normal state, Hb = 0.015 gm/ml

HR [min^{-1}]	Hb [gm/ml]	Coronary flow [ml/min 100 gm]	Venous PO$_2$ [mmHg]	Oxygen extraction [%]	Hypoxic fraction of the myocardium
	0.04	195	16.7	76	–
60	0.07	118	17.6	73	–
	0.15	65	21.0	62	–
	0.04	281	16.4	77	–
90	0.07	167	17.7	73	–
	0.15	84	19.3	68	–
	0.04	300	16	78	0.7
120	0.07	228	17.6	73	–
	0.15	109	18	72	–
	0.04	283	15	81	0.9
150	0.07	257	15.6	79	–
	0.15	144	18	72	–

extraction fraction (Messer, 1962). A 3-D plot of the coronary flow distribution as a function of the heart rate is shown in Figure 6, illustrating the even increase of the blood flow to all the myocardial layers with an increase in the heart rate.

Varying the coronary pressure at constant operating conditions is a well established experiment in coronary physiology. A mathematical simulation of such an experiment is presented in Figure 7. At very low pressures, below the zero flow pressure, no flow occurs in any of the layers. As the coronary pressure increases, the coronary perfusion begins in the epicardial layers. The coronary flow at each layer is relatively steady at the autoregulatory pressure range between 45 and 110 mmHg. When this range is exceeded, the flow to all the layers increases as the coronary pressure increases.

Pathologic states

Anemia
The effect of anemia on the coronary flow was studied here (Table 3), by comparing the two values of abnormal hemoglobin concentrations, Hb = 0.07 gm/ml and Hb = 0.04 gm/ml, to the normal value of 0.15 gm/ml. Anemia is shown here to be associated with increased coronary flow, increased oxygen extraction and a decrease in the oxygen tension in the coronary venous blood. (Jan *et al.*, 1977). It is shown by the model that at hemoglobin values of 0.07 gr/ml and a heart rate of 120 cycles per minute the myocardium is not hypoxic throughout. However, when Hb = 0.04 gm/ml, similar heart rate is associated

Table 4. The effect of hypoxia on the coronary flow

HR min^{-1}	Arterial PO$_2$ [mmHg]	Arterial oxygen saturation [%]	Coronary flow ml (min 100 gm)	Oxygen extraction [%]	Venous PO$_2$ [mmHg]
60	100	97	65	62	21
120			109	72	18
60	80	95	65	63	20.6
120			113	72	18
60	60	90	68	63	20
120			116	72	18
60	40	76	85	60	19
120			159	63	18
60	30	59	135	49	19
120			246	52	18

with subendocardial hypoxia. This will certainly result in a shift to anaerobic metabolism and lactic acid production.

Hypoxemia

Hypoxemia is defined as a state of decreased tension of O$_2$ in the arterial blood. Hypoxemia is caused by a variety of disorders mainly pulmonary diseases. The effect of hypoxemia on the coronary circulation was studied here (Table 4), for two basic heart rates. As seen in Table 4, the coronary flow does not change significantly above a critical arterial PO$_2$ level of 60 mmHg. However, below this value, the decrease in the arterial oxygen content causes a decreased PO$_2$ in the coronary venous blood, a decreased oxygen extraction and a considerable in-

Table 5. Valvular aortic stenosis

Aortic valve diameter [cm]	Aortic valve area (cricular) [cm^2]	Peak aortic flow [ml/s]	Peak gradient (PG) [mmHg]	Ejection fraction [%]	Stroke work [erg 10^7]	Blood pressure [mmHg]	Ejection time [ms]	Wall stress [mmHg]
3	7.06	404	1	67	1.04	135/83	310	96
1	0.78	308	54	67	1.36	129/83	330	141
0.8	0.50	258	95	67	1.55	121/83	370	171
0.6	0.28	180	156	60	1.69	103/83	460	224

Table 6. Compensation (of equal cardiac output) of a valvular stenosis of 0.6 cm diameter

	Peak aortic flow [ml/sec]	Peak gradient (PG) [mmHg]	Ejection fraction [%]	Stroke work [erg 10^7]	Blood pressure [mmHg]	Ejection time [ms]	Wall stress [mmHg]
by preload: end diastolic volume = 114 ml	200	175	59	2.01	105/83	470	265
by contractility F_{max} = 1390 mmHg	204	180	67	2.07	104/83	460	250
by hypertropy: increase in LV muscle volume from 172 to 234 g	201	179	67	2.03	104/83	470	181

crease in the coronary flow needed to compensate these effects. Note that no myocardial hypoxia is associated with the above-mentioned conditions.

Aortic stenosis

Valvular aortic stenosis is a common disorder caused by a variety of diseases and is usually characterized by formation of a jet of blood passing through the valve stenosed orifice. As shown by Hatle (1981, 1982) and Goldberg, (1980), the pressure gradient (PG) across the stenosed valve can be estimated from the kinetic energy losses by:

$$PG = \frac{1}{2} \rho u^2, \tag{5}$$

where ρ is the density of the blood and u the velocity of the jet leaving the stenosed valve with an opening area A_{st}:

$$u = \frac{Q}{A_{st}} \tag{6}$$

Eq. (5) and (6) can be incorporated into the general model discussed here and solved for different values of A_{st}. Table 5 lists the calculated mechanical parameters for different valvular stenosis. Interestingly, the ejection fraction and cardiac output does not change until a critical stenosis is reached. A decrease in the peak flow with increased stenosis is followed by a longer ejection time so as to maintain a constant ejection fraction. The ejection fraction sharply declines once

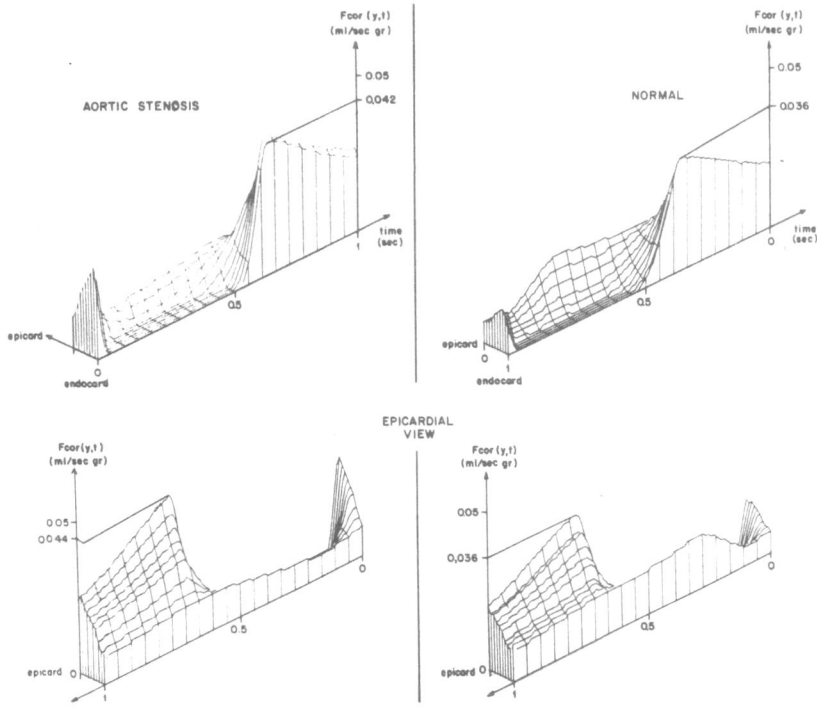

Figure 8. Coronary flow in aortic stenosis compared to normal pattern.

the critical stenosis state is reached. As shown in Table 6, compensation of a stenosed valve, can involve either an acute contractility or preload changes. However, chronic compensation for the increased afterload involves hypertropy of the muscle which tends to attenuate the increased muscle stress in this case.

The blood flow distribution in aortic stenosis is compared in Figure 8 to the normal state. It is shown that, in the case of stenosis, a large portion of the myocardium is not perfused during systole, as compared to the normal situation. This implies that subendocardial hypoxia is more likely to occur in aortic stenosis patients. This theoretically derived conclusion is indeed generally known clinically. Note that the large values of the LV wall stress and pressure are not accompanied by large aortic pressures, and the compressive forces on the coronary bed are increased to a greater extent than the flow driving forces.

Summary

A quantitative approach to assess the interrelationships between the LV mechanics, energetics and blood perfusion is presented and discussed here.

Although the geometrical assumption of axial symmetry limits the analysis, and precludes attacking problems which are associated with regional inhomogeneities, the model provides a powerful tool which enables to study the local interactions between LV mechanics and the energy balance within the myocardium. Furthermore, it yields and excellent tool for the study of the interacting global parameters. Three representative pathologies which are treated here, illustrate the power of the model to give quantitative interrelationships between the different parameters. Aortic stenosis, a clear mechanical perturbation, affects the wall stress and the oxygen consumption via the compressive effects on the microvasculature in the myocardium. Anemia and hypoxemia, each a 'pure' metabolic perturbation, are shown to affect the coronary flow, the coronary reserve and the cardiac reserve. Clearly, the model is applicable to other asymmetrical pathologies such as hypertension, cardiomyopathy and (some) defective homoglobin syndromes.

The theoretical model presented here is, in fact, based on experimental functional physiology. The integrated approach to the cardiac system discussed here, provides a qualitative tool for the study of normal states under different loading conditions, certain pathologies, effects of drugs on the cardiac behavior and other related problems. This study is part of the wide range research program aimed at the dynamic simulation of the cardiac system presently underway in these laboratories.

Acknowledgement

This study was supported by the Michael Kennedy Leigh Fund, London, and sponsored by the MEP Group Women's Division, American Technion Society, N.Y.

Nomenclature

BC	Oxygen binding capacity of hemoglobin (ml O_2/gm HB)
$E_T(y)$	Myocardial energy demand (in ml O_2/s gm)
Hb	Hemoglobin concentration (gm/ml)
$MVO_2(y)$	Oxygen consumption
n	Cooperation number, Hills Eq. (2)
PG	Aortic value pressure gradient
PO_2	Oxygen tension
PVO_2	Venous oxygen tension
P_{50}	Oxygen tension at 50% Hb saturation
$P_w(y, t)$	Intramural pressure
SO_2	Oxygen saturation of hemoglobin

SAO_2	Arterial oxygen saturation of hemoglobin
SVO_2 (y)	Venous oxygen saturation of hemoglobin
$\bar{S}VO_2$	Average venous oxygen saturation
S (y)	Surface area of a spheroid at distance y from the endocard
T_{wf} (y)	Tonus of the coronary resistance vessels
u	Blood velocity (Eq. (5))
y	Radial distance from the endocard
ρ	Blood density
ε	Strain
$\dot{\varepsilon}$	Strain rate
σ	Stress

References

Archie JP (1978a) Minimum left ventricular coronary resistance in dogs. J of Surg Res 25:21–25

Baller D, Bretschneider HJ, Hellige G (1979) Validity of myocardial oxygen consumption parameters. Clin Cardiol 2:317–327

Bellamy RF, Lowersohn JS (1980b) Effect of systole on coronary pressure flow relations in the right ventricles of the dog. Am J Physiol (Heart Circ Physiol 7) 238:H481–H486

Berne RM (1959) Cardiodynamics and the coronary circulation in hypothermia. An NY Acad Sci 80:365–383

Berne RM, Rubio R (1979) Coronary circulations. In: Berne RM, Sperlakis M, Geiger SR (eds) Handbook of Physiology. The Cardiovascular System: The Heart. Am Physiol Soc Bethesda, Maryland, pp 873–952

Beyar R, Sideman S (1984a) A model for left ventricular contraction combining the force length velocity relationship with the time varying elastance theory. Biophys J 45:1167–1177

Beyar R, Sideman S (1984b) A computer study of the left ventricular performance based on the fiber structure, sarcomere dynamics and transmural electrical propagation velocity. Circ Res 55:358–375

Beyar R, Sideman S (1984c) Time dependent coronary blood flow distribution in the left ventricular wall. Submitted for publication

Beyar R, Sideman S (1984d) Spatial energy balance within a structural model of the left ventricle. Submitted for publication

Binak KN, Harmanci N, Sirmaci N, Ataman N, Ogan H (1976) Oxygen extraction rate of the myocardium at rest and on exercise in various conditions, Brit Heart J 29:422–427

Bing RJ, Hammong MM, Handelsman JC, Powers SM, Spencer FC, Eckenhoff JE, Goodale WT, Hafkenshell JH, Kety SS (1949) Measurement of coronary blood flow, oxygen consumption and efficiency of the left ventricle in man. Heart J 38:1–24

Braunwald E (1971) Control of myocardial oxygen consumption: Physiologic and chemical consideration. Am J Cardiol 27:426–432

Bretschneider HJ (1979) Die haemodynamischen Determinanten des myocardialen Sauerstoffverbrauchs in: Dengler HJ, (ed) Die therapeutische Anwendung β-sympathikolitischer Stoffe. Stuttgart p. 45

Burns JW, Covell JW (1972) Myocardial oxygen consumption during isotonic and isovolumic contractions in the intact heart. Am J Physiol 223:6:1491–1497

Cross CE, Rieben PA, Salisbury PF (1970) Coronary driving pressure and vasomotor tonus or determinants of coronary blood flow. Circ Res 9:589–600

348

Diamond G, Forrester JS, Hargis J, Parmley WW, Danzig R, Swan HJC (1971) Diastolic pressure volume relationship in the canine left ventricle. Circ Res 29:267–275

Feigl EO (1983) Coronary physiology. Physio Rev 63:1–204

Feit TS (1979) Diastolic pressure volume relationship and distribution of pressure and fiber extension across the wall of a model left ventricle. Biophys J 28:143–166

Gamble WJ, Lafarge CG, Fyler DC, Weisal J, Monroe RG (1974) Regional coronary venous oxygen saturation and myocardial oxygen tension following abrupt changes in ventricular pressure in the isolated dog heart. Circ Res 34: 672–681

Ghista DN, Hamid MS (1977) Finite element. Stress analysis of the human left ventricle where irregular shape is developed from single plane cineangiogram. Computer programs in biomedicine 7:219–231

Gibbs CL, Chapman JB (1979) Cardiac Energetics, in: Berne RM, Sperelakis N, Geiger SR, (eds) Handbook of Physiology, vol. 1. The Heart. Am Physiol Society, Bethesda, Maryland, pp 755–804

Goldberg SS, Allen HD, Sahn DJ (1980) Pediatric and Adolescent Echocardiography. A Handbook. 2nd ed. Chicago: Year Book Medical, Ch. 3

Graham TP, Covel JW, Sonnenblick EH, Ross J, Braunwald E (1968) Control of myocardial oxygen consumption: relative influence of contractile state and tension development. J Clin Invest 47:376–385

Hatle L, Angelsen BA, Tromsdal A (1982) Noninvasive assessment of aortic stenosis by doppler ultrasound. Br Heart J 43:284

Hatle L (1981) Noninvasive assessment and differentiation of left ventricular outflow obstruction with doppler ultrasound. Circulation 66:381

Hoffman JIE, Buckberg GD (1976) Transmural variations in myocardial perfusion. In: Yu PN, Goodwin JF (eds) Progress in Cardiology. Philadelphia: Lea and Febiger

Hoffman JIE (1978) Determinants and prediction of transmural myocardial perfusion. Circulation 58:281–391

Jan KM, Chien S (1927) Effect of hemotocrit variations on coronary hemodynamics and oxygen utilization. Am J Physiol 233:H106

Janz RF, Grimm AF (1973) Deformation of the diastolic left ventricle I. Non-linear elastic effects. Biophys J 13:689–704

Janz RF, Inbert BR, Moriatry TF (1974) Deformation of the diastolic left ventricle II. Non-linear geometric effects. J Biomech 7:509–516

Johnson EA (1979) Force interval relationship of cardiac muscle. In: Berne RM, Sperelakis N, Geiger SR (eds) Handbook of Physiology Sect 2., Am Physiol Society, Bethesda, Maryland, pp 475–496

Klocke FJ (1976) Coronary blood flow in man. Proc Cardiovasc Dis 1952:117–166

Klocke FJ, Ellis AK (1980) Control of coronary blood flow. Ann Rev Med 31:489–508

McKeever WP, Gregg DE, Ranney PC (1958) Oxygen uptake of the nonworking left ventricle. Circ Res 6:612–623

Messer JV, Wangman RJ, Levie HL, Neill WA, Krasnow N, Gorlin R (1962) Patterns of human myocardial oxygen extraction during rest and exercise. J Clin Invest 41:725–742

Mirsky I (1970) Effects of unisotropy and nonhomogeneity and left ventricular in intact heart. Bull Math Biophysics 32:197–213

Mirsky I, Ghista DN, Sandler H (1974) Cardiac Mechanics Physiological Clinical and Mathematical Considerations. New York: John Wiley & Sons Inc. p 45

Moir TW (1972) Subendocardial distribution of coronary blood flow and the effect of antianginal drugs. Circ Res 30:621–627

Monroe RG, Gamble WG, Kumar AE, Stark J, Plange R, Sanders GL, Phornfutkul C, Davis M (1972) The Anrep effect reconsidered. J Clin Invest 51:2573–2583

Moskowitz SW (1979) On the mechanics of left ventricular diastole. J Biomechanics 13:301–311

Pao YC, Ritman EL, Woods EH (1974) Finite element analysis of left ventricular myocardial stresses. J Biomechanics 7:69–477

Pao YC, Ritman EL (1977) Visceelastic fibrous finite element, dynamic analysis of the beating heart. Proc Symp on Appl Comput Methods, pp 477–486

Pao YC, Mayendra KK, Padiyar RR, Ritman EL (1980) Derivation of myocardial fiber stiffness equation based on theory of laminated composite. Trans ASME 103:202–259

Parmley WW, Tyberg JV (1976) Determination of myocardial oxygen demand. Prog Cardiol 5:19–36

Pierce WH (1981) Body forces and pressures in elastic models of the myocardium. Biophys J 34:35–39

Pollack OH, Krueger JW (1978) Myocardial sarcomere mechanics: some parallels with skeletal muscle. In: Baan Y, Noordegraaf A, Raines J (eds) Cardiovascular System Dynamics, Cambridge, pp 3–10

Ross J, Covel JE, Sonnenblick EH, Braunwald E (1966) Contractile state of the heart characterised by force velocity relations in variably afterloaded and isovolumic beats. Circ Res 18: 149–163

Ruch TC, Patton HD (1974) Physiology and Biophysics. Philadelphia, London: WB Saunders Co., p 329

Sherman IA, Grayson AJ, Bayliss CE (1980) Critical closing and critical opening phenomena in the coronary vasculature of the dog. Am J Physiol (Heart Circ Physiol 7) 238:H533–H538

Skelton CL, Coleman HN, Wildenthal K, Braunwald E (1970) Augmentation of myocardial oxygen consumption in hyperthyroid cats. Circ Res 27:301–309

Skelton CL, Sonnenblick EH (1974) Myocardial energetics. In: Mirsky I, Ghista DN, Sandler H (eds) Cardiac Mechanics, New York: J Wiley & Sonc Inc. pp 112–140

Strauser DE (1979) Myocardial oxygen consumption in chronic heart disease: Rate of wall stress, hypertropy and coronary reserve. Am J Cardiol 44: 730–740

Streeter DD, Ramesh RN, Patel DJ, Spotnitz HM, Ross J, Sonnenblick EH (1970) Stress distribution in the canine left ventricle during diastole and systole. Biophys J 10:345–363

Streeter DD, Vaisnav RN, Patel DJ, Ross J Jr, Sonnenblick EH (1969) Fiber orientation in the canine left ventricle during diastole and systole. Circ Res 24:339–247

Van der Broek JHJM, Van der Broek MHLM (1979) Application of an ellipsoidal heart model in studying left ventricular contractions. J Biomechanics 13:493–503

Weber KT (1979) Seminars on myocardial oxygen utilization physiological and chemical correlates. Am J Cardiol 44:719–721

Weber KT, Janicki JS (1979) The metabolic demand and oxygen supply of the heart: physiological and chemical considerations. Am J Cardiol 44:722–729

Weber KT, Janicki JS (1979) The heart as a muscle pump system and the concept of heart failure. Amer Heart J 98:371–384

Weber KT, Janicki JS (1980) The dynamics of ventricular contraction force length and shortening. Fed Proc 39:188–195

Weiss M, Forrester W (1975) A model for the assessment of left ventricular compliance: the effect of hypertropy and infarction. Cardiovasc Res 9:544–553

Weiss HR, Newbauer JA, Lipp JA, Sinha AK (1978) Quantitative determination of regional oxygen consumption in the dog heart. Circ Res 42:394–401

West ES, Todd WR, Mason HS, Van Brugger JT (1966) Textbook of Biochemistry, Fourth Edition, London: The Maxmillan Co., p 612

Appendix A: The model of the LV mechanics

Figure A1 is a schematic presentation of the geometries of the assumed thick shell LV model in the reference, unstressed, and general states. It is assumed that:

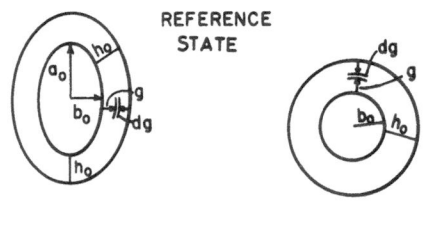

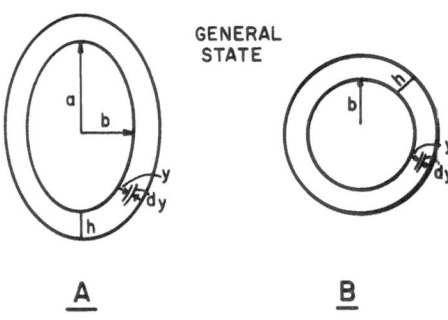

$$a/b = k \tag{A1}$$

throughout the contraction. The LV muscle volume is given by:

$$V_m = \frac{4\pi}{3} \left[(b_0 + h_0)^2 (kb_0 + h_0) - kb_0^3 \right] \tag{A2}$$

A layer of thickness dg at a distance g from the endocard in the reference state, transforms after contraction into dy and y according to:

$$dy = dg \frac{S(g)}{S(y)}, \tag{A3}$$

$$y = \int_0^g \left(\frac{dy}{dg} \right) dg, \tag{A4}$$

where $S(g)$ and $S(y)$ are the surface areas of the spheroidal shell at the corresponding distances. The strain rate of the different layers is obtained by differentiating (A2) (after replacing b_0 and h_0, by b and y), assuming incompressibility of the cardiac muscle:

$$\text{where} \quad \varepsilon_y = - \varepsilon_b \left(\frac{4kb^2 + kby + 2b^2 + 2yb}{2kb^2 + 2ybk + b^2 + 4by + 3y^2} \right), \tag{A5}$$

$$\varepsilon_y = \frac{1}{y} \frac{dy}{dt} \quad \text{and} \quad \varepsilon_b = \frac{1}{b} \frac{db}{dt}. \tag{A5}$$

The circumferential strain rate ε_{cf} is calculated by:

$$\varepsilon_{cf} = \frac{\varepsilon_b}{b + y} \left(b + y \frac{\varepsilon_y}{\varepsilon_b} \right). \tag{A6}$$

The fiber orientation α in the unstressed configuration is assumed to be a linear function of g:

$$\alpha = \frac{\pi}{3} - \frac{2\pi g}{3h_0}. \tag{A7}$$

The circumferential and the meridoinal stresses $\sigma_{\theta\theta}$ and $\sigma_{\varphi\varphi}$ are related to the pressure gradient by:

$$\frac{dP_w(y, t)}{dy} = \left(\frac{\sigma_{\theta\theta}}{r_1} + \frac{\sigma_{\phi\phi}}{r_2} \right), \tag{A8}$$

where r_1 and r_2 are the cavity curvature radii and $P_w(y, t)$ is the tissue intramural pressure. Modifying and integrating Eq. (A8) yields:

$$P_w(y, t) = \int_h^y \frac{\sigma_f}{b + y} \left(\cos^2\alpha + \frac{\sin^2\alpha}{k_1^2} \right) dy, \tag{A9}$$

where σ_f is the stress in the fiber direction and k_1 is given by:

$$k_1 = \frac{a + y}{b + y} \tag{A10}$$

$P_w(y, t)$ is used in the model of the coronary circulation as the tissue pressure. The normalized isometric stress $\bar{\sigma}_f(t)$ (defined as the stress developed by contracting a constant number of fibers) is related to the fiber physiological properties and is given by

$$\bar{\sigma}_f(t) = \begin{cases} (\bar{\sigma}_{f,max}) \sin \left| \frac{t - \tau(y)}{T} \right| \pi + \bar{\sigma}_{fp} & ; \ 0 < t - \tau(y) < T \\ \\ \bar{\sigma}_{fp} & ; \ 0 > t - \tau(y) \text{ and } t - \tau(y) > T \end{cases} \tag{A11}$$

The electrical activation front moves radially from the endocardium to the epicardium at a velocity c, causing a time delay $\tau(y)$ for the corresponding muscle layer

The maximum normalized isometric stress $\bar{\sigma}_{f, max}$ is given by Eq. 10 in the text. The passive stress $\bar{\sigma}_{fp}$ is defined by:

$$\bar{\sigma}_{fp} = \begin{cases} E(e^{D(\lambda-1)} - 1) & ; \quad \lambda > 1 \\ -B(1-\lambda) & ; \quad \lambda < 1 \end{cases} \tag{A12}$$

E, B and D are empirical constants, and λ is given by:

$$\lambda = \frac{SL}{SLP_0} \tag{A13}$$

The stress strain rate relationship is now introduced as:

$$\dot{\varepsilon}_{cf} = -\frac{\dot{\varepsilon}_{cf, max}}{\sigma_0} (\sigma_f - \sigma_0). \tag{A14}$$

The above equations governing LV function are solved in combination with a Windkessel arterial model which is formalized as:

$$P_{ao}(t) = e^{-t/R \cdot C} \left[P_0 - \frac{1}{C} \int_0^t e^{t/R \cdot C} Q(t) \, dt \right], \tag{A15}$$

where $P_{a0}(t)$ and $Q(t)$ are the aortic inlet pressure and flow, are the resistance and capacitance of the arterial system and P_0 is the end diastolic aortic pressure.

The relationship between the force of contraction (the contractility) and the heart rate HR known as the force interval relationship is given by Ref (A-2):

$$\bar{\sigma}_{0HR} = C_{HR}(HR - 60) + \sigma_0 \tag{A16}$$

where $C_{HR} = 10$ (a constant) and σ_0 is the maximum isovolumic stress for HR = 60 cpm.

The relationship between the duration of the activation function (in ms) and the heart rate can be deduced from the duration of the QS_2 interval. As shown in Beyar and Sideman (1984b), the end of systole is close to the peak of the activation function. It is assumed here that the duration of the activation function T is twice the duration of the QS_2 interval.

$$T = 2(418 - 1.8 \, HR) \tag{A17}$$

For more details about the LV model, See Beyar and Sideman (1984b).

Appendix B: The mathematical basis of energy metabolism

The energy demand of the myocardium $E_T(y)$ is approximated by:

$$E_T(y) = E_{bm} + E_{ma} \tag{B1}$$

where E_{bm} relates to basal metabolism and E_{ma} relates to mechanical activity.

The rate of ATP consumption is related to the instantaneous number of actin myosin crossbridges $N_{as}(t)$ given by:

$$N_{as}(t) = F_{ac}(t) \cdot N_{TS} \tag{B2}$$

where $F_{ac}(t)$ is time dependent activation function of the sarcomere and N_{TS} is the maximum number of cross bridges that can possibly be formed in a sarcomere of given length and contractility.

N_{TS} is proportional to the maximum isometric stress $\sigma_{f,max}$:

$$N_{TS} = C_1 \cdot \sigma_{f,\ max} \tag{B3}$$

Combining Eqs (B2 and (B3) yields:

$$N_{as}(t) = F_{ac}(t) \cdot C_1 \cdot \sigma_{f,max} = C_1 \cdot \sigma_f(t), \tag{B4}$$

where $\sigma_f(t)$ is the instantaneous isometric stress.

The rate of ATP consumption is a linear combination of:

(a) active stress formation, proportional to $\dot{N}_{as}(t)$
(b) maintenance of stress, proportional to $N_{as}(t)$
(c) slippage of actin and myosin fibers dictating a rate of reformation of cross bridges proportional to $N_{as}(t) \cdot \dot{\varepsilon}(t)$

Thus E_{ma} is given by a linear combination of the above relations i.e.:

$$E_{ma}(t) = \begin{cases} \alpha_1 \dot{N}_{as}(t) + \alpha_2 N_{as}(t) + \alpha_3 N_{as}(t)\dot{\varepsilon}(t) & ; \quad \dot{N}_{as}(t) > 0 \\ -\alpha_4 \dot{N}_{as}(t) + \alpha_2 N_{as}(t) + \alpha_3 N_{as}(t)\dot{\varepsilon}(t) & ; \quad \dot{N}_{as}(t) < 0 \\ \alpha_2 N_{as}(t) + \alpha_3 N_{as}(t)\dot{\varepsilon}(t) & ; \quad \dot{N}_{as}(t) = 0 \end{cases} \tag{B5}$$

differentiating Eq. B4 yields:

$$N_{as}(t) = C_1 \frac{d(\sigma_{f,max} F_{ac}(t))}{dt} = C_1 [\sigma_{f,max} \cdot \dot{F}_{ac}(t) + F_{ac}(t) \cdot \dot{\sigma}_{f,max}] \tag{B6}$$

Following earlier studies, the activation function $F_{ac}(t)$ is approximated by (half) a sinusoidal wave of the form:

$$F_{ac}(t) = \sin \frac{\pi t}{T_c} \tag{B7}$$

Introducing Eq. (B7) to (B6) yields:

$$N_{as}(t) = C_1 \cdot \sigma_{f,\,max} \cdot \frac{\pi}{T_c} \left(\cos \frac{\pi t}{T_c} \right) + C_1 \left(\sin \frac{\pi t}{T_c} \right) \cdot \dot{\sigma}_{f,\,max} \tag{B8}$$

$\sigma_{f,\,max}$ and $\dot{\sigma}_{f,\,max}$ are given by

$$\sigma_{f,\,max} = \begin{cases} 0 \\ \sigma_0 (SL - 1.65)/0.55 \\ \sigma_0 \\ \sigma_0 (2.95 - SL)/0.55 \end{cases} ; \dot{\sigma}_{f,\,max} = \begin{cases} 0 & ; \quad SL<1.65\,\mu \\ \sigma_0 \cdot SL \cdot \dot{\varepsilon}(t) & ; \quad 1.65<SL<2.2\,\mu \\ 0 & ; \quad 2.2<SL<2.4\,\mu \\ -\sigma_0 \cdot SL \cdot \dot{\varepsilon}(t) & ; \quad 2.4\,\mu<SL \end{cases} \tag{B9}$$

where σ_0 is defined as the maximum isometric stress which develops with an optimal sarcomere length, and SL is the instantaneous sarcomere length of the fiber. Combining Eqs. (B5) and (B8), assuming that ATP consumption is linearly proportional to the oxygen consumption, yields the oxygen demand due to the mechanical activity of the LV:

$$E_{ma}(t) = \varphi + \beta_2 \sigma_f(t) + \beta_3 \sigma_f(t) \cdot \dot{\varepsilon}(t), \tag{B10}$$

where φ is given by:

$$\varphi = \begin{cases} \beta_1 [\sigma_{f,\,max} \dfrac{\pi}{T_c} \cos \dfrac{\pi t}{T_c} + \sin \dfrac{\pi t}{T_c} \dot{\sigma}_{f,\,max}] & ; \quad \dot{N}_{as}>0 \\ -\beta_4 [\sigma_{f,\,max} \dfrac{\pi}{T_c} \cdot \cos \dfrac{\pi t}{T_c} + \sin \dfrac{\pi}{T_c} \cdot \dot{\sigma}_{f,\,max}] & ; \quad \dot{N}_{as}<0 \\ & ; \quad \dot{N}_{as} = 0 \end{cases} \tag{B11}$$

and β_1 to β_4 are linear combinations of the constants α_1 to α_4. Note that while Eqs. (B1) and (B5) are related to the ATP consumption rates, Eqs. (B10) and (B11) are transformed, via the constants β_1 to β_4, to oxygen consumption rates.

The time averaged oxygen consumption in each layer at a distance y from the endocardium $\bar{E}_T(y)$, is given by:

$$\bar{E}_T(y) = E_{bm} + \frac{1}{T} \int_0^T [\varphi + \beta_2 \sigma_f(t) + \beta_3 \sigma_f(t)\dot{\varepsilon}(t)]\,dt \equiv MVO_2 \tag{B12}$$

where T is the total duration the cycle. Finally, the averaged oxygen consumption per unit volume of the LV is given by:

$$E_T = \frac{1}{V_m} \int_0^h \overline{E_T}(y) \cdot S(y) \, dy \equiv \overline{MVO_2}, \qquad (B13)$$

where V_m is the muscle volume of the LV and $S(y)$, the surface area of the (assumed spheroidal) muscle layer in the myocardium at distance y from the endocardium, is given by

$$S(y) = 2\pi \left[(b + y)^2 + \frac{(a + y)^2 (b + y)}{(a + y)^2 - (b + y)^2} \arcsin \sqrt{\frac{(a + y)^2 - (b + y)^2}{(a + y)^2}} \right] \quad (B14)$$

For more details about the parameter values and the calculations see Beyar and Sideman (1984d).

Appendix C: The mathematical basis of the myocardial perfusion

The coronary resistance at each point y is assumed to vary between $R_{min}(y)$ (maximum vasodilatation) and $R_{max}(y)$ (maximum vasoconstriction). A regulatory function. $T_{wf}(y)$, ranging between 0 and 1 represents the tonus of the wall and related to the coronary resistance by:

$$R_{cor}(y) = R_{min}(y) + T_{wf}(y) [R_{max}(y) - R_{min}(y)]. \qquad (C1)$$

The critical closing pressure $P_{cr}(y)$ is assumed to depend on $T_{wf}(y)$ according to:

$$P_{cr}(y) = P_{c\,min} + T_{wf}(y) [P_{c\,max} - P_{c\,min}], \qquad (C2)$$

where $P_{c\,min}$ and $P_{c\,max}$ are the minimum and maximum critical closing pressures respectively.

The zero flow pressure $P_{zf}(y, t)$ is defined by:

$$P_{zf}(y, t) = P_{cr}(y) + P_w(y, t), \qquad (C3)$$

where $P_w(y, t)$ is the pressure distribution within the LV wall.

The total coronary resistance is assumed to be a function of the transmural pressure, i.e.:

$$RT(y, t) = \begin{cases} \infty & ; P_{cor}(t) - P_w(y, t) < P_{cr}(y) \\ R_{cor}(y) \dfrac{\Delta P_T}{P_{cor}(t) - P_w(y, t)} & ; P_{cor}(t) - P_w(y, t) > P_{cr}(y) \end{cases} \tag{C4}$$

where ΔP_T is the transmural pressure corresponding to the given values of $R_{min}(y)$ and $R_{max}(y)$.

The instantaneous local coronary perfusion is given by:

$$F_{cor}(y, t) = \frac{P_{cor}(t) - P_{zf}(y, t)}{RT(y, t)}. \tag{C5}$$

The time averaged coronary flow distribution is given:

$$\overline{F}_{cor}(y) = \frac{1}{T} \int\limits^{T} F_{cor}(y, t)\, dt. \tag{C6}$$

The total average coronary flow is given by:

$$F_{cor}(y) = \frac{1}{T} \int\limits_{0}^{h} \int\limits_{0}^{T} F_{cor}(y, t)\, S(y)\, dt dy, \tag{C7}$$

where $S(y)$ is given in Eq. (B14).

The time dependent total coronary flow of the LV is given by:

$$F_{cor}(t) = \int\limits_{0}^{h} F_{cor}(y, t)\, S(y)\, dy. \tag{C8}$$

For more details see Beyar and Sideman (1984c).

DISCUSSION

MIRSKY: Dr. Beyar, you mentioned that the myocardial oxygen consumption was higher or highest in the endocardial layers. Would you therefore expect the wall stresses to be higher there, and if so, does that agree with your other results? They seem to indicate that the maximum stresses are in the mid wall.

ANS: Although the maximum in the circumferential stresses are achieved towards mid wall, the stresses along the fibers' axis are maximal at the endocardial layers. A linear combination of the stress and strain rate along the fibers yields the local oxygen consumption. At high preload, or high volume, where the endocardial sarcomeres are extended to a much greater extent than the epicardial sarcomeres, they develop a much higher stress according to the classical micro level of the Starling law. That would imply that the endocardial sarcomeres develop higher stresses during high preloads, and lower stresses at lower preloads. This is really a preload dependent variable. My model predicts that unless you assume that there is some kind of twisting, the stresses and the external work are higher for the endocardial sarcomeres. This is why my calculated results of oxygen consumption are highest for the endocardial layers. I would suggest that the effect of twist should really be considered in this simulation. An observation that endocardial/epicardial flow ratio is reduced with increased rates may be explained as follows: Usually, in oxygen consumption experiments, the heart rate is controlled by pacing, but I am not sure whether the end diastolic volume is also measured. It is possible that at high heart rates the preload value decreases, and a decreased preload could be associated with an inverse in the direction of oxygen consumption distribution. We need results from well controlled experiments, looking into the distributed parameters of oxygen consumption in order to be able to relate to the question of the linkage between mechanical distributed parameters and oxygen consumption distribution.

FEIGL: There is accumulating experimental evidence, and I think your model shows thereotical evidence, that torsion, or twist as you call it, is going to be very important as far as the sarcomeres as concerned. A modest amount of torsion will equalize sarcomere length across the ventricular wall. Just looking at a heart, let alone doing a dissection the way Streeter does, would lead one to think that there must be some torsion.

ANS: I agree that torsion tends to equalize the sarcomere length and stress distribution even though it does not completely equalize it. There is more extension and movement of the endocardial sarcomeres than the epicardial ones. Measurements of Yoran and Ross of the sarcomere length at end diastole and end systole show that the endocardial sarcomeres change length to a higher extent than the epicardial sarcomeres, though less than what my calculations show. We shall, of cource, include twist in the next step of our analysis.

FEIGL: If we get very fine resolution, then it will be necessary to consider folding of the inner layer of the endocardium and the trebeculae. That is beyond what anyone wants to do in a model, but folding will also tend to equalize the sarcomere lengths.

SAGAWA: I too agree that the twist is very important to equalize the degree of shortening. The question you briefly mentioned is that there currently seems to be no information as to in which phase of contraction it happens. My feeling in reading the papers by Theo Arts and my colleagues work, Hunter, is that, probably, a greater equalization occurs due to contraction as ejection goes on and the shortening of the various parts of the wall come into equilibrium equalizing the degree of shortening.

FEIGL: But there is a shape change during isovolumic contraction . . . .

SAGAWA: I do not deny that completely.

Physiological factors determining cardiac energy expenditure

COLIN L. GIBBS

Department of Physiology, Monash University, Clayton, Victoria 3168, Australia

Abstract

The factors determining the energy flux in cardiac muscle are outlined. The suggestion is made that the *initial* energy liberated during a contraction can be explained in terms of three major ATPases:– the Na^+–K^+ and Ca^{++}ion transport ATPases and the actin-activated myosin ATPase whilst *recovery* metabolism relates primarily to the process of oxidative phosphorylation restoring the levels of high energy phosphates. It is further suggested that under normal *in vivo* conditions there is considerable temporal overlap of the initial and recovery metabolisms. Total energy flux can be divided into basal and activity-related metabolisms. The difficulty of measuring the former is described and its biochemical basis is considered. Active energy flux per minute depends upon 4 major factors namely; (i) heart rate, (ii) end-diastolic volume, (iii) contractile state and (iv) afterload. The active enthalpy per beat can be subdivided into at least 3 distinct components; (i) an activation term that relates to Ca^{++} release and retrieval, (ii) a work term and (iii) a stress-dependent term. The likely physiological magnitudes of these components are estimated from myothermic data and the way these values change with afterload and preload is shown. Enthalpy: load curves are discussed and the way these curves change with contractility is outlined. A brief mention is made of some of the other mechanical parameters that can be shown to predict myocardial oxygen consumption and attention is paid to a recently introduced index (pressure-volume-area). The reason why this latter index is successful is explained and the relationship between enthalpy:PVA and enthalpy:load curves is discussed. Differences between mechanical and thermodynamic efficiency definitions are explained. If allowances are made for recovery metabolism plus the basal and activation processes it is calculated that the actomyosin mechanical efficiency may exceed 50% whereas the actomyosin thermodynamic efficiency possibly just reaches 40%. There is a brief discussion of current muscle models, particularly those related to the heart, and it is concluded that although it is possible to predict cardiac energy expenditure with a fair degree of accuracy on the basis of present experimental knowledge real progress will only be made when our limited knowledge of (a) the cardiac activation cycle and (b) the cross-bridge mechanism is improved.

Introduction

Upon excitation cardiac muscle responds with the development of force and the performance of work together with the evolution of heat by those chemical reactions that underwrite contraction; this initial phase is followed by the recovery process involving the consumption of oxygen, the generation of carbon dioxide, the restoral of high energy phosphate levels and the evolution of heat associated with the chemical reactions of substrate oxidation.

Cardiac muscle will expend part of its energy as useful work, but the largest energy fraction will appear as heat and will be lost to the heart's surroundings. It should be noted that *in vivo* most of the stroke work component will eventually be degraded to heat in the resistance vessels of the various organs. *In vivo* cardiac heat loss includes convective heat loss to the coronary circulation, conductive heat loss to the endocardial and epicardial surfaces and to endothermic chemical reactions (ten Velden *et al.,* 1982). In the thermopile system, with which I am most familiar, the heat output is lost mainly by conduction along the elements of the thermopile to the metal frame which serves as a heat sink; there are additional heat losses via convection and radiation to the gaseous surroundings, within the muscle chamber. Space prohibits any consideration of thermodynamics as it applies to biological systems but the standard reference work is that of Wilkie (1960) and over the last 10 years my colleagues and I have considered its application to cardiac muscle (Gibbs, 1974; Gibbs and Chapman, 1979; Gibbs, 1983).

An isolated cardiac preparation can be treated thermodynamically as a closed system exchanging energy but not matter with its environment because the thermal consequence of respiratory gas exchange can be ignored. Therefore the measured enthalpy production (heat + work) can be equated to equivalent quantities of the associated chemical reactions such as oxygen consumption or high energy phosphate utilization. The thermodynamic justification for this statement has been provided recently (Gibbs and Chapman, 1979). The ultimate test of consistency between muscle biophysics and muscle biochemistry is the criterion of satisfying the First Law of Thermodynamics and this requires:

(a) complete and specific identification of the appropriate chemical reactions underlying the contractile events and the subsequent recovery.
(b) accurate measurement of (i) the molar enthalpies of all the identified reactions *in vivo*; (ii) the extent of the chemical changes occurring in contracting muscle; (iii) the evolution of heat and performance of work by muscle contracting under conditions similar to those used for the chemical measurements.

Initial and recovery metabolism

The energy expended during cardiac contraction is mainly apportioned among the following 3 enzymes; (a) the Na^+, K^+-ATPase of the sarcolemmal sodium pump activated in response to the altered ionic concentrations resulting from fluxes underlying electrical excitation, (b) the Ca^{++}-ATPase of the sarcoreticular and sarcolemmal calcium pumps activated in response to the flux or release of calcium ions underlying excitation-contraction coupling and (c) the actomyosin ATPase of the contractile mechanism which transforms chemical energy into mechanical work. The combined activity of these three enzymes linked directly with the energy cost of excitation and contraction may be called the *initial metabolism*. The ATP levels available for the reactions of initial metabolism are buffered by the creatine kinase reaction (Bessman and Geiger, 1981).

The distinction between the thermal accompaniment of the initial and recovery processes has been classically described for amphibian skeletal muscle by Hartree and A.V. Hill, (1922) who showed that the *initial heat* appears within the timecourse of a single contraction, whereas the *recovery heat* evolves over the next 20 to 30 min at $0°C$, the two phases being approximately equal in magnitude. This contrasts with the thermal behaviour of mammalian cardiac muscle where there is a rapid phase of heat production followed immediately by a much smaller and slower phase of heat production (Ricchiuti and Gibbs, 1965; Gibbs, 1969; Chapman and Gibbs, 1974; Alpert and Mulieri, 1982). Evidence has been obtained that in heart muscle a variable fraction of the recovery metabolic response is evolved within the timecourse of the mechanical event even at temperatures as low as 20 to $27°C$ although it is only fair to mention, however, that there is some dispute about this point as Alpert and Mulieri (1982) believe that a clear temporal separation can be obtained in rabbit cardiac tissue contracting at $20°C$ with glucose as the only exogenous substrate. At *in vivo* temperatures, normal heart rates and with the usual array of substrates in the blood my colleagues and I believe there can be little doubt that there is considerable overlap of the initial and recovery events. We have calculated (Chapman and Gibbs, 1974) that the recovery heat: initial energy ratio should be about 0.72: the exact value depends upon the substrate being oxidized. Two groups of workers using different experimental protocols have established that the calorific equivalent of oxygen is close to that predicted biochemically i.e. 20 kJ/l, (see Coulson, 1976; Chapman et al., 1982).

Basal metabolism

Even in the absence of mechanical activation all cardiac muscles consume oxygen and produce heat albeit at a rate much lower than when they are working. There are large variations across species in the magnitude of this basal metabolism and it may be surprising to readers to learn that I believe we have no real basis for giving an exact *in vivo* value for any species with certainty. All metabolic values for arrested hearts depend upon how the heart is arrested and several other factors have been shown to influence the measured basal value they include: flow rate, pressure head, substrate supply, temperature, end-diastolic volume, level of activity prior to arrest, time after arrest, blood versus saline arrest, cardioplegic agent e.g. high K^+ or low Ca^{2+}.

In a recent experiment (Gibbs *et al.*, 1980) with arrested hearts from dogs, blood-perfused at a high potassium level 20 mmol. l^{-1}, a basal $m\dot{V}_{O_2}$ of 1.9 ml O_2. 100 g^{-1}. min^{-1}; (equivalent to an energy flux of 6.3 mW.g^{-1}) was obtained. At levels of coronary flow found in the normally working heart it may be that this figure would be somewhat elevated both because of the distending effect of blood within the coronary circulation itself (Arnold *et al.*, 1970) and because of the higher level of Na-K ATPase activity associated with maintaining ionic homeostasis (Gibbs and Chapman, 1979). On dimensional grounds (Gibbs and Loiselle, 1978) it would seem reasonable to believe that the basal value in man would be lower, perhaps in the 1 to 1.5 ml. 100 g^{-1}. min^{-1} range. It is apparent, however, on the basis of our own results and the evidence of heart bypass surgery that it is possible to lower the normal *in vivo* rate perhaps 5–10 fold for two to three hours without destroying cellular integrity.

In recent publications I have considered (Gibbs, 1982, 1983) some of the underlying biochemical processes, particularly Na-K ATPase activity and protein turnover and calculated to what extent they might account for the measured 'normal' values of resting metabolism (about 20 to 50% depending upon assumptions). In order to account for the deficit I have speculated about other alternatives. A paper by Loiselle and Gibbs (1983) details some of the factors that can alter heat estimates of basal metabolism and it reports the surprising fact that the metabolic Q_{10} is about 1.4. In all our measurements the oxygen tension has normally been kept at values where respiration should not have been affected and the quoted energy flux rates include both initial and oxidative components. In arrested whole hearts, without perfusion, it seems likely that the lowered high energy phosphate utilization rate would have to be met by anaerobic high energy phosphate production. Some of the problems encountered in analysing basal metabolism are high-lighted in Figure 1 and some indirect evidence that protein synthesis is involved is shown by the data provided in Figure 2.

Active metabolism

The total active energy flux of the heart over a given time interval is influenced primarily by four factors; (1) heart rate, (2) the initial length or end-diastolic volume (EDV) of the heart, (3) the inotropic state or level of contractility and (4) the mechanical conditions under which the contraction occurs. For a given set of physiological conditions where factors (1), (2), and (3) are kept constant the

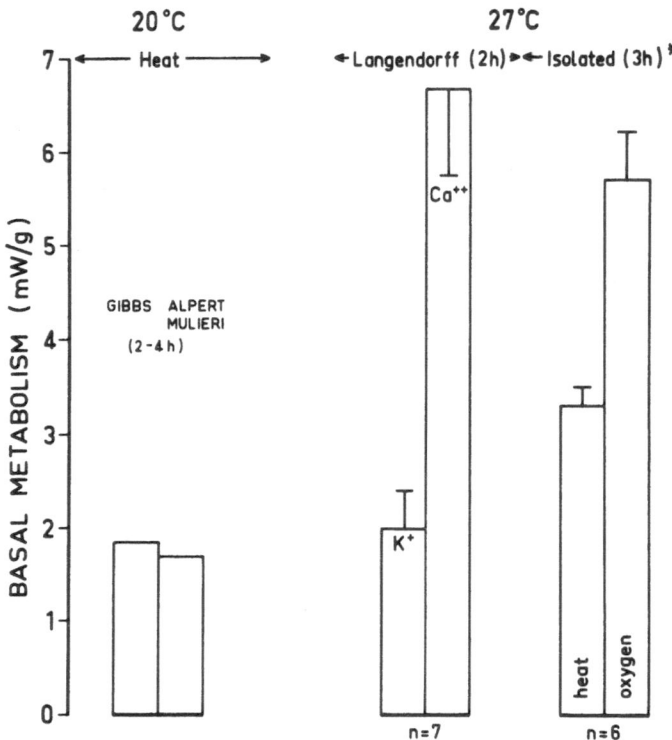

Figure 1. Basal metabolism measured in rabbits by a variety of techniques. On the left are some literature myothermic values recorded at 20° C, in the centre of the diagram are some values obtained at 27° C in whole hearts arrested either with high potassium (20 mmol. l⁻¹) or low calcium (0.1 mmol. l⁻¹, Ca⁺⁺; 10 mmol.l⁻¹, K⁺); the measurements were made 2 h after cardiectomy. On the right are some values recorded from papillary muscles taken from the *same* hearts but now bathed in normal Krebs Henseleit solution. The P_{O_2} in the oxygen electrode study was ~680 torr whilst in the drained myothermic chamber the P_{O_2} was ~450 torr.

energy flux per beat varies with the load. *In vivo* the arterial blood pressure constitutes the load against which the heart expels a volume of blood thereby doing stroke work. If one assumes a simple mechanical model of the heart (Mirsky, 1974) it is possible by making use of the Laplace relationship to relate energy flux to wall stress: physiologically blood pressure and EDV are the prime determinants of wall stress.

Myocardial active enthalpy is made up of two energy terms; (a) stroke work and (b) heat production. Normally in myothermic experiments papillary muscles are made to contract either isometrically or isotonically and their heat production is measured. Usually some 15 to 30 contractions are examined to achieve a stable mechanical response; the experiments are run at low temperatures (20 to 30° C) and at stimulus rates well below those occuring *in vivo* this ensures that tissue oxygenation is adequate; for a detailed discussion, see Loiselle, (1982). A typical record from a cat papillary muscle is shown in Figure 3, the small steps on the heat trace show the initial (rapid) phase of energy flux. In Figure 4 the active energy

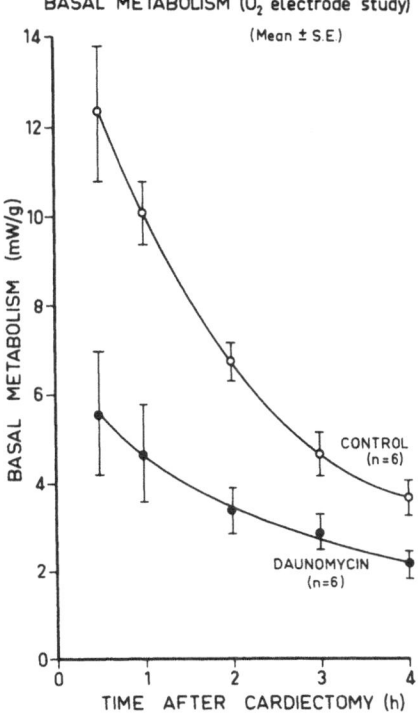

Figure 2. Resting metabolism, measured polargraphically at 27° C, versus time after cardiactomy in control and daunorubian (DNR) treated rabbits. The treated rabbits had received DNR for 6–11 weeks and were in cardiac failure as judged by their systolic-time indices and heart weight: body weight ratios.

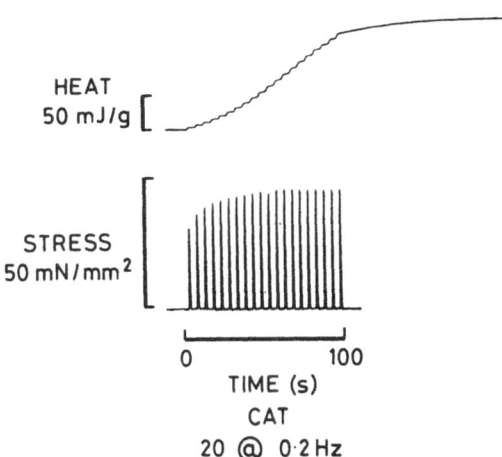

Figure 3. The heat production (top trace) and the force development (bottom trace) in a train of 20 isometric contractions of a cat papillary muscle. The stimulus frequency was 0.2 Hz and the temperature was 27° C.

364

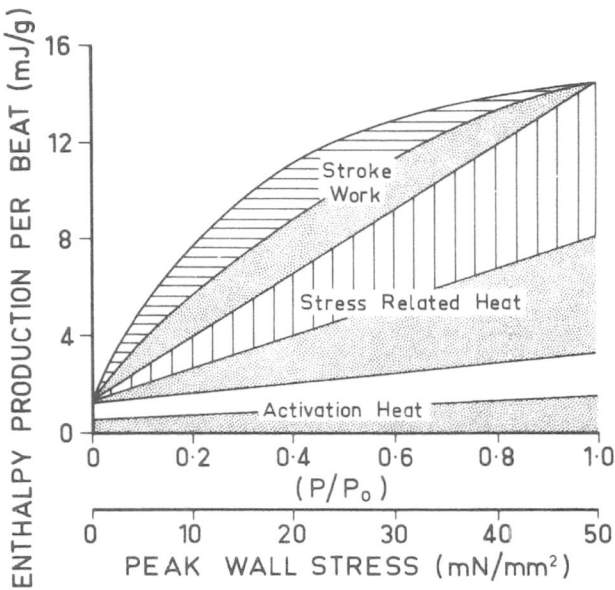

Figure 4. A schematic diagram showing energy output per beat (mJ/g) plotted against stress (mN/mm²) or load, where the load is expressed as a fraction of the maximum force developed for the prevailing conditions of initial length and contractility. The stippled areas represent the recovery heat contribution to the three active enthalpy components. The diagram is not accurately to scale.

output (enthalpy) per contraction (mJ/g of muscle) has been plotted against various loads. Similarly shaped enthalpy-load curves have been obtained by several groups of workers using a variety of different procedures to measure energy production; for a review, (see Gibbs, 1978). In the simplest analysis the *total* active energy can be considered to be the sum of two terms (stroke work + active heat production) but the active heat production term can be further subdivided following the skeletal muscle pattern as elucidated in the experiments of A.V. Hill. Thus in cardiac muscle there is a stress-independent term that is analogous to the activation heat term of Hill (1949). This heat component has it origins in the energy associated with the rise in free calcium ion concentration during sytole: this calcium has to be retrieved by the sarcoplasmic reticulum to produce mechanical relaxation, see Hasselbach (1976) for a review. Its magnitude, which is estimated to range between 2 and 4 mJ/g, will be governed (1) by the inotropic state of the heart and (2) by its end-diastolic volume since calcium release is now known to be continually modulated by fibre length (Jewell, 1977). None of the current experimental methodologies for measuring activation heat are secure in the sense that tissue stretch, tissue shortening or exposure to hypertonic solutions (see Homsher *et al.,* 1974) all influence calcium release or allow calcium pump heat to be contaminated with heat from other sources. A recent experiment which shows that the muscle shortening approach of Gibbs *et*

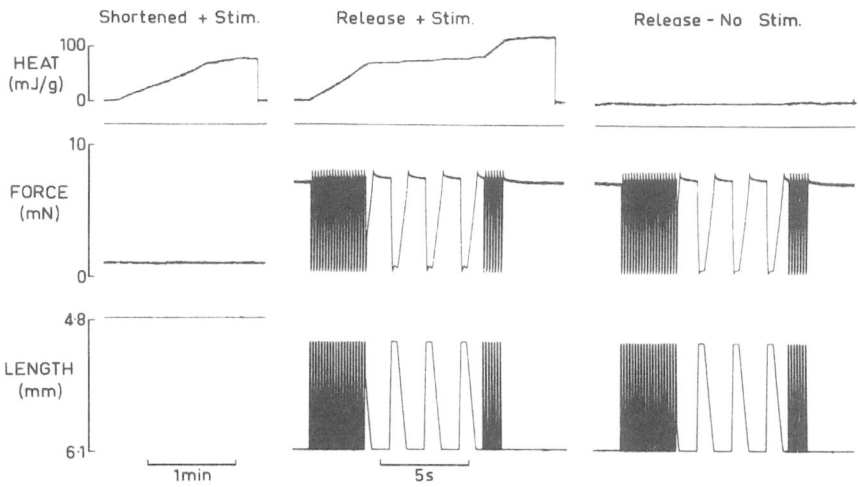

Figure 5. Activation heat recorded from a rabbit papillary muscle at 27°C. The preparation was stimulated 30 times @ 0.5 Hz, the muscle weighed 2.6 mg and l_{max} was 6.1 mm. The first panel shows the heat production when the muscle was pre-shortened to 4.8 mm; the centre panel shows the heat production when the muscle was kept at 6.1 mm before stimulation and was shortened during the latency period to about 5 mm length (notice the small active mechanical response superimposed upon the large fall in passive tension); the third panel constitutes a control series where the muscle was released but not stimulated.

al. (1967) underestimates the magnitude of this component is shown in Figure 5 and some comparative data is provided in Figure 6.

The other major heat component of the balance sheet is associated with the energy liberated by actin-activated myosin ATPase, i.e. the energy flux arising because of cross-bridge turnover. This heat term can be called the stress or tension-dependent term. In isometric studies if total heat production is plotted against peak active stress a curvilinear relationship usually results, (see Gibbs and Gibson, 1969) but in many preparations if the heat production is plotted against the total (active + passive) stress per beat a linear plot can result, see Figure 7, such that $H = A + kS$ where H = heat (mJ/g), A = activation heat and S = wall stress (mN/mm²) the coefficient k has a value of about 0.15. At a wall stress of 20 mN/mm², which is not an unlikely value during ejection against normal blood pressure (Gibbs and Chapman, 1979), this equation would predict a stress-dependent heat component of 3 mJ/g. Under isovolumetric experimental conditions, however, a peak stress of 50 mN/mm² might be developed and the magnitude of this component would then reach 7–8 mJ/g. As mentioned above in the ejecting heart, the stroke work per beat is probably about 3 mJ/g under optimal loading conditions and there must be a recovery heat counterpart of the stroke work term: our data would predict this recovery component to be close to 2 mJ/g giving a total work related metabolism of 5 mJ/g. The total myosin ATPase energy, when the stress dependent heat term is included at the 0.4 P_0 load level,

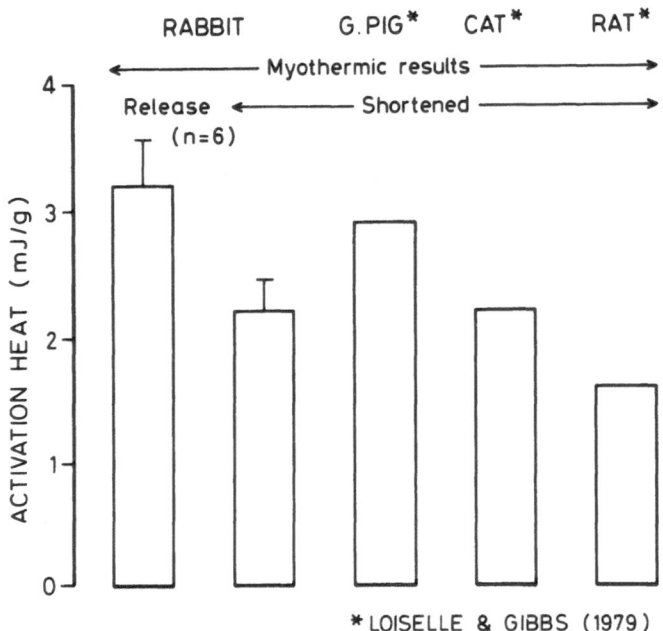

Figure 6. Measurements of activation heat in four different species. All data were collected at 27° C rabbit hearts were stimulated at 0.5 Hz, cats at 0.2 Hz, guinea pigs at 1.0 Hz and rats at 0.16 Hz. These stimulus rates produced force responses at 27° C and l_{max} that were at least 50% of the maximum possible values. Note that the rabbit activation heat has been estimated by the latency release method (see Figure 5) and by the shortening method of Gibbs *et al.* (1967).

would hence be, $3 + 3 + 2 = 8$ mJ/g. In Figure 4 an active enthalpy versus wall stress (or fractional load) diagram was constructed. I must emphasise that it is possible to plot energy output per beat against several other mechanical indices but I am not convinced that much greater predictive accuracy results (a more detailed account of some of these indices will be found in reviews by Gibbs (1978), Chapman and Gibbs (1979) and later I will discuss a very promising new index, PVA, or pressure-volume-area, developed by Khalafbeigui *et al.* (1979).

One's critics always like to suggest that it is dangerous to extrapolate from studies on papillary muscles to the behaviour of the whole heart *in vivo* and amongst several problems they focus on the unphysiological nature of the load produced by normal lever systems, the large experimenter-induced series elasticity caused by tie-damage, the inadequacy of oxygen supply in nonperfused preparations, the difference in activation patterns and cellular architecture of the heart and papillary muscles. Nonetheless the papillary muscle results obtained over many years agree with the early, 1930's, metabolic whole heart data; the later more physiological metabolic studies of Sarnoff and colleagues in the 1950's and with data obtained using the complex blood-perfused working heart preparation of Elzinga and Westerhof (1980). The latter authors have developed an

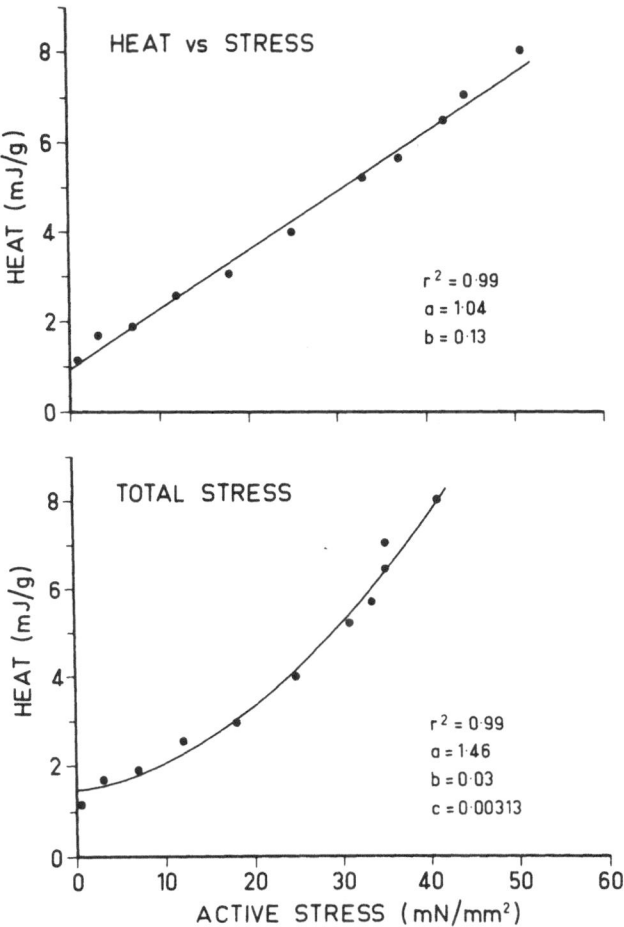

Figure 7. Isometric heat production per beat (mJ/g) plotted against active developed stress; the relationship has a pronounced curviture (bottom panel). The same heat data plotted against total stress (developed + passive) (top panel) is well fitted by a linear relationship. Data obtained from a rabbit papillary muscle at 27° C, stimulus frequency 1.0Hz; data averaged from 30 contractions.

experimental set-up, such that their preparations 'see' an afterload that mimics the complex *in vivo* load.

It seems likely that the *in vivo* load represents 40% (0.4 P_0) or less of the isovolumetric stress that would be achieved at the normal end-diastolic volume if the aortic valve failed to open; such an arrangement would allow the heart to function close to peak mechanical efficiency (Gibbs, 1978; Ford, 1980). The enthalpy: wall stress relationship is not static. Physiologically the curves will be altered by the pre-load (end-diastolic volume or pressure) and by the prevailing level of contractility. I have considered these factors in more detail recently (Gibbs, 1982). There are several physiological mechanisms that will increase contractility, a shift of the curve upwards and to the left, the main ones being; (i)

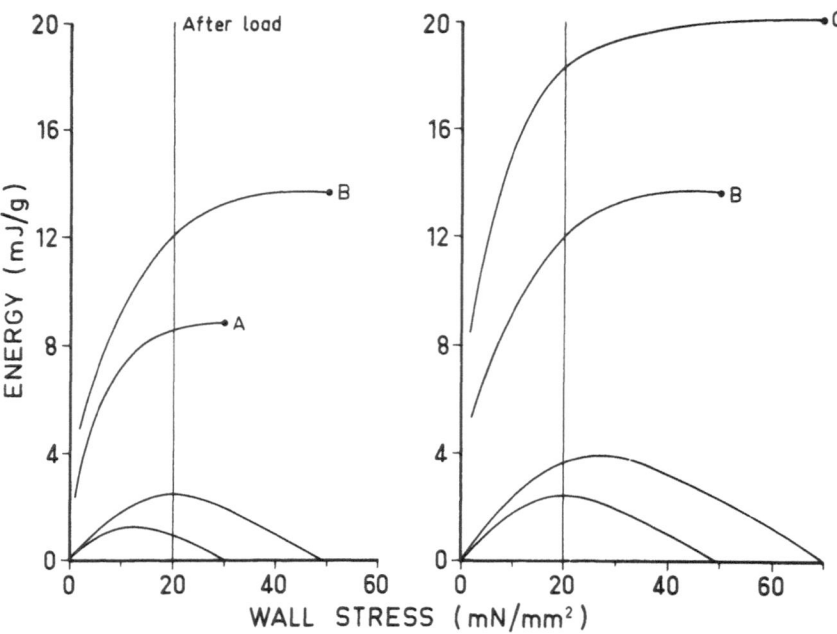

Figure 8. Schematic enthalpy: wall stress relationships showing the effect of (1) increasing pre-load A→B (left panel) and of (11) increasing contractility, B→C (right panel). The solid vertical lines give the approximate wall stress values for the normal after-load situation.

an increased sympathetic drive, (ii) an increase in heart rate, this effect is not necessarily accomplished by an increase in sympathetic outflow as the effect is an intrinsic one and (iii) release of certain circulating hormones e.g. glucagon. Some of the effects produced by altering pre-load, afterload and contractility are summarized schematically in figure 8.

In 1979 Suga and colleagues (Khalafbeigui *et al.*, 1979; Suga *et al.*, 1981) showed that cardiac oxygen usage per heat can be linearly correlated with left ventricular pressure-volume area. This area is shown diagramatically in Figure 9. It is the area bounded by the end-systolic and end-diastolic pressure-volume lines and the systolic segment of the pressure-volume loop. Thus PVA is the sum of; (i) a stroke work term and (ii) a potential energy term. Suga (1979) has shown that under the appropriate experimental conditions it is possible to realise about $^2/_3$ of the potential energy term as actual external work. Because PVA is linearly related to $m\dot{V}_{O_2}$, regardless of the type of contraction, and because it is dimensionally already in energy units, Suga has promoted its use as the mechanical index of choice in predicting energy flux. I have no quarrel with the concept but I think it is interesting to see why this linearity results when the $m\dot{V}_{O_2}$ or enthalpy versus fractional load (P/P_0) plot is curvilinear, see Figures 4 and 8. If PVA is calculated from the left pressure-volume panel of Figure 10 for different afterload levels (in this case different pressure levels) then when PVA, defined as above, is plotted

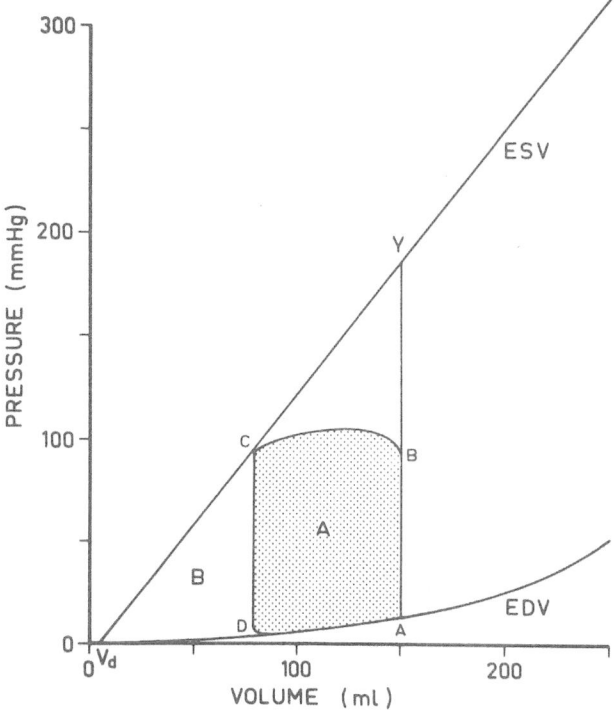

Figure 9. Schematic illustration of the pressure-volume-area (PVA) concept, see text for details. V_d represents the residual blood volume and Y shows the pressure that would be generated, with the heart at end-diostolic volume A, if the aortic value failed to open. The line V_d, C, Y is the end-systolic pressure-volume line. In an ejecting contraction PVA is measured as the sum of areas 'A' and 'B'. In an isovolumetric contraction PVA is given by the area enclosed by V_dYA.

against fractional pressure a curve is generated that is strikingly similar in curviture to an enthalpy versus load curve. I have already indicated that the load or stress axis of the isotonic enthalpy diagram can be replaced by a mean arterial pressure scale (see Gibbs and Chapman, 1979; Gibbs, 1982) this allows extrapolation of the data to the *in vivo* situation. Whether the curviture of the PVA: fractional pressure relationship is identical to that of the enthalpy: load relationship only further studies can tell with certainty. I do think however, that it is clear that they are similar enough to account for the observed linearity of the active enthalpy ($m\dot{V}_{O_2}$) versus PVA relationship.

Efficiency

At a thermodynamic level the usual definition of mechanical efficiency offers no real insights about mechanisms when applied to muscle (Wilkie, 1960, 1974) however some of the problems discussed by Wilkie (1960) are now nearer to being

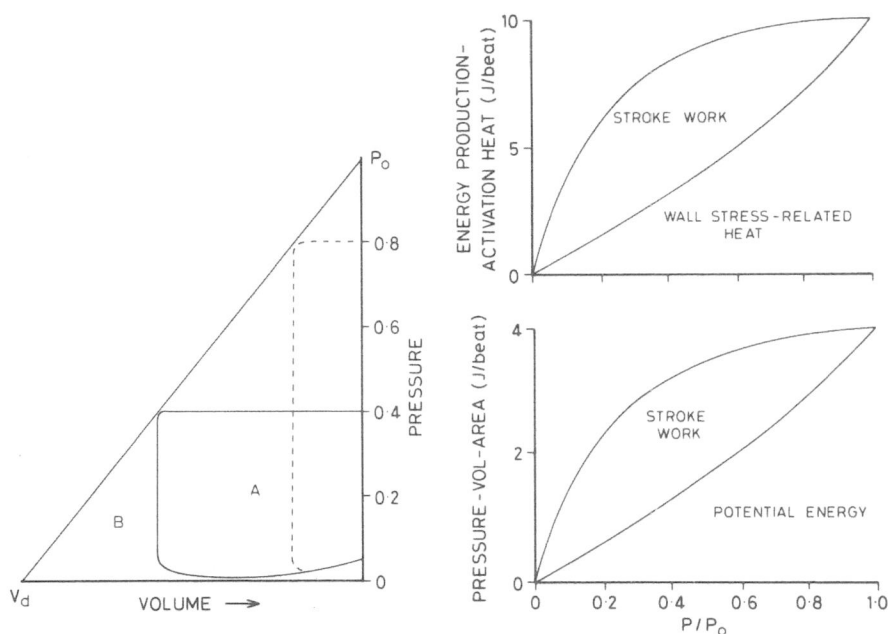

Figure 10. On the left is a pressure-volume diagram. At an after-load pressure of 0.4 P_0, where P_0 is the potential isovolumetric pressure, then PVA is given by the sum of areas 'A' and 'B', see Figure 9. The value of PVA does however depend upon the afterload pressure, the dotted 0.8 P_0 data illustrates this point. On the right, (lowest panel) the relationship between PVA and fractional after-load is shown. Note that the relationship is curvilinear and resembles the enthalpy: fractional load relationships shown in Figures 4 and 8 and the top right panel of this illustration. When the after-load is small stroke work is a large fraction of PVA or enthalpy but at high loads the potential energy or wall-stress term becomes the major countributor.

resolved. Thus the ratio of $\Delta G_{ATP}\, \Delta H_{ATP}$ *in vivo* is now more clearly understood: ΔH_{ATP} is considered to be -48 kJ/mol (Homsher and Kean, 1978) and ΔG_{ATP} to be about -60 kJ/mol (Kammermeier *et al.*, 1982) so that the $\Delta G/\Delta H$ ratio is about 1.25 in cardiac muscle. If we subtract the basal metabolism and examine the active mechanical efficiency, defined as stroke work/active enthalpy i.e. (work + heat), then over the past 18 years my colleages and I have obtained peak mechanical efficiency values, over 0.2 to 0.4 P_0 load range, that approach 30%; see also the earlier balance sheet calculation. Now the total enthalpy term as measured here contains an energy contribution that relates to ATP utilized by the sarcoreticular and sarcolemmal $Ca++$ pumps. This term can be subtracted out (Gibbs, 1974) and my colleague Brian Chapman, has called the resultant efficiency the myosin ATPase mechanical efficiency (J.B. Chapman, 1983) and it peaks at 37.5%. Now this efficiency value relates to the entire cardiac cycle so if we remove the *recovery* part of the cycle and calculate the *initial* myosin ATPase mechanical efficiency we obtain a value of 65%.

Of more fundamental significance is a calculation of the 'thermodynamic efficiency', (Wilkie, 1960; Gibbs, 1983), of the actin-activated myosin ATPase – this tells us what precentage of the free energy made available by ATP hydrolysis can be transduced into work. If we use a $\Delta G/\Delta H$ ratio of 1.25, the resultant *initial* cycle efficiency is 52%. This value, seems high for a chemomechanical transduction process. If a cross-bridge has a linear stress-strain relationships then, $W_{max} = {}^{1}/_{2} . P_0 \, l_{max}$, where P_0 is the maximum cross bridge force of 6pN (Pybus and Tregear, 1973) and the maximum cross-bridge throw, l_{max}, is 12.5 nm (Huxley and Simmons, 1971) then the calculated maximum work would be 0.38×10^{-19}J. If the *in vivo* ΔG_{ATP} is about -60 kJ/mol (Kammermeier *et al.*, 1982) then the free energy available per molecule at ATP split is 10^{-19}J giving a thermodynamic efficiency of 38% which is considerably below the value of 52% calculated above for the papillary muscle data.

Earlier on I referred to the PVA index of myocardial oxygen consumption (Suga *et al.*, 1981) and I have shown, though not explained at the molecular level, why (1) PVA is a good predictor of $m\dot{V}_{O_2}$ regardless of the type of contraction being considered and why (2) the relationship between PVA and $m\dot{V}_{O_2}$ is linear, see Figure 10. Now an additional important experimental observation made by Suga and colleagues was that if the basal and activation metabolisms are subtracted out then the PVA ($m\dot{V}_{O_2}$-activation metabolism) ratio is constant and Suga has called the resulting plot an isoefficiency line, see bottom of Figure 11, and has shown experimentally that it has a value close to 40% for the complete cardiac cycle i.e. initial and recovery metabolism being considered. Note, that when allowance is made for recovery metabolism, Suga's *initial* iso-efficiency value would be 69%: the value is even higher than the papillary muscle estimate! Not only is the isoefficiency line afterload and preload independent but it is not altered by inotropic agents. In Figure 11 I have tried to show in a schematic way how this comes about for the various types of contractions; I hope, in spite of a rather complex schematic, that readers will see that for light to medium loads (equivalent to an energy usage of 0 to 0.4J/beat) the stroke work term dominates the PVA index but from then on the potential energy term becomes the major component of the index. Please note that the energy flux data were obtained from dog hearts and to compare the values of Suga and colleagues with the myothermic values provided earlier in this review the data have to be divided through by the heart weight (approximately 100 g).

Muscle models

In a symposium devoted to imaging and simulation of the cardiac system it is perhaps appropriate that I make a few comments about the various muscle models that exist and their relevance to the cardiovascular system. I will deliberately refrain from covering material already reviewed previously, Gibbs (1978),

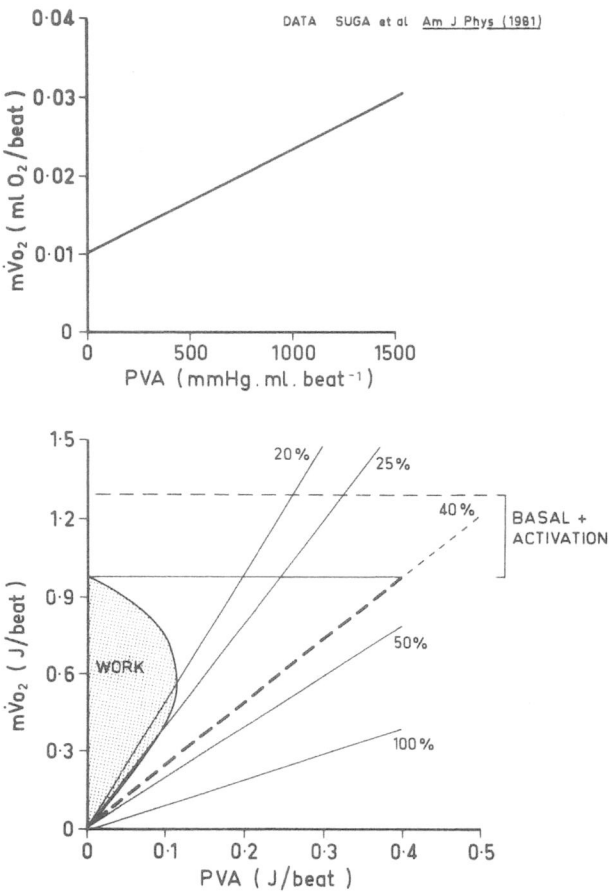

Figure 11. Top plot shows the type of liner relationships that is observed when active oxygen consumption per beat is plotted against PVA in ejecting or isovolumetric whole heart contractions. The bottom plot shows the relationship between active oxygen consumption and PVA when the basal and activation metabolisms are subtracted out. Experimentally it is found that all the data cluster around the 40% isoefficiency line (dotted line). The contribution of stroke work (stippled area) and potential energy terms (clear area) to PVA are shown. If the efficiency values were different for different types of contractions the data would have been widely scattered. The solid lines show various other isoefficiency values.

since in that article I outlined more or less historically the development of muscle models and described in detail the pioneering work of A.F. Huxley (1957). His model which is based on the sliding-filament theory of muscle contraction has cross-bridges which represent actual structures within the muscle. Since 1957 practically all the models developed have used the sliding filament hypothesis of muscle contraction as their starting point and most of the literature debate over the past 15 years has related to producing realistic models of; (i) the activation-relaxation sequence and (ii) the transduction process at the cross-bridge level.

At the present time, although there have been great advances made in our understanding of the activation mechanisms that are at work in cardiac muscle, only a person of great physiological naivity would suggest that there is general agreement about the multiplicity of activation mechanisms (Fabiato, 1983; R. Chapman, 1983); even the several ways in which Ca^{++} can be removed is far from sorted out quantitatively. These activation cycle problems have led most authors from Taylor (1969) and Julian (1969) onwards to adopt a fairly empirical approach to simulating the calcium transient. In the first real energetic model of cardiac muscle Wong (1973) opted to make the activation heat $A = K \int P_m(t)dt$ where $P_m(t)$ was the time-course of muscle tension and K was a constant evaluated from the data of Gibbs and Gibson (1969). In (1980) Panerai developed a more realistic model of excitation-contraction coupling where once again the equations were developed fairly empirically to fit experimental data in the literature. His simulation took into account length-dependent activation effects (Jewell, 1977) and interestingly Panerai's model was more successful, from a mechanical viewpoint, when this length-dependence was achieved by making the binding of calcium to troponin the underlying cause of the effect rather than changing the calcium release from the sarcoplasmic reticulum.

The most important part of the contraction cycle i.e. the crossbridge turnover mechanism, is the least satisfactorily understood part of all the present muscle models. In the two quasi-energetic models of cardiac muscle with which I am most familiar (Wong, 1974; Panerai, 1980) the cross-bridge mechanism of Huxley (1957) is assumed to be operating with appropriate values of g_1, f_1 and g_2 being entered to simulate the mechanical data. In Wong's analysis no assumptions were made about the ATP usage per crossbridge cycle: energy production aside from the work and activation terms was predicted from the myothermic demonstration (Gibbs and Gibson, 1970) that a linear relationship exists between heat production and tension-time integral. Panerai (1980) on the other hand made use of a general energy equation (initial cycle) suggested by Chapman and Gibbs (1972) where

$$E = A + \delta H \int_{t_1}^{t^2} k \cdot n \cdot dt$$

where E = initial enthalpy, A = activation enthalpy (see above), δH = molecular enthalpy of ATP hydrolysis *in vivo*, k = rate constant for disintegration of cross-links between action and myosin, and n = instantaneous numbers of cross links in existence. This model assumes that one ATP molecule will be hydrolysed per cross-bridge cycle and it seems to have produced very acceptable fitting of the data of my colleagues and myself, although the scaling procedure that was adopted by Panerai (1980) was fairly crude and the energetic results are hence expressed in arbitrary units. While I remain convinced that the idea of liberating a constant molecular enthalpy per crossbridge cycle is the simplest way to proceed (at least until there is clear evidence to the contrary) some authors in the skeletal muscle field, where there is an embarrassing amount of energy liberated with shortening under light loads, at least at low temperatures, have felt compelled to postulate that the energy quantum released per crossbridge cycle is less than that liberated in the hydrolysis of one ATP molecule (Chaplain and Frommelt, 1971), and that the affinity of the ATPase reaction decreases as the load is reduced. The cardiac data doesn't seem to necessitate this modification because with light loads enthalpy output decreases very noticeably, see Figure 4.

The essential problem for all muscle models seems to be to produce a cross-bridge cycle that is realistic from a physico-chemical viewpoint. Although the original Huxley (1957) model has been updated to take account of the mechanical-transient data (Huxley and Simmons, 1971) there are several objections to the proposed force generation scheme, see Pollack (1983) for an interesting review: this has caused other authors to draw-up alternative proposals (Iwazumi, 1971; Gray and Gonda 1977; Eisenberg and Hill, 1978). The energetic consequences of such models are yet to be explored in any detailed fashion so it will presumably be sometime before their ability to satisfy the cardiac mechanical and energetic data will be tested.

Acknowledgement

Much of the work mentioned in this article was done with grant support from the National Health and Medical Research Council of Australia, the National Heart Foundation and the Utah Foundation.

References

Alpert NR, Mulieri LA (1982) Increased myothermal economy of isometric force generation in compensated hypertrophy induced by pulmonary artery constriction. Circ Res 50:491–500

Arnold G, Morgenstern C, Lochner W (1970) The autoregulation of the heart work by the coronary perfusion pressure. Pflugers Archiv. 321:34–55

Bessman SP, Geiger PJ (1981) Transport of energy in muscle: the phoshorylcreatine shuttle. Science 211:448–452

Chapman JB (1983) Heat Production. In: Drake AJ, Noble MIM (eds) Cardiac Metabolism, Chichester: Wiley, pp 239–256

Chapman JB, Gibbs CL (1972) An energetic model of muscle contraction. Biophys J 12:227–236

Chapman JB, Gibbs CL (1974) The effect of metabolic substrate on mechanical activity and heat production in papillary muscle. Cardiovas. C. Res. 8:656–667

Chapman JB, Gibbs CL, Gibson WR (1970) Effects of calcium and sodium on cardiac contractility and heat production in rabbit papillary muscle. Circ. Res. 27:601–610

Chapman JB, Gibbs CL, Loiselle DS (1982) Myothermic, polarographic, and flurometric data from mammalian muscles. Correlations and an approach to a biochemical synthesis. Federation Proc. 41:176–184

Chapman RA (1983) Control of cardiac contractility at the cellular level. Am J Physiol 245:H535–H552

Coulson RL (1976) Energetics of isovolumic contractions of the isolated rabbit heart. J Physiol London 260:45–53

Eisenberg E, Hill TL (1978) A cross-bridge model of muscle contraction. Prog Biophys Mol Biol 33:55–82

Elzinga G, Westerhof N (1980) Pump function of the feline left heart: changes with heart rate and its bearing on the energy balance. Cardiovasc Res 14:81–92

Fabiato A (1983) Calcium-induced release of calcium from the sarcoplasmic reticulum. Am J Physiol 245: C1–C14

Ford LE (1980) Effect of afterload reduction on myocardial energetics. Circ Res 46:161–166

Gibbs CL (1969) The energy output of normal and anoxic cardiac muscle. In: McCann FV (ed) Comparative Physiology of the Heart: Current Trends. Basel: Birkhauser Verlag, pp 78–92

Gibbs CL (1974) Cardiac Energetics. In: Langer GA, Brady AJ (eds) The Mammalian Myocardium. New York: Wiley, pp 105–133

Gibbs CL (1982) Modification of the physiological determinants of cardiac energy expenditure by pharmacological agents. Pharmac Ther 18:133–157

Gibbs CL (1983) Thermodynamics and cardiac energetics. In: Dintenfass L, Julian DG, Seaman GV (eds) Heart Perfusion, Energetics and Ischaemia. New York, Plenum, pp 549–576

Gibbs CL and Chapman JB (1979) Cardiac energetics. In: Handbook of Physiology. Cardiovascular System. Sect. 2, vol. 1, Chapt. 22, p. 775–804. Am Physiol Soc Bethesda, M.D.

Gibbs CL, Gibson WR (1969) Effect of ouabain on the energy output of rabbit cardiac muscle. Circ Res 24:951–967

Gibbs CL, Gibson WR (1970) Effect of alterations in the stimulus rate upon energy output, tension development and tension-time integral of cardiac muscle in rabbits. Circ Res 27:611–618

Gibbs CL, Loiselle DS (1978) The energy output of tetanized cardiac muscle: species differences. Pflugers Archiv 373:31–39

Gibbs CL, Mommaerts WFHM, Ricchiuti NV (1967) Energetics of cardiac contractions. J Physiol London 191:25–46

Gibbs CL, Papadoyannis DF, Drake AJ, Noble MIM (1980) Oxygen consumption of the nonworking and potassium chloride-arrested dog heart. Circ Res 47:408–417

Gray BF, Gonda I (1977) The sliding filamont model of muscle contraction. II. The energetic and dynamical predictions of a quantum mechanical transducer model. J Theoret Biol 69:187–230

Hasselbach W (1976) Release and uptake of calcium by the sarcoplasmic reticulum. In: Herlmeyer L, Ruegg JC, Wieland T (eds) Molecular Basis of Motility. New York, Springer-Verlag, pp 81–91

Hartree W, Hill AV (1922) The recovery heat production of muscle. J Physiol London 56:367–381

Hill AV (1949) The heat of activation and the heat of shortening in a muscle twitch. Proc Roy Soc London Ser B, 136:195–211

Homsher E, Briggs FN, Wise RM (1974) Effects of hypertonicity on resting and contracted frog skeletal muscles. Am J Physiol 226:855–863

Homsher E, Kean CJ (1978) Skeletal muscle energetics and metabolisms. Ann Rev Physiol 40:93–131

Huxley AF (1957) Muscle structure and theories of contraction. Prog Biophys Biophys Chem 7:225–318

Huxley AF, Simmons RM (1971) Proposed mechanisms of force generation in striated muscle. Nature London 233:533–538

Iwazumi T (1970) A new field theory of muscle contraction. Ph D Thesis. Ann Arbor, Michigan: Univ. Pennsylvania

Jewell BR (1977) A re-examination of the influence of muscle length on myocardial performance. Circulation 40:221–230

Julian FJ (1969) Activation in a skeletal muscle contraction model with a modification for insect fibrillar muscle. Biophys J 9:547–570

Kammermeier H, Schmidt R, Jungling E (1982) Free energy change of ATP hydrolysis: a causal factor of early hypoxic failure of the myocardium. J Molec Cell Cardiol 14:267–277

Khalafbeigui F, Suga H, Sagawa K (1979) Left ventricular systolic pressure-volume area correlates with oxygen consumption. Am J Physiol 237:H566–H569

Loiselle DS (1982) On the stretch-induced increase in resting metabolism of isolated papillary muscle. Biophys J 38:185–194

Loiselle DS, Gibbs CL (1983) Factors affecting the metabolism of resting rabbit papillary muscle. Pflugers Archiv 396:285–291

Mirsky I (1974) Review of various theories for the evaluation of left ventricular wall stress. In: Mirsky L, Ghista D, Sandler M (eds) Cardiac Mechanics. New York: Wiley, pp 381–409

Panerai RB (1980) A model of cardiac muscle mechanics and energetics. J Biomechanics 13:929–940

Pybus J, Tregear R (1972) Estimates of force and time of actomyosin interaction in an active muscle and of the number interacting at any one time. Cold Spring Harbor Symp Quant Biol 37:655–660

Ricchiuti NV, Gibbs CL (1965) Heat production in a cardiac contraction. Nature 208:897–898

Suga H (1979) External mechanical work from relaxing ventricle. Am J Physiol 236:H494–H497

Suga H, Hayashi T, Shirahata M (1981) Ventricular systolic pressure volume area as predictor of cardiac oxygen consumption. Am J Physiol 240:H39–H44

Taylor CPS (1969) Isometric muscle contraction and the active state: an analog computer study. Biophys J 9:759–780

Ten Velden GHM, Elzinga G, Westerhof N (1982) Left ventricular energetics: heat loss and temperature distribution of canine myocardium. Circ Res 50:67–73

Wilkie DR (1960) Thermodynamic and the interpretation of biological heat measurements. Prog Biophys Biophys Chem 10:260–298

Wilkie DR (1974) The efficiency of muscular contraction. J Mechanochem Cell Motil 2:257–267

Wong AYK (1973) Some proposals in cardiac muscle mechanics and energetics. Bull Math Biol 35:375–399

DISCUSSION

BEYAR: I wonder if you could comment about the temperature distribution in the L$\cdot$ $\cdot$ $\frac{}{k}$ one of the questions raised in the beginning of the conference.

ANS: It is my understanding that the temperature of the endothermic wall is slightly higher. The results that I would believe are those of Elzinga, Westerhof and colleagues, and I know Bruce Smaill and Peter Hunter (Smaill B, Douglas J, Hunter PJ and Anderson I. Steady state heat transfer in the left ventricule in heart perfusion. In: Dintenfass, Julian, Seaman Plenum Press (eds) Energetics and inchaemia, NY, 1983, pp 623–648), in New Zealand have got exactly the same result: the Elzinga et al. data is out in Circulation Research (Ten Velden GHM, Elzinga G and Westerhof, N. Cir Res 50, 63–73 (1982)), I think that the endocardial wall was a little higher in temperature but the mid-wall temperature was 0.4 to 0.5° greater than the endocardial or epicardial temperature. Both sets of workers had similar figures.

FEIGL: There is probably a countercurrent exchange with the coronary circulation which favour a hotter inside than outside.

SAGAWA: Since I heard my correlative work with Suga presented by you much better than I can do, I would like to have you comment, if you will, on this: Suga thinks that potential work portion goes totally into heat during the relaxation period. It should, from an energy balance point of view. Is there any biochemical basis, any study which supports this kind of thinking?

ANS: There must be internal work. There must be cross bridges there to generate a force equal to the afterload that the heart is ejecting against. So there is no question about there being degraded internal work there and I think Suga (Suga H, Am J Physiol 236 H494–H497)has done an experiment getting a fairly large fraction of the potential energy out. Something up to about $^2/_3$ of the potential energy is availble under special experimental conditions. My answer therefore is that I would expect all that potential energy to go into heat, unless you get up to some fancy trick to utilize that internal energy.

BEYAR: Would you also like to comment on what happens at hypoxia levels to the energy metabolism when things become disturbed.

ANS: Dr. Sagawa and Dr. Berkhoff have preliminary data showing that the slope of the PVA energy line decreases, and that is exactly what I would expect because of the coupling of the recovery metabolism to initial metabolism. I did experiments back in 1969 on the energy output of normal and anoxic cardiac muscle, (Gibbs C, In: McCann, FV (ed.) Comparative Physiology of the Heart: Current Trends, Birkhauser Verlag, Basel (1969) pp 78–92, in rabbit papillary muscles in nitrogen and with glycolysis blocked. I showed that the heat: stress relation comes down to practically where you would predict on the basis of the ratio of initial to recovery metabolism. So I think there would be a change in the slope of the PVA:oxygen relationship. The other interesting thing, however, is the tremendous saving that the heart can make on its basal metabolic rate. The heart really has a lot of potential for glycolytic activity and it aso has the ability to shut down a very big fraction of its normal non-beating metabolism. That is why I think it can look after itself for quite some time when arrested without being perfused.

Constraints in the interpretation of dynamic images of metabolic events

JAMES B. BASSINGTHWAIGHTE

Center for Bioengineering WD-12, University of Washington, Seattle, WA 98195, U.S.A.

Abstract

The processes of delivery of substrates to the cells of an organ begin with the local flows, followed by permeation of the capillary membrane, diffusion through the interstitial fluid space, and transport across the sarcolemma. After this the intercellular events such as reaction, binding, or sequestration can occur. The question to be discussed is whether a specific component of the system, such as transsarcolemmal transport, or an intracellular metabolic rate, can be characterized quantitatively with reasonable accuracy from a particular type of experiment.

Introduction

In general, we are concerned with the kinetics of *tracer* transport in a system which is otherwise in steady state. This means that the system can be considered as linear, and so long as the flows and concentrations of non-tracer mother substance are constant, then it is also stationary. When a system is both linear and stationary (non-fluctuating), then superposition applies, which allows the utilization of convolution integration, greatly simplifying mathematical analysis. Applicability of superposition is not an essential feature for eliciting transport or metabolic rates, but it is exceedingly helpful.

We are moving into an era in which such kinetics may be studied noninvasively, but the future approaches are based on older approaches. The standard approach which can be applied invasively or in isolated organs is the multiple indicator dilution technique: a set of tracers of differing molecular characteristics is injected into the inflow while recording from the outflow using rapid sequential sampling. For transmyocardial transport, appropriate rates of sampling are time intervals from one-half to two seconds for the earliest, highest frequency component of the outflow dilution curve, and then at slower rates at later times. The standard set of indicators would contain an intravascular plasma reference indicator, such as albumin (and perhaps a red cell label simultaneously), a solute which remains extracellular but escapes from the vascular space, such as cobaltic EDTA (Bridge *et al.*, 1982) or sucrose to provide a measure of the capillary permeability and the volume of the interstitial space. These 2 (or 3) serve as reference indicators against which the transport rates for a third indicator of interest may have its kinetics evaluated. The third tracer might therefore be one whose sarcolemmal permeability surface area product, or perhaps its first intracellular reaction, is desired. In actuality, the strategy is usually worked the other way. Given the goal to evaluate transport parameters for a particular solute, then the appropriate reference tracers are chosen; the extracellular reference would preferably have the same molecular weight, but be inert so that its volume of distribution would be the same as the solute of interest, and its capillary permeability-surface area product, PS_C, would be precisely the same as that for the solute of interest, given that the transport is through the same routes of passage. (When the solutes are hydrophilic, this is ordinarily understood to be the cleft between endothelial cells.) The intravascular reference would ordinarily be any large molecule which does not escape from the plasma, but when the substance of interest enters red cells, then the red cell reference is also needed in order to account for transport and exchange between red cells and plasma during transcapillary passage. (In this case, three reference tracers are being used.)

The multiple indicator dilution technique is not the only one, and is certainly not to be universally preferred. Techniques for external data acquisition include techniques for recording the content of tracer within an organ. The use of gamma photons of differing energy spectra allows the use of simultaneous tracers. Positron emission tomography allows the use of only one tracer at a time, but has the great advantage of good spatial resolution, providing estimates of residual content in tissue volumes of less than 1 cm³. Currently there are no standard detection systems designed to produce 3-D images from more than one gamma-emittor at a time. Even if there were, the price to be paid for the synchrony of the information would be much lower spatial resolution than by PET. X-ray contrast reconstructive imaging can provide good spatial and temporal resolution but only for one solute at a time, and for an extremely limited class of substances, namely, X-ray absorbing substances such as heavily iodinated compounds, which are not ordinarily of any metabolic interest. NMR, while being useful for high resolution proton imaging, has limited possibilities for tracer substances, since the concentrations must be at substantial levels in order to permit detection. Phosphorous and ¹³C imaging by NMR, while of potential use for metabolized substances, have very poor spatial and temporal resolution at this time.

Consequently, in this presentation I will emphasize the use of the multiple indicator dilution technique, if only because its applications can illustrate all the principles involved, without compromises due to technical limitations. These principles can be applied to the outflow indicator dilution technique and the residue function technique alike, so that translations may be made directly to the residue function approach whenever technical limitations do not intervene.

Theoretical considerations

Delivery to the tissue is via the local blood flow

For a substance whose capillary permeability is less than infinite, an increase in flow diminishes the initial transcapillary extraction. But regions with more flow always receive more indicator. Ordinarily, an estimate of flow is needed in order to estimate the membrane conductances. When it is not measured directly, it can be estimated from the area of the curve and the amount of the injectate using the standard formula:

$$F = q_0 \bigg/ \int_0^\infty C(t)\,dt, \tag{1}$$

where F = flow, cm³/s, q_0 is the amount of indicator injected, moles, and $C(t)$ is the concentration-time curve recorded at the outflow, moles/cm³. The response to a brief pulse injection gives the transport function $h(t) = FC(t)/q_0$. The instantaneous fractional extraction $E(t)$ is calculated by comparison with the intravascular reference curve $h_R(t)$: $E(t) = 1 - h(t)/h_R(t)$. Raising flow, causing diminished extraction is seen experimentally, for example in the potassium outlow dilution curves of Tancredi *et al.* (1975). The influence of changing flow is easy enough to understand, but in a complex system the influences of other parameters on the form of the impulse response is more complicated; it is useful to develop models as formal statements of one's hypothesis of the form of the system and thence to examine the sensitivity functions to the various parameters.

A blood tissue exchange model

Because capillaries in the myocardium are arrayed in densely packed, long-itudinally distributed arrays, the convection-diffusion equations can be simply written when radial diffusion is considered to be instantaneous within each region. Given that there are no interactions between neighboring capillaries, or that they are all alike within a region, then the equations are written as follows for an exchange region consisting of a capillary, endothelial cell, interstitial fluid space and an intracellular space (Bassingthwaighte *et al.*, 1983):
Plasma, pl:

$$\frac{\partial C_{pl}}{\partial t} = \frac{-F_{pl}L}{V_{pl}} \cdot \frac{\partial C_{pl}}{\partial x} - \frac{PS_g}{V'_{pl}}(C_{pl} - C_{isf}) - \frac{PS_{ecl}}{V'_{pl}}(C_{pl} - C_{ec}) + D_{pl}\frac{\partial^2 C_{pl}}{\partial x^2}, \quad (2)$$

Endothelial cell, ec:

$$\frac{\partial C_{ec}}{\partial t} = \frac{-PS_{ecl}}{V'_{ec}}(C_{ec} - C_{pl}) - \frac{PS_{eca}}{V'_{ec}}(C_{ec} - C_{isf}) - \frac{G_{ec}}{V'_{ec}} \cdot C_{ec} \quad (3)$$

Interstitial fluid, isf:

$$\frac{\partial C_{isf}}{\partial t} = \frac{-PS_g}{V'_{isf}}(C_{isf} - C_{pl}) - \frac{PS_{eca}}{V'_{isf}}(C_{isf} - C_{ec}) - \frac{PS_{pc}}{V'_{isf}}(C_{isf} - C_{pc}) - \quad (4)$$

$$\frac{G_{isf}}{V'_{isf}} C_{isf} + D_{isf}\frac{\partial^2 C_{isf}}{\partial x^2},$$

Parenchymal cell, pc:

$$\frac{\partial C_{pc}}{\partial t} = \frac{-PS_{pc}}{V'_{pc}}(C_{pc} - C_{isf}) - \frac{G_{pc}}{V'_{pc}} C_{pc} + D_{pc}\frac{\partial^2 C_{pc}}{\partial x^2}. \quad (5)$$

Conservation expression in absence of consumption and diffusion:

$$\frac{\partial C_{pl}}{\partial t} + v_{pl}\frac{\partial C_{pl}}{\partial x} + \frac{V'_{ec}}{V'_{pl}}\frac{\partial C_{ec}}{\partial t} + \frac{V'_{isf}}{V'_{pl}}\frac{\partial C_{isf}}{\partial t} + \frac{V'_{pc}}{V'_{pl}}\frac{\partial C_{pc}}{\partial t} = 0, \quad (6)$$

where C denotes concentration, D is the diffusion coefficient (D_0 in free (aqueous) solution, D_{pl} – in plasma, D_{isf} in interstitium, D_{pc} intracellular). F_s is flow of solute-containing mother fluid, G represents consumption (a first order clearance or removal without return) by any mechanism, L is the capillary length, PS is the permeability-surface area product of a barrier; V'_r is a virtual volume of distribution, equal to the actual volume V_r times the region-to-plasma partition coefficient; v_p is the plasma velocity in axial direction, x.

Subscripts: eca denotes antiluminal (basilar) surface of endothelial cell, while ecl denotes the luminal surface; g denotes the gap or cleft between endothelial cells providing a diffusional path between plasma and interstitial fluid.

In addition, certain ratios are commonly used in the coding and have useful physiological meanings:

PS_c/F_s is the total capillary permeability-surface area product divided by the total flow of solute-containing mother fluid. PS_{pc}/F_s is the analogous ratio for the cell PS. γ_r is the ratio of volume of distribution in region r to the plasma volume, V'_r/V_{pl}.

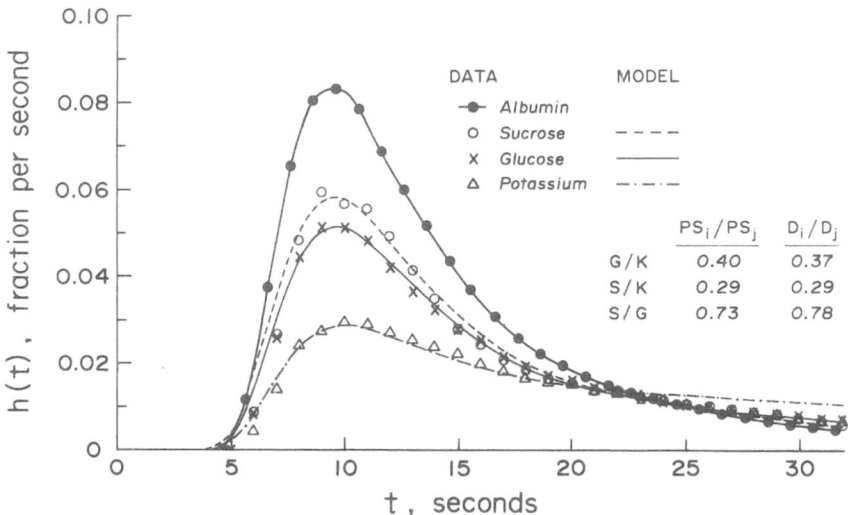

Figure 1. Outflow dilution curves from a blood-perfused isolated dog heart fitted with the axially-distributed capillary-isf model of Bassingthwaighte (1974). Note that the tail of the model potassium curve is too high – the model is inadequate, lacking cellular uptake.

Such a model for the capillary tissue exchange unit is incomplete by itself, and it must be considered to be in series with arterial and venous transport functions:

$$h(t) = h_A(t)*h_c(t)*h_v(t) \tag{7}$$

where the asterisk denotes the process of convolution. Since with superposition applying, convolution is commutative, then the arterial and venous transport functions can be combined as the transport function for the large vessels, h_{LV}, allowing the expression to be:

$$h(t) = h_{LV}(t)*h_c(t) . \tag{8}$$

Estimation of capillary conductance, PS_C

When this model is fitted to a set of indicator dilution curves such as for albumin, sucrose, glucose, and potassium, then the capillary-tissue unit can be considered as consisting only of the plasma space in order to fit the albumin curve, and must have an interstitial space and a finite PS_C for sucrose, glucose, and potassium. A 2-region model suffices to fit sucrose and glucose curves obtained over a 60-s period quite well, but the model fails to fit the simultaneously obtained potassium dilution curve. See Figure 1. For potassium, a third region must be opened up, namely a finite permeability for PS_{pc} and an intracellular volume of distribution.

Estimates of capillary PS_C's obtained by the fitting of the simultaneous sets of outflow dilution curves are useful for characterizing the capillary transport rates. Since it is often the capillary permeability which limits the rate of entry into cells, this parameterization is useful in understanding delivery of substrates or pharmaceutical agents. It also is the best mechanism for determining the routes of transcapillary transport, i.e. via interendothelial cellular clefts or across endothelial cells.

Computational aspects of the model fitting

The process of optimizing the fitting of the models to the observed indicator dilution data is a tedious one using standard procedures. The analytical solution for a 3-region axially distributed model published by Rose *et al.* (1977) is very slow to compute and even then has limitations to its accuracy. To facilitate computation a highly efficient numerical approach has recently been developed (Bassingthwaighte *et al.*, 1984) following the Lagrangian flow approach, sliding a fluid element within the capillary, described earlier by Bassingthwaighte (1974). This numerical method of solution, combined with a new and more rapid optimization technique using sensitivity functions (Levin *et al.*, 1980) greatly speeds up the modeling analysis.

Sensitivity analysis

Sensitivity functions are the partial differentials of the form of the model solution with respect to a perturbation of parameter values: $S_i(t) = \partial h(t)/\partial p_i$, where p_i is the value of ith parameter. These can be obtained for each parameter as shown in Figure 2.

The influences of F and PS are more or less reciprocal as might be expected from the form of the analytical solution which includes the term for the transmitted, non-extracted fraction of indicator as suggested by the derivation of Crone (1963) and Renkin (1959):

$$PS_C/F_s = \log_e (1 - E) . \tag{9}$$

The peaks of the sensitivity functions follow in the same sequential order as does the tracer in going from the arterial inflow into the cell. The relative magnitudes of the influences of each of the parameters on the solutions is dependent on the values for the others, in a particular way. When values for PS_C are high and V'_{isf} are low then the sensitivities to PS_{pc} and V'_{pc} are increased. This is simply to state the obvious, namely that the sensitivity is greatest to the rate limiting feature of the transport.

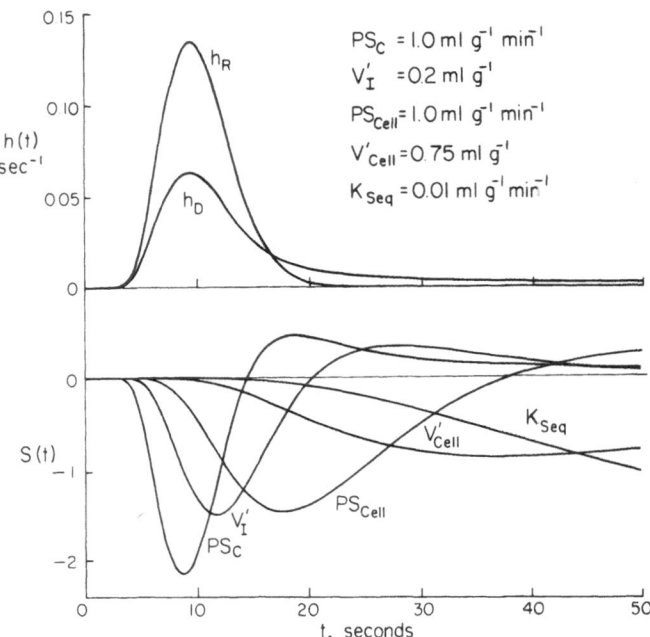

Figure 2. Sensitivity functions for the impulse response for an axially-distributed capillary-interstitial fluid-parenchymal cell model. Their peaks are in the same sequence as for a molecule passing from blood to cell. (Used with permission from Bassingthwaighte and Chaloupka, 1984.)

Estimation of cellular uptake rate, PS_{pc}

This is best determined when there is a nicely paired reference tracer to go along with the solute of interest. An example is the use of L-glucose which is not transported across membranes, as a reference for D-glucose, which is transported by a special mechanism and consumed within the cell, since it is the same molecular weight and therefore the same rate of penetration through the interendothelial cellular clefts, PS_g, and volume of distribution in the interstitial space, V_I'. The estimates of PS_{pc} for D-glucose is then made fairly accurately by virtue of the difference between the tails of the D- and L-glucose curves.

When a specialized transport process is involved, this may be characterized by performing a sequence of studies at different constant levels of non-tracer mother substance while determining the transport rate for tracer, which has a linear transport at each one of these constant levels. The linear transport rate, PS_{pc}, is influenced by the concentration of the mother substance in a particular way, namely that there is competition between the non-tracer and tracer substances for transport: a high concentration of non-tracer mother substance reduced the value of PS_{pc} obtained via the modeling analysis (Bassingthwaighte, 1982),

Estimates of myocardial sarcolemmal permeability, PS_{pc}, are useful for providing unidirectional rates of uptake, for tests of the mechanisms of transport (passive vs. saturable), and for revealing changes in the state of the membrane or of the transporter characteristics or transporter abundances.

Transport across endothelial cell walls

Contrary to the traditional view of the capillary wall as a cellophane lining, the endothelial cell is not merely passively involved in the transport process, but has a direct influence on transport of several substances. Even though this has been long recognized for the brain (Crone, 1963), it has not been recognized more generally as important for the transport of humoral agents (adenosine, serotonin, acetylcholine) or for substrates such as fatty acids. Now it is seen that endothelial transport needs also to be characterized since the transport across the capillary walls occurring through the endothelial cells and in parallel through the clefts between adjacent cells. Thus the total transport out of the blood is governed by the combination of two conductances in parallel:

$$PC_C = PS_g + PS_{ecl} .$$ (10)

The model therefore needs to be extended to account for the permeation at the endothelial cell on its luminal surfaces as well as on its antiluminal surfaces, and, as well, intraendothelial cellular consumption or transformation, and of course the endothelial volume of distribution. The equations for such a system, Eq. (2) to (5), have been solved by Bassingthwaighte *et al.* (1983). The analytical solution is given by them, but is not useful to compute since it contains destabilizing features such as taking the roots of a cubic, which are then used in Bessel functions, and which are in turn included terms in a double convolution integration. Thus the best technique for obtaining accurate and fast solutions is using the Lagrangian flow numerical solutions (Bassingthwaighte *et al.*, 1984). Such solutions have been fitted to data observed for serotonin and adenosine, and for the substrate palmitic acid. In each case a molecule of comparable molecular weight is used to characterize the rate of transport, PS_g, through the interendothelial cellular clefts.

As for PS_{ecl}, the mechanism of permeation through the endothelial luminal surface can be characterized by changing the background concentration of mother substances. When it is passive, concentration changes have no influence on PS_{ecl}, but when a facilitated transport is involved, then raising concentration reduces the apparent PS_{ecl}. Facilitated transport has been identified for adenosine (Gorman *et al.*, 1983).

The influences of flow heterogeneity on parameter estimation and on the distribution of deposition densities in the tissue

Because the heart has been recognized to have a moderate heterogeneity of flows, the range being from about 30% to 200% of the mean flow, it is important to recognize that this heterogeneity has an influence on the estimation of the transmembrane transport coefficients. The relative dispersions of regional flows, the standard deviation of flows per gram of tissue divided by the mean, is about 25 to 35% in awake intact baboons (King *et al.*, 1985), in isolated blood perfused dog hearts (Yipintsoi *et al.*, 1973), and in Krebs-Ringer perfused isolated rabbit hearts. The accounting for this heterogeneity has taken various forms, since there are a large variety of possible models for flow heterogeneity, and only in a few instances has there been an attempt to estimate the influence of this heterogeneity on the transport parameters. Rose and Goresky (1976) have utilized a model in which flow is considered to occur through non-dispersive large vessels and non-dispersive capillaries in series: the organ is represented by a large set of such units in parallel. This model has not been fully assessed, either in terms of its reality or in terms of the impact on the use of the model versus a single capillary tissue model, but it should be recognized that the need for the model was felt because curves were better fitted by use of this multi-capillary model than by a single capillary model, when the flows were considered to be non-dispersive. What might be a more realistic model for regional flow distributions is that given by Levin *et al.* (1980), who considered single large vessel dispersive functions, $h_A(t)$ and $h_V(t)$ combined to form $h_{LV}(t)$, in series with a set of parallel, dispersive capillary units. The model is given by the equation:

$$h(t) = h_{LV}(t) * \sum_{i=1}^{i=N} w_i f_i \Delta f_i h_{C_i}(t), \tag{10}$$

where the $w_i f_i \Delta f_i$ is the weighting function of relative regional flows w_i times the relative regional flow f_i providing the relative amount of indicator delivered to each region. The error in estimates of transport parameters and of volumes of distribution have been estimated by Goresky and Bassingthwaighte (1984) showing that PS_C is underestimated increasingly strongly if a single capillary representation is used instead of multi-capillary representations of increasing heterogeneity. The same study reveals that the errors in estimates of PS_{pc} are in the opposite direction and are larger, particularly when the values for PS_{pc} are large.

Improved models for accounting for heterogeneity may have to include the dispersion in distributed sets of large vessels, in addition to the intravascular dispersion along small vessels and the dispersion produced by parallel flows of unequal velocity. That is to say it is unlikely that either the model of Levin *et al.* (1980) or of Rose and Goresky (1976) will be the most realistic model to be worked out as a descriptor of the real system. A factor which may simplify such future efforts in this direction is the use of similarity of transport function through the vascular system, as described by Knopp *et al.* (1976). Similarity of transport functions means that the impulse responses superimpose when normalized with respect to their mean transit times, showing that they have the same relative dispersions, skewness, etc., and differ only in their mean transit times. Since this is a generally observed phenomenon for any particular rheological condition, it is rational to base heterogenous large vessel models on this phenomenon.

The most important features of these modeling efforts have been the incorporation of realistic capillary exchange units, of incorporating heterogeneity of flows, of fitting the multiple sets of data obtained simultaneously with sets of equations which utilize similar parameters where that is possible (for permeabilities or volumes), and account for the axially distributed nature of the system along with the heterogeneity of regional flows.

All of the principles demonstrated in these multiple outflow indicator dilution techniques are applicable to the residue function techniques.

Next developments

The next stages of development toward applications of this technologic approach to the analysis of images of metabolized substances are not easy. Perhaps amongst the simplest are the developments of the coding for fast computation of multi-capillary models for describing small but still heterogenous regions. Optimization algorithms must be speeded up yet further when hundreds or thousands of local concentration-time curves are simultaneously available, using for example positron emission tomography. Even though only modest modifications are needed in the theory of application of these models to residue function rather than outflow data, much consideration must be given to the use of residue data, whose 'noise' is different and the weighting of information at different times is different from that for outflow data. Since residue data provide a much higher weighting of information on the tail of the impulse response, that is, the deeper parameters of the system, this is likely to be the preferred approach for estimating sarcolemmal permeabilities and more particularly, intracellular reactions.

One of the perils of any modeling analysis is the failure to obtain the input function to the system under study. For both single photon and PET imaging of the heart, the left ventricular cavity blood pool concentration-time curve gives the appropriate information when it is convoluted with the vascular transport function between the ventricular cavity and the coronary artery inflow. (Low order differential operators can be used to describe purely intravascular dispersive transport.)

Positron tomography's advantage in spatial resolution is compromised by the inability to record concentrations of a few tracers simultaneously. An approach being tested by Raichle's group (Mintun *et al.*, 1984) is to record at separate times the residue curves for an intravascular indicator (e.g. ^{11}CO-hemoglobin) for regional flow or vascular volume, or a flow-limited (or nearly so) indicator (H_2^{15}O-water) to estimate regional flow and water space, and the solute of interest (a receptor-ligand or a substrate). What need working out are the kinds of error in parameter estimation occurring when there are shifts in flow or other feature in the intervals between the recordings.

NMR offers the possibility of seeing chemical transformation of tracer-labeled substances (e.g. ^{13}C-labeled substrate), or of changes in chemical composition of natural substances (phosphorous in various high energy phosphates; phosphocreatine and free phosphate). The recording time required for good spectra is minutes, rather than the seconds adequate for on-line gamma recording, so that NMR can be considered for slow changes or steady states, or, with gating, regularly fluctuating steady states, but without much hope for anything but very gross spatial resolution for metabolic substrates and tracers. In contrast, PET is good for spatial and potentially temporal localization of tracers but provides no indicator of chemical transformation except via the kinetics.

Summary

New developments in imaging single gamma photons, positron emittors, and NMR-detectable substrates and receptor agonists are paving the way for informative non-invasive approaches to understanding physiological processes and their degradation in clinical disorders. The instrumental technologies are advancing rapidly, and now much effort must be put into developing the analytical approaches to identifying the information contained in the data.

Acknowledgment

The efforts of Geraldine Crooker and Jean-Vi Lenthe in the preparation of the manuscript are greatly appreciated.

References

Bassingthwaighte JB (1974) A concurrent flow model for extraction during transcapillary passage. Circ Res 35: 483–503

Bassingthwaighte JB (1982) Overview of symposium: Measuring cellular transport *in vivo*. Fed Proc 41: 3031–3032

Bassingthwaighte JB, Chaloupka M, Wang CY (1983) Transport by endothelial cells *in vivo*: model analysis from indicator dilution after single transcapillary passage. (abstr) Fed Proc 42: 580

Bassingthwaighte JB, Lenhoff AM, Stephenson JL (1984) A sliding-element algorithm for rapid solution of spatially distributed convection-permeation models. (abstr) Biophys J 45: 175a

Bassingthwaighte JB, Goresky CA (1984) Modeling in the analysis of solute and water exchange in the microvasculature. In: Handbook of Physiology. Sec. 2 The Cardiovascular System. Vol. 4, The Microcirculation, EM Renkin and CC Michel, eds, pp. 549–626.

Bridge JHB, Bersohn MM, Gonzalez G, Bassingthwaighte JB (1982) Synthesis and use of radiocobaltic EDTA as an extracellular marker in rabbit heart. Am J Physiol 242:H671–H676

Crone C (1963) The permeability of capillaries in various organs as determined by the use of the 'indicator diffusion' method. Acta Physiol Scand 58:292–305

Gorman MW, Bassingthwaighte JB, Olsson RA, Sparks HV (1983) Endothelial cell uptake of adenosine in canine skeletal muscle. (abstr) Fed Proc 42:1261

King RB, Bassingthwaighte JB, Hales JRS, Rowell LB (1985) Stability of heterogeneity of myocardial blood flow in normal awake baboons. Circ Res: (under review)

Knopp JT, Dobbs WA, Greenleaf FJ, Bassingthwaighte JB (1976) Transcoronary intravascular transport functions obtained via a stable deconvolution technique. Ann Biomed Eng 4:44–59

Levin M, Kuikka J, Bassingthwaighte JB (1980) Sensitivity analysis in optimization of time-distributed parameters for a coronary circulation model. Med Prog Technol 7:119–124

Mintun MA, Raichle ME, Martin WRW, Herscovitch P (1984) Brain oxygen utilization measured with 0–15 radiotracers and positron emission tomography. J Nucl Med 25:177–187

Renkin EM (1959) Exchangeability of tissue potassium in skeletal muscle. Am J Physiol 197:1211–1215

Rose CP, Goresky CA (1976) Vasomotor control of capillary transit time heterogeneity in the canine coronary circulation. Circ Res 39:541–554

Rose CP, Goresky CA, Bach GG (1977) The capillary and sarcolemmal barriers in the heart – An exploration of labeled water permeability. Circ Res 41:515–533

Tancredi RG, Yipintsoi T, Bassingthwaighte JB (1975) Capillary and cell wall permeability to potassium in isolated dog hearts. Am J Physiol 229:537–544

Yipintsoi T, Dobbs Jr WA, Scanlon PD, Knopp TJ, Bassingthwaighte JB (1973) Regional distribution of diffusible tracers and carbonized microspheres in the left ventricle of isolated dog hearts. Circ Res 33:573–587

DISCUSSION

SIDEMAN: I was intrigued by a side point regarding the L- and D-glucose. We here have developed a system for glucose transport between maternal and fetal circulation. Would it be useful to use L-glucose against which to compare D-glucose transport across a live placenta?

ANS: From my point of view, very definitely. In order to actually paramaterize the carrier mediated transport of D-glucose, we have found it very important to utilize reference non-transported molecule of the same weight. Therefore D- and L-glucose are an ideal pair. Obviously, one could use other hexoses as a reference. But when the cellular uptake plays a role in the transport from maternal to fetal blood across the placenta, the solute is traversing a complex membrane composed of several sets of cells; each cell may be both transporting and consuming glucose, not merely acting as an inert obstruction, so I would think that the use of a reference like L-glucose would be very valuable.

SIDEMAN: Thank you. May I ask you another general question? In this meeting we have multi-leveled problems, going from the micro to the macro. How would you tailor your cellular approach to a larger macro scale application?

ANS: One of the things I didn't emphasize here was how little we know about an important feature of the macro scale, the characterization of the heterogeneity within an organ. For example, dr. Feigl mentioned diffusional shunting of hydrogen. None of the heterogeneity models that I showed thus far will account for both hydrophilic solute transport and heat or hydrogen transport such as that shown by Roth and Feigl (1981). Their observations, and ours (Bassingthwaighte, Yipintsoi and Knopp, 1984) suggest an approach to a more global assessment. If one uses a large set of tracers of differing diffusivity, the differing degrees of interactions between regions may be quantitated, and one may be able to end up with a proper characterization of that vascular network, in terms of the flow profiles, in a more global way through the tissue. We are not very close to that yet. We do need something more realistic in that heterogeneity field.

Another approach that may help to define studies at the macro level is the use of sensitivity functions for deciding whether you have the right experiment or not. Commonly, one explores model behaviour to get a feeling for the system and designing experiments. Actually instead of, or in addition to, manipulating parameters, you can calculate sensitivity functions. Their form gives an answer to the question of whether the experiment is going to give information on each particular parameter. This is an example of a nice technique that is increasingly useful as a model becomes more complex.

Discussion References

Bassingthwaighte JB, Yipintsoi T, Knopp TJ (1984) Diffusional arteriovenous shunting in the heart. Microvasc Res 28:233–253

Roth AC, Feigl EO (1981) Diffusional shunting in the canine myocardium. Circ Res 48:470–480

Flux analysis of ^{13}C NMR metabolite enrichments in perfused rat hearts using FACSIMILE

JOHN R. WILLIAMSON, STEVEN H. SEEHOLZER and
EDWIN M. CHANCE*
*Dept. of Biochemistry and Biophysics, University of Pennsylvania, Philadelphia,
PA 19104, and * Dept. of Biochemistry, University of London, United Kingdom
WC1 6BT.*

Abstract

The fractional ^{13}C enrichments in specific carbon sites of key metabolites in perchloric acid extracts of perfused rat hearts were measured as a function of time after addition of ^{13}C labeled substrates. Accurate quantitation of ^{13}C fractional enrichments in glutamate, aspartate, and alanine, which are in exchange with their respective α-ketoacids, is made possible by the relative large pool size of these metabolites. A detailed mathematical flux model of the citric acid cycle and ancillary reactions has been constructed with the FACSIMILE program and used to solve unknown flux parameters by optimization techniques using nonlinear least squares analysis of the simultaneous differential equations required to describe the reactions. Parameters calculated from the quantitative analysis of the resonance line splitting caused by ^{13}C-labeling of one or more adjacent carbon atoms in the same molecule were found to be in excellent agreement with the corresponding parameters derived from the mathematical model. The quality of this agreement serves as an important cross-check for the appropriateness of the model's topology as well as the general validity of the calculated flux parameters. The present results adumbrate the practicality of ^{13}C NMR when used in conjunction with mathematical modeling for the assessment of metabolic networks and the measurements of metabolic flux parameters in living systems.

Introduction

Our studies with ^{13}C NMR in relation to cardiac metabolism have focussed primarily on the development of a mathematical model that allows flux parameters to be calculated from a knowledge of the specific carbon enrichments of metabolic intermediates resolvable by high resolution ^{13}C NMR spectroscopy (Chance et al., 1983). The concentrations of most intermediates in tissues are below the level necessary for adequate detection of the ^{13}C resonances, even when the carbon atoms are ^{13}C-enriched by administration of ^{13}C-labeled substrates. Therefore, available data for model building consists mainly of values for the fractional enrichment of the individual carbon atoms of glutamate, aspartate, and alanine, since in heart these are the most abundant tissue metabolites. However, because these amino acids are in isotopic exchange with their respective α-ketoacids, which are themselves key metabolites of the citric acid cycle (α-ketoglutarate and oxalacetate) or the end product of aerobic glycolysis (pyruvate), the information is sufficient to model the major aspects of energy metabolism in heart. Metabolic flux information is given from measurements of the increases of the ^{13}C fractional enrichments of the different carbon atoms of the intermediates visible by NMR following replacement of unlabeled substrates with the same concentration of ^{13}C labeled substrate. The pool sizes of all tissue intermediates thus remain constant, and there is a replacement of ^{12}C isotope with ^{13}C isotope.

In this paper we report studies that are a continuation of our previously reported work (Chance *et al.*, 1983) and all ^{13}C NMR spectra were obtained using tissue extracts prepared after rapidly freezing hearts perfused for different periods of time up to steady state isotopic equilibrium following replacement of normal substrates with ^{13}C labeled substrates. With this approach, a large number of scans can be accumulated (typically 2000 with a repetition time of 2 s) and high resolution of the line splittings due to [13]C–[13]C spin coupling between adjacent carbon atoms is obtained. The primary purpose of these studies was to extend our previous mathematical flux model (Chance *et al.*, 1983) by use of additional data with different ^{13}C labeled substrates. In addition, the line splittings of the noncarboxyl carbons of glutamate and aspartate for the different experiments have been quantitated in order to compare independently determined experimental values for the relative contributions of different isoptomers in the carbon resonances with corresponding values calculated from the model. The agreement was generally excellent and provides an important criterion for model validation. The present model gives well determined values of citric acid cycle flux for the different substrate conditions. The importance of malic enzyme activity in the regulation of the pool sizes of cycle intermediates and related amino acids is illustrated by the use of ^{13}C labeled pripionate as substrate.

Methods

Heart perfusions

Hearts from male, Sprague-Dawley rats (350–400 g) fed *ad libitum* were perfused without recirculation at 37°C using the Langendorff technique and a perfusion pressure of 95 cm H_2O (Pearce *et al.*, 1979). The pulmonary artery was cannulated for measurement of the coronary flow rate and the effluent oxygen tension. All hearts were paced at a rate of 300 beats/min and the aortic pressure was recorded. The perfusion fluid was Krebs bicarbonate medium containing 1.25 mM $CaCl_2$ equilibrated with 95% O_2 and 5% CO_2. Substrates were present throughout, and after 20 min of perfusion to stabilize the preparation, they were replaced with the corresponding ^{13}C-enriched substrate at the same concentration, and perfusion was continued for different times up to 34 min. Perfusion was terminated by rapid freezing the heart with tongs cooled in liquid N_2.

Sample preparation and analytical techniques

The frozen tissue from three hearts for each time point was separately powdered in a mortar and pestle at dry ice temperature. An aliquot was removed for dry/wet weight ratio determination and the remainder of the frozen powder was extracted in 3.0 ml of 6% (w/v) perchloric acid/g of heart, wet weight. After centrifugation, the supernatant was neutralized to pH 6.5 with 3 N KOH after addition of 10 μmol/ml K_2PO_4. The supernatants obtained from each time of heart perfusion were dried *in vacuo* and reconstituted in 1 ml of 33% D_2O/200 mg of heart, dry weight. ^{13}C NMR spectra were obtained after making final adjustments of the pH to 6.50, and metabolic intermediates in the extracts were measured by standard spectrophotometric (Bergmeyer, 1974) or fluorometric (Williamson and Corkey, 1969) techniques.

^{13}C NMR Techniques

^{13}C NMR spectra were obtained on a Bruker WH 360 spectrometer operating at 90.55 MHz. The tissue extracts (2 ml) were placed in a 10 mm NMR tube at 4°C with a coaxial capillary tube containing 20% (v/v) dioxane in 30% D_2O as an external standard (67.4 ppm). Data were accumulated using radiofrequency 45° pulses (7 μs), 16 K data points, 2 s pulse delay with composite pulse proton decoupling (1.4 W), and were Fourier transformed with 16K of zero filling. Quantitative measurements of the ^{13}C content of each resonance were made by normalizing to the dioxane resonance and correcting for the effect of saturation and nuclear Overhauser enhancement. Standardization of the dioxane capillary was determined separately under identical conditions used for obtaining tissue extracts, using 50 mM glutamate in 0.1 M KCl and 10 mM KH_2PO_4 (pH 6.5) and a value of 1.108% for the ^{13}C natural abundance. The correction factors were determined by gated decoupling with a 12 s delay time (Harris and Newman, 1976).

Model construction

The basic construction of the mathematical model using simplified metabolic networks to describe the reactions of the citric acid cycle and associated trans-amination reactions between pyruvate and alanine, oxalacetate and aspartate and α-ketoglutarate and glutamate, and the use of the FACSIMILE program (Chance *et al.*, 1977) to solve the rather large number of simultaneous differential equations generated by the model was the same as previously described (Chance *et al.*, 1983). For the present experiments the model was expanded to include an input flux at the level of succinate to represent propionate metabolism to succinyl-CoA, and a dilution of the aspartate pool to represent net proteolysis. These input fluxes required an output flux of carbon from the citric acid cycle in order to maintain a steady state carbon balance, for which the conversion of malate to pyruvate via malic enzyme was chosen. The model calculates the unknown flux parameters to provide a minimum least squares fit of the ^{13}C fractional enrich-ments of specific carbon atoms of metabolic intermediates as measured by ^{13}C NMR spectroscopy.

Results and discussion

Perfusion with [3-^{13}C] pyruvate

A ^{13}C NMR spectrum of a tissue extract prepared from three pooled hearts perfused for 21 min with 5 mM glucose and 1 mM [3-^{13}C] pyruvate is shown in Figure 1. The bottom part of the figure shows the spectrum from 15 to 57 ppm with resonances corresponding to alanine C–3, lactate C–3, glutamate C–2, C–3 and C–4, aspartate C–2 and C–3, malate C–3 and citrate C–2 plus C–4. Singlets of the C–1 and C–2 of taurine at 48.4 and 36.5 ppm, respectively, and small lines arising from glutamine C–2, C–3, and C–4 are also seen. The inserts at the top of the figure show the line splittings of the glutamate and aspartate carbons more clearly. The number and relative size of the individual lines gives information about the relative abundance of isoptomers containing adjacent ^{13}C-labeled carbons. A detailed interpretation of the line-splittings will be given in a later section.

Figure 2 shows the time courses of changes in the ^{13}C fractional enrichments of specific carbon atoms of alanine (YAl_3), glutamate (YG_4, YG_3, YG_2) and aspar-tate (YA_3, YA_2) in hearts perfused under conditions similar to those of Figure 1. Experimentally determined values for YG_2 and YG_3 were similar, as were those for YA_2 and YA_3, and have been averaged in Figure 2. The lines shown are those calculated by the mathematical model using the network shown in Figure 3. Mean values for the calculated flux parameters are shown in Figure 3 and are presented in more detail with 5% and 95% confidence limits in Table 1.

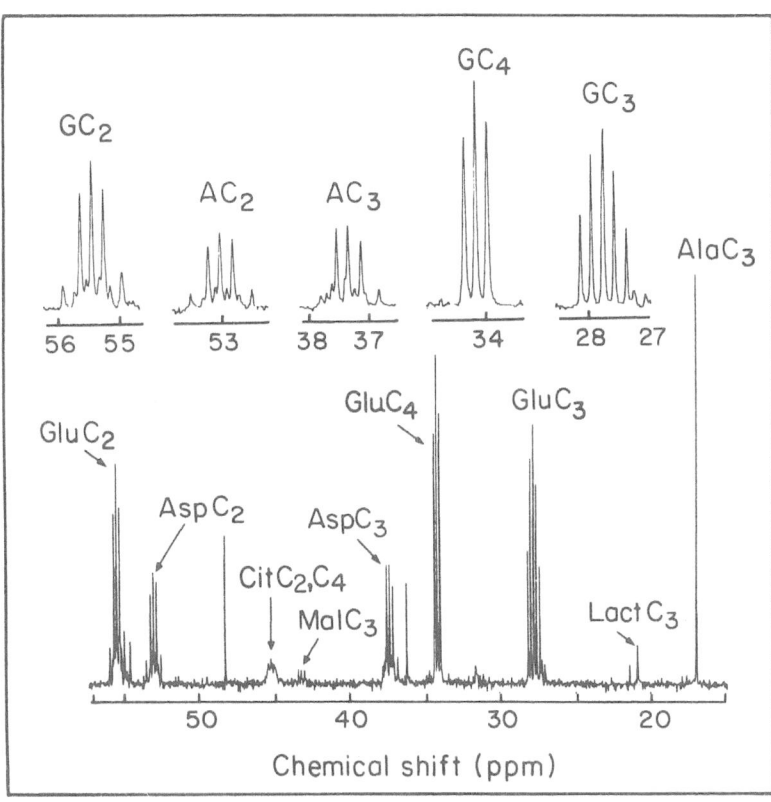

Figure 1. ^{13}C NMR spectrum of a neutralized perchloric acid extract prepared from three pooled rat hearts each perfused for 21 min with 5 mM glucose and 1 mM [3-^{13}C] pyruvate. The spectrum represents the accumulation of 2000 scans obtained at 90.55 MHz using composite pulse proton decoupling, 45° pulse, and a 2 s recycling time. Abbreviations used are: Glu C_2 (GC$_2$), glutamate C-2; Glu C_3 (GC$_3$), glutamate C-3; Glu C_4 (GC$_4$), glutamate C-4; Asp C_2 (AC$_2$), aspartate C-2; Asp C_3 (AC$_3$), aspartate C-3; Ala C_3, alanine C-3; Cit C_2, C_4, citrate C-2 plus citrate C-4; Mal C_3, malate C-3.

From Figure 2 it is evident that alanine C–3 and glutamate C–4 become labeled relatively quickly and prior to the appearance of ^{13}C label into other intermediates. The half times for ^{13}C incorporation into alanine C–3 and glutamate C–4 were both about 3 min, but the maximum extent of labeling was different, being 87% for alanine 70% for glutamate. Glutamate C–2 and C–3 become labeled with a half time of 8 min, while ^{13}C incorporation into aspartate C–2 and C–3 increased more rapidly with a half time of 6 min. Values calculated from the mathematical model for these parameters once a steady state had been reached after about 30 min gave a common ^{13}C enrichment of 63%. The different steady state ^{13}C fractional enrichments of YA1$_3$, YG$_4$ and YG$_2$, YG$_3$, YA$_2$, YA$_3$ reflect different dilutions of several primary intermediates reacting with the citric acid cycle, namely pyruvate, acetyl–CoA and oxalacetate. Alanine C–3 is produced by

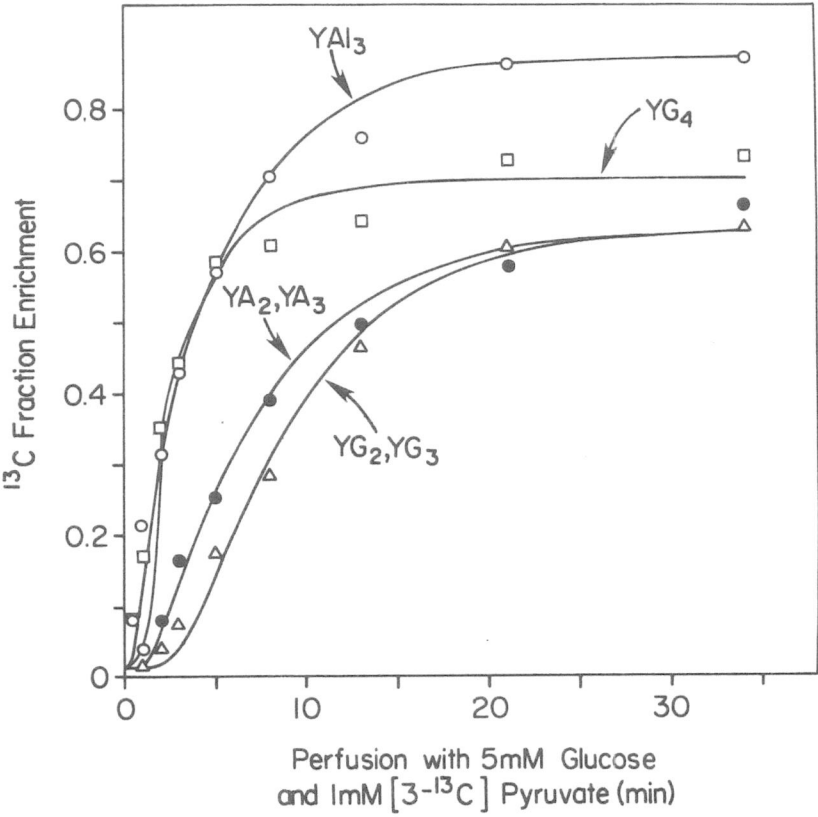

Figure 2. Time course of the change in the ^{13}C fractional enrichment of glutamate, aspartate, and alanine carbon atoms in hearts perfused with 5 mM glucose and 1 mM [$3-^{13}C$] pyruvate. The experimentally determined values for the ^{13}C fractional enrichment of alanine C-3 (YAL_3) is represented by the open circles, that of glutamate C-4 (YG_4) is represented by the open squares, while mean values for those of glutamate C-2 and C-3 (YG_2, YG_3) are represented by open triangles, and mean values for those of aspartate C-2 and C-3 (YA_2, YA_3) are represented by closed circles. The lines shown are derived from the optimized fit of the mathematical model to the data points.

exchange with pyruvate C–3 via alanine aminotransferase and is diluted mainly because the [$3-^{13}C$] pyruvate used as substrate was only 90% enriched. The small further dilution arises because of conversion of malate to pyruvate via malic enzyme (F_{MP} in Figure 3) from a percursor pool of malate of lower specific enrichment than the [$3-^{13}C$] pyruvate used as substrate.

Initial attempts to model these data using a simple citric acid cycle network gave large nonrandom errors and poorly determined values for the flux parameters since the model predicted a common steady state value for YG_4, YG_3, YG_2, YA_3 and YA_2. In order to allow convergence with a reasonable standard error, it was necessary to assume the presence of a small isotopically non-exchangeable pool of aspartate. The size of this pool was allowed to be an unknown parameter,

Table 1. Flux parameters calculated from the model

Flux parameter	Mean value	Confidence limits	
		5%	95%
		μmol/g dry wt.min	
Cycle flux (F)	12.12	11.35	12.93
FP	9.16	8.44	9.93
FAc	2.33	1.79	3.04
FA = FMP	0.63	0.39	1.01
FPAc	9.79	8.94	10.71
FOA	97.1	11	844
FAO	97.7	11	837
FALP = FPAL	1.48	1.25	1.75

Values shown are calculated for hearts perfused with 1 mM [3–^{13}C] pyruvate and 5 mM glucose. The abbreviations used for the flux parameters are the same as those given in the legend to Figure 3. The overall standard deviation for the computer fit was 3% with 48 degrees of freedom.

and was calculated by iterative procedures to be about 10% of the total aspartate content (Chance *et al.*, 1983). In addition some of the experimental YG$_4$ values gave large nonrandom residuals and it was not clear whether this represented error in the data points or a poor model. Consequently, the network was modified according to the scheme shown in Figure 3. The primary goal was to provide an alternative method of diluting the ^{13}C labeling in aspartate C–2 and C–3, independently of the glutamate C–4 labeling, by a biochemically acceptable mechanism. The input flux of unlabeled aspartate, denoted by FA in Figure 3, represents proteolysis since it is known that normal Langendorff perfused hearts are in a state of net negative protein balance (Takala *et al.*, 1980; Chua *et al.*, 1978). For this purpose the simplification was made that the overall net production of the different amino acids could be represented by a single input flux of aspartate as far as dilution of the isotopically labeled citric acid cycle intermediates was concerned. Since in the steady state any input of carbon intermediates into the citric acid cycle must be balanced by an equal output of carbon, this was assumed to occur via malic enzyme activity, which is known to be active in heart (Frenkel, 1972; Lin and Davis, 1974; Andres *et al.*, 1980; Nagel *et al.*, 1980; Penhkurinen, 1982). Finally, in order to provide a carbon balance for a transamination flux of aspartate plus α-ketoglutarate to oxalacetate plus glutamate, a net glutamate dehydrogenase flux (FGK) equal to both FA and FMP in the direction of glutamate deamination to α-ketoglutarate must be postulated. Again, this enzyme is known to be present in cardiac muscle, albeit at a much lower concentration than in liver (Takala *et al.*, 1980; Nuutinen *et al.*, 1981). With these modifications to the network, an excellent fit for all the data was obtained with an overall standard deviation of 3%. As shown in Table 1, the flux parameters of the

Flux Parameters With $[3-^{13}C]$ Pyruvate

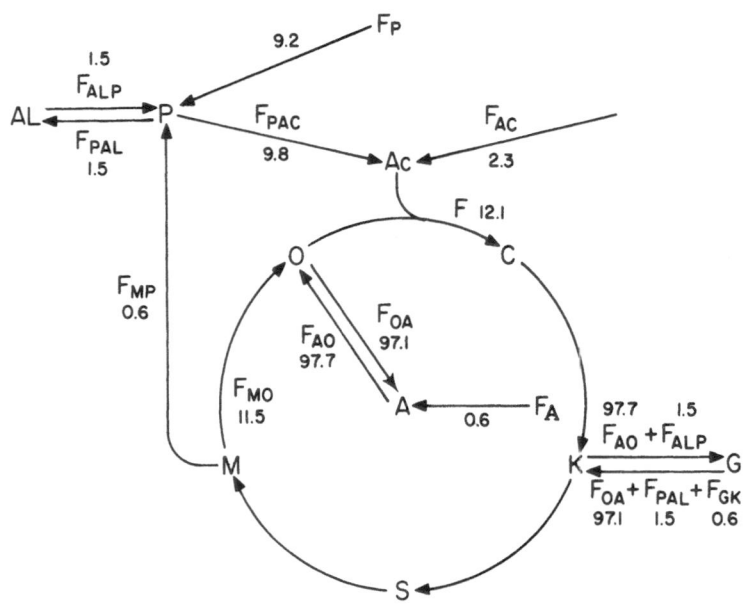

Figure 3. Metabolic network used for calculating the indicated flux parameters from the data in Figure 2. Abbreviations used are as follows: P, pyruvate; AL, alanine; AC, acetyl-CoA; C, citrate; K, α-ketoglutarate; G, glutamate; S, succinate; M, malate; O, oxalacetate; A, aspartate; Fp, influx of $[3-^{13}C]$ pyruvate; F_{ALP}, and F_{PAL}, forward and reverse fluxes, respectively, through alanine aminotransferase; F_{PAC}, pyruvate dehydrogenase flux; F_{AC}, flux of acetyl-CoA units derived from β-oxidation of fatty acids; F, citric acid cycle flux; F_{GK}, glutamate dehydrogenase flux; F_A, input flux of unlabeled aspartate from proteolysis; F_{MO}, malate dehydrogenase flux; F_{MP}, flux through malic enzyme.

model were all well determined except for the forward and reverse fluxes of aspartate aminotransferase. Interestingly, the primary flux parameters calculated with the modified network were similar to those of the previous model, e.g. 12.1 versus 11.9 μmol/g dry weight.min for citric acid cycle flux, 8.4 versus 9.1 μmol/g dry weight.min for pyruvate uptake (FP) and 2.33 versus 2.84 μmol/g dry weight.min for the input of unlabeled acetyl-CoA from β-oxidation (FAc). This latter flux determines dilution of acetyl-CoA C–2 relative to pyruvate C–3 in order to account for the lower values of YG_4 compared with $YA1_3$. This is accounted for by the fact that the 2-carbon of acetyl-CoA is the sole source for ^{13}C labeling in glutamate C–4, as described by the equation $YG_4/YA1_3 = 1 - FAc/F$, where F is the citric acid cycle flux and FAc is the rate of acetyl-CoA production from β-oxidation.

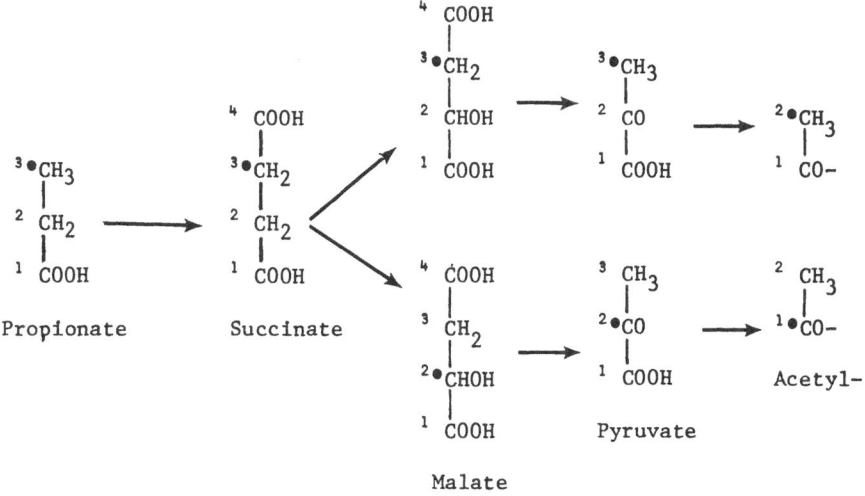

Figure 4. Metabolic scheme showing how ^{13}C label from [3–^{13}C] propionate forms equal proportions of [1–^{13}C] and [2–^{13}C] acetyl-CoA.

Perfusion with [3–^{13}C] propionate

In order to test the model with the modified network using a higher flux through malic enzyme, a series of hearts were perfused with 2 mM 90% enriched [3–^{13}C] propionate and 5 mM glucose. Propionate is known to be metabolized by rat hearts (Davis & Quastel, 1964; Davis *et al.*, 1972; Penhkurinen, 1982) and enters the citric acid cycle as succinyl-CoA after a carboxylation step to methylmalonyl-CoA. As shown in Figure 4, ^{13}C from propionate C–3 labels succinate C–3 (which in the mathematical model is not formally treated as a symmetrical molecule) and is randomized through fumarate to produce ^{13}C labeled malate C–3 and malate C–2 in equal amounts. Pyruvate labeled with ^{13}C in the C–3 or C–2 positions is then formed via malic enzyme activity, and acetyl-CoA labeled with ^{13}C in the C–2 or C–1 positions is subsequently formed as the product of pyruvate de-hydrogenase activity. Thus, a major difference between the use of [3–^{13}C] pyruvate and [3–^{13}C] propionate as metabolic substrate for the perfused heart is that with propionate equal amounts of ^{13}C–labeled acetyl-CoA C–2 and C–1 are formed with subsequent oxidation by the reactions of the citric acid cycle, together with equal proportions of ^{13}C–labeled oxalacetate C–3 and C–2.

The nature of the major ^{13}C-labeled isoptomers of intermediates formed by consecutive turns of the citric acid cycle are illustrated in Figure 5A for condensation of various labeled oxalacetate species with acetyl-CoA C–2 (Ac_2) and in Figure 5B for reactions involving acetyl-CoA C–1 (Ac_1). Consequently, these reaction schemes illustrate the sequential formation of multiply-labeled inter-mediates, where C refers to citrate, K to α-ketoglutarate (which in the steady

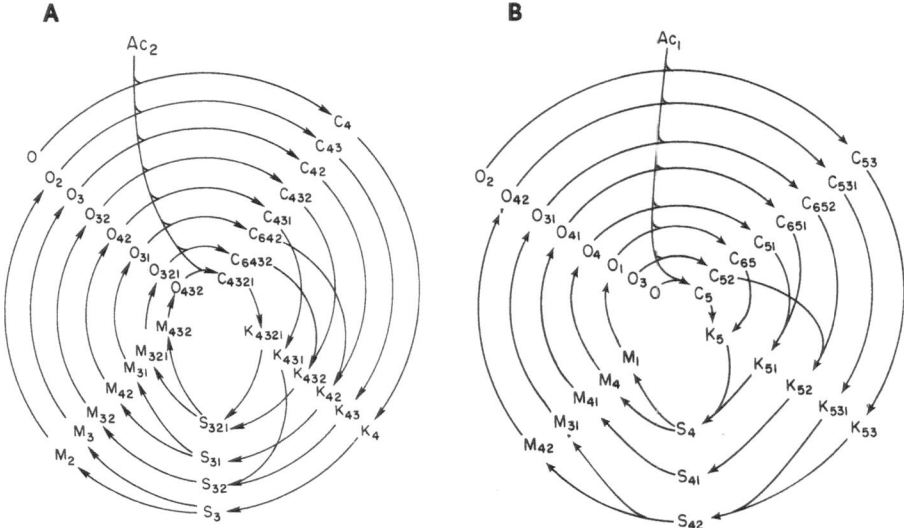

Figure 5. Schematic diagrams of the sequential labeling of the individual carbon atoms of different intermediates of the citric acid cycle. *A* shows reactions of acetyl-CoA C-2 (Ac_2) and *B* shows reactions of acetyl-CoA C-1 (Ac_1) with ^{13}-C-labeled and unlabeled isoptomers of oxalacetate. The abbreviations used to denote the different intermediates are: O, C, K, S, and M, for oxalacetate, citrate, α-ketoglutarate, succinate and malate, respectively.

state is in isotopic equilibrium with glutamate), S refers to succinate, M to malate and O to oxalacetate (in isotopic equilibrium with aspartate). Entry of ^{13}C substrate as Ac_2 produces a preponderance of glutamate isoptomers that are multiply labeled in adjacent carbon atoms, with G_{432} being twice as great as G_{4321} in the final steady state, as previously illustrated from time courses of the appearance of ^{13}C labeled glutamate species calculated from the mathematical model (1). Consequently, with [3-^{13}C] pyruvate as substrate there is a considerable degree of line splitting of the glutamate carbon resonances, as illustrated by the data in Figure 1. Likewise, the dominant species of aspartate will be A_{321} and A_{432}, with ^{13}C enrichment in the C–3 and C–2 positions being equal and twice that in the C–1 and C–4 positions, which also have equal ^{13}C enrichments. The high proportion of multiply labeled isoptomers of glutamate and aspartate accounts for the high degree of line splitting observed in the spectra of Figure 1 since these are caused by ^{13}C–^{13}C spin coupling between adjacent carbon atoms (London *et al.*, 1975a; 1975b; Tran-Dinh *et al.*, 1974). In contrast, as shown in Figure 5B, reaction of Ac_1 with unlabeled oxalacetate, O_2 and O_3 and further oxalacetate species generated by subsequent turns of the citric acid cycle produces glutamate labeled in the C–5 position plus G_{51}, G_{52}, G_{531}, and G_{53}, together with singly labeled aspartate isoptomers and A_{42}, A_{31}, andd A_{41}. These multiply labeled isoptomers do not have adjacent ^{13}C labeled carbon atoms, and therefore will not contribute to line splitting of the carbon resonances.

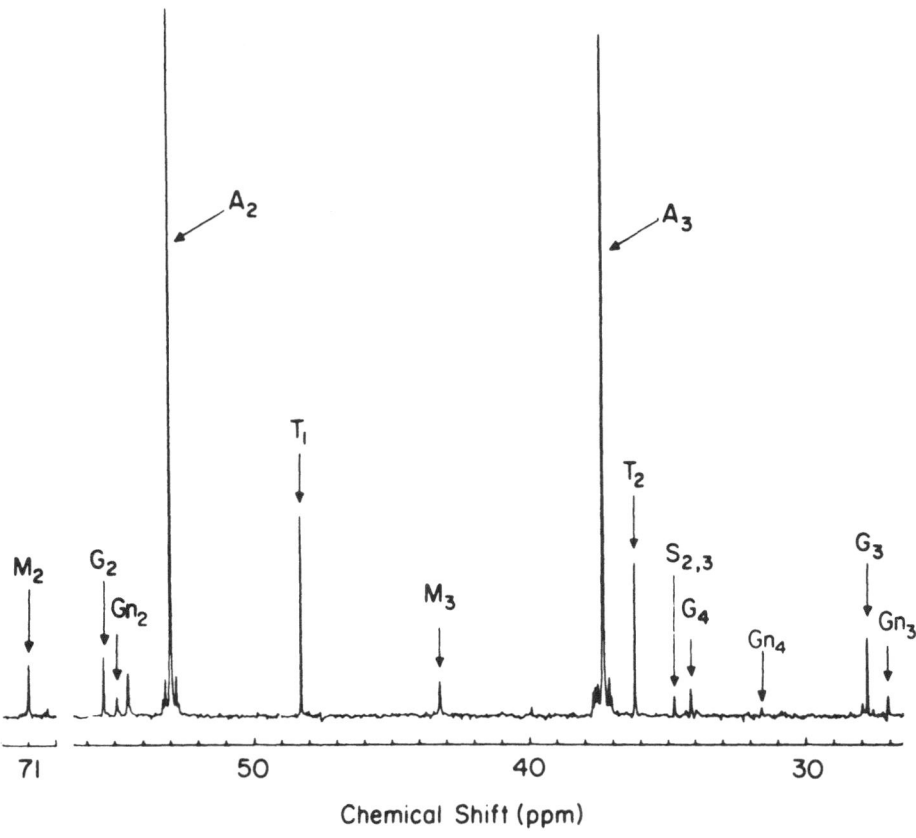

Figure 6. ^{13}C NMR spectrum of a neutralized perchloric acid extract prepared from three pooled rat hearts each perfused for 34 min with 5 mM glucose and 2 mM 90% enriched [3–^{13}C] propionate. The spectrum was obtained under the same conditions as that of Figure 1. Abbreviations in addition to those defined in Figure 1 are: Gn_4, Gn_3 and Gn_2, glutamine C-4, C-3, and C-2, respectively; T_1 and T_2, taurine C-1 and taurine C-2, respectively, M_3, M_2, malate C-3 and malate C-2, respectively; $S_{2,3}$, succinate C-2 plus C-3.

The ^{13}C NMR spectrum of a tissue extract prepared from hearts perfused for 34 min with 2 mM [3–^{13}C] propionate and 5 mM glucose is shown in Figure 6. Perfusion of hearts with propionate greatly increases the pool size of aspartate from 7 μmol/g dry weight for hearts perfused with glucose alone to 38 μmol/g dry weight for hearts perfused with glucose plus propionate, while the glutamate content decreases from 20 to 3.5 μmol/g dry weight. Consequently, the spectrum shown in Figure 6 is dominated by aspartate C–2 (A_2) and aspartate C–3 (A_3) resonances. Resonances attributable to glutamate C–2, C–3, and C–4 are also seen, together with malate C–2 and C–3 (M_2 and M_3) and succinate C–2 + C–3 ($S_{2,3}$). Also shown are the two resonances of natural abundant taurine (T_1 and T_2) and small peaks attributable to glutamine. The exchange of ^{13}C between glutamate and glutamine is very slow in heart muscle, and the glutamine resonances seen in the spectra are largely derived from natural abundant glutamine (1.1% of

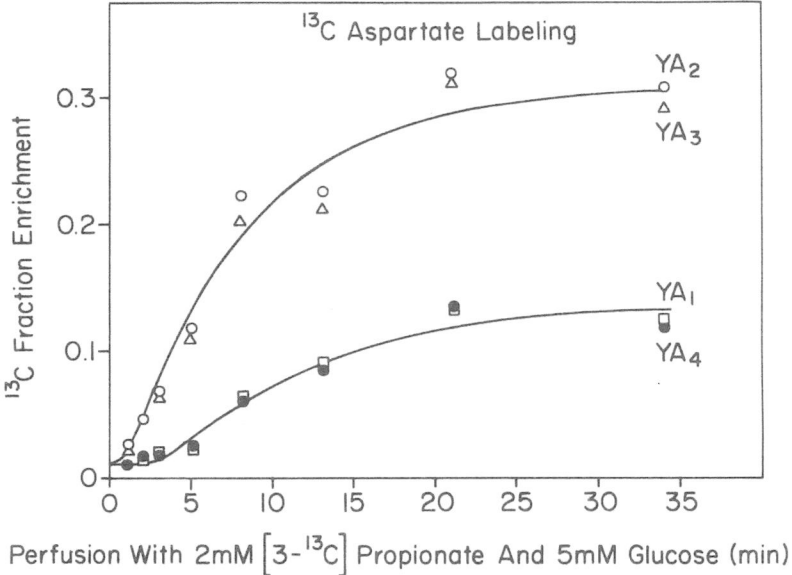

Figure 7. Time course of the change in the fractional enrichment of ^{13}C-aspartate specific carbons in hearts perfused with 5 mM glucose and 2 mM 90% enriched [3–^{13}C] propionate. The experimentally determined values for the ^{13}C fractional enrichment of aspartate C-1 (YA_1) is represented by the closed circles, that for aspartate C-2 (YA_2) is represented by the open circles, that for aspartate C-3 (YA_3) is represented by the open triangles, and that for aspartate C-4 (YA_4) is represented by the open squares. The lines shown are derived from the optimized fit of the mathematical model to the data points.

total carbon) which are visible because of the large glutamine pool size (20–25 nmol/g dry weight). Apart from the different relative levels of glutamate and aspartate in the heart extracts, the most notable difference between the spectra shown in Figure 1 and in Figure 6 is the small extent of line splitting of the aspartate resonances with the propionate-perfused hearts.

The time course of ^{13}C fractional enrichments in the different carbon atoms of aspartate after perfusion of hearts with [3–^{13}C] propionate is shown in Figure 7. The experimentally determined values for YA_2 and YA_3 were approximately the same, as were those for YA_1 and YA_4. Because of the large pool size of aspartate in this experiment compared with those of other metabolites, the C–1 and C–4 carboxyl carbons of aspartate at 175.1 ppm and 178.3 ppm, respectively, could be accurately quantitated. As seen from Figure 7, YA_2 and YA_3 increased after a short lag and reached a steady state ^{13}C enrichment of about 30% with a half time of 6 min. There was a larger lag of 2–3 min before YA_1 and YA_4 started to increase; the steady state ^{13}C enrichment was 13% with a half time of 9 min. These data were used to calculate flux parameters from the mathematical model, and the lines shown in Figure 7 are those derived from the minimum least squares fit.

Flux Parameters With $\left[3-{}^{13}C\right]$ Propionate

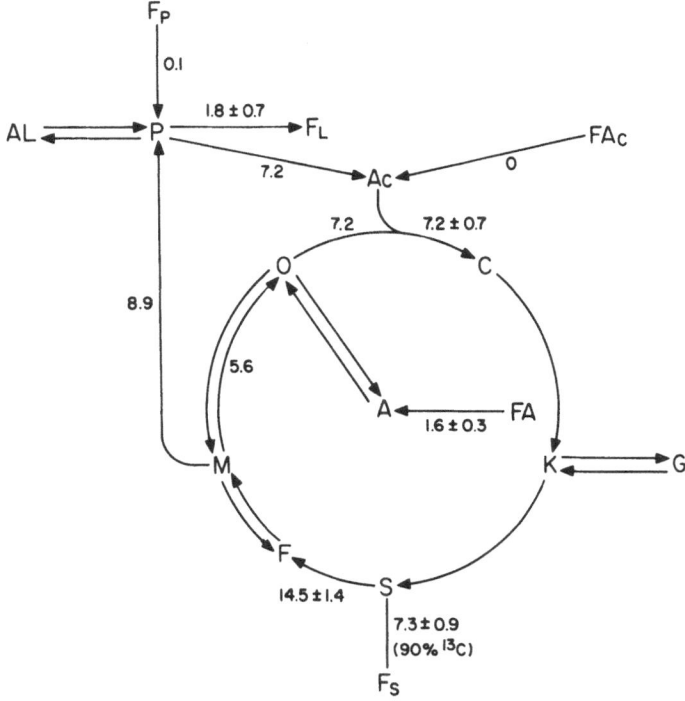

Figure 8. Metabolic network used for calculating the indicated flux values from the data in Figure 7. Abbreviations additional to those defined in Fig. 6 are: F_L, efflux of lactate; F, fumarate; F_s, influx of ${}^{13}C$-propionate.

The calculated flux parameters for this experiment are shown in Figure 8 superimposed on the metabolic network used for curve fitting. It must be noted, however, that this must be regarded as a preliminary analysis since the only experimental parameters used were the aspartate ${}^{13}C$ fractional enrichments. In this model, F_s represents the rate of input of 90% enriched $[3-{}^{13}C]$ propionate into the citric acid cycle at the level of succinate (S). Well determined flux parameters are shown with standard errors, and it is seen that the rate of propionate metabolism is approximately the same as the citric acid cycle flux. This was calculated to be equal to pyruvate dehydrogenase flux, while input of unlabeled pyruvate from glycolysis (F_p) and unlabeled acetyl-CoA from β-oxidation (FAc) were calculated to be very small. However, since the experimental parameter of YG_4 is a primary determinant of FAc, it is not surprising that during flux parameter iterations with the model this flux could not be calculated. The measured ${}^{13}C$ fractional enrichments in glutamate for this series of experiments were unfortunately unreliable because of a partial hydrolysis of glutamine to glutamate during preparation of the tissue extracts. As with the $[3-{}^{13}C]$ pyruvate

Line Splitting Of Aspartate C-2
^{13}C NMR Resonance

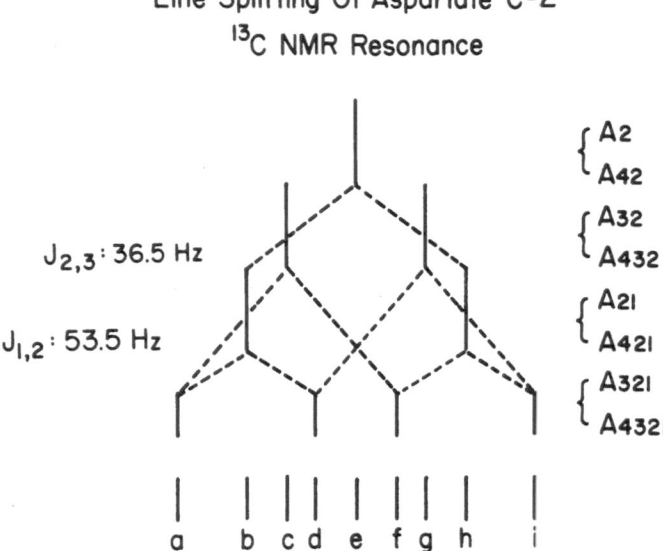

$J_{2,3}$: 36.5 Hz

$J_{1,2}$: 53.5 Hz

{ A2
  A42

{ A32
  A432

{ A21
  A421

{ A321
  A4321

a   b c d   e   f g   h   i

Figure 9. Schematic representation of the different possibilities for line splitting of the aspartate C-2 resonance caused by incorporation of one or two ^{13}C atoms adjacent to the ^{13}C in aspartate C-2. The isoptomers which contain ^{13}C in carbon 2 are listed beside the lines to which they contribute.

experiments, the topology of the citric acid cycle together with isotope exchange between oxalacetate and aspartate and α-ketoglutarate and glutamate via the transaminases requires that YA_2, YA_3 and YG_2, YG_3 should be approximately the same in the final steady state. More recent studies show that this is indeed the case, but YG_4 is enriched with ^{13}C to only about 10% (compared with 30% enrichment for YG_2 and YG_3) suggesting a significant dilution of acetyl–CoA C–2. The more complete data for this experiment have not yet been used for flux modeling.

Analysis of ^{13}C resonance line splittings

Line splittings of individual ^{13}C carbon resonances are caused by interactions between adjacent ^{13}C-labeled carbon atoms. The patterns that may be obtained are illustrated in Figure 9 with respect to aspartate C–2, but similar principles hold for all the noncarboxyl carbons of aspartate and glutamate. If aspartate is ^{13}C labeled only in the C–2 position (A_2), a single line denoted by *e* is observed at 53.2 ppm (*cf* Figure 7). The effect of non-adjacent ^{13}C-labeled carbon atoms on each other is very small, hence the A_{42} isoptomer also produces a single line at position *e*. When the C–3 position is also ^{13}C–labeled due to the presence of A_{32} and A_{432} species, the line at *e* is split into two lines at *c* and *g* with a characteristic coupling constant (measured by the separation of the lines $J_{2,3}$ of 36.5 Hz). If the carboxyl

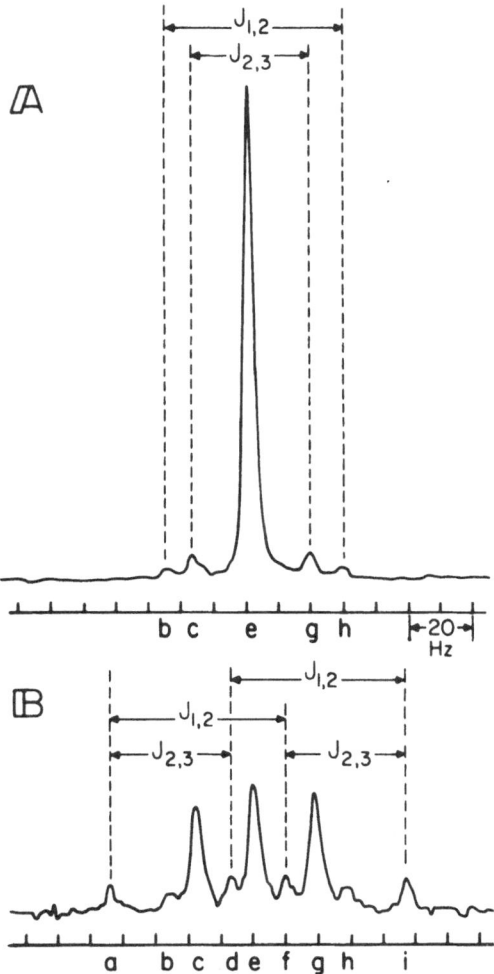

Figure 10. Aspartate C-2 resonances in tissue extracts from (A): hearts perfused for 21 min with 5 mM glucose plus 2 mM [3–^{13}C] propionate and (B): hearts perfused for 21 min with 5 mM glucose plus 2 mM [3–^{13}C] pyruvate. The magnitude of the coupling constants $J_{1,2}$ and $J_{2,3}$, as well as the positions of the J-coupled peaks are indicated by the dashed lines.

carbon is labeled in the C–1 position, the coupling constant $J_{1,2}$ is larger (53.5 Hz) and the central resonance of aspartate C-2 will be split into two lines at *b* and *h* in accordance with the proportion of A_{21} and A_{421} isoptomers. If aspartate contains ^{13}C in adjacent carbon atoms represented by $^{13}C_1$ - $^{13}C_2$ - and - $^{13}C_2$ - $^{13}C_3$ -, a quintet of lines will be seen (*b*, *c*, *e*, *g*, and *h*). When the carbon atom under observation (e.g. aspartate C-2) has two nearest neighbors containing ^{13}C, as denoted by isoptomers A_{321} and A_{4321}, additional line splittings occur to produce a further four lines, namely *a*, *d*, *f*, and *i* to give a resonance containing a total of nine separate lines.

Table 2. Comparison of the relative proportions of aspartate isoptomers measured from ^{13}C resonance line splittings with those calculated from the model

Substrate and data source	Aspartate isoptomer groups						
	$A_2(s)$	$A_3(s)$	$A_{2.1}$	$A_{2.3}$	$A_{3.4}$	$A_{2.3.1}$	$A_{3.4.2}$
	% contribution to total ^{13}C aspartate						
[3–^{13}C] Propionate							
Observed	84	85	6	10	6		
Model	84		4	12	4		
[3–^{13}C] Pyruvate							
Observed	20	19	11	42	14	26	27
Model	24		10	43	10	23	23
[3–^{13}C] Pyruvate + [1–^{13}C] Propionate							
Observed	47	46	6	35	6	12	12
Model	45		9	34	9	12	12

Rat hearts were perfused with ^{13}C labeled substrate for 34 min, rapidly frozen and ^{13}C NMR spectra were obtained at 90.55 MHz using neutralized perchloric acid extracts. The abbreviations used to describe the aspartate isoptomer groups are defined below, and the numbers shown represent the fractional contribution of the different isoptomers to the overall ^{13}C resonance signal of aspartate C-2 ($\bar{z} A_2$) and aspartate C-3 ($\bar{z} A_3$). Experimentally and as calculated from the model the total ^{13}C incorporation into the C-2 and C-3 positions of aspartate are the same. $A_2(s)$ refers to the C-2 aspartate singlet containing A_2 and A_{42} isoptomers; $A_3(s)$ contains A_3 and A_{31} isoptomers. The other isoptomer groups expressed as fractional contributions are: $A_{2.1} = (A_{21} + A_{421})/\bar{z} A_2$, $A_{2.3} = (A_{32} + A_{432})/\bar{z} A_2$ or $(A_{32} + A_{321})/\bar{z} A_3$, $A_{3.4} = (A_{43} + A_{431})/\bar{z} A_3$, $A_{2.3.1} = (A_{321} + A_{4321})/\bar{z} A_2$, $A_{3.4.2} = (A_{432} + A_{4321})/\bar{z} A_3$. Including unlabeled aspartate, there are maximally 16 possible aspartate isoptomers.

Illustrations of the observed line splittings of the aspartate C-2 resonance in tissue extracts for hearts perfused for 21 min with 2 mM [3–^{13}C] propionate plus 5 mM glucose are shown in Figure 10A and for hearts perfused for 21 min with 1 mM [3–^{13}C] pyruvate plus 5 mM glucose in Figure 10 B. As previously noted, very little line splitting occured with the ^{13}C propionate perfused hearts, and besides the large singlet peak (e), arising from isoptomers $A_2 + A_{42}$, only small peaks at b, c, g, and h can be observed (Figure 10A). With reference to Figure 5 and Figure 9 this pattern indicates the presence of a relatively small amount of ($A_{32} + A_{432}$) and ($A_{21} + A_{421}$) isoptomers. The absence of further peaks indicates negligible amounts of ($A_{321} + A_{4321}$) isoptomers. In constrast, with the ^{13}C pyruvate perfused hearts, which have a greater proportion of their acetyl-CoA input as Ac_2, the central peak e in Figure 10B no longer dominates the aspartate C-2 resonance. The spectrum consists mainly of three peaks (c, e and g) corresponding to isoptomers containing - $^{13}C_2$ - $^{13}C_3$ - coupling, as well as a smaller but significant contribution from isoptomers containing $^{13}C_1$ - $^{13}C_2$ - and $^{13}C_1$ - $^{13}C_2$ - $^{13}C_3$ - coupling patterns which give rise to peaks a, b, d, f h, and i in Figure 10B. These small peaks were not observed in the spectra at early times of perfusion; the gradual accumulation of multiply labeled isoptomers may also be deduced by following the labeling pattern spiral in Figure 5A.

Since the resonance line splittings provide information about the relative proportion of ^{13}C labeled isoptomers contributing to the overall ^{13}C enrichment of specific carbon atoms in different metabolites, these may be quantitated and compared with corresponding values calculated from the flux model. With reference to Figure 10A where only five lines are observed, the aspartate C-2 resonance is measured from the sum of the integrals of lines b, c, e, g, and h, ($\bar{z} A_2$). The contribution of the large singlet peak e (representing mainly the A_2 isoptomer but with a low content of the A_{42} isoptomer) to the overall aspartate C-2 resonance is given by the ratio of the integral of line e to $\bar{z} A_2$. Likewise, the contribution of the - $^{13}C_2$ - $^{13}C_3$ - isoptomers A_{32} and A_{432} to the aspartate C-2 resonance is given by the ratio of the integrals of lines $c + g$ to $\bar{z} A_2$, and the contribution of the $^{13}C_1$ - $^{13}C_2$ - isoptomers A_{21} and A_{421} is given by the ratio of the integrals of lines $b + h$ to $\bar{z} A_2$.

Table 2 shows the relative proportions of isoptomers contributing to the aspartate singlets A_2 and A_3, calculated as above, compared with the corresponding values calculated from the mathematical model for the aspartate C-2 and aspartate C-3 resonances for hearts perfused for 34 min. The results from three separate experiments are shown, namely hearts perfused with 2 mM [3–^{13}C] propionate and 5 mM glucose, with 1 mM [3–^{13}C] pyruvate and 5 mM glucose and with 1 mM [3–^{13}C] pyruvate and 1 mM [1–^{13}C] propionate. In general, data obtained from the ^{13}C resonance line splittings and from the model were in very good agreement despite large differences between the relative proportions of singly and multiply labeled aspartate isoptomers in the different experiments.

The results of similar calculations for the resonances of ^{13}C labeled glutamate C-2, glutamate C-3, and glutamate C-4 are shown in Table 3 for three experiments in which hearts were perfused for 34 min with 1 mM [3–^{13}C] pyruvate and 5 mM glucose, for 34 min with 1 mM [3–^{13}C] pyruvate and 1 mM [1–^{13}C] propionate or for 41 min with 5 mM [2–^{13}C] acetate and 5 mM glucose. The differences between the two sets of values calculated for the relative distribution of the different isoptomers are rather greater for the glutamate carbons than for the aspartate carbons, suggesting that some further improvements of the model or of the resolution of the ^{13}C carbon resonances may be required. Nevertheless, the overall agreement for the numerous different parameters is sufficiently good that it provides general confidence in the validity of the model.

Conclusions

There are relatively few other studies in which the ^{13}C enrichment into metabolic intermediates of intact cardiac muscle have been measured by ^{13}C NMR spectroscopy. These include studies by Bailey *et al.* (1981) with perfused rat heart and

Table 3. Comparison of the relative proportions of glutamate isoptomers measured from ^{13}C resonance line splittings with those calculated from the model

Substrate and data source	Glutamate isoptomer groups							
	$G_{2(s)}$	$G_{3(s)}$	$G_{4(s)}$	$G_{2,1}$	$G_{2,3}$	$G_{4,3}$	$G_{2,3,1}$	$G_{3,4,2}$
	% contribution to total ^{13}C glutamate							
[3–^{13}C] Pyruvate								
Observed	19	8	29	9	46	71	26	55
Model	24	10	36	10	48	61	23	46
[3–^{13}C] pyruvate +[1–^{13}C] propionate								
Observed	57	23	64	0[a]	43	35	0[a]	20
Model	46	20	59	9	34	33	12	29
[2–^{13}C] Acetate								
Observed	12	1	20	7	45	80	36	72
Model	11	3	19	7	48	81	33	66

[a] Below the limit for quantitation

Rat hearts were perfused with ^{13}C-labeled substrate for 34 min or 41 min ([2–^{13}C] acetate experiment only), rapidly frozen and ^{13}C NMR spectra were obtained at 90.55 MHz using neutralized perchloric acid extracts. The format for the data presentation and the meaning of the abbreviations used for the isoptomer groups are similar to those used for Table 2 except they apply to the glutamate C-2, C-3 and C-4 resonances. For the sake of clarity all possible glutamate isoptomer groups are not presented in the table, and isoptomers containing glutamate C-5 labeling are not present unless acetyl-CoA C-1 becomes labeled. The glutamate carbon used for measured values is given by the first number in the isoptomer notation. Including unlabeled glutamate, there are maximally 32 possible glutamate isoptomers.

Neurohr *et al.* (1983) with guinea pig heart *in vivo.* In both these studies the lack of a mathematical analysis of the data severely limited the interpretation of the data in relation to metabolic fluxes. Studies reported here and in our earlier paper (Chance *et al.*, 1983) illustrate that a mathematical model built around rather simple metabolic networks, together with solution of large systems of differential equations and curve fittings by nonlinear least squares analysis using a suitable computer program such as FACSIMILE (Chance et al., 1977), can be used to determine primary flux parameters including those at metabolic branch points. The network coding as well as the FACSIMILE program can be stored on magnetic tape for transportation and used with any large main frame computer having a compatible operating system. Solutions for unknown flux parameters can be determined either from a knowledge of the steady state ^{13}C fractional enrichments of the specific carbons of alanine, glutamate, and/or aspartate together with a primary input flux for substrate utilization, or from the kinetics of the specific carbon ^{13}C fractional enrichments when all fluxes are unknown parameters. The lack of readily usable metabolic flux models is likely to have been a major factor in inhibiting many investigators from exploring the use of ^{13}C NMR for metabolic studies, and it was on the basis of this perceived need that the present model was developed.

During development of the model it was important that stringent criteria were applied to assess whether the particular metabolic network used for the flux calculations was adequate. These criteria are: (1) that the overall standard deviation for the minimum least squares data fitting is within the error of the primary data, (2) that the distribution of the residuals is random and (3) that the calculated flux parameters are statistically well determined (Clore and Chance, 1978). In addition, further constraints can be applied from a knowledge of the oxygen consumption of the heart since that is the major determinant of citric acid cycle flux in cardiac tissue (Randle and Tubbs, 1979). The ^{13}C resonance line splitting data, when available, also provides independent criteria for model validation as illustrated from the present study. Our studies to date have also illustrated that although a solution of primary fluxes can be obtained from the model with a rather small number of measured parameters, the final decision concerning acceptability of a particular network or calculated fluxes is greatly strengthened by using as many independently measured parameters as possible for the computer generated solutions. The present paper represents a progress report on our studies, and since we have not yet achieved a completely satisfactory analysis of all the available data, conclusions of a metabolic significance from the ^{13}C NMR studies with perfused rat hearts will be reported separately in a further publication.

Acknowledgement

This work was supported by NIH Grant HL 29691.

References

Andres A, Satrustegui J, Machado A (1980) Development of NADPH-producing pathways in rat heart. Biochem J 186: 799–803

Bailey IA, Gadian DG, Mathews PM, Radda GK, Seeley PJ (1981) Studies of metabolism in the isolated perfused rat heart using ^{13}C NMR. FEBS Lett 123: 315–318

Bergmeyer UH (1974) Methods of enzymatic analysis. Academic Press New York

Chance EM, Seeholzer SH, Kobayashi K, Williamson JR (1983) Mathematical analysis of isotope labeling in the citric acid cycle with applications to ^{13}C NMR studies in perfused rat hearts. J Biol Chem 258: 13785–13794

Chance EM, Curtis AR, Jones IP, Kirby CR (1977) FACSIMILE: A computer program for flow and chemistry simulation and general initial value problems. Rep No R8775. United Kingdom Atomic Energy Authority HM Stationery Office London

Chua B, Kao R, Rannels DE, Morgan HE (1978) Hormonal and metabolic control of proteolysis. Biochem Soc Symp 48: 1–15

Clore GM, Chance EM (1978) The mechanism of reaction of fully reduced membrane-bound cytochrome oxidase with oxygen at 176K. Biochem J 173: 799–810

Davis EJ, Lin RC, Chao D (1972) Sources and disposition of aerobically generated intermediates in heart muscle. In: Mehlman MA, Hansen R (eds) Energy Metabolism and Regulation of Metabolic Processes in Mitochondria. New York, Academic Press pp 211–238

Davis EJ, Quastel JH (1964) The effects of short chain fatty acids and starvation on the metabolism of glucose and lactate by the perfused guinea pig heart. Canad. J Biochem 42: 1605–1621

Frenkel R (1972) Bovine heart malic enzyme. J Biol Chem 247: 5569–5572

Harris RK, Newman RH (1976) Choice of pulse spacings for accurate T_1 and NOE measurements in NMR spectroscopy. J Magn Res 24: 449–456

Lin RC, Davis EJ (1974) Malic enzymes of rabbit heart mitochondria. J Biol Chem 249: 3867–3875

London RE, Kollman VH, Matwiyoff NA (1975a) The quantitative analysis of carbon-carbon coupling in the ^{13}C nuclear magnetic resonance spectra of molecules biosynthesized from ^{13}C enriched precursors. J Am Chem Soc 97: 3565–3573

London RE, Matwiyoff NA, Kollman VH (1975b) Differential nuclear overhauser enhancement for ^{13}C siglet and ^{13}C-^{13}C multiplet resonances of a carboxyl carbon. J Magn Res 18: 555–557

Nagel WO, Dauchy RT, Sauer LA (1980) Mitochondrial malic enzymes. J Biol Chem 255: 3849–3854

Neurohr KJ, Barrett EJ, Shulman RG (1983) in vivo carbon-13 nuclear magnetic resonance studies of heart metabolism. Proc Natl Acad Sci USA 80: 1603–1607

Nuutinen EM, Hiltunen JK, Hassinen IE (1981) The glutamate dehydrogenase system and the redox state of mitochondrial free nicotinamide adenine dinucleotide in myocardium. FEBS Lett 128: 356–360

Pearce FJ, Deleeuw G, Forster J, Williamson JR, Tutwiler GF (1979) Inhibition of fatty acid oxidation in normal and hypoxic perfused rat hearts by 2-Tetradecylglycidic acid. J Mol Cell Cardiol 11: 893–915

Peuhkurinen KJ (1982) Accumulation and disposal of tricarboxylic acid cycle intermediates during propionate oxidation in the isolated perfused rat heart. Biochem. Biophys. Acta 721: 124–134

Randle PJ, Tubbs PK (1979) Carbohydrate and fatty acid metabolism. In: Berne, RM, Spherelakis N, Geiger SR (eds) Handbook of Physiology, The Cardiovascular System. Bethesda: pp 804–844

DISCUSSION

SIDEMAN: How do you foresee a larger model and where do you think it will lead? I mean in the practical sense of application and utilization.

ANS: As far as basic heart metabolism is concerned the model is already rather large and is able to provide well-determined estimates of the citric acid cycle flux from knowledge of the specific carbon enrichments of glutamate, provided that these parameters are accurately measured. Problems arise when the number of metabolic branch points is increased, as is needed to model the more complex metabolic situation in liver. More complex and, therefore, more metabolically realistic models require additional flux or carbon enrichment data for curve fitting. Thus, with the heart model it was interesting that when accurate enrichment patterns for glutamate, aspartate, and alanine were available, a better fit to the overall data was obtained by expansion of the network and model to include proteolysis and malic enzyme activity. In the long run we anticipate that it will be possible to construct an adequate in vivo model of cardiac metabolism using a combination of ^{31}P and ^{13}C NMR data. The necessary NMR technology is advancing at a rapid rate, and quite a number of ^{31}P NMR studies have been reported using surface coils for live animals. Studies with ^{13}C NMR in vivo are not as far advanced, but this area will become more attractive when the cost of the isotopes decreases.

The future of the interface between medicine and engineering

MERVYN S. GOTSMAN and DAN SAPOZNIKOV

Department of Cardiology, Hadassah-Hebrew University Medical Center, Jerusalem, Israel

Introduction

The human being is a biological organism whose function can be described by simple physical and chemical processes. Human creation, with all its intellectual complexity, was a magnificent feat. The world was created from nothingness but the original Jewish commentators – Rashi and Ramban – argue whether it was created at once or during the course of 7 days. Whatever point of view may be correct, the well designed architecture of the body and in particular, the heart and the brain are unique and have an almost unfathomable physiology.

It is appropriate that this meeting should be held in Israel – 'from Zion goes forth knowledge'. Jewish learning has always added fresh layers of thought. Our Talmud, for example, shows didactic summary in the Mishna, learned classroom discussion in the Gemorrah and unlimited exegesis in the early and late commentators. It has created the unique climate of Jewish thought – law or Pentateuch – as it was received and written and the oral tradition as it has been handed down from generation to generation and gradually modified. Jewish epistimology – the theory of learning – defines learning from divine inspiration; learning from intuition and learning from experience and experiment. We all have basic divine inspiration and intuition but each one at this meeting has added knowledge through experience and experiment.

The human body is a unique functioning organ but the physician in the past has been a pragmatic practitioner who based his art and science on observation and recording. Osler wrote: 'Observe and treat your patients and record your findings during the day – at night, peruse the literature, think on the problems and come to new conclusions'. The early physicians were men of action and practical doctors – Hales, Jenner, Heberden and others. Lewis and Wiggers were the first persons to understand cardiology in the laboratory, while A.V. Hill, Dale and the other great British physiologists and pharmacologists tried to explain the facts of medicine in physiological terms.

Lewis married modern cardiology and science, but Paul Wood compared physical examination with clinical measurements. He took physical examination into the catheterization laboratory and interpreted the results at the bedside. He would interrogate and examine a patient, record the physical findings carefully and meticulously, predict the results of cardiac catheterization, make the invasive study and then compare the findings of his procedures with the results of his physical examination and, if there were inconsistencies, resolve the differences.

Today mathematical reasoning and in particular, electronic and structural engineering, solid state physics and computer techniques have exploded. Moreover, the climate of medicine has changed – the older professor of internal medicine was appointed because of his clinical acumen and skill, his intellectual ability and his talented use of language and rhetoric. Modern medical leaders are chosen because of their profound insight, intellectual depth of thought, prowess in production and execution of research, and organizational ability. Braunwald, Earl Wood, Guyton and others, in the USA, founded a new school of cardiovascular thought in which science formed the basis of clinical practice. Their students and disciples have spread widely throughout the world and there has been a proliferation of academic cardiac units. Europe, too, has emerged from the ashes of the second world war, and after a latent period of 30 years has moulted and retooled and is now leading in medical engineering.

The future

Cardiology has advanced by quantum leaps. We can measure invasively – pressure (transducers), flow (velocity probes) and volume (angiography) – but all these techniques are invasive and can be applied to man only under specific conditions. Today, we have the echo-cardiogram, the gamma camera, the Doppler velocity probe, digital angiography, computed axial tomography, nuclear magnetic resonance and positron emission tomography; they have added more and more complicated, sophisticated and expensive hardware, in which the prices increase from tens of thousands to millions of dollars. The techniques are simple and permit repeated non-invasive measurement: studies can be made frequently, atraumatically and repetitively in all circumstances, and it has been become possible to measure details of the functional physiology of the heart and the cardiovascular system in health and disease.

There also has been an explosion of therapeutic possibilities: both medical and surgical. Witness the growth of closed heart surgery from closure of a patent ductus arteriosus and repair of coarctation of the aorta and mitral valvulotomy, profound hypothermia for atrial septal defect closure and pulmonary stenosis, open heart surgery, with cross-circulation and later extracorporeal circulation for valve repair and replacement, repair of complex congenital malformations and coronary artery bypass surgery and more recently the development of less invasive procedures such as balloon dilatation of the coronary arteries and valve stenosis, catheter closure of patent ductus arteriosus and atrial septal defect and streptokinase infusion to open obstructed coronary arteries.

Congenital heart disease has been conquered. Most of the operations are corrective: pulmonary valvulotomy and closure of atrial and ventricular septal defects. New areas of development include; the simpler pump oxygenators with non-thrombotic, non-turbulent and non-traumatic surfaces, controlled automatically by microprocessors and suitable for use in very small babies and infants. Complete correction can then be undertaken immediately after birth. There is the need for durable and pliable prosthetic materials for replacing the interatrial septum in common atrium, refashioning the intraventricular septum in common ventricle, replacing valves where the orificial diameter is very small and the manufacture of new conduits which will not provoke excessive endothelial proliferation or calcification. There is the need for early operation to prevent the development of pulmonary hypertension and new non-clottable substances for aorto-pulmonary anastomosis when pulmonary blood flow is low. The material and hydraulic engineers have a great contribution to make in the field of pediatric cardiovascular surgery.

Rheumatic fever has been controlled in the western world by a vigorous program of primary and secondary prophylaxis, particularly in susceptible communities but the ravages of subtle infections and uncontrolled epidemics in the third world countries makes scarred valves a common problem in adult life. Valve repair is usually inadequate, since valvular tissue is thickened, fibrosed and often calcified: pericardium, dacron and dura mater are inadequate valve tissue substitutes, while homograft and heterograft valves have not proved durable. There is the need for new durable and pliable plastic substances to replace valve tissue, substances that do not need anticoagulants or subsequent replacement.

Coronary artery disease remains the main killer. The mortality from coronary artery disease has decreased by 28% in the last 20 years. A first acute myocardial infarction had mortality of 28% in 1963 and today it is about 7%. The price of life has become more and more valuable. We are only on the threshold of understanding the pathogenic and biological principles of the generation of atheroma, but once established, obstructive lesions need coronary artery dilatation, coronary artery bypass or arterial replacement. The saphenous vein is an excellent bypass conduit but its life expectancy is 3 to 10 years only until it thromboses, or becomes atheromatous and is blocked or obliterated by cholesterol filled intima or clot. The internal mammary artery is ideal but flow is too small to sustain adequate flow to the entire heart. Here too, there is the need for new non-thrombogenic materials to reconstruct artificial arteries, substances which are durable, non-thrombotic and do not promote atherogenesis. There is also the need for simple, non-invasive techniques to measure coronary blood flow and the anatomy of the coronary arteries to plan subsequent surgical procedures.

Acute myocardial infarction can be limited by streptokinase which dissolves fresh clots and opens the artery, but muscle death and necrosis causes a mechanical defect. Subsequent infarcts cause further muscle death and ultimately lead to defective ventricular function and cardiac failure. There is the need for simple alarm systems to detect acute myocardial infarction and less traumatic invasive procedures to dissolve the clot and dilate the artery immediately. Coronary arteries ramify and branch in 3-dimensional space and the present generation of balloon catheters for percutaneous transluminal coronary angioplasty carries a small but definite risk. New, non-traumatic guidewires, low profile dilatation systems and more powerful dilatation balloons which will not rupture the artery are needed.

Cardiac transplantation blossomed in the late 1960's. The operation is relatively simple and involves excising and detaching the recipient heart with a circumferential incision around the atria, pulmonary artery and aorta. The donor heart needs to be compatible in size and is implanted by opening the atria, completing a periatrial suture line, reattaching the interatrial septum and anastamosing the main pulmonary artery and aorta of donor and recipient. The major problems are denervation, two atria beating independently and most important, rejection. Donors are in short supply and exact histo-compatability is essential.

Attention has been shifted to simpler procedures and these include myocardial preservation to paralyze the heart, permit more complex intracardiac procedures and thereby permit myocardial protection and recovery.

Mechanical devices are important and these include intra-aortic balloon pump and the development of the total artificial heart as exemplified by the Jarvik Mark 7. The artificial heart is placed inside the thorax, sutured to the recipient atria, pulmonary artery and aorta. It is completely mechanical with inlet and outlet valves, a smooth non-thrombogenic inner surface, elastic pumping balloons and an external power source. Difficulties include prolonged valve function, an appropriate non-clottable endocardial lining, a durable elastic pumping membrane, a reliable power source, a portable external power supply and infection of the machine-man interface.

Medical treatment has now improved greatly and new drugs have been introduced – nitrates, beta receptor agonists and antagonists, afterload reducing drugs and calcium channel blocking agents. Management of the arrhythmias has undergone a revolution – new drugs, sophisticated electrocardiographic monitoring systems including telemetry, telephone transmission, Holter monitoring and computer-aided systems of temporal and spatial analysis and programmed stimulation of the atria and ventricles. Witness the proliferation of new defibrillators, pacemakers, cardiac assist devices (the balloon pump) and finally total mechanical heart assist devices and cardiac transplantation. All these developments have occurred in the last 30 years.

Research, education and communication

In this setting, what are the priorities, how do we educate patients and physicians, how do we set our goals, who will pay the bill and who will judge the results of the research?

Education starts in the medical school but it has two quite distinct aspects. Formal education with lectures, workshops and training exercises and clear didactic instruction. Formal courses include mathematics, logic, statistics, physics, physical chemistry, and computer science including hardware, firmware, data structures, software engineering, picture processing and artificial intelligence. Peer directed instruction needs a cadre of educated clinical staff with sufficient education in engineering and computer science to integrate engineering principles with bedside teaching and engineers who are familiar with clinical problems. Postgraduate education includes formal training of physicians in engineering and computer science and the education of engineers and computer specialists in biological and medical laboratories.

Long-term postdoctoral education is often haphazard. Books, textbooks or monographs are out of date before they are written, but they provide excellent formal surveys of the field. Journals reflect editorial thought, but are determined mainly by the taste of the research workers who prepare the articles. Large international conferences are too big and cumbersome, while small specialist conferences and workshops bring together the leaders in the field but forget the young research worker who cannot afford to travel, or the unknown researcher who is working alone, quietly and anonymously in a small unit.

We need a new form of electronic literature distribution, where the researcher can introduce his data immediately, where peer review is concurrent and there is instant transmission of the data, results and interpretation for study by others on a computer terminal or television set. This electronic data bank can be supplemented by scientific news programs on television, and video tape recordings.

What are our goals and how will they be set and monitored?

The National Institute of Health in the United States has set up a national research machine. It chooses the leaders in the field and gives them time to gel their thoughts. They implement large programs which have included: the importance of lipids and lipid lowering drugs in coronary artery disease (the Lipid Clinic Research project), which has shown that cholestyramine can decrease serum cholesterol by 15% and reduce the incidence of new myocardial events by 25%, the role of the Coronary Care Unit in the management of acute myocardial infarction which has reduced hospital mortality from 30 to 10% (MIRU project), the importance of diagnostic tools in cardiovascular disease (SCORE) and the value of coronary artery bypass surgery (CASS) study. These studies are large, multicentred, and have budgets of millions of dollars. They invite interested centers to participate and set up, in addition, data collection centers, monitoring centers, statistical centers and appropriate centers for supervision. The research is expensive and the results are important but the individual workers are stultified by adhering to rigidly established research guidelines.

Research is expensive. It needs buildings and floor space, equipment hardware and software, research workers and technical and paratechnical staff. Who pays the bill – the government, research departments, NIH and the Medical Research Council, philanthropic research foundations, individual donors and finally the researcher himself who devotes his life and time and inspires the program with intellectual creativity?

Usefulness and cost effectiveness cannot be judged immediately. Only history will judge the importance and relevance of each stride. All new ideas stand or fall in the test of time. Echocardiography was first introduced in 1958. It became popular only in 1968 but since 1978 a machine can be found in every hospital, cardiac department and doctors' offices.

I am a proponent of free research. I define my problem, ask the appropriate questions, design a protocol, set up and make the experiment, record the observations, analyze the results, make a decision tree and publish the report. Monitoring is performed by peers who review the final article. My goals are directed by personal intuition and thought, clinical observation and questioning; the nature of my laboratory, my staff; and finally by financial support available to undertake the study.

My initial research studies started in 1962 with observations made in children with congenital heart disease who were studied by cine-angiography, a technique then confined to only a few institutions. We studied the structure and function of the pulmonary and aortic valves, the nature of post-stenotic dilatation of the pulmonary artery in pulmonary stenosis and the dynamics of right ventricular outflow tract obstruction in Fallot's tetralogy (Gotsman, 1964). Artificial valves were introduced in 1963 and it became obvious that certain patients failed to improve after valve replacement surgery. These patients have a large heart on X-ray and severe left ventricular hypertrophy on ECG (Gotsman et al., 1967; 1968). We noted that on left ventricular angiography, the ventricle was dilated and contracted poorly. We measured left ventricular end-diastolic and end-systolic volumes and ejection fraction and showed that patients with large ventricular volumes and a low ejection fraction responded poorly after valve replacement surgery (Lewis and Gotsman, 1973; 1974). Congestive cardiomyopathy was a common condition in South Africa and provided an excellent clinical example of severe global left ventricular dysfunction. We studied the function of the left ventricle during isovolumic contraction using isovolumic indices such as V_{max} and V_{ce} and also simpler non-invasive indices such as systolic time intervals (Lewis et al., 1973; Gotsman et al., 1973). Contrictive pericarditis was an example of failure of left ventricular compliance (Lewis and Gotsman, 1973b). This was studied and a model of diastolic ventricular failure developed and applied to other disorders such as coronary artery disease and mitral and aortic incompetence, particularly acute aortic valve rupture (Lewis *et al.*, 1975; Lewis and Gotsman, 1975).

Myocardical ischemia produces reversible ventricular paresis, so that our next studies were extended to include regional ventricular dysfunction (Bakst, 1973; Lewis *et al.*, 1974), atrial pacing, examining ventricular function by cineangiocardiography and in particular by non-invasive nuclear angiography (Rozenman *et al.*, 1984; Zivoni *et al.*, 1981).

We have also studied the distribution of coronary artery atheroma in a series of 300 patients to determine which factors were responsible and have shown that the usual risk factors, proximality of the lesion and presence of bifurcations are the most important causative factors (Halon *et al.*, 1983). Since coronary artery disease is more common, we have studied regional ventricular function by frame-by-frame analysis of cineangiograms and are able to show the pattern of contraction on a 3-dimensional reference axis which takes into account the position on the ventricular circumference, time of the cardiac cycle and extent of contraction. This can be converted into a simple contour map which shows the 3-dimensional picture in a 2-dimensional plane (Sapoznikov *et al.*, 1983).

What will happen in the future? Will we study at a macro, a micro or a micro-micro level? The left ventricle is a pump; the functional unit the sarcomere, the energy factory the mitochondrion, and repair occurs through DNA and RNA synthesis. These all operate through different channels. Each function is important but I predict that the micro-micro world will become more and more important.

What causes damage to endothelial cells, how do platelets and monocytes adhere to arterial wall, how is cell damage repaired? What causes medial myocytic migration into the intima, how and why does cholesterol enter some cells and not others, how does endothelium rupture, why and how does clot accrete and dissolve? What is the time course of myocardial cell anoxia, destruction and recovery and how does this affect myocardial infarction.

We need to ask the appropriate questions, make the relevant experiments and obtain the correct replies. Let each man seek his own field, ask intelligent questions, experiment and record and then think about the meaning of the conclusions and finally, in the words of King Solomon realise that 'A good name is better than good balsam and the day of death better than the day of birth' – because when a man is born, who knows how he will succeed, but when he dies his record is there for all to see.

Acknowledgement

This study was supported by the Joseph and Ceil Mazer Foundation.

References

Bakst A, Lewis BS, Gotsman MS (1973) Isolated obstruction of the left anterior descending coronary artery. South African Med J 47: 1534–1540

Gotsman MS (1964) The relative value of cineangiography in the diagnosis and assessment of congenital heart disease in infancy and childhood. MD Thesis, University of Cape Town

Gotsman MS, Beck W, Barnard CN, Schrire V (1967) Changes in the appearances of the chest radiograph after a repair or replacement operation on the mitral valve. Brit J Radiology 40: 724–739

Gotsman MS, Beck W, Barnard CN, Schrire V (1968) Changes in the chest X-ray after aortic valve replacement. Brit H J 30: 219–225

Gotsman MS, Lewis BS, Mitha AS, Bakst A (1973) Left ventricular performance in congestive cardiomyopathy. In: Bajuz E, Rona Co. (eds), Cardiomyopathies Vol. 2 of Recent Advances in Cardiac Structure & Metabolism, pp 677–698, University Park Press, Baltimore

Halon D, Sapoznikov D, Lewis BS, Gotsman MS (1983) The localisation of lesions in the coronary circulation. Amer J Cardiology 52: 921–926

Lewis BS, Gotsman MS (1973a(Left ventricular function in systole and diastole in aortic stenosis. South African Med J 47: 2064–2070

Lewis BS, Gotsman MS (1973b) Left ventricular function in systole and diastole in constrictive pericarditis. Amer H J 86: 23–41

Lewis BS, Armstrong TG, Samson RI, Everson RC, Van Der Horst RL, Gotsman MS (1973) Non-invasive techniques in assessing left ventricular performance in congestive cardiomyopathy. In: Ed. Bajuz E, Rona G (eds) Cardiomyopathies, Vol. 2 of Recent Advances in Cardiac Structure & Metabolism pp 699–715, University Park Press, Baltimore

Lewis BS, Gotsman MS (1974) Left ventricular function during systole and diastole in mitral incompetence. Amer J Cardiology 34: 635–643

Lewis BS, Bakst A, Gotsman MS (1974) Relationship between regional ventricular asynergy and the anatomical lesion in coronary artery disease. Amer H J 88: 211–218

Lewis BS, Gotsman MS (1975) Cardiac hypertrophy and left ventricular end-diastolic stress. Israel J Med Sci 11: 299–303

Lewis BS, Mitha AS, Gotsman MS (1975) Left ventricular function in systole and diastole in aortic incompetence. Israel J Med Sci 11: 420–434

Rozenman Y, Weiss AT, Atlan H, Gotsman MS (1984) Left ventricular volumes and function during atrial pacing in coronary artery disease: A radionuclide angiographic study. Amer J Cardiology 53: 497–503

Sapoznikov D, Halon DA, Lewis BS, Gotsman MS (1983) Frame by frame analysis of left ventricular function. Quantitative assessment of regional and temporal function. Cardiology 70: 61–72

Tzivoni D, Weiss AT, Salomon J, Warshaw D, Rod JL, Gotsman MS, Atlan H (1981) Diagnosis of coronary artery disease by multigated radionuclide angiography during right atrial pacing. Chest 80: 562–565

Closing session

SIDEMAN: I would like to start, with your permission, the closing session with a paragraph from a letter defining the purpose of the workshop. The letter reads:

'In view of the tremendous efforts and the intensity of research in the numerous aspects of the cardiac vascular field, it is desired to develop an integrated view of the various interrelated parameters in the areas of hemodynamics, coronary circulation, coronary metabolism, cardiac mechanics, electrocardiography, imaging techniques and related topics. An international workshop aimed at reviewing and discussing the state of the heart from the various points of view is therefore highly desired for efficient and meaningful future developments, both in research and clinical applications. This meeting of the world renown scholars, each a leader in his specific discipline, will bring together the most updated information which will be used as guidelines for future research programs.'

This sums up why we are here. The question, then, is did we succeed? I did not make a slip of the tongue when I said in the welcoming address that this is the *First* Henry Goldberg Workshop. There is no question in my mind that one session, long as it might be, can not encompass everything. I have a very good feeling that we have accomplished one important thing. We heard each other and viewed the various aspects of this complicated problem from different points of view. By doing that we have accomplished a lot, and I hope it will be used wisely.

SAGAWA: There are two kinds of people. There are those who really like to watch the natural phenomenon, measure, document, think a little bit, but primarily, learn about the heart by observation of nature. And there is the other kind, who, of course, does that too, but who really like to spend time in integrating information, searching for abstract governing principles and then trying out how the generalized view applies to new innovations. Both kinds are necessary. However, as a member of the former group, I would like to show two slides in order to remind you of the soft nature of the socalled experimental facts in biology. In physics, a field of hard science, one performs an experiment to find out a crucial result which serves as the final judge between two alternative hypotheses. The situation is not so clear cut in biological sciences.

Shown in Figure A is a set of pressure-volume loops obtained against a constant aterial impedence at four different preloads. Isochronous sets of pressure-volume points on the loops were collected together and a linear regression analysis was applied. You can see that the regression line, something like a volume elastance, is changing with time and a reasonable description of the whole chamber contraction can be given by this time-varying volume elastance. This is what we found in isolated canine hearts years ago and we do still find the same thing whenever we load the ventricle in this fashion. When we performed another set of experiments in which the ventricle was made to contract from the same end-diastolic volume, but against drastically different afterload impedances, and determined similar isochrones pressure-volume regression lines, Figure B, we found them to be parallel, shifting from left to right, rather than changing the slope steeper with time, sometimes even

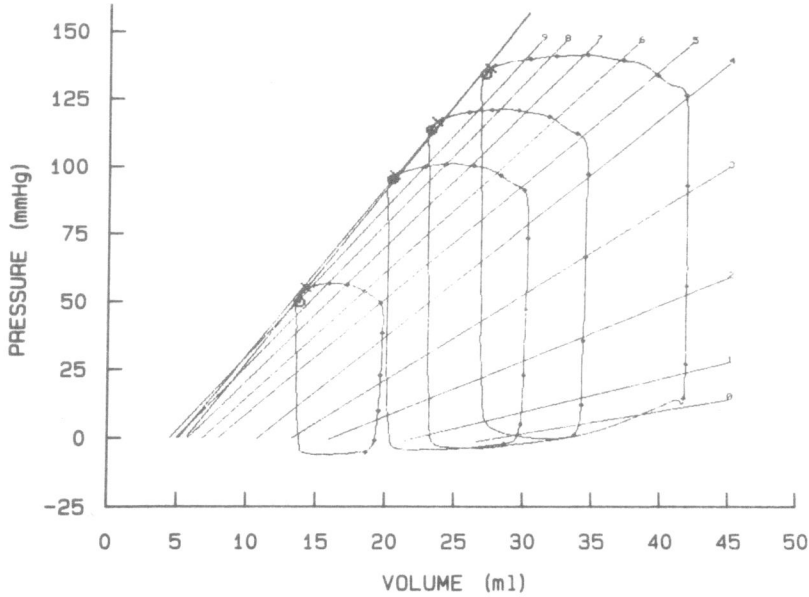

Figure A. Pressure-volume loops and isochrones obtained against constant arterial impedance for different preloads.

being initially steeper and then getting flatter. We observed the former and latter kind in the same hearts under the same contractile state, simply by changing the loading pattern. Although just one example, this observation leads to deeper insights. We come across this kind of provocative observation by trying one experiment after another in an untiring search; we certainly could not forsee it.

When I read a model simulation paper and come across a happy positive note that the simulated results fitted the experimental data very nicely, I get uneasy and attempt to think of alternative tests for the model; particularly when the facts used by the modeller come from our own experimental results. I feel the need to inform the modeller of all the diverse results that we can get by slightly changing experimental parameters, but could not describe in the publication for one reason or another. Therefore, a most important function of this meeting lies in the unorganized part of the meeting where this type of intimate communications can happen.

GESELOWITZ: I made a couple of comments, some of which could be interpreted as taking pot shots at models or modellers. I guess I go against the general tenor. I have spent a lot of my life defending models and modellers in the life sciences, medicine and biology. This has been a tough road to convince the life scientist that models do play a role. I have done it most in my life and here I've taken an opposite point of view. I want to pursue this briefly. I was very much taken by Professor Sideman's personal remarks about his initial exposure to biomedical engineering in terms of being sought to solve a problem. What I am concerned about is the opposite sort of thing. That is to beware of the solution looking for a problem. It seems that a lot of these modelling-engineers have techniques, and they go ahead merrily applying the techniques, but are not concerned with the problem that is of interest to the physician and the physiologist.

SIDEMAN: As chairman of the Department of Biomedical Engineering, I had to defend, not models but the place of the Biomedical Engineering discipline. One of the questions is 'do we need people with a special outlook in this biomedical field,' or 'can we just take a good electrical engineer, or a good mechanical engineer, or a good chemical engineer and let them do relevant biomedical work, each on his own.' I think that the time for this approach has passed. It is now generally

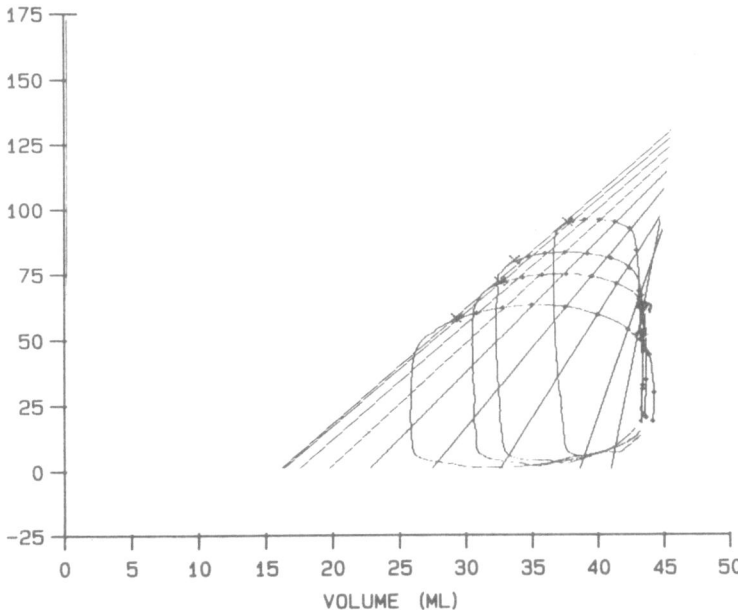

Figure B. Pressure-volume loops and isochrones obtained against drastically different afterload impedances.

understood, and accepted, that the disciplines of Biology, Medicine, Engineering Science and Medical Science, somehow fall together to make up the Biomedical Engineering discipline. We have a Medical School as part of our science and engineering program, giving a good example for the interaction between these fields. I do not have, in this distinguished audience, to emphasize this point. I also do not have to defend whether we should have models or whether we should have experiments. What we should have are good models and good experiments, and strong interactions between them. With this kind of approach, if we do a good job, the arguments whether we should or should not have models will end.

RITMAN: I am quite sorry that this meeting is coming to an end. There's a certain sadness about it. It's really been good fun. As I briefly mentioned earlier, what happens if you have a good model? What are you going to do with it? It is unlikely that we will ever have a perfect model. It will probably have to be extremely complicated, if it is going to be near perfect. That is unrealistic. The question is how are you going to improve a model from time to time. I think you are going to have to do experiments and always be in touch with people who try to apply this model. If you want to pursue modelling, it is very important that an integral part of your organization are people who can do the blood and guts of it.

BASSINGTHWAIGHTE: The question is not the man of engineering in contrast, or in collaboration, with the man of medicine, but rather the blending of the arts of experimentation and of analysis, no matter who does them. The analysis, or the experiment, might be very 'local', dealing with a specific and small element of our broad science, or it might be very global. What the Technion bioengineering group have presented, for example, is a very global approach; it is going to be very difficult to implement if it must contain all of the detailed elements. No one person is going to be able to do all of the experiments, perform all of the intricate analyses that would go into the global model. I would like to see individuals who will be able to handle both the experimentation *and* the analysis defining the components of such systems; Dr. Beyar's global modelling should show where those components can be integrated into a more composite view, and where they can not. Whenever elements of the system are shown to be self contradictory, then new experiments must be done, new analyses performed, new viewpoints developed. That to me is the potential strength of the integrated viewpoint that has been taken by the group here at the Technion. It has the potentialities to force new developments, but very careful blending of experimentation and analysis at all of the hierarchical levels within the global model are required before new insight will emerge.

MIRSKY: The experience I gained in the aerospace industry really stood me in good stead when I embarked on a research career in medicine. I worked for a company that built rocket engines and the parent company built the missile structure. I was amazed at their success with the rocket engines which had about a .999 reliability. But the reason they had success was because of the team effort, involving experts from many different disciplines. Let me say that this workshop, as far as I am concerned, is 17 years late in coming because as a basic scientist I was really isolated initially from the cardiologist and physiologist who at that time were skeptical of the mathematical modeling approach to cardiac mechanics. This is the first workshop that I have been involved in where there have been so many experts from different disciplines.

Getting back to the question of mathematical modelling, and reemphasizing some of the remarks Dr. Gotsman made, my best advice to the young investigator interested in mathematical modelling, is that he should cultivate relationships between the physiologist and the cardiologist very early, and to always keep in mind the possibility of testing their models in the physiological setting and ultimately their clinical application. It has been my experience that oversimplified models have no clinical value and that sophisticated computer models are research tools not meant to have clinical utility. However, by employing the classical mathematical approach along with judicious simplifications, models can help elucidate a number of problems that are controversial in cardiology today. One problem that comes to my mind relates to the mechanisms involved in what cause the dramatic shifts in the diastolic pressure-volume relationship following certain drug interventions. Each investigator has his own mechanism and if you remember the slide I showed the other day with regard to chamber stiffness, the simple mathematical expression incorporated all the important factors. From that model I was able to quantitate these various factors. Of course, a multiplicity of factors are generally involved in most biological problems. That simple model was able to explain a number of the controversies and has since been validated experimentally. I guess that the single component aproach which has worked beautifully in aerospace research may well be successful in cardiovascular research.

SKORTON: Another aspect of this conference that I thought was an eye opener for me, and for some others, was the realization that certain experimental problems or certain questions are being asked by different groups. The answers are being published in different literatures. I know that at least three or four times in the conference I noticed people from biological or physiological disciplines being surprised at information that was well known to those in the biomedical engineering literature and vice versa. I learnt two important things that I didn't know about, and I have communicated informally a couple of things that people who are going into this area should know before they go any further. This conference certainly was a good start in bringing together different people from different disciplines. (I could see an argument for having a conference at least this long on any one of the aspects that we talked about.) It would be a lot to accomplish the goal of bringing everyone up to date on what other people are doing, and to try to answer the same question, or find the answer to the same problem, but from different points of view. Perhaps one good use of such a conference might be put to is to try to bring across information in narrow, well circumscribed areas from many different disciplines that one finds very hard to assimilate within the constraints of one's professional life and time.

SIDEMAN: When we thought about this meeting we hoped, and we were not disappointed, that by bringing together the experts from the different aspects of the cardiac system, we would not only enjoy a personal experience, but also gain an insight into the various approaches to the cardiac system. The pros and cons of this or that. I think we got it. Whatever we are trying to accomplish here, we do not want to reinvent the wheel! What we would like to do is to take what you are doing and put it together in a quantitative comprehensive and uncomplicated way, so that we can understand it from all points of view. The combination of Dr. Gibb's with Dr. Sagawa's lectures is a good example of how ideas can be interrelated from different points of view. I hope that this meeting is just an opener for future communication between all of us. Dr. Ritman asked what would we have if we do get a working model. We don't want just a model, per se. We want understanding and insight; we want to know what we are all talking about. What we would like to do is to try to translate, or incorporate, available physiological knowledge into something quantitative and be able to learn from it all. This is basically what we are trying to accomplish here. If we succeed in learning and understanding, we may eventually contribute to preventive medicine. Towards this end I would like to throw a challenge your way. I can't ask you all to come and stay with us. You are too busy, although a sabbatical may be in order. It would be an excellent idea if you would send one of your young colleagues over here for a year to work with us, to bring his expertise, or maybe his ignorance, and join us in what we are doing. This could be a very good way to get a dialogue going between our respective efforts. Please consider us as a home, as partners to whatever we can do and send your students to help out. This will open up a very wide road of cooperation and understanding.

Another aspect is communication by computers. We are all hooked to the Big Daddy and shortly, we will probably have a complete hook-up to everywhere all over the world. It is completely reasonable to expect that we may soon be connected directly to some Center of specialty that we may want to test, and use on-line information. This is a very powerful tool and may help us overcome the enormous task of chasing the literature. I would like you to be aware of this possibility of communication not only by travel, but also by the computer. It can be done and it will soon become part of the routine. Finally, we come to the closing moments and I would like to ask forgiveness for being a little rushed, and ringing the bell when you were all enthused and ready to continue with your lecture. Please consider it as part of a beautiful melody we played together. I would like to apologize, too, to those who were not invited, and the list is huge. Please help me with my friends and tell them that the room was really small and the work was hard . . . I want to thank all the chairmen who held the whip and kept time and all the lecturers who came a long way and did a beautiful job. We were very fortunate with the presentations, with all the lecturers being really good so that it was all very pleasant, not only interesting, to listen to the well delivered lectures. I would also like to thank our students, Eitan Kimmel and Arye Horowitz, for their very quiet and efficient attention to detail. I also wish to thank the people who made the travel arrangements, my secretaries, Mrs. Dalia Zalman and Mrs. Rachel Brett.

GESELOWITZ: On behalf of the participants I want to thank you all for organizing this meeting. From a scientific standpoint it turned out to be an excellent one, and from the social and gastronomic viewpoints it was really superbe.

SIDEMAN: Thank you all!

List of contributors

Adam, D., MD, Department of Biomedical Engineering, The Julius Silver Institute, Technion – IIT, Haifa 32000, Israel

Ameling, W., Department of Electrical Engineering and Computer Science, Rheinisch-Westfälische Technische Hochschule, D-5100 Aachen, FRG

Barr, R.C., Department of Biomedical Engineering, Duke University, Durham NC 277706, USA

Bassingthwaighte, J.B., Center for Bioengineering WD 12, University of Washington, Seattle WA 98195, USA

Berne, R.M., Department of Physiology, School of Medicine, University of Virginia, Charlottesville VA 22908, USA

Beyar, R., Department of Biomedical Engineering, The Julius Silver Institute, Technion – IIT, Haifa 32000, Israel

Brennecke, R., Department of Pediatric Cardiology and Biomedical Engineering, University of Kiel, Clinic der Christian Albrechts, Froebel Street, Kiel, FRG

Bürsch, J.H., Department of Pediatric Cardiology and Biomedical Engineering, University of Kiel, Clinic der Christian Albrechts, Froebel Street, Kiel, FRG

Chance, E.M., Department of Biochemistry, University of London, London WC1 6BT, United Kindom

Chandran, K.B., Cardiovascular Center, Departments of Internal Medicine, Biomedical Engineering, Electrical and Computer Engineering and Radiology, University of Iowa and VA Medical Center, Iowa City IA 52242, USA

Collins, S.M., Cardiovascular Center, Departments of Internal Medicine, Biomedical Engineering, Electrical and Computer Engineering and Radiology, University of Iowa and VA Medical Center, Iowa City IA 52242, USA

Dinnar, U., Department of Biomedical Engineering, The Julius Silver Institute, Technion – IIT, Haifa 32000, Israel

Feigl, E.O., Department of Physiology and Biophysics, University of Washington, School of Medicine, Seattle WA 98195, USA

Geselowitz, D.B., Bioengineering Program, Pennsylvania State University, 254

Hammond Building, University Park PA 16802, USA

Gibbs, C.L., Department of Physiology, Monash University, Clayton, Victoria 3168, Australia

Gotsman, M.S., Department of Cardiology, Hadassah-Hebrew University Medical Center, Jerusalem, Israel

Hahne, H.J., Department of Pediatric Cardiology and Biomedical Engineering, University of Kiel, Clinic der Christian Albrechts, Froebel Street, Kiel, FRG

Heethaar, J., Interuniversity Cardiology Institution, Catharijnesingel 101, 3511 GV Utrecht, The Netherlands

Heethaar, R.M., Departments of Cardiology and Medical Physics, University Hospital Utrecht, Catharijnesingel 101, 3511 GV Utrecht, The Netherlands and Department of Biomedical Engineering, University of Technology, Twente, The Netherlands

Heintzen, P.H., Department of Pediatric Cardiology and Biomedical Engineering, University of Kiel, Clinic der Christian Albrechts, Froebel Street, Kiel, FRG

Hoffman, E.A., Department of Physiology and Biophysics and Division of Cardiovascular Diseases and Internal Medicine, Mayo Foundation, Rochester MN 55905, USA

Horowitz, A., Departments of Mechanical and Biomedical Engineering, Technion – Israel Institute of Technology, Haifa 32000, Israel

Huyghe, J.M., Department of Biomedical Engineering, University of Technology, Twente, The Netherlands

Iwasaki, T., Department of Physiology and Biophysics and Division of Cardiovascular Diseases and Internal Medicine, Mayo Foundation, Rochester MN 55905, USA

Janicki, J.S., Cardiovascular Research Institute, Department of Medicine, Michael Reese Hospital and Medical Center, Chicago ILL 60616, USA

Kerber, R.E., Cardiovascular Center, Departments of Internal Medicine, Biomedical Engineering, Electrical and Computer Engineering and Radiology, University of Iowa and VA Medical Center, Iowa City IA 52242, USA

Levy, M.N., Division of Investigative Medicine, The Mount Sinai Medical Center, Case Western Reserve University, University Circle, Cleveland OH 44106, USA

McPherson, D.D., Cardiovascular Center, Departments of Internal Medicine, Biomedical Engineering, Electrical and Computer Engineering and Radiology, University of Iowa and VA Medical Center, Iowa City IA 52242, USA

Maughan, L., Department of Biomedical Engineering, The Johns Hopkins Medical School, Baltimore MD 21205, USA

Mirsky, I., Department of Medicine, Harvard Medical School and Brigham and Women's Hospital, 75 Francis Street, Boston MA 92115, USA

Moldenhauer, K., Department of Pediatric Cardiology and Biomedical Engineering, University of Kiel, Clinic der Christian Albrechts, Froebel Street, Kiel, FRG

Nerem, R.M., Physiological Fluid Mechanics Laboratory, Department of Mechanical Engineering, University of Houston, Houston TX 77004, USA

Neufeld, H., The Heart Center and the Division of Cardiology, The Sheba Medical Center, Tel Hashomer, Israel

Noel, M.P., Cardiovascular Center, Departments of Internal Medicine, Biomedical Engineering, Electrical and Computer Engineering and Radiology, University of Iowa and VA Medical Center, Iowa City, IA 52242, USA

Olshansky, B., Cardiovascular Center, Departments of Internal Medicine, Biomedical Engineering, Electrical and Computer Engineering and Radiology, University of Iowa and VA Medical Center, Iowa City IA 52242, USA

Onnasch, D.W.G., Department of Pediatric Cardiology and Biomedical Engineering, University of Kiel, Clinic der Christian Albrechts, Froebel Street, Kiel, FRG

Pao, Y.C., Department of Engineering Mechanics, University of Nebraska, 311 Bancroft Hall, Loncoln NE 68588, USA

Perl, M., Departments of Mechanical and Biomedical Engineering, Israel Institute of Technology, Technion, Haifa 32000, Israel

Petree, L.P., Cardiovascular Center, Departments of Internal Medicine, Biomedical Engineering, Electrical and Computer Engineering and Radiology, University of Iowa and VA Medical Center, Iowa City, IA 52242, USA

Plonsey, R., Department of Biomedical Engineering, Duke University, Durham NC 27706, USA

Ritman, E.L., Department of Physiology and Biophysics and Division of Cardiovascular Diseases and Internal Medicine, Mayo Foundation, Rochester MN 55905, USA

Rooz, E., Physiological Fluid Mechanics Laboratory, Department of Mechanical Engineering, University of Houston, Houston TX 77004, USA

Rudy, Y., Department of Biomedical Engineering, Case Western University, Cleveland OH 44106, USA

Sagawa, K., Department of Biomedical Engineering, The Johns Hopkins Medical School, 720 Rutland Avenue, Baltimore MD 21205, USA

Sapoznikov, D., Haddassah Heart Center and Hebrew University, Jerusalem, Israel

Schwartz, R.S., Department of Physiology and Biophysics and Division of Cardiovascular Diseases and Internal Medicine, Mayo Foundation, Rochester MN 55905, USA

Seeholzer, S.H., Department of Biochemistry and Biophysics, University of Pennsylvania, Philadelphia PA 19104, USA

Shroff, S.G., Cardiovascular Research Institute, Department of Medicine, Michael Reese Hospital and Medical Center, Chicago ILL 60616, USA

Sideman, S., Department of Biomedical Engineering, The Julius Silver Institute, Technion – IIT, Haifa 32000, Israel

Sinak, L.J., Cardiovascular Center, Departments of Internal Medicine, Biomedical Engineering, Electrical and Computer Engineering and Radiology, University of Iowa and VA Medical Center, Iowa City 52242, USA

Skorton, D.J., Department of Internal Medicine, University of Iowa Hospital, Iowa City IA 52242, USA

Sunagawa, K., Department of Biomedical Engineering, The Johns Hopkins Medical School, Baltimore MD 23205, USA

Weber, K.T., Cardiovascular Research Institute, Department of Medicine, Michael Reese Hospital and Medical Center, Chicago ILL 60616, USA

Welkowitz, W., Department of Electrical Engineering, Rutgers State University, P.O. Box 909, Piscataway NJ 08854, USA

Wiesner, T.F., Physiological Fluid Mechanics Laboratory, Department of Mechanical Engineering, University of Houston, Houston TX 77004, USA

Williamson, J.S., Department of Biochemistry and Biophysics, University of Pennsylvania Medical Center, Philadelphia PA 19104, USA

Index